Contents in Brief

*3x5 index card w/ notes
Ch. 1 and 3 Review
for extra credit*

GARY A. THIBODEAU, PhD
Chancellor Emeritus and Professor Emeritus of Biology
University of Wisconsin—River Falls
River Falls, Wisconsin

KEVIN T. PATTON, PhD
Professor of Life Science
St. Charles Community College
Cottleville, Missouri

14th EDITION

STRUCTURE & FUNCTION
of the Body

ELSEVIER

ELSEVIER
MOSBY

3251 Riverport Lane
St. Louis, Missouri 63043

STRUCTURE & FUNCTION OF THE BODY   ISBN: 978-0-323-07722-4

Notices

Knowledge and best practice in this field are constantly changing. As new research and experience broaden our understanding, changes in research methods, professional practices, or medical treatment may become necessary.

Practitioners and researchers must always rely on their own experience and knowledge in evaluating and using any information, methods, compounds, or experiments described herein. In using such information or methods they should be mindful of their own safety and the safety of others, including parties for whom they have a professional responsibility.

With respect to any drug or pharmaceutical products identified, readers are advised to check the most current information provided (i) on procedures featured or (ii) by the manufacturer of each product to be administered, to verify the recommended dose or formula, the method and duration of administration, and contraindications. It is the responsibility of practitioners, relying on their own experience and knowledge of their patients, to make diagnoses, to determine dosages and the best treatment for each individual patient, and to take all appropriate safety precautions.

To the fullest extent of the law, neither the Publisher nor the authors, contributors, or editors, assume any liability for any injury and/or damage to persons or property as a matter of products liability, negligence or otherwise, or from any use or operation of any methods, products, instructions, or ideas contained in the material herein.

Library of Congress Cataloging-in-Publication Data

Thibodeau, Gary A., 1938-
  Structure & function of the body / Gary A. Thibodeau, Kevin T. Patton. -- 14th ed.
    p.   cm.
  Includes bibliographical references and index.
  ISBN 978-0-323-07721-7 (hardcover : alk. paper) -- ISBN 978-0-323-07722-4 (pbk. : alk. paper)
1. Human physiology--Textbooks. 2. Human anatomy--Textbooks. I. Patton, Kevin T. II. Anthony, Catherine Parker, 1907- Structure & function of the body. III. Title. IV. Title: Structure and function of the body.
  QP34.5.T5 2012
  612--dc23

                                                            2011030968

Executive Editor: Kellie White
Managing Editor: Rebecca Swisher
Editorial Assistant: Emily Thomson
Publishing Services Manager: Deborah Vogel
Project Manager: Brandilyn Tidwell
Designer: Margaret Reid

Printed in the United States of America

Last digit is the print number: 9 8 7 6 5 4 3 2 1

About the Authors

Gary Thibodeau has been teaching anatomy and physiology for more than three decades. Since 1975, *Structure & Function of the Body* has been a logical extension of his interest and commitment to education. Gary's teaching style encourages active interaction with students, and he uses a variety of teaching methodologies—a style that has been incorporated into every aspect of this edition. He is considered a pioneer in the introduction of collaborative learning strategies to the teaching of anatomy and physiology. His focus continues to be successful, student-centered learning—leveraged by text, Web-based, and ancillary teaching materials. Gary is active in numerous professional organizations, including the Human Anatomy and Physiology Society (HAPS), the American Association of Anatomists, and the American Association for the Advancement of Science (AAAS). His biography is included in numerous publications, including *Who's Who in America, Who's Who in American Education, Outstanding Educators in America, American Men and Women of Science,* and *Who's Who in Medicine and Healthcare.* While earning master's degrees in both zoology and pharmacology, and a PhD in physiology, Gary says that he became "fascinated by the connectedness of the life sciences." That fascination has led to this edition's unifying themes, which focus on how each concept fits into the "big picture" of the human body.

To my parents, M.A. Thibodeau and Florence Thibodeau, who had a deep respect for education at all levels and who truly believed that you never give up being a student.

To my wife, Emogene, an ever-generous and uncommonly discerning critic, for her love, support, and encouragement over the years.

To my children, Douglas and Beth, for making it all worthwhile.

Gary A. Thibodeau

Kevin Patton has taught anatomy and physiology to high school, community college, and university students from various backgrounds for three decades. This experience has helped him produce a text that will be easier to understand for all students.

He has earned several citations for teaching anatomy and physiology, including the Missouri Governor's Award for Excellence in Teaching. "One thing I've learned," says Kevin, "is that most of us learn scientific concepts more easily when we can *see* what's going on." His talent for using imagery to teach is evident throughout this edition, with its extensively revised illustration program. Kevin's interest in promoting excellence in teaching anatomy and physiology has led him to take an active role in the Human Anatomy and Physiology Society (HAPS). He serves as HAPS President Emeritus and was the founding Director of HAPS Institute (HAPS-I), a professional continuing education program for anatomy and physiology teachers. Kevin also produces several online resources for A&P students and teachers, including *theAPstudent.org* and *theAPprofessor.org.* Like Gary, Kevin found that the work that led him to a PhD in vertebrate anatomy and physiology instilled in him an appreciation for the "big picture" of human structure and function.

To my family and friends, who never let me forget the joys of discovery, adventure, and good humor.

To the many teachers who taught me more by who they were than by what they said.

To my students, who help me keep the joy of learning fresh and exciting.

Kevin T. Patton

The true quality of a textbook is best measured by how well it supports, promotes, and encourages both good teaching and effective learning. The 14th edition of *Structure & Function of the Body* is a new text with a long tradition of excellence. It is based on profound respect for both the teacher and the student. That respect is coupled with an excitement for the subject matter honed by both authors during decades of teaching anatomy and physiology. We have listened carefully to input from users of previous editions. We know that teachers use different techniques to convey ideas, present difficult concepts, or explain how applications of principles of anatomy and physiology can affect, for example, health, diverse personal interests of students in the class, or other areas of biology. Students, of course, learn in different ways, at different paces, and for different reasons. Success for some is largely predicated on readability of the text, others are more visual in their learning and rely heavily on excellent illustrations; still others learn best in groups and by verbal review of concepts. A good text must be flexible enough to help accommodate, not hinder, these differing needs of both teacher and student.

In the 21st century, success in both teaching and learning is, in many ways, determined by how effective we are at transforming information into knowledge. This is especially true in anatomy and physiology, where both student and teacher are now being confronted with an enormous accumulation of factual information. *Structure & Function of the Body* is intended to help transform that information into a coherent knowledge base. It was written at an appropriate level to help students with divergent needs and learning styles to unify information, stimulate critical thinking, and hopefully acquire a taste for knowledge about the wonders of the human body. The new edition is designed for ease of use and will encourage students to explore, question, and look for relationships not only between related facts in a single discipline but also among fields of academic inquiry and personal experience.

This 14th edition of *Structure & Function of the Body* retains many features that have proved successful in several decades of classroom use; however, as an updated text, it presents a wealth of carefully selected new content in both anatomy and physiology, as well as pedagogical enhancements that will better serve the needs of today's instructors and students. The writing style and depth of coverage are intended to challenge, reward, and reinforce introductory students as they grasp and assimilate important concepts.

During the revision of this text, each change in content and organization was evaluated by anatomy and physiology teachers working in the field—teachers currently assisting students to learn about human structure and function for the first time. The result is a text that students will read, one designed to help the teacher teach and the student learn. It is particularly suited to introductory anatomy and physiology courses in nursing and allied health-related programs. Emphasis is on material required for entry into more advanced courses, completion of professional licensing examinations, and successful application of information in a practical, work-related environment.

UNIFYING THEMES

Structure & Function of the Body is dominated by two major unifying themes. First, structure and function complement one another in the normal, healthy human body. Second, nearly all structure and function in the body can be explained in terms of keeping conditions in the internal environment relatively constant—in homeostasis. Repeated emphasis of these principles encourages students to integrate otherwise isolated factual information into a cohesive and understandable whole. As a result, anatomy and physiology emerge as living and dynamic topics of personal interest and importance to the student.

ORGANIZATION AND CONTENT

The 21 chapters of *Structure & Function of the Body* present the core material of anatomy and physiology most important for introductory students. The selection of appropriate information in both disciplines eliminates the confusing mix of nonessential and overly specialized material that unfortunately accompanies basic information in many introductory textbooks. Information is presented in a way that makes it easy for students to know and understand what is important. Further, pedagogical aids in each chapter identify learning objectives and then reinforce successful mastery of this clearly identified core material. The sequencing of chapters in the book follows a course organization most commonly used in teaching at the undergraduate level. However, because each chapter is self-contained, instructors have the flexibility to alter the sequence of material to fit personal teaching preferences or the special content or time constraints of their courses or students.

At every level of organization, both within and among chapters, care has been taken to couple structural information with important functional concepts. In each chapter of the text, appropriate physiological content balances the anatomical information that is presented. As a result, the student has a more integrated understanding of human structure and function. Throughout the text, examples that stress the complementarity of structure and function have been consciously selected to emphasize the importance of homeostasis as a unifying concept.

Acquiring and using the terms so necessary for the study of anatomy and physiology can be difficult for many students. To assist students in this area, new terms are introduced, defined, and incorporated into a working vocabulary. The organization of chapters and paragraphs allows students to both "read" and "raid" this book easily to learn essential concepts of human structure and function. Every chapter also uses skillfully designed visuals to reinforce written information with sensory input.

The style of presentation of material in this text and its readability, accuracy, and level of coverage have been carefully developed to meet the needs of undergraduate students taking an introductory course in anatomy and physiology. *Structure & Function of the Body* remains an introductory textbook—a teaching book rather than a reference text. No textbook can replace the direction and stimulation provided by an enthusiastic teacher to a curious and involved student. A good textbook, however, can and should be enjoyable to read and helpful to both.

PEDAGOGICAL FEATURES

Structure & Function of the Body is a student-oriented text. Written in a very readable style, it has numerous pedagogical aids that maintain interest and motivation. Every chapter contains the following elements that facilitate learning and the retention of information in the most effective manner.

Chapter outline: An overview outline introduces each chapter and enables the student to preview the content and direction of the chapter at the major concept level before the detailed reading.

Chapter objectives: The opening page of each chapter contains several measurable objectives for the student. Each objective clearly identifies for the student, before he or she reads the chapter, what the key goals should be and what information should be mastered.

Study tips: Each chapter includes a list of specific tips and hints on how to most effectively study the concepts of that chapter. Prepared by the authors and Ed Calcaterra, these tips are a unique and useful feature that make this text even more student friendly.

Key terms and pronunciation guide: Key terms, when introduced and defined in the text body, are identified in boldface to highlight their importance. A pronunciation guide follows each new term that students may find difficult to pronounce correctly. A listing of these new terms is recapped at the end of each chapter. You can also find an audio glossary on the accompanying Evolve website.

Quick Check questions: The popular Quick Check feature provides a way for students to check their basic reading comprehension at the end of each passage that they have read. Quick Checks each consist of a few questions and are scattered at appropriate points throughout the text of each chapter. The questions are *simple,* meant only to check whether the student read and understood the main points of each passage.

AnimationDirect: In each chapter, boxes with a CD icon point the reader to animations of important principles available in AnimationDirect, which has been included on the

CD. AnimationDirect features brief animated sequences that demonstrate concepts that are not easily illustrated in static diagrams. This edition features more than thirty additional animations in the collection. These animations help put a student's understanding in motion and thus help solidify learning.

Boxed inserts and essays: Boxed information appears in every chapter. We have grouped these boxed features into four categories: Health and Well-Being; Clinical Application; Research, Issues, & Trends; and Science Application. The boxed features increase student interest. They also help students apply information learned in the course to help them develop critical thinking skills.

Carefully selected clinical examples are included in each chapter of the book to help students understand that the disease process is a disruption in homeostasis and a breakdown of the normal integration of form and function. We use clinical examples to reinforce the concepts of how disease affects normal function and how therapies can restore normal function. We have found in our own teaching that such examples stimulate student interest.

Boxed information highlighting health and wellness issues reinforces the basic concepts of human structure and function by applying them in practical ways to current problems in public health, athletics, and fitness.

Select boxed essays on issues and trends in research and medicine will spark an interest in the dynamic fields of science, technology, and ethics that underlie the modern arena of human biology.

Science Applications feature possible career paths that use the concepts taught in this text. These career paths are mentioned in the context of the work of an important figure in the history of scientific endeavor. Such information will further motivate learning by illustrating its practical applications and will stimulate students to think about their own career choices.

Outline summaries: Extensive and detailed end-of-chapter summaries in outline format provide excellent guides for students as they review the text materials when preparing for examinations. Many students also find these detailed guides useful as a chapter preview in conjunction with the chapter outline. Audio chapter summaries are also available on the accompanying Evolve website.

Review questions: Subjective review questions at the end of each chapter allow students to use a narrative format to discuss concepts and synthesize important chapter information for review by the instructor. The answers to these review questions are available in the Instructor's Resource Manual that accompanies the text.

Critical thinking questions: Review questions that encourage students to use critical thinking skills are highlighted at the end of each chapter. Answers to these questions are also found in the Instructor's Resource Manual.

Chapter tests: Objective-type chapter test questions are included at the end of each chapter. They serve as quick checks for the recall and mastery of important subject matter. They are also designed as aids to increase the retention of information. Answers to all chapter test questions are provided at the end of the text.

Body mass index (BMI) appendix: A brief overview of the body mass index and how it is used to assess risk for weight-related health conditions is included as a separate appendix that can be used in the introduction to the body in Chapter 1, the study of tissues in Chapter 3, the study of nutrition and metabolism in Chapter 16, or anywhere else the student or teacher finds it useful.

Additional learning and study aids at the end of the text include Common Medical Abbreviations, Prefixes, and Suffixes; an extensive Glossary to assist students in mastering the vocabulary of anatomy and physiology; and a detailed Index that serves as a ready reference for locating information.

ILLUSTRATIONS

A major strength of *Structure & Function of the Body* has always been the exceptional quality, accuracy, and beauty of the illustration program. This edition features a complete refreshing of the art program. The truest test of any illustration is how effectively it can complement and strengthen written information found in the text and how successfully it can be used by the student as a learning tool. Extensive use has been made of full-color illustrations, micrographs, and dissection photographs throughout the text. Each illustration is carefully referred to in the text and is designed to support the text discussion. Many new and enhanced illustrations appear in this edition of the textbook. Each was carefully designed in a collaboration among the authors, editors, and illustration creators with the goal of enhancing learning.

Continuing in this edition of *Structure & Function of the Body* is the careful use of anatomical rosettes in all anatomical illustrations (see the Anatomical Directions page at the beginning of the book for an illustration of this useful element). These rosettes, like the compass rosettes found on geographical maps, orient the user to the direction, or orientation, of the figure by pointing which way is left and which way is right—directions that in anatomy may appear backward to the beginning student. As with map users, the need for these rosettes will diminish as one becomes more familiar with "the territory" of the human body.

Clear View of the Human Body

We are particularly excited to once again present a full-color, semitransparent model of the body called the *Clear View of the Human Body.* Located around Chapter 4 in the textbook, this feature permits the virtual dissection of male and female human bodies along several different planes. Developed by Kevin Patton and Paul Krieger, this tool helps learners assimilate their knowledge of the complex structure of the human body. It also helps students visualize human anatomy in the manner of today's clinical and scientific body-imaging technology.

COMPANION CD-ROM

The CD-ROM included in the back of the book contains two programs built to help students visualize concepts presented in the text.

AnimationDirect features over 75 three-dimensional animations (31 added for this edition), categorized by chapter, helping students visualize anatomical structures and physiological processes in a uniquely engaging way.

Each animation contained on the CD is referenced within the body of the text so that students can easily connect the major concepts described in the body of the chapter with these state-of-the-art multimedia depictions.

The CD-ROM also includes the newly updated **Body Spectrum Electronic Coloring Book,** which offers 80 anatomy illustrations that the student can color online or print out to color and study offline.

SUPPLEMENTS

The supplements package has been carefully planned and developed to assist instructors and to enhance their use of the text. Each supplement, including the test items and Study Guide, has been thoroughly reviewed by many of the same instructors who reviewed the text.

Anatomy & Physiology Online

This complete, interactive online course includes audio and visual elements that complement the most important concepts presented in *Structure & Function of the Body,* 14th Edition. **Anatomy & Physiology Online** is organized into modules that correspond with key chapters in the core text. Within each module resides a set of lessons for specific anatomical and physiological concepts. With hundreds of step-by-step animations and interactive exercises, **Anatomy & Physiology Online** demonstrates complex processes in a clear and concise way!

- 800 full-color images of anatomical structures, physiological concepts, and disease processes are included.

- Hundreds of state-of-the-art animations clarify anatomical and physiological processes and provide a realistic foundation of underlying structures and functions—such as air flow through the respiratory tract, pulmonary circulation, events of the cardiac cycle, and sensory and motor pathways of the central nervous system.
- Essential information is highlighted and easy to read, with extensive use of diagrams and illustrations.
- More than 250 interactive exercises include a variety of engaging activities such as crossword puzzles, labeling, and sequencing.
- Immediate feedback is provided for self-assessment questions and lesson exams in each module, allowing students to measure their comprehension.
- A complete glossary defines key terms and concepts, and includes audio pronunciations.

TEACH Instructor Resource

The **TEACH Instructor Resource** provides text adopters with substantial support in teaching from the text. The following features are found in every chapter:

- Chapter synopsis of major components and principles
- Learning objectives with rationales for review of chapter objectives
- Lecture outline to parallel textbook summary
- Suggestions for student activities and assignments
- Information resources for distribution to students
- Answers to the Review Questions and Case Study Questions found in the text

The **TEACH Lesson Plans** link all parts of the *Structure & Function of the Body* educational package by providing customizable lesson plans and lecture outlines based on learning objectives drawn from the text. Each lesson plan features:

- Teaching Focus summaries that identify essential lesson goals
- Lesson preparation checklists that make planning your class quick and easy
- Pretests and background assessment questions that gauge student readiness
- Critical thinking questions to focus and motivate students

- Teaching resources that cross-reference all of Mosby's curriculum solutions
- Class activities designed to engage students in the learning process
- Practical, concise talking points that complement the PowerPoint slides

Instructor's Electronic Resource

The **Instructor's Electronic Resource CD-ROM** was written and developed specifically for this new edition of *Structure & Function of the Body*. It includes the **TEACH Instructor Resource,** a **PowerPoint** presentation of over 600 slides, and an **Electronic Image Collection,** featuring nearly 400 full-color illustrations and photographs, labeled and unlabeled, for you to use in enhancing your lectures.

Study Guide

Written by Linda Swisher, this guide provides students with additional self-study aids, including chapter overviews, topic reviews, application and labeling exercises (including matching, crossword puzzles, fill in the blank, and multiple choice), and answers to the questions in the Study Guide.

Evolve ℮volve

The **updated Evolve website for instructors includes:**

- A **Computerized Test Bank** with over 3500 multiple choice, true/false, short answer, and challenge questions
- **iClicker** content for your Classroom Response System
- **Image Collection** of over 400 illustrations and photographs, labeled and unlabeled
- **TEACH Instructor Resource**
- **PowerPoint** presentation of over 600 slides
- **Revision Notes** with a detailed listing of new or revised content for each chapter
- **Conversion Guide**

Student resources include the following:
- NEW **Audio Chapter Summaries**
- **Audio Glossary** with definitions and pronunciations for hundreds of key terms from the textbook
- **Frequently Asked Questions**
- **Online Tutoring** that offers help from experts in the field of anatomy and physiology

- **Panorama of Anatomy & Physiology** features quizzes, video clips, fun facts, and information on careers in the field of health sciences
- **Quick Check Answers**
- **Post Test Questions**
- **Weblinks**

A WORD OF THANKS

Many people have contributed to the development and success of *Structure & Function of the Body.* We extend our thanks and deep appreciation to the various students and classroom instructors who have provided us with helpful suggestions following their use of earlier editions of this text.

A special thank you to Ed Calcaterra for his many previous contributions to this text. A specific thank you goes to the following clinicians, researchers, and instructors who critiqued in detail the previous editions of this text or various drafts of the revision. Their invaluable comments were instrumental in the development of this new edition.

Bert Atsma
Union County College
Cranford, New Jersey

Ethel J. Avery
Trenholm State Technical College
Montgomery, Alabama

Gail Balser, RN, BSN, MSN
Lakeland, Florida

Joan I. Barber, PhD
Delaware Technical & Community College
Newark, Delaware

Barbara Barger
Clarion County Career Center
Shippenville, Pennsylvania

Rachel Beecham, PhD
Mississippi Valley State University
Itta Bena, Mississippi

Kristi Bertrand, MPH, CMA (AAMA), CPC, PBT (ASCP)
The Medical Institute of Kentucky
Lexington, Kentucky

Jackie Brittingham
Simpson College
Indianola, Iowa

Kristin Bruzzini, PhD
Maryville University
St. Louis, Missouri

Donna J. Burleson, RN, MS, MSN
Cisco Junior College
Abilene, Texas

Ed Calcaterra, BS, MEd
Instructor, DeSmet Jesuit High School
Creve Coeur, Missouri

Jeanne Calvert, BA, MS
University of Saint Francis
Fort Wayne, Indiana

Dale Charles, MS, RN, ACLS, CPR
Spencerian College
Louisville, Kentucky

Lydia R. Chavana
South Texas Vo-Tech Institute
McAllen, Texas

Linda C. Cole, RN, MSN, CS, FNP
Saint Charles Community College
Cottleville, Missouri

Maria Conn
Mayo State Vo-Tech School
Pikeville, Kentucky

Jane Corbitt, RN, MLS
Central Georgia Technical College
Milledgeville, Georgia

Joseph Devine
Allied Health Careers
Austin, Texas

Edna M. Dilmore
Bessemer State Technical College
Bessemer, Alabama

Camille DiLullo, PhD
Philadelphia College of Osteopathic Medicine
Philadelphia, Pennsylvania

Kathleen Reilly Dolin, MS, RN
Northampton Community College
Bethlehem, Pennsylvania

Marian Doyle, MS
Northampton Community College
Fogelsville, Pennsylvania

Cammie Emory
Bossier Parish Community College
Benton, Louisiana

David Evans, PhD, FRES
Penn College
Williamsport, Pennsylvania

Sally Flesch, PhD, RN
Black Hawk College
Moline, Illinois

Michael Harman, MS
Lone Star College – North Harris
Houston, Texas

Ann Henninger, PhD
Wartburg College
Waverly, Iowa

Elizabeth Hodgson, MS
York College of Pennsylvania
York, Pennsylvania

Denise L. Kampfhenkel
Schreiner College
Kerrville, Texas

Patricia Laing-Arie
Meridian Technology Center
Stillwater, Oklahoma

Anne Lilly
Santa Rosa Junior College
Santa Rosa, California

Melanie S. MacNeil, MS, PhD
Brock University
St. Catharines, Ontario, Canada

Evie Mann
National College
Florence, Kentucky

Dan Matusiak, PhD
St. Dominic High School
O'Fallon, Missouri

Richard E. McKeeby
Union County College
Cranford, New Jersey

Michael Murrow
George Washington University
Annapolis, Maryland

Amy Obringer, PhD
University of Saint Francis
Fort Wayne, Indiana

Susan Caley Opsal, MS
Illinois Valley Community College
Oglesby, Illinois

Keith R. Orloff
California Paramedical and Technical College
Long Beach, California

Christine Payne
Sarasota County Technical Institute
Sarasota, Florida

Roberta Pohlman, PhD
Wright State University
Dayton, Ohio

Ann Senisi Scott
Nassau Tech VOCES
Westbury, New York

Gerry Silverstein, PhD
University of Vermont
Burlington, Vermont

Kathleen Stockman
Delaware Technical & Community College
Newark, Delaware

Anna M. Strand
Gogebic Community College
Ironwood, Michigan

Kent R. Thomas, PhD
Wichita State University
Wichita, Kansas

Karin Vanmeter, PhD
Iowa State University
Ames, Iowa

Eugene R. Volz
Sacramento City College
Sacramento, California

Amy Way
Lock Haven University
Clearfield, Pennsylvania

Margaret Weck, D.A.
St. Louis College of Pharmacy
St. Louis, Missouri

Iris Wilkelhake
Southeast Community College
Lincoln, Nebraska

Thanks are due to all the people at Elsevier who have worked with us on this new edition. We wish especially to acknowledge the support and efforts of Sally Schrefer, Executive Vice President, Nursing & Health Professions; Tom Wilhelm, Vice President, eSolutions; Becky Swisher, Managing Editor; Joe Gramlich, Developmental Editor; Emily Thomson, Editorial Assistant; Deborah Vogel, Publishing Services Manager; Brandi Tidwell, Project Manager; and Maggie Reid, Designer; all of whom were instrumental in bringing this edition to successful completion.

Gary A. Thibodeau
Kevin T. Patton

Contents

OBJECTIVES

AFTER YOU HAVE COMPLETED THIS CHAPTER, YOU SHOULD BE ABLE TO:

1. Define the terms *anatomy* and *physiology*.
2. Describe the scientific method.
3. List and discuss in order of increasing complexity the levels of organization of the body.
4. Define the term *anatomical position*.
5. List and define the principal directional terms and sections (planes) used in describing the body and the relationship of body parts to one another.
6. List the nine abdominopelvic regions and the abdominopelvic quadrants.
7. List the major cavities of the body and the subdivisions of each.
8. Discuss and contrast the axial and the appendicular subdivisions of the body. Identify a number of specific anatomical regions in each area.
9. Explain the meaning of the term *homeostasis* and give an example of a typical homeostatic mechanism.

An Introduction to the Structure and Function of the Body

There are many wonders in our world, but none is more wondrous than the human body. This is a textbook about that incomparable structure. It deals with two very distinct and yet interrelated sciences: **anatomy** and **physiology.**

As a science, anatomy is often defined as the study of the structure of an organism and the relationships of its parts. The word *anatomy* is derived from two Greek words that mean "a cutting up." Anatomists learn about the structure of the human body by cutting it apart. This process, called **dissection,** is still the principal technique used to isolate and study the structural components or parts of the human body.

Physiology, on the other hand, is the study of the functions of living organisms and their parts. It is a dynamic science that requires active experimentation. In the chapters that follow, you will see again and again that anatomical parts have structures that allow them to perform specific functions. Each has a particular size, shape, form, or position in the body related directly to its ability to perform a unique and specialized activity.

THE SCIENTIFIC METHOD

What we call the **scientific method** is merely a systematic approach to discovery. Although there is no single method for scientific discovery, many scientists follow the steps outlined here (and in Figure 1-1) to discover the concepts of human biology discussed in this textbook.

First, one makes a tentative explanation, called a **hypothesis.** A hypothesis is a reasonable guess based on previous informal observations or on previously tested explanations.

After a hypothesis has been proposed, it must be tested. This testing process is called **experimen-**

STUDY TIPS

A number of topics are introduced in this chapter that will be important throughout the rest of the course.

1. The most important topic in this chapter is probably *homeostasis*. The word itself tells you what it means: *homeo* means "the same," *stasis* means "staying." Homeostasis is the balance the body tries to maintain by keeping its internal environment "staying the same." Make sure you understand this concept.
2. Become familiar with the directional terms used in this text. You will see them in almost every diagram in the text and in the names of a number of body structures (e.g., *superior vena cava*, *distal convoluted tubule*). These terms consist of opposite pairs, so if you know the definition of one term, then you almost automatically know its opposite. Flash cards will help you learn them. Table 1-2 and Appendix B are helpful resources to keep in mind when you see an unfamiliar term.
3. This chapter also introduces you to levels of organization. This organizational structure should help you understand the big picture as you go through the rest of the text.
4. In your study groups try to come up with examples of negative feedback loops that help maintain a balance. Be creative. Do not just use the furnace example.
5. Go over your directional flash cards or photocopy Figure 1-3 and blacken out the terms and then use it to quiz each other.
6. Go over the questions in the back of the chapter and discuss possible test questions.

tation. Scientific experiments are designed to be as simple as possible, to avoid the possibility of errors. Often, *experimental controls* are used to ensure that the test situation is not affecting the results. For example, if a new cancer drug is being tested, half of the test subjects will get the drug and half of the subjects will be given a harmless substitute. The group getting the drug is called the *test group,* and the group getting the substitute is called the

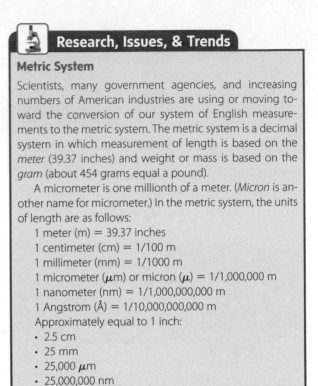

FIGURE 1-1 **The scientific method.** In this classic example, initial observations or results from other experiments may lead to formation of a new hypothesis. As more testing is done, eliminating outside influences or biases and ensuring consistent results, scientists begin to have more confidence in the principle and call it a theory or law.

control group. If both groups improve, or if only the control group improves, the drug's effectiveness hasn't been demonstrated. If the test group improves, but the control group does not, the hypothesis that the drug works is tentatively accepted as true. Experimentation requires accurate measurement and recording of data, along with logical interpretations of the data.

If the results of experimentation support the original hypothesis, it is tentatively accepted as true, and the researcher moves on to the next step. If the data do not support the hypothesis, the researcher tentatively rejects the hypothesis. Knowing which hypotheses are untrue is as valuable as knowing which hypotheses are true.

Initial experimental results are published in scientific journals so that other researchers can benefit from them and verify them. If experimental results cannot be reproduced by other scientists, then the hypothesis is not widely accepted. If a hypothesis withstands this rigorous retesting, the level of confidence in the hypothesis increases. A hypothesis that has gained a high level of confidence is called a **theory** or **law.**

The facts presented in this textbook are among the latest theories of how the body is built and how it functions. As methods of imaging the body and measuring functional processes improve, we find new data that cause us to replace old theories with newer ones.

STRUCTURAL LEVELS OF ORGANIZATION

Before you begin the study of the structure and function of the human body and its many parts, it is important to think about how those parts are organized and how they might logically fit together into a functioning whole. Examine Figure 1-1. It illustrates the differing levels of organization that influence body structure and function. Note that the levels of organization progress from the least complex (chemical level) to the most complex (body as a whole, or organism level).

Science Application

Modern Anatomy
Andreas Vesalius (1514-1546)

Anatomists study the structure of the human body. Modern anatomy started during the Renaissance in Europe with the Flemish scientist Andreas Vesalius (left) and his contemporaries. Vesalius was the first to apply a scientific method (see the text on pp. 1-2) to the study of the human body. Most anatomists still dissect *cadavers* (preserved human remains). However, today many anatomists also use imaging technologies such as x-rays, computerized scans, and even digitized photographs of thin slices of the body as you can see in the figure from the National Library of Medicine's Visible Human Project. Such digitized images can be reconstructed into dissectible, three-dimensional body views by computers.

Applications of modern anatomy are also found in the fields of forensic science, anthropology, medicine and allied health professions, sports and athletics, dance, and even art and computerized animation.

Organization is one of the most important characteristics of body structure. Even the word *organism,* used to denote a living thing, implies organization.

Although the body is a single structure, it is made up of trillions of smaller structures. Atoms and molecules are often referred to as the *chemical level* of organization. The existence of life depends on the proper levels and proportions of many chemical substances in the cells of the body.

Many of the physical and chemical phenomena that play important roles in the life process are reviewed in Chapter 2. Such information provides an understanding of the physical basis for life and for the study of the next levels of organization so important in the study of anatomy and physiology—cells, tissues, organs, and systems.

Cells are considered to be the smallest "living" units of structure and function in our body. Although long recognized as the simplest units of living matter, cells are far from simple. They are extremely complex, a fact you will discover in Chapter 3.

Tissues are somewhat more complex than cells. By definition a tissue is an organization of many cells that act together to perform a common function. The cells of a tissue may be of several types but all are working together in some way to pro-

duce the structural and functional qualities of the tissue. Cells of a tissue are often held together and surrounded by varying amounts and varieties of gluelike, nonliving intercellular substances.

Organs are larger and more complex than tissues. An organ is a group of several different kinds of tissues arranged in way that allow them to act as a unit to perform a special function. For instance, the heart shown in Figure 1-2 is an example of organization at the organ level. Unlike microscopic molecules and cells, some tissues and most organs are gross (large) structures that can be seen easily without a microscope.

Systems are the most complex units that make up the body. A system is an organization of varying numbers and kinds of organs that can work together to perform complex functions for the body. All of the organs of the cardiovascular system shown in Figure 1-2 allow blood to carry nutrients, oxygen, and wastes to and from the tissues of the body. The heart and each of the blood vessels are the organs that pump blood and carry it throughout the body as it performs its functions.

The *body as a whole* is all the atoms, molecules, cells, tissues, organs, and systems that you will study in subsequent chapters of this text. Although capable of being dissected or broken down into many parts, the body is a unified and complex

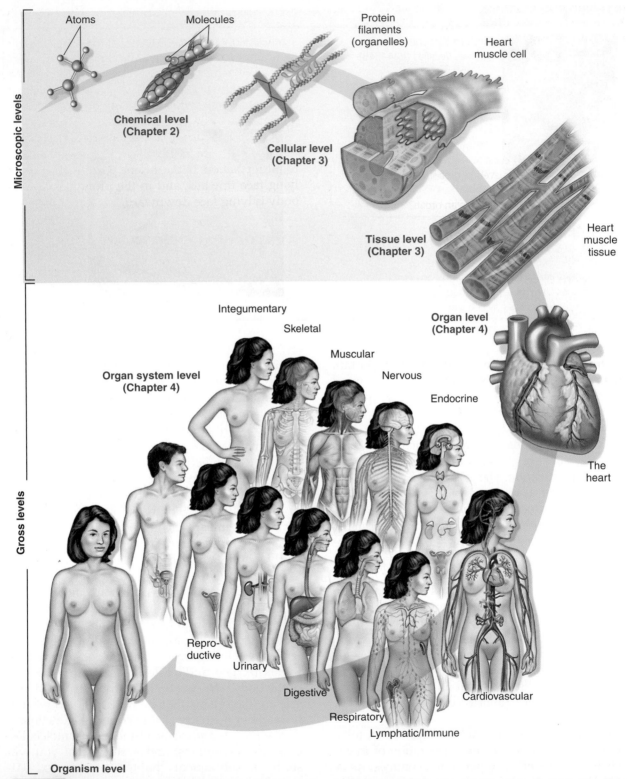

FIGURE 1-2 **Structural levels of organization in the body (see opposite page).** Atoms, molecules, and cells can ordinarily be seen only with a microscope, but the gross (large) structures of tissues, organs, systems, and the whole organism can be seen easily with the unaided eye.

assembly of structurally and functionally interactive components, each working together to ensure healthy survival.

 For a brief 3D tour of each of the body's organ systems, go to AnimationDirect on your CD-ROM.

✓ QUICK CHECK

1. What is *anatomy*? What is *physiology*?
2. What are the major levels of organization in the body?
3. How is a tissue different than an organ?

ANATOMICAL POSITION

Discussions about the body, the way it moves, its posture, or the relationship of one area to another assume that the body as a whole is in a specific position called the **anatomical position.** In this reference position (Figure 1-3) the body is in an erect or standing posture with the arms at the

FIGURE 1-3 **Anatomical position.** The body is in an erect or standing posture with the arms at the sides and the palms forward. The head and feet also point forward. The anatomical compass rosette is explained in the text on pp. 6-7.

sides and palms turned forward. The head and feet also point forward. The anatomical position is a reference position that gives meaning to the directional terms used to describe the body parts and regions. In other words, you need to know the anatomical position so that you know how to apply directional terms correctly no matter what position the body being described is in.

Supine and **prone** are terms used to describe the position of the body when it is not in the anatomical position. In the supine position the body is lying face upward, and in the prone position the body is lying face downward.

ANATOMICAL DIRECTIONS

When studying the body, it is often helpful to know where an organ is in relation to other structures. The following **directional terms** are used in describing relative positions of body parts. To help you understand them better, they are listed in sets of opposite pairs.

1. **Superior** and **Inferior** (Figure 1-4)—*superior* means "toward the head," and *inferior* means "toward the feet." *Superior* also means "upper" or "above," and *inferior* means "lower" or "below." For example, the lungs are located superior to the diaphragm, whereas the stomach is located inferior to it. (Check Figure 1-8 on p. 9 if you are not sure where these organs are.)
2. **Anterior** and **posterior** (see Figure 1-4)—*anterior* means "front" or "in front of." *Posterior* means "back" or "in back of." In humans, who walk in an upright position, *ventral* (toward the belly) can be used in place of anterior, and *dorsal* (toward the back) can be used for posterior. For example, the nose is on the anterior surface of the body, and the shoulder blades are on its posterior surface.
3. **Medial** and **lateral** (see Figure 1-4)—*medial* means "toward the midline of the body." *Lateral* means "toward the side of the body or away from its midline." For example, the great toe is at the medial side of the foot, and the little toe is at its lateral side. The heart lies medial to the lungs, and the lungs lie lateral to the heart.
4. **Proximal** and **distal** (see Figure 1-4)—*proximal* means "toward or nearest the trunk of the body, or nearest the point of origin of one

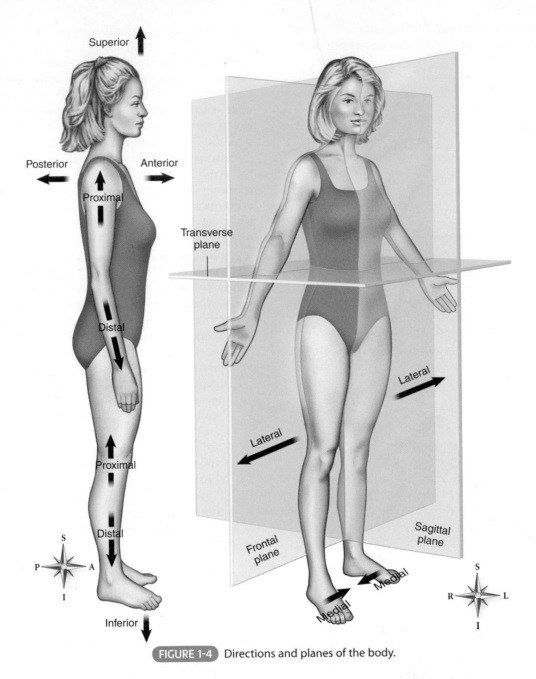

FIGURE 1-4 Directions and planes of the body.

of its parts." *Distal* means "away from or farthest from the trunk or the point of origin of a body part." For example, the elbow lies at the proximal end of the lower arm, whereas the hand lies at its distal end.

5. **Superficial** and **deep**—*superficial* means nearer the surface. *Deep* means farther away from the body surface. For example, the skin of the arm is superficial to the muscles below

it, and the bone of the upper arm is deep to the muscles that surround and cover it.

To make the reading of anatomical figures a little easier for you, we have used an anatomical compass rosette throughout this book. On many figures, you will see a small compass rosette like you might see on a geographical map. Instead of being labeled **N, S, E,** or **W,** the anatomical rosette is labeled with abbreviated anatomical directions.

For example, in Figure 1-3, the rosette is labeled **S** (for superior) on top and **I** (for inferior) on the bottom. Notice that in Figure 1-3 the rosette shows **R** (right) on the subject's right, not your right. Here are the directional abbreviations used with the rosettes in this book:

	A =	Anterior
	D =	Distal
	I =	Inferior
(opposite M) L =	Lateral
(opposite R) L =	Left
	M =	Medial
(opposite A) P =	Posterior
(opposite D) P =	Proximal
	R =	Right
	S =	Superior

 For a review of anatomical directions, go to AnimationDirect on your CD-ROM.

✓ QUICK CHECK

1. What is the anatomical position?
2. Why are the anatomical directions listed in pairs?

PLANES OR BODY SECTIONS

To facilitate the study of individual organs or the body as a whole, it is often useful to subdivide or "cut" it into smaller segments. To do this, body **planes** or **sections** have been identified by special names. Read the following definitions and identify each term in Figure 1-4.

1. **Sagittal**—a sagittal cut or section is a lengthwise plane running from front to back. It divides the body or any of its parts into right and left sides. The sagittal plane shown in Figure 1-4 divides the body into two *equal halves*. This unique type of sagittal plane is called a **midsagittal plane.**
2. **Frontal**—a frontal *(coronal)* plane is a lengthwise plane running from side to side. As you can see in Figure 1-4, a frontal plane divides the body or any of its parts into anterior and posterior (front and back) portions.
3. **Transverse**—a transverse plane is a horizontal or crosswise plane. Such a plane (see Figure 1-4) divides the body or any of its parts into upper and lower portions.

BODY CAVITIES

Contrary to its external appearance, the body is not a solid structure. It is made up of open spaces or cavities that in turn contain compact, well-ordered arrangements of internal organs. The two major body cavities are called the **ventral** and **dorsal body cavities.** The location and outlines of the body cavities are illustrated in Figure 1-5.

The upper part of the ventral cavity includes the **thoracic cavity,** a space that you may think of as your chest cavity. Its midportion is a subdivision of the thoracic cavity, called the **mediastinum.** Its other subdivisions are called the right and left **pleural cavities.** The lower part of the ventral cavity in Figure 1-5 includes an **abdominal cavity** and a **pelvic cavity.** Actually, they form only one cavity, the **abdominopelvic cavity,** because no physical partition separates them. In Figure 1-5 a dotted line shows the approximate point of separation between the abdominal and pelvic subdivisions. No-

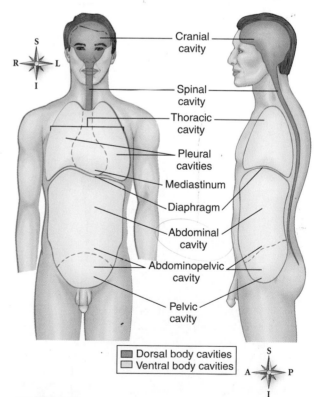

FIGURE 1-5 **Body cavities.** Location and subdivisions of the dorsal and ventral body cavities as viewed from the front (anterior) and from the side (lateral).

tice, however, that an actual physical partition separates the thoracic cavity from the abdominal cavity. This muscular sheet is the **diaphragm.** It is dome-shaped and is the most important muscle for breathing.

To make it easier to locate organs in the large abdominopelvic cavity, anatomists have divided the abdominopelvic cavity into four **quadrants:**

1. Right upper (or right superior) quadrant
2. Right lower (or right inferior) quadrant
3. Left upper (or right superior) quadrant
4. Left lower (or right inferior) quadrant

As you can see in Figure 1-6, the midsagittal and transverse planes, which were described in the previous section, pass through the navel (umbilicus) and divide the abdominopelvic region into the four quadrants. This method of subdividing the abdominopelvic cavity is frequently used by health professionals and is useful for locating the origin of pain or describing the location of a tumor or other abnormality.

Another and perhaps more precise way to divide the abdominopelvic cavity is shown in Figure 1-7. Here, the abdominopelvic cavity is subdivided into nine regions defined as follows:

1. **Upper abdominopelvic regions**—the **right** and **left hypochondriac regions** and the **epigastric region** lie above an imaginary line across the abdomen at the level of the ninth rib cartilages.
2. **Middle regions**—the **right** and **left lumbar regions** and the **umbilical region** lie below an imaginary line across the abdomen at the level of the ninth rib cartilages and above an imaginary line across the abdomen at the top of the hip bones.
3. **Lower regions**—the **right** and **left iliac** (or *inguinal*) **regions** and the **hypogastric region** lie below an imaginary line across the abdomen at the level of the top of the hip bones.

The dorsal cavity shown in Figure 1-5 includes the space inside the skull that contains the brain. It

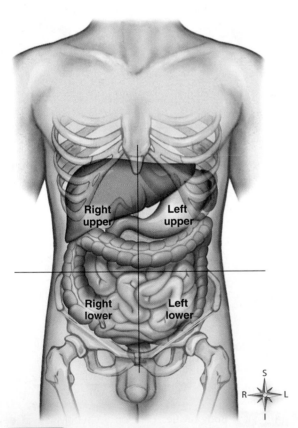

FIGURE 1-6 Division of the abdominopelvic cavity into four quadrants. Diagram showing relationship of internal organs to the four abdominal quadrants.

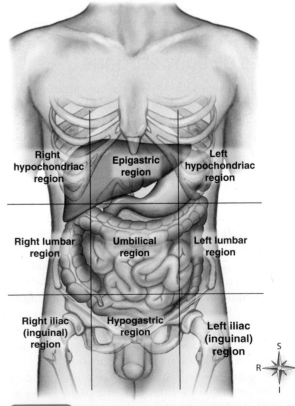

FIGURE 1-7 The nine regions of the abdominopelvic cavity. The most superficial organs are shown. Look at Figure 1-8 (p. 9). Can you identify the deeper structures in each region?

is called the **cranial cavity.** The space inside the spinal column is called the **spinal cavity.** It contains the spinal cord. The cranial and spinal cavities are *dorsal cavities,* whereas the thoracic and abdominopelvic cavities are *ventral cavities.*

Some of the organs in the largest body cavities are visible in Figure 1-8 and are listed in Table 1-1. Find each body cavity in a model of the human body if you have access to one. Try to identify the organs in each cavity, and try to visualize their locations in your own body. Study Figures 1-5 and 1-8.

> **QUICK CHECK**
>
> 1. What is meant by a *section* of the body?
> 2. What are the two major cavities of the body?
> 3. What is the difference between the *abdominal cavity* and the *abdominopelvic cavity*?

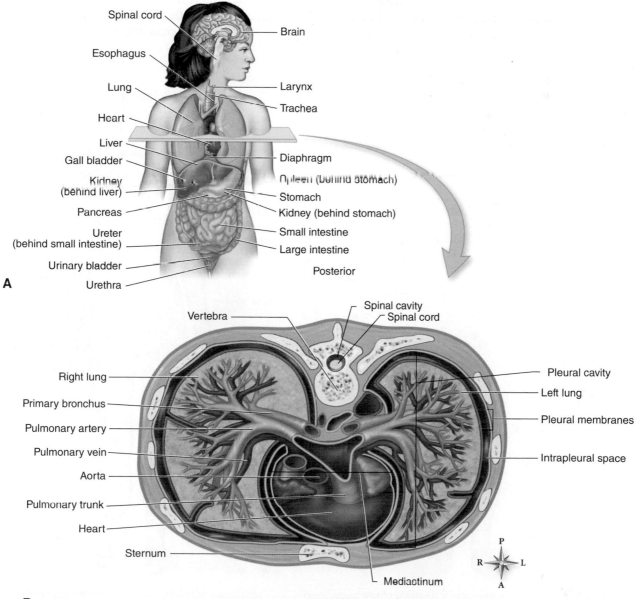

FIGURE 1-8   Organs of the major body cavities. **A,** A view from the front. **B,** Transverse section viewed from above.

TABLE 1-1	
Body Cavities	
BODY CAVITY	**ORGAN(S)**
Ventral Body Cavity	
Thoracic cavity	
Mediastinum	Trachea, heart, blood vessels
Pleural cavities	Lungs
Abdominal cavity	Liver, gallbladder, stomach, spleen, pancreas, small intestine, parts of large intestine
Pelvic cavity	Lower (sigmoid) colon, rectum, urinary bladder, reproductive organs
Dorsal Body Cavity	
Cranial cavity	Brain
Spinal cavity	Spinal cord

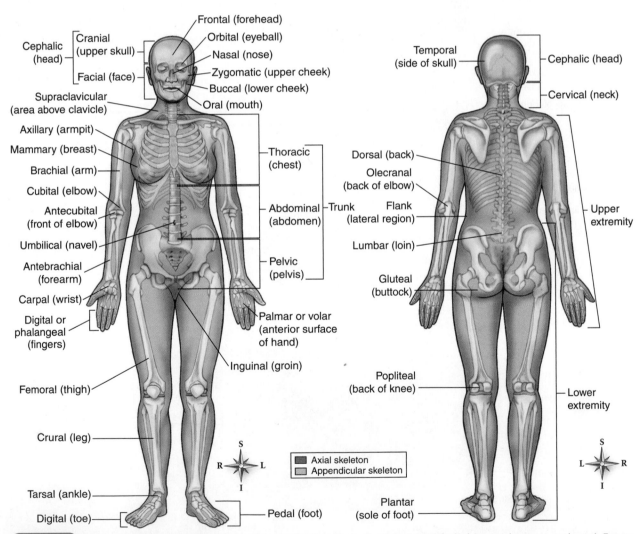

FIGURE 1-9 **Axial and appendicular divisions of the body.** Specific body regions are labeled (examples in parentheses). For example, the cephalic region includes the head. Notice how the axial and appendicular regions of the body frame are distinguished by contrasting colors.

BODY REGIONS

To recognize an object, you usually first notice its overall structure and form. For example, a car is recognized as a car before the specific details of its tires, grill, or wheel covers are noted. Recognition of the human form also occurs as you first identify overall shape and basic outline. However, for more specific identification to occur, details of size, shape, and appearance of individual body areas must be described. Individuals differ in overall appearance because specific body areas such as the face or torso have unique identifying characteristics. Detailed descriptions of the human form require that specific regions be identified and appropriate terms be used to describe them.

The ability to identify and correctly describe specific body areas is particularly important in the health sciences. For a patient to complain of pain in the head is not as specific and therefore not as useful to a physician or nurse as a more specific and localized description. Saying that the pain is facial provides additional information and helps to more specifically identify the area of pain. By using correct anatomical terms such as forehead, cheek, or chin to describe the area of pain, attention can be focused even more quickly on the specific anatomical area that may need attention. Familiarize yourself with the more common terms used to describe specific body regions identified in Figure 1-9 and listed in Table 1-2.

The body as a whole can be subdivided into two major portions or components: **axial** and **appendicular.** The axial portion of the body consists of the head, neck, and torso or trunk. The appendicular portion consists of the upper and lower extremities. Each major area is subdivided as shown in Figure 1-9. Note, for example, that the

TABLE 1-2

Descriptive Terms for Body Regions

AREA OR BODY REGION	EXAMPLE	AREA OR BODY REGION	EXAMPLE
Abdominal (ab-DOM-i-nal)	Anterior torso below diaphragm	**Femoral** (FEM-or-al) **region**	Thigh
Antebrachial (an-tee-BRAY-kee-al)	Forearm	**Gluteal** (GLOO-tee-al) **region**	Buttock
Antecubital (an-tee-KYOO-bi-tal)	Depressed area just in front of elbow	**Inguinal** (ING-gwi-nal) **region**	Groin
		Lumbar (LUM-bar) **region**	Lower back between ribs and pelvis
Axillary (AK-si-lair-ee)	Armpit	**Mammary** (MAM-er-ee) **region**	Breast
Brachial (BRAY-kee-al)	Arm	**Occipital** (ok-SIP-i-tal) **region**	Back of lower skull
Buccal (BUK-al) **region**	Cheek	**Olecranal** (oh-LEK-ra-nal) **region**	Back of elbow
Carpal (KAR-pal) **region**	Wrist	**Palmar** (PAHL-mar) **region**	Palm of hand
Cephalic (seh-FAL-ik) **region**	Head	**Pedal** (PEED-al) **region**	Foot
Cervical (SER-vi-kal) **region**	Neck	**Pelvic** (PEL-vik) **region**	Lower portion of torso
Cranial (KRAY-nee-al) **region**	Skull		
Crural (KROOR-al) **region**	Leg	**Perineal** (pair-i-NEE-al) **region**	Area (perineum) between anus and genitals
Cubital (KYOO-bi-tal) **region**	Elbow*		
Cutaneous (kyoo-TAYN-ee-us) region	Skin (or body surface)	**Plantar** (PLAN-tar) **region**	Sole of foot
Digital (DIJ-i-tal) **region**	Fingers or toes	**Popliteal** (pop-li-TEE-al) **region**	Area behind knee
Dorsal (DOR-sal) **region**	Back	**Supraclavicular** (soo-prah-klah-VIK-yoo-lar) **region**	Area above clavicle
Facial (FAY-shal) **region**	Face		
Frontal (FRON-tal) **region**	Forehead	**Tarsal** (TAR-sal) **region**	Ankle
Nasal (NAY-zal) **region**	Nose	**Temporal** (TEM-poh-ral) **region**	Side of skull
Oral (OR-al) **region**	Mouth	**Thoracic** (thoh-RAS-ik) **region**	Chest
Orbital (OR-bi-tal) **region** or **ophthalmic** (op-THAL-mik) region	Eyes	**Umbilical** (um-BIL-i-kul) **region**	Area around navel or umbilicus
Zygomatic (zye-goh-MAT-ik) region	Upper cheek	**Volar** (VOH-lar) **region**	Palm or sole

*The term *cubital* may also be used to refer to the forearm.

torso is composed of thoracic, abdominal, and pelvic areas, and the upper extremity is divided into arm, forearm, wrist, and hand components. Although most terms used to describe gross body regions are well understood, misuse is common. The word *leg* is a good example: it refers to the area of the lower extremity between the knee and ankle and not to the entire lower extremity.

The structure of each person's body is unique. Even identical twins have some variations in the size, shape, and texture of various tissues and organs. The structure of the body also changes in many ways and at varying rates during a lifetime. Before young adulthood, the body develops and grows. After young adulthood, the body gradually undergoes changes related to aging. For example, with the reduced activity of the body as one advances through older adulthood, many body organs and tissues decrease in size and therefore change in their functions. A degenerative process that results from disuse is called **atrophy.** In many cases, atrophy can be reversed with therapy. Some tissues simply lose their elasticity or ability to regenerate as we get older. Nearly every chapter of this book refers to a few of the changes that occur through the life cycle.

> ✓ **QUICK CHECK**
>
> 1. What is the difference between the *axial* portion of the body and the *appendicular* portion of the body?
> 2. What are some of the regions of the upper extremity and lower extremity?

THE BALANCE OF BODY FUNCTIONS

Although they may have very different structures, all living organisms maintain mechanisms that ensure survival of the body and success in propagating its genes through its offspring.

Survival depends on the body maintaining relatively constant conditions within the body. **Homeostasis** is what physiologists call the relative constancy of the internal environment. The cells of the body live in an internal environment made up mostly of water combined with salts and other dissolved substances. Like fish in a fishbowl, the cells are able to survive only if the conditions of their watery environment remain relatively stable—that is, only if conditions stay within a narrow range. The temperature, salt content, acid level (pH), fluid

volume and pressure, oxygen concentration, and other vital conditions must remain within acceptable limits. To maintain a narrow range of water conditions in a fishbowl, one may add a heater, an air pump, and filters. Likewise, the body has mechanisms that act as heaters, air pumps, and the like, to maintain the relatively stable conditions of its internal fluid environment.

Because the activities of cells and external disturbances are always shifting the conditions inside the body, fluctuations occur frequently. Therefore, the body must constantly work to maintain or restore stability, or homeostasis. For example, the heat generated by muscle activity during exercise may cause the body's temperature to rise above normal. The body must then release sweat, which evaporates and cools the body back to a normal temperature. To accomplish such self-regulation, a highly complex and integrated communication control system is required. The basic type of control system in the body is called a **feedback loop.**

The idea of a feedback loop is borrowed from engineering. Figure 1-10, *A*, shows how an engineer would describe the feedback loop that maintains stability of temperature in a building. Cold winds outside a building may cause a decrease in building temperature below normal. A **sensor,** in this case a thermometer, detects the change in temperature. Information from the sensor *feeds back* to a **control center**—a thermostat in this example—that compares the actual temperature with the normal temperature and responds by activating the building's furnace. The furnace is called an **effector** because it has an effect on the controlled condition (temperature). Because the sensor continually feeds information back to the control center, the furnace will be automatically shut off when the temperature has returned to normal.

As you can see in Figure 1-10, *B*, the body uses a similar feedback loop in restoring body temperature when a person becomes chilled. Nerve endings that act as temperature sensors feed information to a control center in the brain that compares actual body temperature to normal body temperature. In response to a chill, the brain sends nerve signals to muscles that shiver. Shivering produces heat that increases our body temperature. We stop shivering when feedback information tells the brain that body temperature has increased to normal.

Feedback loops such as those shown in Figure 1-10 are called **negative feedback loops** because

FIGURE 1-10 **Negative feedback loops. A,** An engineer's diagram showing how a relatively constant room temperature (controlled condition) can be maintained. A thermostat (control center) receives feedback information from a thermometer (sensor) and responds by counteracting a change from normal by activating a furnace (effector). **B,** A physiologist's diagram showing how a relatively constant body temperature (controlled condition) can be maintained. The brain (control center) receives feedback information from nerve endings called cold receptors (sensors) and responds by counteracting a change from normal by activating shivering by muscles (effectors).

they oppose, or negate, a change in a controlled condition. Most homeostatic control loops in the body involve negative feedback because reversing changes back toward a normal value tends to stabilize conditions, and this is exactly what homeostasis is all about. Think about the opposite circumstance of that shown in Figure 1-10, as when we become overheated during hot weather. Temperature receptors detect a body temperature higher than normal, and the brain sends signals to the sweat glands to cool us down through evaporation. Thus the conditions are reversed and balance is restored.

Another example of a negative feedback loop occurs when decreasing blood oxygen concentration caused by muscles using oxygen during exercise is counteracted by an increase in breathing to bring the blood oxygen level back up to normal. An additional example is the excretion of larger than usual volumes of urine when the volume of fluid in the body is greater than the normal, ideal amount.

Although not common, **positive feedback loops** exist in the body and are also involved in normal function. Positive feedback control loops are stimulatory. Instead of opposing a change in the internal environment and causing a "return to normal," positive feedback loops temporarily amplify the change that is occurring. This type of feedback loop causes an ever-increasing rate of events to occur until something stops the process. An example of a positive feedback loop includes the events that cause rapid increases in uterine contractions before the birth of a baby. Another example is the increasingly rapid sticking together of blood cells called *platelets* to form a plug that begins formation of a blood clot. In each of these cases, the process increases rapidly until the positive feedback loop is stopped suddenly by the birth of a baby or the formation of a clot. In the long run, such normal positive feedback events also help maintain constancy of the internal environment.

It is important to realize that homeostatic control mechanisms can only maintain a *relative* constancy. All homeostatically controlled conditions in the body do not remain absolutely constant. Rather, conditions normally fluctuate near a normal, ideal value. Thus body temperature, for example, rarely remains exactly the same for very long. It usually fluctuates up and down near a person's normal body temperature.

Because all organs function to help maintain homeostatic balance, we will be discussing negative and positive feedback mechanisms often throughout the remaining chapters of this book.

Before leaving this brief introduction to physiology, we must pause to state an important principle: the ability to maintain the balance of body functions is related to age. During childhood, homeostatic functions gradually become more and more efficient and effective. They operate with maximum efficiency and effectiveness during young adulthood. During late adulthood and old age, they gradually become less and less efficient

and effective. Changes and functions occurring during the early years are called *developmental processes*. Those occurring after young adulthood are called *aging processes*. In general, developmental processes improve efficiency of functions. Aging processes usually diminish them.

Health and Well-Being

Exercise Physiology

Exercise physiologists study the effects of exercise on the body organ systems. For example, many are interested in the complex control mechanisms that preserve or restore homeostasis during or immediately after periods of strenuous physical activity. Exercise, defined as any significant use of skeletal muscles, is a normal activity with beneficial results. However, exercise disrupts homeostasis. For example, when muscles are worked, the core body temperature rises and carbon dioxide levels in the blood increase. These and many other body functions quickly deviate from "normal ranges" that exist at rest. Complex control mechanisms must then "kick in" to restore homeostasis.

As a scientific discipline, exercise physiology attempts to explain many body processes in terms of how they maintain homeostasis. Exercise physiology has many practical applications in therapy and rehabilitation, athletics, occupational health, and general wellness. This specialty concerns itself with the function of the whole body, not just one or two body systems.

QUICK CHECK

1. Why is *homeostasis* also called "balance" of body function?
2. What is a *feedback loop* and how does it work?
3. How does *negative feedback* differ from *positive feedback*?

OUTLINE SUMMARY

THE SCIENTIFIC METHOD

A. Science involves logical inquiry based on experimentation (see Figure 1-1)
  1. Hypothesis — idea or principle to be tested in experiments
  2. Experiment — series of tests of a hypothesis; a controlled experiment eliminates biases or outside influences
  3. Theory or law — a hypothesis that has been proved by experiments to have a high degree of confidence
B. The process of science is active and changing as new experiments add new knowledge

STRUCTURAL LEVELS OF ORGANIZATION

A. Organization is the most important characteristic of body structure
B. The body as a whole is a unit constructed of the following smaller units (see Figure 1-2):
   1. Chemical level — atoms and molecules
   2. Cells — the smallest structural units; organizations of various chemicals
   3. Tissues — organizations of similar cells
   4. Organs — organizations of different kinds of tissues
   5. Systems — organizations of many different kinds of organs

ANATOMICAL POSITION

A. Reference position in which the body stands erect with the arms at the sides and palms turned forward (see Figure 1-3)
B. Anatomical position gives meaning to directional terms

ANATOMICAL DIRECTIONS

A. Superior — toward the head, upper, above
   Inferior—toward the feet, lower, below
B. Anterior — front, in front of (same as ventral in humans)
   Posterior — back, in back of (same as dorsal in humans)
C. Medial — toward the midline of a structure
   Lateral — away from the midline or toward the side of a structure
D. Proximal — toward or nearest the trunk, or nearest the point of origin of a structure
   Distal — away from or farthest from the trunk, or farthest from a structure's point of origin
E. Superficial — nearer the body surface
   Deep — farther away from the body surface

PLANES OR BODY SECTIONS (See Figure 1-4)

A. Sagittal plane — lengthwise plane that divides a structure into right and left sections
B. Midsagittal — sagittal plane that divides the body into two equal halves
C. Frontal (coronal) plane — lengthwise plane that divides a structure into anterior and posterior sections
D. Transverse plane — horizontal plane that divides a structure into upper and lower sections

BODY CAVITIES (See Figure 1-5)

A. Ventral cavity
   1. Thoracic cavity
      a. Mediastinum — midportion of thoracic cavity; heart and trachea are located in mediastinum
      b. Pleural cavities — right lung is located in right pleural cavity, left lung is in left pleural cavity
   2. Abdominopelvic cavity
      a. Abdominal cavity contains stomach, intestines, liver, gallbladder, pancreas, and spleen
      b. Pelvic cavity contains reproductive organs, urinary bladder, and lowest part of intestine
      c. Abdominopelvic regions
         (1) Four quadrants (see Figure 1-6)
         (2) Nine regions (see Figure 1-7)
B. Dorsal cavity
   1. Cranial cavity contains brain
   2. Spinal cavity contains spinal cord

BODY REGIONS (See Figure 1-9)

A. Axial region — head, neck, and torso or trunk
B. Appendicular region — upper and lower extremities
C. Body structure and function vary among individuals and also throughout an individual's life span; atrophy (decrease in size) occurs when an organ is not used

THE BALANCE OF BODY FUNCTIONS

A. Survival of the individual and of the genes that make up the body is of the utmost importance
B. Survival depends on the maintenance or restoration of homeostasis (relative constancy of the internal environment; see Figure 1-10)
   1. The body uses negative feedback loops and, less often, positive feedback loops to maintain or restore homeostasis
   2. Feedback loops involve a sensor, a control center, and an effector
C. All organs function to maintain homeostasis
D. Ability to maintain balance of body functions is related to age. Peak efficiency occurs during young adulthood, and diminishing efficiency of many functions begins after young adulthood

NEW WORDS

abdominopelvic cavity	spinal	dissection	organ
abdominopelvic	thoracic	effector	system
quadrants (4)	ventral	epigastric (region)	physiology
abdominopelvic	control center	experimentation	planes or sections
regions (9)	diaphragm	feedback loop	sagittal
anatomical position	directional terms	homeostasis	midsagittal
anatomy	superior	hypochondriac (region)	frontal
appendicular	inferior	hypogastric (region)	transverse
atrophy	anterior	hypothesis	positive feedback loop
axial	posterior	iliac (region)	prone
cavities	ventral	lumbar (region)	quadrants
abdominal	dorsal	negative feedback loop	scientific method
abdominopelvic	medial	organization (structural	sensor
cranial	lateral	levels)	supine
dorsal	proximal	chemical	theory (law)
mediastinum	distal	cell	umbilical (region)
pelvic	superficial	tissue	
pleural	deep		

REVIEW QUESTIONS

1. Define anatomy and physiology.
2. Describe the process used to form scientific theories.
3. List and explain the levels of organization in a living thing.
4. Describe the anatomical position.
5. Name and explain the three planes or sections of the body.
6. List two organs of the mediastinum, two organs of the abdominal cavity, and two organs of the pelvic cavity.
7. From the upper left to the lower right, list the nine regions of the abdominopelvic cavity.
8. Name the two subdivisions of the dorsal cavity. What structures does each contain?
9. Explain the difference between the terms *lower extremity*, *thigh*, and *leg*.
10. List four conditions in the cell that must be kept in homeostatic balance.
11. List the three parts of a negative feedback loop and give the function of each.

CRITICAL THINKING

11. Name a structure that is inferior to the heart, superior to the heart, anterior to the heart, posterior to the heart, and lateral to the heart.
12. The maintenance of body temperature and the birth of a baby are two body functions that are regulated by feedback loops. Explain the different feedback loops that regulate each process.
13. If a person complained of a pain in the epigastric region, what organs could be involved?

CHAPTER TEST

1. _____ is a term derived from two Greek words meaning "cutting up."
2. _____ means the study of the function of living organisms and their parts.
3. A hypothesis that has been rigorously tested can be called a or _____.
4. _____, _____, _____, _____, and _____ are the five organizational levels of a living thing.
5. _____ and _____ are terms used to describe the body position when it is not in anatomical position.
6. A _____ section cuts the body or any of its parts into upper and lower portions.
7. A _____ section cuts the body or any of its parts into front and back portions.
8. A _____ section cuts the body or any of its parts into left and right portions.
9. If the body is cut into equal right and left sides, the cut is called a _____ section or plane.
10. The body portion that consists of the head, neck, and torso is called the _____ portion.
11. The body portion that consists of the upper and lower extremities is the _____ portion.
12. The two major cavities of the body are the:
    a. thoracic and abdominal
    b. abdominal and pelvic
    c. dorsal and ventral
    d. anterior and posterior
13. The structure that divides the thoracic cavity from the abdominal cavity is the:
    a. mediastinum
    b. diaphragm
    c. lungs
    d. stomach

14. The epigastric region of the abdominopelvic cavity:
    a. is inferior to the umbilical region
    b. is lateral to the umbilical region
    c. is medial to the umbilical region
    d. none of the above
15. The hypogastric region of the abdominopelvic cavity is:
    a. inferior to the umbilical region
    b. lateral to the left iliac region
    c. medial to the right iliac region
    d. both a and c
16. Which of the following is an example of a positive feedback loop:
    a. Maintaining a constant body temperature
    b. Contractions of the uterus during childbirth
    c. Maintaining a constant volume of water in the body
    d. Both a and c

Match each of the directional terms in Column B with its opposite term in Column A.

COLUMN A	COLUMN B
17. _____ superior	a. posterior
18. _____ distal	b. superficial
19. _____ anterior	c. medial
20. _____ lateral	d. proximal
21. _____ deep	e. inferior

OBJECTIVES

AFTER YOU HAVE COMPLETED THIS CHAPTER, YOU SHOULD BE ABLE TO:

1. Define the terms *atom, element, molecule,* and *compound.*
2. Describe the structure of an atom.
3. Compare and contrast major types of chemical bonding.
4. Distinguish between organic and inorganic chemical compounds.
5. Discuss the chemical characteristics of water.
6. Explain the concept of pH.
7. Discuss the structure and function of the following types of organic molecules: carbohydrate, lipid, protein, and nucleic acid.

Chemistry of Life

Life is chemistry. It is not quite that simple, but the more we learn about human structure and function, the more we realize that it all boils down to interactions among chemicals. The digestion of food, the formation of bone tissue, and the contraction of a muscle are all chemical processes. Thus the basic principles of anatomy and physiology are ultimately based on principles of chemistry. A whole field of science, **biochemistry,** is devoted to studying the chemical aspects of life. To truly understand the human body, it is important to understand a few basic facts about biochemistry, the chemistry of life.

LEVELS OF CHEMICAL ORGANIZATION

Matter is anything that occupies space and has mass. Biochemists classify matter into several levels of organization for easier study. In the body, most chemicals are in the form of **molecules.** Molecules are particles of matter that are composed of one or more smaller units called **atoms.** Atoms are considered to be the basic units of matter. So a good place to start is with the atom.

Atoms

Atoms are so small that until recently they could not be seen by scientists. Modern tools such as *tunneling microscopes* and *atomic force microscopes (AFMs)* can produce pictures of atoms (Figure 2-1). Atoms are composed of several kinds of *subatomic particles:* **protons, electrons,** and **neutrons.**

At the core of each atom is a **nucleus** composed of positively charged protons and uncharged neutrons. The number of protons in the nucleus is an atom's **atomic number.** The number of protons and neutrons combined is the atom's **atomic mass.**

Negatively charged electrons surround the nucleus at a distance. In an electrically neutral atom, there is one electron for every proton. Electrons keep darting about within certain limits called **orbitals.** Each orbital can hold two electrons. Even though the name *orbital* implies that their electrons move around in elliptical orbits, and they are even

FIGURE 2-1 **Atoms.** A group of cloudlike atoms in a crystal as pictured by atomic force microscopy (AFM). Added colors highlight different kinds of atoms.

pictured that way in some atomic models, electrons actually move about in chaotic, unpredictable paths.

Orbitals are arranged into **energy levels** (shells), depending on their distance from the nucleus. The farther an orbital extends from the nucleus, the higher its energy level is. The energy level closest to the nucleus has one orbital, so it can hold two electrons. The next energy level has up to four orbitals, so it can hold eight electrons. Figure 2-2 shows a carbon (C) atom. Notice that the first energy level (the innermost shell) contains two electrons and the outer energy level contains four electrons. The outer energy level of a carbon atom could hold up to four more electrons (for a total of eight). The number of electrons in the outer energy level of an atom determines how it behaves chemically (that is, how it may unite with other atoms).

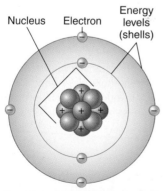

FIGURE 2-2 **A model of the atom.** The nucleus—protons (+) and neutrons—is at the core. Electrons inhabit outer regions called *energy levels*. This is a carbon atom, a fact that is determined by the number of its protons. All carbon atoms (and only carbon atoms) have six protons. (One proton and two neutrons in the nucleus are not visible in this illustration.)

This behavior, called *chemical bonding,* is discussed later in this chapter.

Elements, Molecules, and Compounds

Substances can be classified as **elements** or **compounds.** Elements are pure substances, composed of only one of more than a hundred types of atoms that exist in nature. Four kinds of atoms (*oxygen, carbon, hydrogen,* and *nitrogen*) make up about 96% of the human body, but there are traces of about 20 other elements in the body. Table 2-1 lists some of the elements in the body. Table 2-1 also gives for each element its universal chemical *symbol*—the abbreviation used by chemists worldwide.

Atoms usually unite with each other to form larger chemical units called *molecules.* Some molecules are made of several atoms of the same element. **Compounds** are substances whose molecules have more than one element in them. The *formula* for a compound contains symbols for all the elements present in each molecule. The number of atoms of each element in the molecule is expressed as a subscript after the elemental symbol. For example, each molecule of the compound *carbon dioxide* has one carbon (C) atom and two oxygen (O) atoms; thus its molecular formula is CO_2.

TABLE 2-1		
Important Elements in the Human Body		
ELEMENT	SYMBOL	**NUMBER OF ELECTRONS IN OUTER SHELL***
Major Elements (Greater Than 96% of Body Weight)		
Oxygen	O	6
Carbon	C	4
Hydrogen	H	1
Nitrogen	N	5
Trace Elements (Examples of More Than 20 Trace Elements Found in the Body)		
Calcium	Ca	2
Phosphorus	P	5
Sodium (Latin *natrium*)	Na	1
Potassium (Latin *kalium*)	K	1
Chlorine	Cl	7
Iodine	I	7

*Maximum is eight, except for hydrogen. The maximum for that element is two.

To learn more about molecule formation, go to AnimationDirect on your CD-ROM.

✓ QUICK CHECK

1. What kinds of particles make up matter?
2. What is a compound? An element?
3. Describe an energy level.

CHEMICAL BONDING

Chemical bonds form to make atoms more stable. An atom is said to be chemically stable when its outer energy level is "full" (that is, when its energy shells have the maximum number of electrons they can hold). All but a handful of atoms have room for more electrons in their outermost energy level. A basic chemical principle states that atoms react with one another in ways to make their outermost energy level full. To do this, atoms can share, donate, or borrow electrons.

For example, a hydrogen atom has one electron and one proton. Its single energy shell has one electron but can hold two, so it is not full. If two hydrogen atoms "share" their single electrons with each other, then both will have full energy shells, making them more stable as a molecule than either would be as an atom. This is one example of how atoms *bond* to form molecules. Other atoms may donate or borrow electrons until the outermost energy level is full.

Ionic Bonds

One common way in which atoms make their outermost energy level full is to form **ionic bonds** with other atoms. An ionic bond forms between an atom that has only one or two electrons in the outermost level (that would normally hold eight) and an atom that needs only one or two electrons to fill its outer level. The atom with one or two electrons simply "donates" its outer shell electrons to the one that needs one or two.

For example, as you can see in Table 2-1, the sodium (Na) atom has one electron in its outer level and the chlorine (Cl) atom has seven. Both need to have eight electrons to fill their outer shell. Figure 2-3 shows how sodium and chlorine form an ionic bond when sodium "donates" the electron in its outer shell to chlorine. Now both atoms have full outer shells (although sodium's outer shell is now one energy level lower). Because the sodium atom lost an electron, it now has one more proton than it has electrons. This makes it a positive *ion*, an electrically charged atom. Chlorine has

Clinical Application

Radioactive Isotopes

Each element is unique because of the number of protons it has. In short, each element has its own *atomic number*. However, atoms of the same element can have different numbers of neutrons. Two atoms that have the same atomic number but different atomic masses are **isotopes** of the same element. An example is hydrogen. Hydrogen has three isotopes: ^1H (the most common isotope), ^2H, and ^3H. The figure shows that each different isotope has only one proton but different numbers of neutrons.

Some isotopes have unstable nuclei that radiate (give off) particles. Radiation particles include protons, neutrons, electrons, and altered versions of these normal subatomic particles. An isotope that emits radiation is called a **radioactive isotope.**

Radioactive isotopes of common elements are sometimes used in *nuclear medicine* to evaluate the function of body parts. Radioactive iodine (^{125}I) put into the body and taken up by the thyroid gland gives off radiation that can be easily measured. Thus the rate of thyroid activity can be determined. Images of internal organs can be formed by radiation scanners that plot out the location of injected or ingested radioactive isotopes. For example, radioactive technetium (^{99}Tc) is commonly used to image the liver and spleen. The radioactive isotopes ^{13}N, ^{15}O, and ^{11}C are often used to study the brain in a technique called the *PET scan*.

Radiation can damage cells. Exposure to high levels of radiation may cause cells to develop into cancer cells. Higher levels of radiation completely destroy tissues, causing *radiation sickness*. Low doses of radioactive substances are sometimes given to cancer patients to destroy cancer cells. The side effects of these treatments result from the unavoidable destruction of normal cells with the cancer cells.

^1H ^2H ^3H

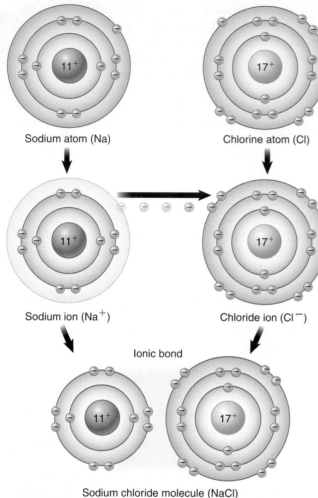

Sodium atom (Na)

Chlorine atom (Cl)

Sodium ion (Na⁺)

Chloride ion (Cl⁻)

Ionic bond

Sodium chloride molecule (NaCl)

FIGURE 2-3 Ionic bonding. The sodium atom donates the single electron in its outer energy level to a chlorine atom having seven electrons in its outer level. Now both have eight electrons in their outer shells. Because the electron/proton ratio changes, the sodium atom becomes a positive sodium ion. The chlorine atom becomes a negative chloride ion. The positive-negative attraction between these oppositely charged ions is called an *ionic bond*.

received an electron to become a negative ion called the *chloride* ion. Because oppositely charged particles attract one another, the sodium and chloride ions are drawn together to form a sodium chloride (NaCl) molecule—common table salt. The molecule is held together by an *ionic bond*.

Ionic molecules usually dissolve easily in water because water molecules are attracted to ions and wedge between the ions, thus forcing them apart. When this happens, we say the molecules **dissociate** (dis-SOH-see-ayt) to form free ions.

Molecules that form ions when dissolved in water are called **electrolytes** (eh-LEK-troh-lytes).

The formula of an ion always shows its charge by a superscript notation after the chemical symbol. Thus the sodium ion is Na⁺, and the chloride ion is Cl⁻. Calcium (Ca) atoms lose two electrons when they form ions, so the calcium ion formula is Ca⁺⁺.

Because the body's internal environment is mostly water, we find many dissolved ions in the body. Specific ions have important roles to play in muscle contraction, nerve signaling, and other vital functions. Table 2-2 lists some of the more important ions present in body fluids. Many of these ions will be discussed in later chapters. Chapter 18 describes mechanisms that maintain the homeostasis of the electrolytes throughout the body.

Covalent Bonds

Atoms may also fill their energy levels by sharing electrons rather than donating or receiving them. When atoms share electrons, then a **covalent** (koh-VAY-lent) **bond** forms. For example, Figure 2-4 shows how two hydrogen atoms may move together closely so that their energy levels overlap. Each energy level contributes its one electron to the sharing relationship. This way, both outer levels have access to both electrons. Because atoms involved in a covalent bond must stay close to each other, it is not surprising that covalent bonds are not easily broken. Covalent bonds normally do not break apart in water.

Covalent bonds are found in many molecules of the body. These bonds hold large molecules together in the watery internal environment. Without covalent bonds, the proteins and carbohydrates of your body would fall apart!

TABLE 2-2

Important Ions in Human Body Fluids

NAME	SYMBOL
Sodium	Na⁺
Chloride	Cl⁻
Potassium (Latin *kalium*)	K⁺
Calcium	Ca⁺⁺
Hydrogen	H⁺
Magnesium	Mg⁺⁺
Hydroxide	OH⁻
Phosphate	PO₄≡

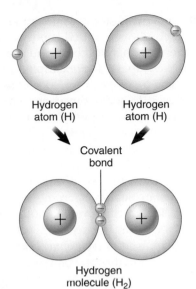

FIGURE 2-4 Covalent bonding. Two hydrogen atoms move together, overlapping their energy levels. Although neither gains or loses an electron, the atoms share the electrons, forming a covalent bond.

Hydrogen Bonds

A kind of weak attraction that helps hold your body's substance together is the **hydrogen bond.** Slight electrical charges may develop in different regions of a molecule when tiny hydrogen atoms are not able to equally share their electrons in a covalent bond. Oppositely charged ends of various molecules then electrically attract one another (Figure 2-5).

FIGURE 2-5 Hydrogen bonds. Because the tiny hydrogen atoms in water cannot share their electrons equally with a large oxygen atom, the water molecule develops slightly different charges at each end. Like weak magnets, the water molecules form temporary attachments (hydrogen bonds) that give liquid water its slightly gluelike properties.

Hydrogen bonds do not form new molecules, but instead provide subtle forces that help a large molecule stay in a particular shape. They may also help hold together neighboring molecules. For example, hydrogen bonds help hold proteins in their complex folded shapes (see Figure 2-12 on p. 28). Hydrogen bonds also keep water molecules loosely joined together, giving water a weak gluelike quality that helps hold your body together (see Figure 2-5).

> To learn more about chemical bonding, go to AnimationDirect on your CD-ROM.

✓ **QUICK CHECK**

1. How is an ion formed?
2. What is meant by an electrolyte *dissociating* in water?
3. What is covalent chemical bonding?
4. Why are hydrogen bonds important?

INORGANIC CHEMISTRY

In living organisms, there are two kinds of compounds: **organic** and **inorganic.** Organic compounds are composed of molecules that contain carbon-carbon (C–C) covalent bonds, carbon-hydrogen (C–H) covalent bonds, or both. Few inorganic compounds have carbon atoms in them, and none has C–C or C–H bonds. Organic molecules are generally larger and more complex than inorganic molecules. The human body has both kinds of compounds because both are equally important to the chemistry of life. We will discuss the chemistry of inorganic compounds first and then move on to some of the important types of organic compounds.

Water

One of the compounds that is most essential to life—water—is an inorganic compound. Water is the most abundant compound in the body, found in and around each cell. Its slightly gluelike properties help hold the tissues of the body together.

Water is the **solvent** in which most other compounds or **solutes** are dissolved. When water is the solvent for a *mixture* (a blend of two or more kinds of molecules), the mixture is called an **aqueous solution.** An aqueous solution containing common salt (NaCl) and other molecules forms the "internal sea" of the body.

Water molecules not only compose the basic internal environment of the body but also participate in many important *chemical reactions*. Chemical reactions are interactions among molecules in which atoms regroup into new combinations.

Dehydration synthesis is a common type of chemical reaction in the body. In any kind of synthesis reaction, the **reactants** combine to form a larger **product.** In dehydration synthesis, reactants combine only after two hydrogen (H) atoms and an oxygen (O) atom are removed. These leftover H and O atoms come together, forming H_2O, or water. As Figure 2-6 shows, the result is both the large product molecule and a water molecule. Just as dehydration of a cell is a loss of water from the cell and dehydration of the body is loss of fluid from the entire internal environment, dehydration synthesis is a reaction in which water is lost from the reactants.

Another common reaction in the body, **hydrolysis** (hye-DROL-i-sis), also involves water. In this reaction, water *(hydro-)* disrupts the bonds in large molecules, causing them to be broken down into smaller molecules *(lysis)*. Hydrolysis is virtually the reverse of dehydration synthesis, as Figure 2-6 shows.

All of the major types of organic compounds discussed later in this chapter are formed in water and use water (dehydration synthesis). And all four organic molecule types are broken apart in water and use water (hydrolysis). Clearly, water is an important substance in the body!

Chemical reactions always involve energy transfers. Energy is required to build the molecules.

Some of that energy is stored as potential energy in the chemical bonds. The stored energy can then be released when the chemical bonds in the molecule are later broken apart. For example, a molecule called *adenosine triphosphate (ATP)* breaks apart in the muscle cells to yield the energy needed for muscle contraction (see Figure 2-15 on p. 30).

Chemists often use a *chemical equation* to represent a chemical reaction. In a chemical equation, the reactants are separated from the products by an arrow ($\longrightarrow$) showing the "direction" of the reaction. Reactants are separated from each other and products are separated from each other by addition signs (+). Thus the reaction *potassium and chloride combine to form potassium chloride* can be expressed as the equation:

$$K^+ \; + \; Cl^- \longrightarrow KCl$$

The single arrow ($\longrightarrow$) is used for equations that occur in only one direction. For example, when hydrochloric acid (HCl) is dissolved in water, all of it dissociates to form H^+ and Cl^-:

$$HCl \longrightarrow H^+ + Cl^-$$

The double arrow ($\longleftrightarrow$) is used for reactions that happen in "both directions" at the same time. When carbonic acid (H_2CO_3) dissolves in water, some of it dissociates into H^+ (hydrogen ion) and HCO_3^- (bicarbonate), but not all of it. As additional ions dissociate, previously dissociated ions bond together again, forming H_2CO_3:

$$H_2CO_3 \longleftrightarrow H^+ \; HCO_3^-$$

FIGURE 2-6   **Water-based chemistry.** Dehydration synthesis *(left)* is a reaction in which small molecules are assembled into large molecules by removing water (H and O atoms). Hydrolysis *(right)* operates in the reverse direction. H and O from water are added as large molecules are broken down into small molecules.

In short, the double arrow indicates that at any instant in time both reactants and products are present in the solution at the same time.

Acids, Bases, and Salts

Besides water, many other inorganic compounds are important in the chemistry of life. For example, acids and bases are compounds that profoundly affect chemical reactions in the body. As explained in more detail at the beginning of Chapter 19, a few water molecules dissociate to form the H^+ ion and the OH^- (hydroxide) ion:

$$H_2O \longleftrightarrow H^+ + OH^-$$

In pure water, the balance between these two ions is equal. However, when an acid such as hydrochloric acid (HCl) dissociates into H^+ and Cl^-, it shifts this balance in favor of excess H^+ ions. In the blood, carbon dioxide (CO_2) forms carbonic acid (H_2CO_3) when it dissolves in water. Some of the carbonic acid then dissociates to form H^+ ions and HCO_3^- (bicarbonate) ions, producing an excess of H^+ ions in the blood. Thus high CO_2 levels in the blood make the blood more acidic.

Bases, or **alkaline** compounds, on the other hand, shift the balance in the opposite direction. For example, sodium hydroxide (NaOH) is a base that forms OH^- ions but no H^+ ions. In short, acids are compounds that produce an excess of H^+ ions, and bases are compounds that produce an excess of OH^- ions (or a decrease in H^+).

The relative H^+ concentration is a measure of how acidic or basic a solution is. The H^+ concentration is usually expressed in units of **pH.** The formula used to calculate pH units gives a value of 7 to pure water. A higher pH value indicates a low relative concentration of H^+—a base. A lower pH value indicates a higher H^+ concentration—an acid. Figure 2-7 shows a scale of pH from 0 to 14. Notice that when the pH of a solution is less than 7, the scale "tips" toward the side marked "high H^+." When the pH is more than 7, the scale "tips" toward the side marked "low H^+." pH units increase or decrease by factors of 10. Thus a pH 5 solution has 10 times the H^+ concentration of a pH 6 solution. A pH 4 solution has 100 times the H^+ concentration of a pH 6 solution.

A *strong acid* is an acid that completely, or almost completely, dissociates to form H^+ ions. A *weak acid*, on the other hand, dissociates very little and therefore produces few excess H^+ ions in solution.

When a strong acid and a strong base mix, excess H^+ ions may combine with the excess OH^- ions to form water. That is, they may neutralize each other. The remaining ions usually form neutral ionic compounds called *salts*. For example:

$$\underset{\text{acid}}{HCl} + \underset{\text{base}}{NaOH} \rightarrow H^+ + Cl^- + Na^+ + OH^- \rightarrow \underset{\text{water}}{H_2O} + \underset{\text{salt}}{NaCl}$$

The pH of body fluids affects body chemistry so greatly that normal body function can be maintained only within a narrow range of pH. The body can remove excess H^+ ions by excreting them in the urine (see Chapter 17). Another way to remove acid is by increasing the loss of CO_2 (an acid) by the respiratory system (see Chapter 14). A

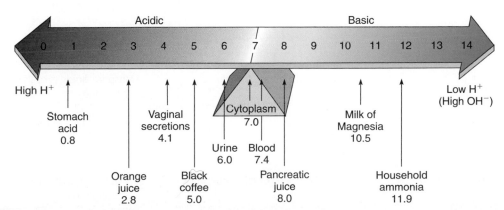

FIGURE 2-7 The pH scale. The H^+ concentration is balanced with the OH^- concentration at pH 7. At values above 7 (low H^+), the scale tips in the basic direction. At values below 7 (high H^+), the scale tips toward the acid side.

third way to adjust the body's pH is the use of **buffers**—chemicals in the blood that maintain pH. Buffers maintain pH balance by preventing sudden changes in the H^+ ion concentration. Buffers do this by forming a chemical system that neutralizes acids and bases as they are added to a solution. The mechanisms by which the body maintains pH homeostasis, or acid-base balance, are discussed further in Chapter 19.

> ✓ **QUICK CHECK**
> 1. Define an organic compound.
> 2. What is the difference between dehydration synthesis and hydrolysis?
> 3. Does an acid have a low pH or a high pH? A base?

ORGANIC CHEMISTRY

Organic compounds are much more complex than inorganic compounds. In this section, we will describe the basic structure and function of each major type of organic compound found in the body: **carbohydrates, lipids** (fats), **proteins,** and **nucleic acids.** Table 2-3 summarizes the structure and the function of each type. Refer to this table as you read through the descriptions that follow.

Carbohydrates

The name *carbohydrate* literally means "carbon (C) and water (H_2O)," signifying the types of atoms that form carbohydrate molecules. The basic unit of carbohydrate molecules is called a *monosaccharide* (mon-oh-SAK-er-yde) (Figure 2-8). Glucose (dextrose) is an important monosaccharide in the body. Cells use it as their primary source of energy (see Chapter 16). A molecule made of two saccharide units is a double sugar, or *disaccharide*. The disaccharides sucrose (table sugar) and lactose (milk sugar) are important dietary carbohydrates. After they are eaten, the body breaks them apart to form monosaccharides that can be used as cellular fuel.

Many saccharide units joined together form *polysaccharides*. Examples of polysaccharides are **glycogen** (GLYE-koh-jen), stored in the human body, and *starch,* found in plants that we eat. Each glycogen molecule is a chain of glucose molecules joined together. Liver cells and muscle cells form

TABLE 2-3

Major Types of Organic Compounds

EXAMPLE	COMPONENTS	FUNCTIONS
Carbohydrate		
Monosaccharide (glucose, galactose, fructose)	Single monosaccharide unit	Used as a source of energy; used to build other carbohydrates
Disaccharide (sucrose, lactose, maltose)	Two monosaccharide units	Can be broken into monosaccharides
Polysaccharide (glycogen, starch)	Many monosaccharide units	Used to store monosaccharides (thus to store energy)
Lipid		
Triglyceride	One glycerol, three fatty acids	Stores energy
Phospholipid	Phosphorus-containing unit, two fatty acids	Forms cell membranes
Cholesterol	Four carbon rings at core	Transports lipids; is basis of steroid hormones
Protein		
Structural proteins	Amino acids	Form structures of the body (fibers)
Functional proteins (enzymes, hormones)	Amino acids	Facilitate chemical reactions; send signals; regulate functions
Nucleic Acid		
Deoxyribonucleic acid (DNA)	Nucleotides (contain deoxyribose)	Contains information (genetic code) for making proteins
Ribonucleic acid (RNA)	Nucleotides (contain ribose)	Serves as a copy of a portion of the genetic code

Carbohydrates

Monosaccharide

Disaccharide

Polysaccharide

FIGURE 2-8 **Carbohydrates.** Monosaccharides are single carbohydrate units joined by dehydration synthesis to form disaccharides and polysaccharides. The detailed chemical structure of the monosaccharide glucose is shown in the inset.

glycogen when there is an excess of glucose in the blood, thus putting them into "storage" for later use. When we eat plants, we can break apart their starch molecules to get glucose.

Carbohydrates have potential energy stored in their bonds. When the bonds are broken in cells, the energy is released and then trapped by the cell's chemistry to do work. Chapter 16 explains more about the process by which the body extracts energy from carbohydrates and other food molecules.

Lipids

Lipids are fats and oils. Fats are lipids that are solid at room temperature, such as the fat in butter and lard. Oils, such as corn oil and olive oil, are liquid at room temperature. There are several important types of lipids in the body:

1. **Triglycerides** (try-GLISS-er-ydz) are lipid molecules formed by a *glycerol* unit joined to three *fatty acids* (Figure 2-9). Like carbohydrates, their bonds can be broken apart to yield energy (see Chapter 16). Thus triglycerides are useful in storing energy in cells for later use.

2. **Phospholipids** are similar to triglycerides but, as their name implies, have phosphorus-containing units in them. The phosphorus-containing unit in each molecule forms a "head" that attracts water. Two fatty acid "tails" repel water. Figure 2-10, *A*, shows the

FIGURE 2-9 **Triglyceride.** Each triglyceride is composed of three fatty acid units attached to a glycerol unit.

A

Head (attracts water)   Tail (repels water)

B

FIGURE 2-10 **Phospholipids. A,** Each phospholipid molecule has a phosphorus-containing "head" that attracts water and a lipid "tail" that repels water. **B,** Because the tails repel water, phospholipid molecules often arrange themselves so that their tails face away from water. The stable structure that results is a bilayer sheet forming a small bubble.

head and tail of the phospholipid molecule. This structure allows them to form a stable *bilayer* in water that forms the foundation for the cell membrane. In Figure 2-10, *B*, the water-attracting heads face the water and the water-repelling tails face away from the water (and toward each other).

3. **Cholesterol** is a *steroid* lipid (a multiple ring structure) that performs several important functions in the body. It combines with phospholipids in the cell membrane to help stabilize its bilayer structure. As explained in Chapter 10, the body also uses cholesterol as a starting point in making *steroid hormones* such as estrogen, testosterone, and cortisone (cortisol) (Figure 2-11).

FIGURE 2-11 **Cholesterol.** Cholesterol *(left)* has a steroid structure, represented here as four yellow rings. Changes to the side groups can convert cholesterol to cortisol *(shown)* or other steroid hormones.

Proteins

Proteins are very large molecules composed of basic units called **amino acids.** In addition to containing carbon, hydrogen, and oxygen, amino acids contain nitrogen (N). By means of a process described fully in Chapter 3, a particular sequence of amino acids is strung together and held by **peptide bonds.** Positive-negative attractions between different atoms in the long amino acid strand cause it to coil on itself again and again to form its highly complex shape. Folded proteins may combine with other folded proteins to form even larger, more complicated shapes. The complex, three-dimensional molecule that results is a protein molecule (Figure 2-12).

The folded shape of a protein molecule determines its role in body chemistry. *Structural proteins* are shaped in ways that allow them to form essential structures of the body. Collagen, a protein with a fiber shape, holds most of the body tissues together. Keratin, another structural protein, forms a network of waterproof fibers in the outer layer of the skin. *Functional proteins* have shapes that enable them to participate in chemical processes of

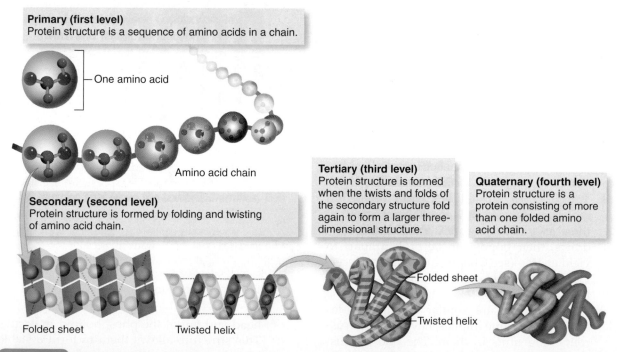

Primary (first level)
Protein structure is a sequence of amino acids in a chain.

One amino acid

Amino acid chain

Secondary (second level)
Protein structure is formed by folding and twisting of amino acid chain.

Tertiary (third level)
Protein structure is formed when the twists and folds of the secondary structure fold again to form a larger three-dimensional structure.

Quaternary (fourth level)
Protein structure is a protein consisting of more than one folded amino acid chain.

Folded sheet

Folded sheet   Twisted helix

Twisted helix

FIGURE 2-12 **Protein.** Protein molecules are large, complex molecules formed by one or more twisted and folded strands of amino acids. Each amino acid is connected to the next amino acid by covalent peptide bonds. This diagram shows how amino acids form strands that fold, and then fold again, into highly complex shapes.

the body. Functional proteins include some of the hormones, growth factors, cell membrane channels and receptors, and enzymes.

Enzymes are chemical catalysts. This means that they help a chemical reaction occur but are not reactants or products themselves. They participate in chemical reactions but are not changed by the reactions. Enzymes are vital to body chemistry. No reaction in the body occurs fast enough unless the specific enzymes needed for that reaction are present.

Figure 2-13 illustrates how shape is important to the function of enzyme molecules. Each enzyme has a shape that "fits" the specific molecules it works on much as a key fits specific locks. This explanation of enzyme action is sometimes called the **lock-and-key model.**

Proteins can bond with other organic compounds and form "mixed" molecules. For example, *glycoproteins* (described in Chapter 3) embedded in cell membranes are proteins with sugars attached. *Lipoproteins* are lipid-protein combinations (as described in the Blood Lipoproteins box).

Nucleic Acids

The two forms of nucleic acid are *deoxyribonucleic acid (DNA)* and *ribonucleic acid (RNA)*. As outlined in Chapter 3, the basic building blocks of nucleic

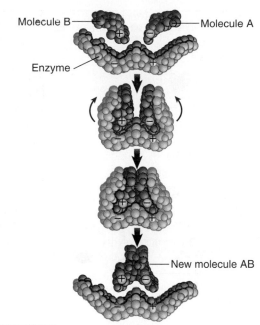

FIGURE 2-13 **Enzyme action.** Enzymes are functional proteins whose molecular shape allows them to catalyze chemical reactions. Molecules *A* and *B* are brought together by the enzyme to form a larger molecule, *AB*.

acids are called **nucleotides.** Each nucleotide consists of a *phosphate unit*, a sugar (*ribose* or *deoxyribose*), and a *nitrogen base*. DNA nucleotide bases include *adenine, thymine, guanine,* and *cytosine*. RNA uses the same set of bases, except for the substitution of *uracil* for thymine (Table 2-4).

Nucleotides bind to one another to form strands or other structures. In the DNA molecule, nucleotides are arranged in a twisted, double strand called a **double helix** (Figure 2-14).

The sequence of different nucleotides along the DNA double helix is the "master code" for assembling proteins and other nucleic acids. *Messenger*

 Clinical Application

Blood Lipoproteins

A lipid such as cholesterol can travel in the blood only after it has attached to a protein molecule, forming a lipoprotein. Some of these molecules are called *high-density lipoproteins (HDLs)* because they have a high density of protein (more protein than lipid). Another type of molecule contains less protein (and more lipid), so it is called *low-density lipoprotein (LDL)*.

The cholesterol in LDLs is often called "bad" cholesterol because high blood levels of LDL are associated with **atherosclerosis,** a life-threatening blockage of arteries. LDLs carry cholesterol to *cells*, including the cells that line blood vessels. HDLs, on the other hand, carry "good" cholesterol *away from cells* and toward the liver for elimination from the body. A high proportion of HDL in the blood is associated with a low risk of developing atherosclerosis. Factors such as cigarette smoking decrease HDL levels and thus contribute to risk of atherosclerosis. Factors such as exercise increase HDL levels and thus decrease the risk of atherosclerosis.

TABLE 2-4

Components of Nucleotides

NUCLEOTIDE	DNA	RNA
Sugar	Deoxyribose	Ribose
Phosphate	Phosphate	Phosphate
Nitrogen base	Cytosine	Cytosine
	Guanine	Guanine
	Adenine	Adenine
	Thymine	Uracil

To learn more about DNA structure and how it encodes genetic information, go to AnimationDirect on your CD-ROM.

FIGURE 2-14 DNA. Deoxyribonucleic acid (DNA), like all nucleic acids, is composed of units called *nucleotides*. Each nucleotide has a phosphate, a sugar, and a nitrogen base. In DNA, the nucleotides are arranged in a double helix formation as you can see in the simple structural models on the left.

A modified nucleotide called **adenosine triphosphate (ATP)** plays an important energy-transfer role in the body. As Figure 2-15 shows, adenosine (a base and a sugar) has not just one phosphate, as in a standard nucleotide, but instead three phosphates. The "extra" phosphates have relatively unstable "high-energy" bonds that require a great amount of energy (from nutrients) to form, and release, great energy when broken. When a phosphate breaks off—forming *adenosine diphosphate (ADP)*—the energy released is used to do work in cells. Thus ATP acts as a sort of energy-transfer "battery" that picks up energy from nutrients and then quickly makes the energy available to cellular processes. Chapter 16 outlines details of how ATP works in the cells.

RNA (mRNA) molecules have a sequence that forms a temporary "working copy" of a portion of the DNA code called a *gene*. The code in nucleic acids ultimately directs the entire symphony of living chemistry.

QUICK CHECK

1. Which types of organic molecules do these subunits form? Monosaccharides? Fatty acids? Amino acids? Nucleotides?
2. Why is the structure of protein molecules important?
3. What is the role of DNA in the body?
4. What is the role of ATP in the body?

FIGURE 2-15 ATP. **A,** Structure of adenosine triphosphate (ATP). Because the adenosine group is made up of a sugar (ribose) and a base (adenine), ATP is really a nucleotide with added phosphates. **B,** The role of ATP in transferring energy from nutrient molecules to cellular processes.

Science Applications

Biochemistry
Rosalind Franklin (1920-1958)

British scientist Rosalind Franklin was one of the leading biochemists of the modern age. Franklin used x rays to cast shadows through DNA to analyze its structure. When she was only 32 years old, she discovered the unusual helical (spiral) structure of the DNA molecule and how the sugars and phosphates form an outer backbone to the molecule (see Figure 2-14). Her breakthrough helped James Watson, Francis Crick, and Maurice Wilkins finally work out the structure and function of DNA in 1953 and thus crack the "code of life." The three men received a Nobel Prize for their achievement in 1962, but Franklin's early death from cancer in 1958 prevented her from sharing in the credit for one of the greatest discoveries of all time.

Biochemists continue to make important discoveries that increase our understanding of human structure and function. Aided by laboratory technicians and assistants, biochemists also find ways to help other professionals apply biochemistry to solve everyday problems. For example, clinical laboratory professionals analyze samples from the bodies of patients for signs of health or disease. Others who use biochemistry as a basis for their work include nuclear medicine technicians, pharmacists and pharmacy technicians, dietitians, forensic investigators, genetic counselors, and even science journalists.

OUTLINE SUMMARY

LEVELS OF CHEMICAL ORGANIZATION
A   Atoms (see Figures 2-1 and 2-2)
   1. Nucleus — central core of atom
      a. Proton — positively charged particle in nucleus
      b. Neutron — noncharged particle in nucleus
      c. Atomic number — number of protons in the nucleus; determines the type of atom
      d. Atomic mass — number of protons and neutrons combined
   2. Energy levels — regions surrounding atomic nucleus that contain electrons
      a. Electron — negatively charged particle
      b. May contain up to eight electrons in each level
      c. Energy increases with distance from nucleus
B. Elements, molecules, and compounds
   1. Element — a pure substance; made up of only one kind of atom
   2. Molecule — a group of atoms bound together in a group
   3. Compound — substances whose molecules have more than one kind of atom

CHEMICAL BONDING
A. Chemical bonds form to make atoms more stable
   1. Outermost energy level of each atom becomes full
   2. Atoms may share electrons, or donate or borrow them to become stable
B. Ionic bonds (see Figure 2-3)
   1. Ions form when an atom gains or loses electrons in its outer energy level to become stable
      a. Positive ion — has lost electrons; indicated by superscript positive sign(s), as in Na^+ or Ca^{++}
      b. Negative ion — has gained electrons; indicated by superscript negative sign(s), as in Cl^-
   2. Ionic bonds form when oppositely charged ions attract each other because of electrical attraction
   3. Electrolyte — molecule that dissociates (breaks apart) in water to form individual ions; an ionic compound
C. Covalent bonds (see Figure 2-4)
   1. Covalent bonds form when atoms share their outer energy to fill up and thus become stable
   2. Covalent bonds do not ordinarily easily dissociate in water

D. Hydrogen bonds
1. Weak forces that hold molecules in folded shapes (see Figure 2-12) or in groups (see Figure 2-5)
2. Do *not* form new molecules

INORGANIC CHEMISTRY

A. *Organic* molecules contain carbon-carbon covalent bonds or carbon-hydrogen covalent bonds; *inorganic* molecules do not
B. Examples of inorganic molecules: water and some acids, bases, and salts
C. Water
1. Water is essential to life
2. Water's slightly gluelike nature helps hold the body together
3. Water is a solvent (liquid into which solutes are dissolved), forming aqueous solutions in the body
4. Water is involved in chemical reactions (see Figure 2-6)
   a. Dehydration synthesis — chemical reaction in which water is removed from small molecules so they can be strung together to form a larger molecule
   b. Hydrolysis — chemical reaction in which water is added to the subunits of a large molecule to break it apart into smaller molecules
   c. All the major organic molecules are formed through dehydration synthesis and are broken apart by hydrolysis
   d. Chemical reactions always involve energy transfers, as when energy is used to build ATP molecules
   e. Chemical equations show how reactants interact to form products; arrows separate the reactants from the products
D. Acids, bases, and salts
1. Water molecules dissociate to form equal amounts of H^+ (hydrogen ion) and OH^- (hydroxide ion)
2. Acid — substance that shifts the H^+/OH^- balance in favor of H^+; opposite of base
3. Base — substance that shifts the H^+/OH^- balance against H^+; also known as an alkaline; opposite of acid

4. pH — mathematical expression of relative H^+ concentration in an aqueous solution (see Figure 2-7)
   a. pH 7 is neutral (neither acid nor base)
   b. pH values above 7 are basic; pH values below 7 are acidic
5. Neutralization occurs when acids and bases mix and form salts
6. Buffers are chemical systems that absorb excess acids or bases and thus maintain a relatively stable pH

ORGANIC CHEMISTRY

A. Carbohydrates — sugars and complex carbohydrates (see Figure 2-8)
1. Contain carbon (C), hydrogen (H), oxygen (O)
2. Made up of six-carbon subunits called *monosaccharides* or single sugars (e.g., glucose)
3. Disaccharide — double sugar made up of two monosaccharide units (e.g., sucrose, lactose)
4. Polysaccharide — complex carbohydrate made up of many monosaccharide units (e.g., glycogen made up of many glucose units)
5. Function of carbohydrates is to store energy for later use
B. Lipids — fats and oils
1. Triglycerides (see Figure 2-9)
   a. Made up of one glycerol unit and three fatty acids
   b. Store energy for later use
2. Phospholipids (see Figure 2-10)
   a. Similar to triglyceride structure, except with only two fatty acids, and with a phosphorus-containing group attached to glycerol
   b. The head attracts water and the double tail does not, thus forming stable double layers (bilayers) in water
   c. Form membranes of cells
3. Cholesterol (see Figure 2-11)
   a. Molecules have a steroid structure made up of multiple rings
   b. Cholesterol stabilizes the phospholipid tails in cellular membranes and is also converted into steroid hormones by the body

C. Proteins
   1. Very large molecules made up of amino acids held together in long, folded chains by peptide bonds (see Figure 2-12)
   2. Structural proteins
      a. Form various structures of the body
      b. Collagen is a fibrous protein that holds many tissues together
      c. Keratin forms tough, waterproof fibers in the outer layer of the skin
   3. Functional proteins
      a. Participate in chemical processes of the body
      b. Examples: hormones, cell membrane channels and receptors, enzymes
      c. Enzymes (see Figure 2-13)
         (1) Catalysts — help chemical reactions occur
         (2) Lock-and-key model — each enzyme fits a particular molecule that it acts on as a key fits into a lock
   4. Proteins can combine with other organic molecules to form glycoproteins or lipoproteins

D. Nucleic acids
   1. Made up of nucleotide units, each made up of:
      a. Sugar (ribose or deoxyribose)
      b. Phosphate
      c. Nitrogen base (adenine, thymine or uracil, guanine, cytosine)
   2. DNA (deoxyribonucleic acid) (see Figure 2-14)
      a. Used as the cell's "master code" for assembling proteins
      b. Uses deoxyribose as the sugar and A, T (not U), C, and G as bases
      c. Forms a double helix shape
   3. RNA (ribonucleic acid)
      a. Used as a temporary "working copy" of a gene (portion of the DNA code)
      b. Uses ribose as the sugar and A, U (not T), C, and G as bases
   4. By directing the formation of structural and functional proteins, nucleic acids ultimately direct overall body structure and function
   5. ATP (adenosine triphosphate) is a modified nucleotide used to transfer energy from nutrients to cellular processes, thus acting as an energy-transfer "battery" (see Figure 2-15)

NEW WORDS

adenosine triphosphate (ATP)	cholesterol	hydrolysis	organic compound
alkaline	compound	inorganic compound	peptide bond
amino acid	covalent bond	ionic bond	pH
aqueous solution	dehydration synthesis	isotope	phospholipid
atherosclerosis	dissociate	lipid	product
atom	double helix	lock-and-key model	protein
atomic mass	electrolyte	matter	proton
atomic number	electron	molecule	radioactive isotope
base	element	neutron	reactant
biochemistry	energy level	nucleic acid	solute
buffer	enzyme	nucleotide	solvent
carbohydrate	glycogen	nucleus	triglyceride
	hydrogen bond	orbital	

REVIEW QUESTIONS

1. Define the following terms: *element, compound, atom, molecule.*
2. Name and define three kinds of particles within an atom.
3. What is an energy level?
4. What is a chemical bond?
5. What are the major types of chemical bond?
6. What is an electrolyte? An ion?
7. Define the terms *organic compound* and *inorganic compound.*
8. What is a solvent? A solute?
9. Explain the concept of pH.
10. What is an acid? A base?
11. Briefly describe the structure of each of these: *protein, lipid, carbohydrate, nucleic acid.*
12. Briefly state the principle functions of each of these: *carbohydrate, protein, lipid, nucleic acid.*

CRITICAL THINKING

13. Compare and contrast how ionic bonds and chemical bonds solve the problem of achieving stability in atoms.
14. A certain protein molecule is hydrolyzed by an enzyme. How would you explain that statement to someone unfamiliar with chemical terminology?
15. If your blood normally has a pH of around 7.4, is your blood alkaline, acid, or neutral?
16. A newly discovered protein is found to regulate how hormones influence the functions of cells in the body. Is this protein a structural protein or a functional protein?
17. What mechanism does DNA use to regulate all of the body's structures and function?
18. How would you explain the difference between ^1H, ^2H, and ^3H?

CHAPTER TEST

1. _____ is anything that occupies space and has mass.
2. Molecules are made up of particles called _____.
3. Positively charged particles within the nucleus of an atom are called _____.
4. Electrons inhabit regions of the atoms called _____ levels.
5. Substances with molecules having more than one kind of atom are called _____.
6. A(n) _____ chemical bond occurs when atoms share electrons.
7. The symbol K^+ represents the potassium _____.
8. A compound that dissociates in water to form ions is called a(n) _____.
9. Molecules that have a carbon-carbon bond in them are classified as _____ compounds.
10. In saltwater, salt is the solute and water is the _____.
11. When water is used to build up small molecules into larger molecules, the process is called _____.
12. _____ are solutions that have an excess of hydrogen ions.
13. Blood contains chemicals called _____ that maintain a stable pH.

Match each type of compound in Column B with the corresponding example given in Column A.

COLUMN A	COLUMN B
14. _____ glycogen	a. salt
15. _____ collagen	b. acid
16. _____ RNA	c. base
17. _____ cholesterol	d. carbohydrate
18. _____ NaCl	e. lipid
19. _____ NaOH	f. protein
20. _____ HCl	g. nucleic acid

21. An ion is formed when
    a. electrons are shared
    b. electrons remain in place
    c. electrons are gained or lost
    d. neutrons are added to the nucleus

CHAPTER TEST—cont'd

22. In the equation $H_2O + CO_2 \longrightarrow H^+ + HCO_3^-$, which of these is a reactant?
   a. CO_2
   b. HCO_3^-
   c. O_2
   d. $\longrightarrow$

23. Which of these chemical subunits is found in DNA?
   a. uracil
   b. ribose
   c. amino acid
   d. deoxyribose

24. Which of these represents an acid?
   a. pH 7.5
   b. pH 6.1
   c. pH 9.0
   d. pH 7.0

25. Steroid hormones are
   a. carbohydrates
   b. proteins
   c. lipids
   d. nucleic acids

OBJECTIVES

AFTER YOU HAVE COMPLETED THIS CHAPTER, YOU SHOULD BE ABLE TO:

1. Identify and discuss the basic structure and function of the three major components of a cell.
2. List and briefly discuss the functions of the primary cellular organelles.
3. Compare the major passive and active transport processes that act to move substances through cell membranes.
4. Compare and discuss DNA and RNA and their function in protein synthesis.
5. Discuss the stages of mitosis and explain the importance of cellular reproduction.
6. Explain how epithelial tissue is grouped according to shape and arrangement of cells.
7. List and briefly discuss the major types of connective and muscle tissue.
8. List the three structural components of a neuron.

Cells and Tissues

3

About 300 years ago Robert Hooke looked through his microscope, one of the very early, somewhat primitive ones, at some plant material. What he saw must have surprised him. Instead of a single magnified piece of plant material, he saw many small spaces created by cell walls. Because they reminded him of miniature storerooms or "cells," that is what he called them: *cells*. Since Hooke's time, thousands of individuals have examined thousands of plant and animal specimens and found them all, without exception, to be composed of cells. This fact, that cells are the smallest structural units of living things, has become the foundation of modern biology. Many living things are so simple that they consist of just one cell. The human body, however, is so complex that it consists not of a few thousand or millions or even billions of cells but of many trillions of them. This chapter discusses cells first and then groups of similar cells, which are called *tissues*.

CELLS

Size and Shape

Human cells are microscopic in size; that is, they can be seen only when magnified by a microscope. However, they vary considerably in size. An ovum (female sex cell), for example, has a diameter of about 150 micrometers, whereas red blood cells have a diameter of only 7.5 micrometers. Cells differ even more notably in shape than in size. Some are flat, some are brick-shaped, some are threadlike, and some have irregular shapes.

Composition

Cells contain cytoplasm (SYE-toh-plaz-em), or "living matter," a substance that exists only in cells. The term *cyto-* is a Greek combining form and denotes a relationship to a cell. Each cell in the body is surrounded by a thin membrane, the *plasma membrane*. This membrane separates the cell contents from the dilute saltwater solution called **interstitial** (in-ter-STISH-al) **fluid,** or simply *tissue fluid,* which bathes every cell in the body. Numerous specialized structures called *organelles* (or-gah-NELZ), which are described in subsequent sections of this chapter, are contained within the cytoplasm of each cell. A small, circular body called the *nucleus* (NOO-klee-us) is also inside the cell.

Parts of the Cell

The three main parts of a cell are:
1. Plasma membrane
2. Cytoplasm
3. Nucleus

The plasma membrane surrounds the entire cell, forming its outer boundary. The cytoplasm is all the living material inside the cell (except the nucleus). The nucleus is a large, membrane-bound structure in most cells that contains the genetic code.

Plasma Membrane

As the name suggests, the **plasma membrane** is the membrane that encloses the cytoplasm and forms the outer boundary of the cell. It is an incredibly delicate structure—only about 7 nm (nanometers) or 3/10,000,000 of an inch thick! Yet it has a precise, orderly structure (Figure 3-1). Two layers of phosphate-containing fat molecules called *phospholipids* form a fluid framework for the plasma membrane. Another kind of fat molecule called *cholesterol* is also a component of the plasma membrane. Cholesterol helps stabilize the phospholipid molecules to prevent breakage of the plasma membrane.

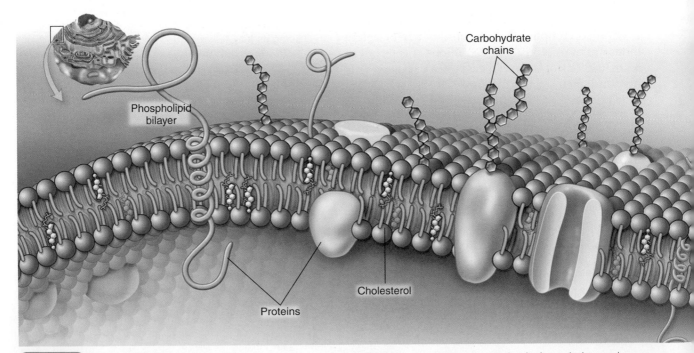

Carbohydrate chains

Phospholipid bilayer

Cholesterol

Proteins

FIGURE 3-1 **Structure of the plasma membrane.** Note that protein molecules may penetrate completely through the two layers of phospholipid molecules.

Note in Figure 3-1 that protein molecules dot the surfaces of the membrane and extend all the way through the phospholipid framework.

Despite its seeming fragility, the plasma membrane is strong enough to keep the cell whole and intact. It also performs other life-preserving functions for the cell. It serves as a well-guarded gateway between the fluid inside the cell and the fluid around it. Certain substances move through it, by way of transporter channels and carriers, but it bars the passage of other substances.

The plasma membrane even functions as a communication device. How? Some of the proteins on the membrane's outer surface serve as receptors for certain other molecules when these other molecules contact the proteins. In other words, certain molecules bind to certain receptor proteins. For example, some hormones (chemicals secreted into blood from ductless glands) bind to membrane receptors, and a change in cell functions follows.

We might therefore think of such hormones as chemical messages, communicated to cells by binding to their cytoplasmic membrane receptors.

The plasma membrane also identifies a cell as being part of one particular individual. Some of its surface proteins serve as positive identification tags because they occur only in the cells of that individual. A practical application of this fact is made in *tissue typing*, a procedure performed before an organ from one individual is transplanted into another. Carbohydrate chains attached to the surface of cells often play a role in the identification of cell types.

Cytoplasm

Cytoplasm is the internal living material of cells. It fills the space between the plasma membrane and the nucleus, which can be seen in Figure 3-2 as a round or spherical structure in the center of the cell. Numerous small structures are part of the

FIGURE 3-2 General characteristics of the cell. Artist's interpretation of cell structure.

cytoplasm, along with the fluid that serves as the interior environment of each cell. As a group, the small structures that make up much of the cytoplasm are called **organelles.** This name means "little organs," an appropriate name because they function for the cell just as organs function for the body.

In Figure 3-2 you can see small threadlike structures scattered around in the cytoplasm. You can see only a few of the many threads that make up the **cytoskeleton,** or "cell skeleton." Thin thread-like filaments in this framework are called *microfilaments*. Tiny, hollow tubes called *microtubules* are also important. Like the body's framework of bones and muscles, the cytoskeleton provides support and movement. The various organelles are not just floating around randomly. They are instead being held (or moved) by the fibers and *molecular motors* of the cytoskeleton. When a cell moves, or when organelles within a cell move, it is actually the parts of the cytoskeleton that are pulling or pushing membranes and organelles.

Look again at Figure 3-2. Notice how many different kinds of structures you can see in the cytoplasm of this cell. A little more than a generation ago, most of these organelles were unknown. We now know of many types of organelles, only a few of which are shown here. They are so small that they are invisible even when magnified 1,000 times by a light microscope. The advent of electron microscopes finally brought them into view by magnifying them many thousands of times. Next we briefly discuss the following organelles, which are found in cytoplasm (Table 3-1):

1. Ribosomes
2. Endoplasmic reticulum
3. Golgi apparatus
4. Mitochondria
5. Lysosomes
6. Centrosome
7. Cell extensions

Ribosomes

Organelles called **ribosomes** (RYE-boh-sohmz), shown as dots in Figure 3-2, are tiny particles found throughout the cell. They are each made up of two tiny subunits constructed mostly of a special kind of RNA called *ribosomal RNA (rRNA)*. Some ribosomes are found temporarily attached to a network of membranous canals called *endoplasmic reticulum (ER)*. Ribosomes may also be free in the cytoplasm. Ribosomes perform a very complex function: they make enzymes and other protein compounds. Thus they are nicknamed "protein factories."

Endoplasmic Reticulum

An **endoplasmic reticulum** (en-doh-PLAS-mik reh-TIK-yoo-lum) (ER) is a system of membranes forming a network of connecting sacs and canals that wind back and forth through a cell's cytoplasm, from the nucleus almost to the plasma membrane. The tubular passageways or canals in the ER carry proteins and other substances through the cytoplasm of the cell from one area to another.

There are two types of ER: *rough* and *smooth*. Rough ER gets its name from the many ribosomes that are attached to its outer surface, giving it a rough texture similar to sandpaper. As ribosomes make their proteins, they may attach to the rough ER and drop the protein into the interior of the ER. The ER then begins folding the new proteins and transports them to areas in which chemical processing takes place. These areas of the ER are so full of molecules that ribosomes have no room into which they can pass their proteins and so they do not attach. The absence of attached ribosomes gives this type of ER a smooth texture. Fats, carbohydrates, and proteins that make up cellular membrane material are manufactured in smooth ER. Thus the smooth ER makes a new membrane for the cell. To sum up: rough ER receives, folds, and transports newly made proteins, and smooth ER makes a new membrane.

Golgi Apparatus

The **Golgi** (GOL-jee) **apparatus** consists of tiny, flattened sacs stacked on one another near the nucleus. Little bubbles, or sacs, break off the smooth ER and carry new proteins and other compounds to the sacs of the Golgi apparatus. These little sacs, also called **vesicles,** fuse with the Golgi sacs and allow the contents of both to mingle.

The Golgi apparatus chemically processes the molecules from the ER by continuing the folding of proteins begun in the ER and combining them with other molecules to form quaternary proteins (see Figure 2-12, p. 28) or combinations such as glycoproteins (carbohydrate/protein combinations). The Golgi apparatus then packages the processed molecules into new little vesicles that break away from the Golgi apparatus and move

TABLE 3-1 ✐

Structure and Function of Some Major Cell Parts

CELL PART	STRUCTURE	FUNCTION(S)
Plasma membrane	Phospholipid bilayer studded with proteins	Serves as the boundary of the cell; protein and carbohydrate molecules on the outer surface of plasma membrane perform various functions; for example, they serve as markers that identify cells of each individual or as receptor molecules for certain hormones
Ribosomes	Tiny particles, each made up of rRNA subunits	Synthesize proteins; a cell's "protein factories"
Endoplasmic reticulum (ER)	Membranous network of interconnected canals and sacs, some with ribosomes attached (rough ER) and some without attachments (smooth ER)	Rough ER receives and transports reticulum (ER) synthesized proteins (from ribosomes); smooth ER synthesizes lipids and certain carbohydrates
Golgi apparatus	Stack of flattened, membranous sacs	Chemically processes, then packages substances from the ER
Mitochondria	Membranous capsules containing a large, folded internal membrane encrusted with enzymes	ATP synthesis; a cell's "power plants" or "battery chargers"
Lysosome	"Bubble" of hydrolysis enzymes encased by membrane	A cell's "digestive bag," it breaks apart large molecules
Centrosome	Area near nucleus without a visible boundary; contains centrioles	Organizes microtubules of the cytoskeleton
Centrioles	Pair of hollow cylinders, each made up of tiny tubules within the centrosome	Help organize and move chromosomes during cell reproduction
Microvilli	Tiny cell surface extensions supported internally by microfilaments	Increase surface area of plasma membrane for efficiency of absorption
Cilia	Hairlike cell surface extensions supported by an internal cylinder made of microtubules (longer than microvilli)	Sensory "antennae" to detect conditions outside the cell; some cilia also move substances over surface of the cell
Flagellum	Long whiplike projection on the sperm; similar to a cilium but much longer	The only example in humans is the "tail" of a sperm cell, propelling the sperm through fluids
Nucleus	Double-membraned, spherical envelope containing DNA strands	Contains DNA, which dictates protein synthesis, thereby playing an essential role in other cell activities such as transport, metabolism, growth, and heredity
Nucleolus	Dense region of the nucleus	Makes subunits that form ribosomes

slowly outward to the plasma membrane. Each vesicle fuses with the plasma membrane, opens to the outside of the cell, and releases its contents. An example of a Golgi apparatus product is the slippery substance called *mucus*. If we wanted to nickname the Golgi apparatus, we might call it the cell's "chemical processing and packaging center."

Mitochondria

Mitochondria (my-toh-KON-dree-ah) are another kind of organelle in all cells. Mitochondria are so tiny that a lineup of 15,000 or more of them would fill a space only about 2.5 cm (1 inch long). Two membranous sacs, one inside the other, compose a single mitochondrion. The inner membrane forms folds that look like miniature incomplete partitions. Within a mitochondrion's fragile membranes, complex, energy-converting chemical reactions occur continuously. Because these reactions supply most of the power for cellular work, mitochondria have been nicknamed the cell's "power plants."

Enzymes (molecules that promote specific chemical reactions), which are found in mitochondrial membranes and inner substance, break down products of glucose and other nutrients to release energy. The mitochondrion uses this released energy to "recharge" **ATP (adenosine triphosphate)** molecules, the "batteries" required for cellular work (see p. 30). This energy-transferring process is called *cellular respiration*.

Each mitochondrion has its own DNA molecule, sometimes called a *mitochondrial chromosome*, which contains information for building and running the mitochondrion.

Lysosomes

The **lysosomes** (LYE-so-sohmz) are membranous-walled organelles that in their active stage look like small sacs, often with tiny particles in them (see Figure 3-2). Because lysosomes contain enzymes that promote hydrolysis, they can break apart (digest) large food molecules. Therefore, they have the nickname "digestive bags." Lysosomal enzymes can also digest substances other than foods. For example, they can digest and thereby destroy microbes that invade the cell. Thus lysosomes can help to protect cells against destruction by microbes.

Formerly, scientists thought lysosomes were involved in programmed cell death. Now, however, we know a different set of mechanisms is responsible for "cell suicide," or **apoptosis** (ap-op-TOH-sis), which makes space for newer cells.

Centrosome

The **centrosome** (SEN-troh-sohm) is a region of cytoplasm near the nucleus of each cell. It serves as the microtubule-organizing center of the cell, thus playing an important role in organizing and moving the structures within the cell.

Centrioles (SEN-tree-olz) are paired organelles found within the centrosome. Two of these rod-shaped structures exist in every cell. They are arranged so that they lie at right angles to each other (see Figure 3-2). Each centriole is composed of microtubules that play an important role in moving chromosomes during cell division.

Cell Extensions

Most cells have various indentations and extensions that serve many different functions. Here we describe three of the major types of cell extensions (Figure 3-3).

Microvilli (my-kroh-VILL-eye) are small, fingerlike projections of the plasma membrane of some cells. These projections increase the surface area of the cell and thus increase its ability to absorb substances. For example, cells that line the small intestine are covered with microvilli that in-

FIGURE 3-3 Cell extensions. **A,** Microvilli *(light blue)* are small, fingerlike extensions of the plasma membrane that increase the surface area for absorption. Cilia *(darker blue)* are longer than microvilli and move back and forth, pushing fluids along the surface. **B,** The tail-like flagellum that propels each sperm cell is so long that it does not fit into the photograph at this magnification.

crease the absorption rate of nutrients into the blood. Microvilli have microfilaments inside them that produce wobbly movement and thus make absorption more efficient.

Cilia (SIL-ee-ah) are extremely fine, almost hairlike extensions on the exposed or free surfaces of cells. Cilia are larger than microvilli and possess inner microtubules that support them and enable them to move. Every cell has at least one cilium. All cilia act like an insect's antenna, allowing the cell to sense its surroundings. For example, the hairlike cilia in the taste buds of the mouth can detect different chemicals by taste. Some specialized cells have hundreds of cilia capable of moving together in a wavelike fashion over the surface of a cell. By moving as a group in one direction, they propel mucus over the cells that line the respiratory or reproductive tubes.

A **flagellum** (flah-JEL-um) is a single projection extending from the cell surface. Flagella are structurally similar to cilia but much longer. Like cilia, flagella can move. The cylinder of microtubules inside the flagellum moves in a way that whips the flagellum around like a propeller, pushing the cell forward. In a human, the only example of a flagellum is the "tail" of the male sperm cell. Wiggling movements of the flagellum make it possible for sperm to "swim" or move toward the ovum after they are deposited in the female reproductive tract.

Nucleus

Viewed under a light microscope, the **nucleus** of a cell looks like a very simple structure—just a small sphere in the central portion of the cell. However, its simple appearance belies the complex and critical role it plays in cell function. The nucleus contains most of the cell's genetic information, which ultimately controls every organelle in the cytoplasm. It also controls the complex process of cell reproduction. In other words, the nucleus must function properly for a cell to accomplish its normal activities and be able to duplicate itself.

Note that the cell nucleus in Figure 3-2 is surrounded by a *nuclear envelope* made up of two sepa-rate membranes. The nuclear envelope has many tiny openings called *nuclear pores* that permit large molecules to move into and out of the nucleus. The nuclear envelope encloses a special type of cell material in the nucleus called **nucleoplasm.** Nucleoplasm contains a number of specialized structures, and two of the most important are shown in Figure 3-2. They are the nucleolus (noo-KLEE-oh-lus) and the chromatin (KROH-mah-tin) granules.

Nucleolus. The **nucleolus** is a dense region of the nuclear material that is critical in protein formation because it is where the cell makes the subunits that form ribosomes. The ribosome subunits then migrate through the nuclear envelope into the cytoplasm of the cell to form ribosomes, which produce proteins.

Chromatin and Chromosomes. Chromatin granules in the nucleus are made of proteins around which are wound segments of the long, threadlike molecules called *DNA,* or *deoxyribonucleic* (dee-OK-see-rye-boh-noo-KLEE-ik) *acid.* DNA is the ge-

---

Science Applications

Microscopy
Antoni van Leeuwenhoek (1632-1723)

Until the very hour of his death in 1723, the Dutch drapery merchant Antoni van Leeuwenhoek *(left)* spent most of his 91 years pursuing adventures with the hundreds of microscopes he had built or collected. Using what were, even then, very simple lenses or combinations of lenses, van Leeuwenhoek discovered a whole world of tiny structures he called "animalcules" in body fluids. Although scientists a century later would declare that all living organisms are made up of cells, van Leeuwenhoek was the first to see and describe human blood cells (see Figure 3-20), human sperm cells, and many other cells and tissues of the body. He was also the first to observe many microscopic organisms that live on or in the human body, many of which are capable of producing disease.

Scientists today use light microscopes that are much more advanced than those of van Leeuwenhoek's time. Some of the most modern microscopes, called *electron microscopes,* use electron beams instead of light to produce images of very high magnification (see Figure 3-15). Both cell biologists and *histologists* (tissue biologists) use microscopes to research the fine structure and function of the human body. A wide variety of professions have found practical applications for microscopy. Most health professionals use microscopes, or at least images produced with microscopes, to perform routine duties. For example, clinical laboratory technicians and pathologists frequently use microscopes to assess the health of human cells and tissues. Outside of the health sciences, professionals such as law enforcement investigators, archaeologists, anthropologists, and paleontologists often use microscopes to further their study of human and animal tissues.

netic material often described as the chemical "cookbook" of the body. Because it contains the code for building both structural proteins and functional proteins, DNA determines everything from gender and metabolic rate to body build and hair color in every human being. During cell division, DNA molecules become tightly coiled. They then look like short, compact structures and are called **chromosomes.** Each cell of the body contains a total of 46 different DNA molecules in its nucleus and one copy of a 47th DNA molecule in each of its mitochondria. The importance and function of DNA is explained in greater detail in the section on cell reproduction later in this chapter.

Relationship of Cell Structure and Function

Every human cell performs certain functions. Some maintain the cell's survival, and others help maintain the body's survival. In many instances, the number and type of organelles within cells cause cells to differ dramatically in terms of their specialized functions. For example, cells that contain large numbers of mitochondria, such as heart muscle cells, are capable of sustained work. Why? Because the numerous mitochondria found in these cells supply the necessary energy required for rhythmic and ongoing contractions of the heart. Movement of the flagellum of a sperm cell is another example of the way a specialized organelle has a specialized function. The sperm's flagellum propels it through the reproductive tract of the female, thus increasing the chances of successful fertilization. This is how and why organizational structure at the cellular level is so important for function in living organisms. Examples in every chapter of the text illustrate how structure and function are intimately related at every level of body organization.

 To learn more about cell structures and their functions, go to AnimationDirect on your CD-ROM.

✓ QUICK CHECK

1. What is the molecular structure of the plasma membrane of the cell?
2. What is cytoplasm? What does it contain?
3. List five of the major structures of the cell and briefly describe their functions.
4. Which two kinds of cell structures contain DNA?

MOVEMENT OF SUBSTANCES THROUGH CELL MEMBRANES

The plasma membrane in every healthy cell separates the contents of the cell from the tissue fluid that surrounds it. At the same time the membrane must permit certain substances to enter the cell and allow others to leave. Heavy traffic moves continuously in both directions through cell membranes. Molecules of water, foods, gases, wastes, and many other substances stream in and out of all cells in endless procession. A number of processes allow this mass movement of substances into and out of cells. These transport processes are classified under two general headings:

1. Passive transport processes
2. Active transport processes

As implied by the name, active transport processes require the expenditure of energy by the cell, and passive transport processes do not. The energy required for active transport processes is obtained from **ATP.** ATP is produced in the mitochondria using energy from nutrients and is capable of releasing that energy to do work in the cell. For active transport processes to occur, the breakdown of ATP and the use of the released energy are required.

The details of active and passive transport of substances across cell membranes are much easier to understand if you keep in mind the following two key facts: (1) in passive transport processes, no cellular energy is required to move substances from a high concentration to a low concentration; and (2) in active transport processes, cellular energy is required to move substances from a low concentration to a high concentration.

Passive Transport Processes

The primary passive transport processes that move substances through the cell membranes include the following:

1. Diffusion
   a. Osmosis
   b. Dialysis
2. Filtration

Scientists describe the movement of substances in passive systems as going "down a concentration gradient." This means that substances in passive systems move from a region of high concentration to a region of low concentration until they reach equal proportions on both sides of the membrane. As you read the next few paragraphs, refer to Table 3-2, which summarizes important information about passive transport processes.

Diffusion

Diffusion is a good example of a passive transport process. Diffusion is the process by which substances scatter themselves evenly throughout an available space. The system does not require additional energy for this movement. To demonstrate diffusion of particles throughout a fluid, perform this simple experiment the next time you pour yourself a cup of coffee or tea. Place some sugar on a teaspoon and lower it gently to the bottom of the cup. Let it stand for 2 or 3 minutes, and then, holding the cup steady, take a sip off the top. It will taste sweet. Why? Because some of the sugar molecules will have diffused from the area of high concentration near the mound of sugar at the bottom of the cup to the area of low concentration at the top of the cup.

Assume that the tea is brewed using a tea bag made of shredded tea leaves inside a pouch of porous filter paper. One can easily watch the diffusion of dark pigment particles from a concentrated area inside the tea bag to the less concentrated area in the water outside the tea bag. Thus the pigment particles moved through a membrane (the paper) by diffusion, that is, the tendency to spread out and create a uniform concentration or *equilibrium*.

The key to diffusion across a membrane is the presence of pores big enough for the particles to pass through. In cell membranes, most molecules cannot pass through the membrane unless there are gateways that permit it. Various protein channels act as gated doorways that permit certain molecules to diffuse through them. Other protein structures act as carriers that bind to the particles and carry them through to the other side of the membrane. Without these transporters, most *solutes* (substances dissolved in the water) could not diffuse through cell membranes.

TABLE 3-2			
Passive Transport Processes			
PROCESS	**DESCRIPTION**		**EXAMPLES**
Diffusion	Movement of particles through a membrane from an area of high concentration to an area of low concentration—that is, down the concentration gradient	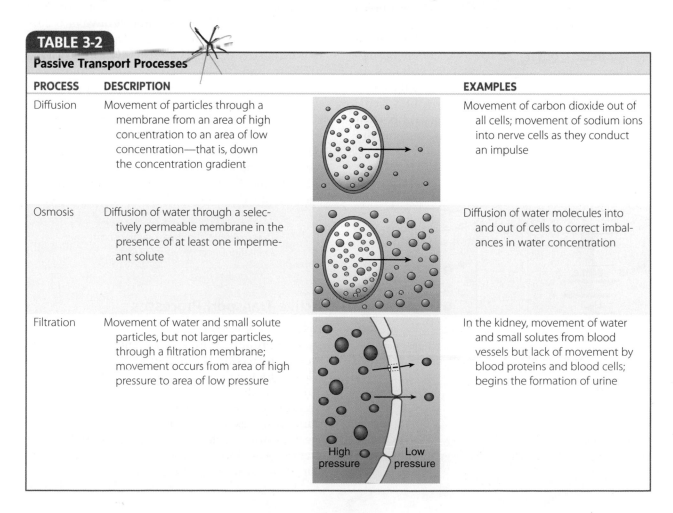	Movement of carbon dioxide out of all cells; movement of sodium ions into nerve cells as they conduct an impulse
Osmosis	Diffusion of water through a selectively permeable membrane in the presence of at least one impermeant solute		Diffusion of water molecules into and out of cells to correct imbalances in water concentration
Filtration	Movement of water and small solute particles, but not larger particles, through a filtration membrane; movement occurs from area of high pressure to area of low pressure		In the kidney, movement of water and small solutes from blood vessels but lack of movement by blood proteins and blood cells; begins the formation of urine

The process of diffusion is shown in Figure 3-4. Note that both substances diffuse rapidly through the porous membrane in both directions. However, as indicated by the purple arrows, more of the solute (dissolved substance) moves out of the 20% solution, where the concentration is higher, into the 10% solution, where the concentration is lower, than in the opposite direction. This is an example of movement down a concentration gradient. Simultaneously, more water moves from the 10% solution, where there are more water molecules, into the 20% solution, where there are fewer water molecules. This is also an example of movement down a concentration gradient. Water moves from high to low concentration. The result? Equilibration (balancing) of the concentrations of the two solutions occurs after an interval of time. After this equilibrium is reached, equal amounts of solute will diffuse in both directions, as will equal amounts of water.

Osmosis and Dialysis. Osmosis (os-MOH-sis) and **dialysis** (dye-AL-i-sis) are specific examples of diffusion. In both cases, diffusion occurs across a selectively permeable membrane. The plasma membrane of a cell is said to be selectively permeable because it permits the passage of certain substances but not others. That is, it has specific channels and carriers to allow diffusion of specific kinds of molecules. This is a necessary property if the cell is to permit some substances, such as nu-

trients, to gain entrance to the cell while excluding others. Osmosis is the diffusion of *water* through water channels in a selectively permeable membrane when some of the *solute* cannot cross the membrane (because there are no open channels or carriers for that solute).

However, in the case of dialysis, some solutes move across a selectively permeable membrane by diffusion and other solutes do not. Thus, dialysis results in an uneven distribution of various solutes.

Filtration

Filtration is the movement of water and solutes through a membrane as a result of a pushing force that is greater on one side of the membrane than on the other side. The force is called *hydrostatic pressure*, which is simply the force or weight of a fluid pushing against some surface (an example is blood pressure, in which blood pushes against vessel walls).

A principle concerning filtration that is of great physiological importance is that it always occurs *down* a hydrostatic pressure gradient. This means that when two fluids have unequal hydrostatic pressures and are separated by a membrane, water and diffusible solutes or particles (those to which the membrane is permeable) will filter out of the solution that has the higher hydrostatic pressure into the solution that has the lower hydrostatic pressure. Filtration is one of the processes responsible for urine formation in the kidney. Wastes are filtered out of the blood into the kidney tubules because of a difference in hydrostatic pressure.

To learn more about passive transport, go to AnimationDirect on your CD-ROM.

Active Transport Processes

Active transport is the uphill movement of a substance through a living cell membrane. *Uphill* means "up a concentration gradient" (that is, from a lower to a higher concentration). The energy required for this movement is obtained from ATP. Because the formation and breakdown of ATP require complex cellular activity, active transport mechanisms can take place only through living membranes. Table 3-3 summarizes active transport processes.

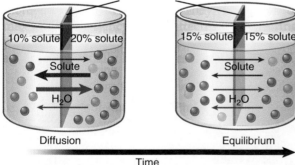

FIGURE 3-4 Diffusion. Note that the membrane is permeable to the purple solute particles and to water molecules and that it separates a 10% solution of purple solute particles from a 20% solution of purple particles. The container on the left shows the two solutions separated by the membrane at the start of diffusion. The container on the right shows the result of diffusion over time.

TABLE 3-3

Active Transport Processes

PROCESS	DESCRIPTION		EXAMPLES
Ion pump	Movement of solute particles from an area of low concentration to an area of high concentration (up the concentration gradient) by means of a carrier protein structure		In muscle cells, pumping of nearly all calcium ions to special compartments—or out of the cell
Phagocytosis	Movement of cells or other large particles into cell by trapping it in a section of plasma membrane that pinches off inside the cell		Trapping of bacterial cells by phagocytic white blood cells
Pinocytosis	Movement of fluid and dissolved molecules into a cell by trapping them in a section of plasma membrane that pinches off inside the cell		Trapping of large protein molecules by some body cells

Ion Pumps

A specialized cellular component called the *ion pump* makes possible a number of active transport mechanisms. An ion pump is an example of a protein structure in the cell membrane called a *carrier*. The ion pump uses energy from ATP to actively move ions across cell membranes *against* their concentration gradients. *Pump* is an appropriate term because it suggests that active transport moves a substance in an uphill direction just as a water pump, for example, moves water uphill.

An ion pump is specific to one particular kind of ion. Therefore, different ion pumps are required to move different types of ions. For example, sodium pumps move sodium ions only. Likewise, calcium pumps move calcium ions, and potassium pumps move potassium ions.

Some ion pumps are "coupled" to one another so that two or more different substances may be moved through the cell membrane at one time. For example, the **sodium-potassium pump,** shown in Figure 3-5, pumps sodium ions out of a cell while it pumps potassium ions into the cell. Because both ions are moved against their concentration

FIGURE 3-5 Sodium-potassium pump. Three sodium ions (Na$^+$) are pumped out of the cell and two potassium ions (K$^+$) are pumped into the cell during one pumping cycle of this carrier molecule. ATP is broken down in the process so that the energy freed from ATP can be used to pump the ions.

gradients, this pump creates a high sodium concentration outside the cell and a high potassium concentration inside the cell. Such a pump is required to remove sodium from the inside of a nerve cell after it has rushed in as a result of the passage of a nerve impulse. Some ion pumps are coupled with other specific carriers that transport glucose, amino acids, and other substances. However, there are no transporter pumps for moving water. Water can move only passively by osmosis.

Phagocytosis and Pinocytosis

Phagocytosis (fag-oh-sye-TOH-sis) is another example of how a cell can actively move an object or substance through the plasma membrane and into the cytoplasm. The term *phagocytosis* comes from a Greek word meaning "to eat." The word is appropriate because this process permits a cell to engulf and literally "eat" relatively large particles. Certain white blood cells can use phagocytosis to destroy invading bacteria and chunks of debris from tissue damage. During this process the cytoskeleton extends the cell's plasma membrane to form a pocket around the particles to be moved into the cell and thus encloses the material in a vesicle. Movements of the cytoskeleton pull the vesicle deeper into the cell. Once inside the cytoplasm, the vesicle fuses with a lysosome and the particles are broken apart (Figure 3-6).

Pinocytosis (pin-oh-sye-TOH-sis) is an active transport mechanism used to incorporate fluids or dissolved substances into cells by trapping them in a pocket of plasma membrane that pinches off inside the cell. Again, the term is appropriate because the word part *pino-* comes from the Greek word meaning "drink."

Because the cytoskeleton uses energy from ATP to produce the movements of both pinocytosis and phagocytosis, these processes are active transport mechanisms.

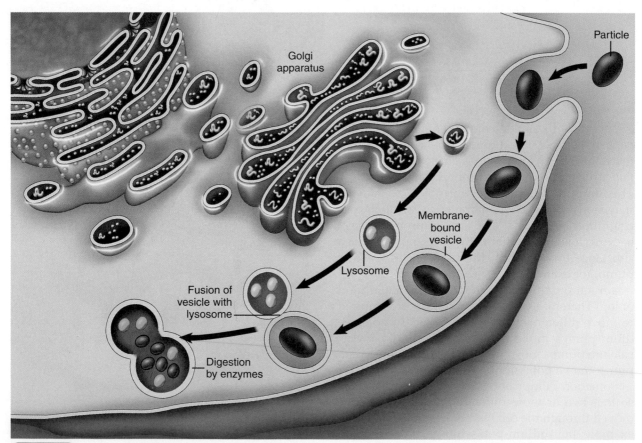

FIGURE 3-6 **Phagocytosis.** The cell's cytoskeleton reaches out and engulfs a particle, forming a vesicle. Cytoskeletal movements pull the vesicle containing the particle into the cytoplasm, where it fuses with a lysosome. Enzymes from the lysosome break down (digest) the particle. Pinocytosis works in a similar way, except that fluids (not large particles) are engulfed and brought into the cell.

Clinical Application

Tonicity

A salt (NaCl) solution is said to be isotonic (*iso* = equal) if it contains the same concentration of salt normally found in a living red blood cell, which measures 0.9% NaCl. Salt particles (Na$^+$ and Cl$^-$ ions) do not cross the plasma membrane easily, so salt solutions that differ in concentrations from the cell's fluid will promote the osmosis of water one way or the other. A solution that contains a higher level of salt than the cell does (above 0.9%) is said to be hypertonic (*hyper* = above) to the cell and one containing less salt (below 0.9%) is hypotonic (*hypo* = below) to the cell. With what you now know about filtration, diffusion, and osmosis, can you predict what would occur if red blood cells were placed in isotonic, hypotonic, and hypertonic solutions?

Examine the figures. Note that red blood cells placed in isotonic solution remain unchanged because there is no effective difference in salt or water concentrations. The movement of water into and out of the cells is about equal. This is not the case with red cells placed in hypertonic salt solution. They immediately lose water from their cytoplasm into the surrounding salty solution, and they shrink. This process is called crenation.

The opposite occurs if red cells are placed in a hypotonic solution. They swell as water enters the cell from the sur-

rounding dilute solution. Eventually the cells break or **lyse,** and the hemoglobin they contain is released into the surrounding solution.

Hypotonic solution (cells lyse)

Isotonic solution

Hypertonic solution (cells crenate)

To learn more about active transport, go to AnimationDirect on your CD-ROM.

✓ QUICK CHECK

1. What is the difference between a passive transport process and an active transport process?
2. What is osmosis?
3. How does an ion pump work? Is it active or passive?
4. Describe the process of phagocytosis.

CELL REPRODUCTION AND HEREDITY

All human cells that reproduce do so by a process called **mitosis** (my-TOH-sis). During this process a cell divides to multiply. That is, one cell divides to form two cells and thus the number of cells multiply. Cell reproduction, and, ultimately, the transfer of heritable traits, is closely tied to the production of proteins. The two *nucleic acids* **ribonucleic acid (RNA)** and **deoxyribonucleic acid (DNA)** play crucial roles in protein synthesis.

DNA Molecule and Genetic Information

Chromosomes, which are composed largely of DNA, make heredity possible. The "genetic information" contained in segments of the DNA molecules that are called **genes** ultimately determines the transmission and expression of inherited traits such as skin color and blood type from each generation of parents to their children (Figure 3-7).

Structurally, the DNA molecule resembles a long, narrow ladder made of a pliable material. It is twisted round and round its axis, taking on the shape of a double helix (see Figure 2-14, p. 30). Each DNA molecule is made of many smaller units, each made up of a sugar, a phosphate, and a base (Table 3-4). The bases are adenine, thymine, guanine, and cytosine. These nitrogen-containing chemicals are called *bases* because by themselves they have a high pH, and chemicals with a high pH are called "bases" (see pp. 25-26 for a discussion of acids and bases). As you can see in Figure 2-14 (p. 30), each step in the DNA ladder consists of a pair of bases. Only two combinations of bases occur, and the same two bases *always* pair off with

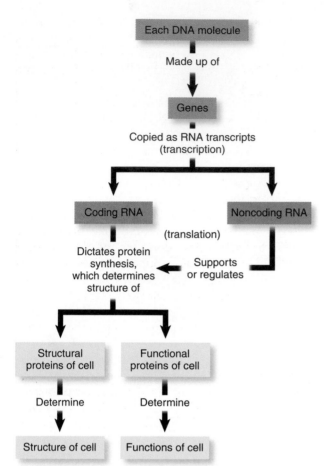

FIGURE 3-7 **Function of genes.** Genes copied from DNA are copied to RNA in a process called transcription. The RNA transcripts are then used in a process called translation, in which a code that determines the sequence of amino acids is translated to form a protein. The structure of the resulting protein determines the role of the protein in body structure and function—and ultimately, the structure and function of the body.

TABLE 3-4		
Components of Nucleotides		
NUCLEOTIDE	**DNA**	**RNA**
Sugar	Deoxyribose	Ribose
Phosphate	Phosphate	Phosphate
Nitrogen base	Cytosine	Cytosine
	Guanine	Guanine
	Adenine	Adenine
	Thymine	Uracil

each other in a DNA molecule. Adenine always binds to thymine, and cytosine always binds to guanine. This characteristic of DNA structure is called *complementary base pairing.*

A *gene* is a specific segment of base pairs in a chromosome. Although the types of base pairs in all chromosomes are the same, the order or *sequence* of base pairs is not the same. This fact has tremendous functional importance because it is the sequence of base pairs in each gene of each chromosome that determines heredity. Most genes direct the synthesis of at least one kind of protein molecule. Each protein may function, for example, as an enzyme, a structural component of a cell, or a specific hormone. Or it may combine other protein molecules, or even with carbohydrates or lipids, to form any number of large, complex molecules such as quaternary proteins, glycoproteins, or lipoproteins.

In humans having 46 nuclear chromosomes and one kind of mitochondrial chromosome in each body cell, DNA has a content of genetic information totaling about 3 *billion* base pairs in perhaps 25,000 protein-coding genes. That means that over a billion bits of information are inherited from each of our two biological parents. Is it any wonder, then, with all of this genetic information packed into each of our cells, that we are such complex organisms?

Genetic Code

How do genes bring about heredity? There is, of course, no short and easy answer to that question. We know that the genetic information contained in each gene is capable of "directing" the synthesis of a specific protein. The unique sequence of a thousand or so base pairs in a gene determines the sequence of specific building blocks required to form a particular protein. This store of information in each gene is called the *genetic code.*

Some genes instead encode the structures of regulatory types of RNA molecules. Regulatory RNA molecules act as functional molecules that affect some of the chemical processes in a cell. For example, ribosomal RNA (rRNA) molecules form most of the ribosome's protein-synthesizing structure and other RNA molecules that serve as temporary working copies of genetic code.

To summarize simply, we can state that the coded information in genes controls RNA production and thus also protein synthesis. These proteins include the enzymes and other functional molecules that facilitate cellular chemical reactions.

These cellular chemical reactions determine cell structure and function and therefore the traits passed to us by heredity.

To learn more about DNA structure and how it encodes genetic information, go to AnimationDirect on your CD-ROM.

RNA Molecules and Protein Synthesis

Most of the DNA, with its genetic code that dictates directions for protein synthesis, is contained in the nucleus of the cell. The actual process of protein synthesis, however, occurs at ribosomes in the cytoplasm and on ER. Another nucleic acid, RNA, copies this genetic information from the nucleus and carries it to the cytoplasm. RNA may also be an end product formed in the nucleus using the DNA code and transported out to the cytoplasm, where it regulates various functions of the cell. (NOTE: If you are not familiar with the chemical structure of proteins or nucleic acids, you may want to review Chapter 2 before reading further.)

Both RNA and DNA are composed of *nucleotide* subunits made up of a sugar, a phosphate, and one of four bases. RNA subunits, however, contain a different sugar and base component. In RNA nucleotide subunits, the base uracil substitutes for the base thymine. The types of RNA discussed here are all single-stranded molecules, not double-stranded like DNA. However, short, double-stranded RNA molecules also exist in nature.

The process of transferring genetic information from the nucleus into the cytoplasm, where proteins are actually produced, requires completion of two steps: **transcription** and **translation.**

Transcription. During **transcription** the double-stranded DNA molecule separates or unwinds, and a type of RNA called **messenger RNA (mRNA)** is formed (Figure 3-8, *Step 1*). Each strand of mRNA is a duplicate or copy of a particular gene sequence along one of the newly separated DNA spirals. The messenger RNA is said to have been "transcribed" or copied from its DNA mold or template. The mRNA molecules pass from the nucleus to the cytoplasm to direct protein synthesis in the ribosomes and ER (Figure 3-8, *Step 2*).

To see how transcription works, go to AnimationDirect on your CD-ROM.

Translation. **Translation** is the synthesis of a protein by ribosomes, which attach to the mRNA molecules in the cytoplasm. The ribosomes "read" the information contained in an mRNA molecule to direct the choice and sequencing of the appropriate chemical building blocks called *amino acids.*

First, the two subunits of a ribosome attach at the beginning of the mRNA molecule (Figure 3-8, *Step 3*). Recall that ribosomes are made mostly of RNA-ribosomal RNA (rRNA). The ribosome then moves down the mRNA strand as amino acids are assembled into their proper sequence (Figure 3-8, *Step 4*). **Transfer RNA (tRNA)** molecules assist the process by bringing specific amino acids in to "dock" at each **codon** along the mRNA strand. A codon is a series of three nucleotide bases, a "triplet," that acts as a code representing a specific amino acid. Each gene encoded in the mRNA is made up of a series of codons that tell the cell the sequence of amino acids to string together to form a protein strand.

The strand of amino acids formed during translation then folds on itself and perhaps even combines with another strand to form a complete protein molecule (see Figure 2-12, p. 28). The specific, complex shape of each type of protein molecule

Research, Issues, & Trends

Human Genome

All of the DNA in each cell of the body is called the genome (JEE-nohm). Intense, coordinated effort by scientists has mapped all the gene locations in the human genome. Efforts at reading the different genetic codes possible at each location are still under way. Much of the work of mapping the human genome was done as part of the Human Genome Project (HGP), which was started in 1990. Besides producing a complete human genetic map and developing tools of genetic mapping, a field called *genomics*, HGP also addresses the ethical, legal, and social issues that may arise—a notable first for such a massive scientific research effort. HGP is sponsored by the Department of Energy (DOE) and the National Institutes of Health (NIH), and its first director was James Watson, one of the scientists credited with originally discovering the structure of the DNA molecule in 1953. With the human genome already mapped, many scientists are working to fill in the details of the many genes and gene variants found in the human genome. Many are also working in the emerging field of *proteomics*, the study of all the proteins encoded by each of the genes of the human genome.

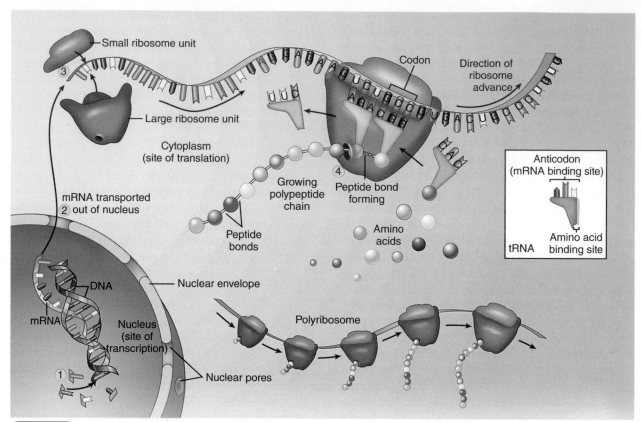

FIGURE 3-8 **Protein synthesis. 1,** Protein synthesis begins with transcription, a process in which an mRNA molecule forms along one gene sequence of a DNA molecule within the cell's nucleus. As it is formed, the mRNA molecule separates from the DNA molecule. **2,** The mRNA transcript then leaves the nucleus through the large nuclear pores. **3,** Outside the nucleus, ribosome subunits attach to the beginning of the mRNA molecule and begin the process of translation. **4,** In translation, transfer RNA (tRNA) molecules bring specific amino acids, encoded by each mRNA codon, into place at the ribosome site. As the amino acids are brought into the proper sequence, they are joined together by peptide bonds to form long strands called polypeptides. Several polypeptide chains may be needed to make a complete protein molecule.

allows the molecule to perform specific functions in the cell. It is clear that because DNA directs the shape of each protein, DNA also directs the function of each protein in a cell (see Figure 3-7).

 To see how translation works, go to AnimationDirect on your CD-ROM.

Cell Division

The process of cell reproduction involves the division of the nucleus (mitosis) and the cytoplasm. After the process is complete, two daughter cells

result. Both have the same genetic material as the cell that preceded them. As you can see in Figure 3-9, the specific and visible stages of cell division are preceded by a period. When a cell is not dividing, but instead going about its usual functions, it is in a period called **interphase** (IN-ter-fayz). Interphase includes the initial growing stages of a newly formed cell, followed by a period during which the cell prepares for possible cell division. During this preparatory part of interphase, the cell is said to be "resting." However, it is resting only from the standpoint of active cell division. In all other aspects it is exceedingly active. During interphase and just before mitosis begins, the DNA of

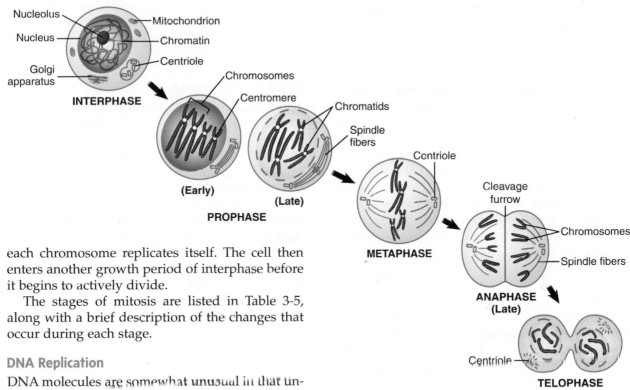

each chromosome replicates itself. The cell then enters another growth period of interphase before it begins to actively divide.

The stages of mitosis are listed in Table 3-5, along with a brief description of the changes that occur during each stage.

DNA Replication

DNA molecules are somewhat unusual in that unlike most molecules in nature, they can make copies of themselves—a process called *DNA replication*. Before a cell divides to form two new cells,

FIGURE 3-9 **Mitosis.** For simplicity, only four chromosomes are shown in the diagram.

each DNA molecule in its nucleus forms another DNA molecule just like itself. When a DNA molecule is not replicating, it has the shape of a tightly coiled double helix. As it begins replication, short segments of the DNA molecule uncoil and the two strands of the molecule pull apart between their base pairs. The separated strands therefore contain unpaired bases. Each unpaired base in each of the two separated strands attracts its complementary base (in the nucleoplasm) and binds to it. Specifically, each adenine attracts and binds to a thymine, and each cytosine attracts and binds to a guanine. These steps are repeated over and over throughout the length of the DNA molecule. Thus each half of a DNA molecule becomes a whole DNA molecule identical to the original DNA molecule. After DNA replication is complete, the cell

TABLE 3-5	
Stages of Cell Division	
STAGE	**CHARACTERISTICS**
Prophase	The chromatin condenses into visible chromosomes
	Chromatids become attached at the centromere
	Spindle fibers appear
	The nucleolus and nuclear envelope disappear
Metaphase	Spindle fibers attach to each chromatid
	Chromosomes align across the center of the cell
Anaphase	Centromeres break apart
	Chromosomes move away from the center of the cell
	The cleavage furrow appears
Telophase	The nuclear envelope and both nuclei appear
	The cytoplasm and organelles divide equally
	The process of cell division is completed

continues to grow until it is ready for the first phase of mitosis.

Prophase

Look at Figure 3-9 and note the changes that identify the first stage of mitosis, **prophase** (PROH-fayz). The chromatin becomes "organized." Chromosomes in the nucleus have formed two strands called **chromatids** (KROH-mah-tidz). Note that the two chromatids are held together by a beadlike structure called the **centromere** (SEN-troh-meer). In the cytoplasm the centrioles are moving away from each other as a network of tubules called **spindle fibers** forms between them. These spindle fibers serve as "guidewires" and assist the chromosomes to move toward opposite ends of the cell later in mitosis.

Metaphase

By the time **metaphase** (MET-ah-fayz) begins, the nuclear envelope and nucleolus have disappeared. Note in Figure 3-9 the chromosomes have aligned themselves across the center of the cell. Also, the centrioles have migrated to opposite ends of the cell, and spindle fibers are attached to each chromatid.

Anaphase

As **anaphase** (AN-ah-fayz) begins, the beadlike centromeres, which were holding the paired chromatids together, break apart. As a result, the individual chromatids, identified once again as chromosomes, move away from the center of the cell. Movement of chromosomes occurs along spindle fibers toward the centrioles. Note in Figure 3-9 that chromosomes are being pulled to opposite ends of the cell. A **cleavage furrow** that begins to divide the cell into two daughter cells can be seen for the first time at the end of anaphase.

Telophase

During **telophase** (TEL-oh-fayz), cell division is completed. Two nuclei appear, and chromosomes become less distinct and appear to break up. As the nuclear envelope forms around the chromatin, the cleavage furrow completely divides the cell into two parts. Before division is complete, each nucleus is surrounded by cytoplasm in which organelles have been equally distributed. By the end of telophase, two separate daughter cells, each having identical genetic characteristics, are formed. Each cell is fully functional and will perhaps itself undergo mitosis in the future.

 To learn more about the steps of cell division, go to AnimationDirect on your CD-ROM.

Results of Cell Division

Mitotic cell division results in the production of identical new cells. During developmental years, the addition of cells helps tissues and organs grow in size. During such periods of body growth, mitosis also allows groups of similar cells to **differentiate,** or develop into different *tissues.* In the adult, mitosis replaces cells that have become less functional with age or have been damaged or destroyed by illness or injury.

If the body loses its ability to control mitosis, an abnormal mass of proliferating cells develops. This mass is a **neoplasm** (NEE-oh-plaz-em). Neoplasms may be relatively harmless growths called **benign** (bee-NYNE) **tumors** or dangerous and **malignant** (mah-LIG-nant) cancerous growths.

 To learn more about neoplasms, go to AnimationDirect on your CD-ROM.

✓ QUICK CHECK

1. How do genes determine the structure and function of the body?
2. Where in the cell is genetic information stored?
3. What are the main steps to making a protein in the cell?
4. What are the four phases of mitotic cell division?

TISSUES

The four main kinds of tissues that compose the body's many organs follow:

1. Epithelial tissue
2. Connective tissue
3. Muscle tissue
4. Nervous tissue

Tissues differ from each other in the size and shape of their cells, in the amount and kind of material between the cells, and in the special functions they perform to help maintain the body's survival. In Tables 3-6 through 3-8, you will find a listing of the four major tissues and the various subtypes of each. The tables also include the structure of each subtype along with examples of the location of the tissues and a primary function of each tissue type.

Epithelial Tissue

Epithelial (ep-i-THEE-lee-al) **tissue** covers the body and many of its parts (Table 3-6). It also lines various parts of the body. Because epithelial cells are packed close together with little or no intercellular material between them, they form continuous sheets that contain no blood vessels. Examine Figure 3-10. It illustrates how this large group of tissues can be subdivided according to the *shape* and *arrangement* of the cells found in each type.

Shape of Cells

If classified according to shape, epithelial cells are identified as:

1. Squamous (flat and scalelike)
2. Cuboidal (cube-shaped)
3. Columnar (higher than they are wide)
4. Transitional (varying shapes that can stretch)

Arrangement of Cells

If categorized according to arrangement of cells, epithelial tissue can be classified as:

1. Simple (a single layer of cells of the same shape)
2. Stratified (many layers of cells; named for the shape of cells in the outer layer)

Several types of epithelium are described in the paragraphs that follow and are illustrated in Figures 3-7 to 3-12.

Simple Squamous Epithelium

Simple squamous (SKWAY-muss) **epithelium** consists of a single layer of very thin and irregularly shaped cells. Because of the structure of simple squamous epithelium, substances can readily pass through its cells, making transport its special function. Absorption of oxygen into the blood, for example, takes place through the simple squamous epithelium that forms the tiny air sacs in the lungs (see Figure 3-11).

Stratified Squamous Epithelium

Stratified squamous epithelium (see Figure 3-12) consists of several layers of closely packed cells, an arrangement that makes this tissue especially adept at protection. For instance, stratified squamous epithelial tissue protects the body against invasion by microorganisms. Most microbes cannot work their way through a barrier of stratified squamous tissue such as that which composes the surface of skin and of mucous membranes.

TABLE 3-6			
Epithelial Tissues			
TISSUE	**STRUCTURE**	**LOCATION(S)**	**FUNCTION(S)**
Simple squamous	Single layer of flattened cells	Alveoli of lungs	Diffusion of respiratory gases between alveolar air and blood
		Lining of blood and lymphatic vessels	Diffusion, filtration, and osmosis
Stratified squamous	Many layers; outermost layer(s) are flattened cells	Surface of lining of mouth and esophagus	Protection
		Surface of skin (epidermis)	Protection
Simple columnar	Single layer of tall, narrow cells	Surface layer of lining of stomach, intestines, parts of respiratory tract	Protection, secretion, transport (absorption)
Stratified transitional	Many layers of varying transitional shapes, capable of stretching	Urinary bladder	Protection
Pseudostratified	Single layer of tall cells that wedge together to appear as if there are two or more layers	Surface of lining of trachea	Protection
Simple cuboidal	Single layer of cells that are as tall as they are wide	Glands, kidney tubules	Secretion, absorption

CELL SHAPES

Squamous

Cuboidal

Columnar

SIMPLE

(Simple squamous)

(Simple cuboidal)

(Simple columnar)

Cilia

Basement membrane

Connective tissue

(Pseudostratified)

STRATIFIED

(Stratified squamous)

(Transitional, relaxed)

(Transitional, stretched)

FIGURE 3-10 Classification of epithelial tissues. The tissues are classified according to the shape and arrangement of cells.

Simple squamous epithelial cell

Simple cuboidal epithelial cell

Basement membrane

Free edge

Nucleus

FIGURE 3-11 Simple squamous and simple cuboidal epithelium. A, Photomicrograph shows thin simple squamous epithelium forming some tubules *(arrow)* and simple cuboidal epithelium forming the walls of other tubules. B, Sketch of photomicrograph.

Superficial squamous   Basal   Basement
epithelial cell   epithelial cell   membrane

FIGURE 3-12   **Stratified squamous epithelium. A,** Photomicrograph. **B,** Sketch of the photomicrograph. Note the many layers of epithelial cells and the flattened (squamous) cells in the outer layers.

One way of preventing infections, therefore, is to take good care of your skin. Do not let it become cracked from chapping, and guard against cuts and scratches.

Simple Columnar Epithelium

Simple columnar epithelium can be found lining the inner surface of the stomach, intestines, and some areas of the respiratory and reproductive tracts. In Figure 3-13 the simple columnar cells are arranged in a single layer lining the inner surface of the colon or large intestine. These epithelial cells are taller than they are wide, and the nuclei are located toward the bottom of each cell. The "open spaces" among the cells are **goblet cells** that produce mucus. The regular columnar-shaped cells specialize in absorption.

Stratified Transitional Epithelium

Stratified transitional epithelium is typically found in body areas subjected to stress and must be able to stretch. An example is the wall of the urinary bladder. In many instances, up to 10 layers of differently shaped cells of varying sizes are present in the absence of stretching. When stretching occurs, the epithelial sheet expands, the number of cell layers decreases, and cell shape changes

from roughly cuboidal to nearly squamous (flat) in appearance. This ability of transitional epithelium keeps the bladder wall from tearing under the pressures of stretching. Stratified transitional epithelium is shown in Figures 3-10 and 3-14.

Pseudostratified Epithelium

Pseudostratified epithelium, illustrated in Figure 3-10, is typical of that which lines the trachea or windpipe. Look carefully at the illustration. Note that each cell actually touches the gluelike **basement membrane** that lies under all epithelial tissues. Although the epithelium in Figure 3-10 (pseudostratified) appears to be two cell layers thick, it is not. This is why it is called *pseudo* (or false) stratified epithelium. The cilia that extend from the cells are capable of moving in unison. In doing so, they move mucus along the lining surface of the trachea, thus affording protection against entry of dust or foreign particles into the lungs.

Cuboidal Epithelium

Simple cuboidal epithelium does not form protective coverings but instead forms tubules or other groupings adapted for secretory activity (Figure 3-15). These secretory cuboidal cells usually function in clusters or tubes of secretory cells

FIGURE 3-13   Simple columnar epithelium. **A,** Photomicrograph. **B,** Sketch of the photomicrograph. Note the oblong nuclei in all the cells and the goblet or mucus-producing cells that are present.

FIGURE 3-14   Stratified transitional epithelium. **A,** Photomicrograph of tissue lining the urinary bladder wall. **B,** Sketch of the photomicrograph. Note the many layers of epithelial cells of various shapes.

commonly called **glands.** Glands of the body may be classified as **exocrine** if they release their secretion through a duct or as **endocrine** if they release their secretion directly into the bloodstream. Examples of glandular secretions include saliva produced by the salivary glands, digestive juices, sweat or perspiration, and hormones such as those secreted by the pituitary or thyroid glands. Simple cuboidal epithelium also forms the tubules that form urine in the kidneys.

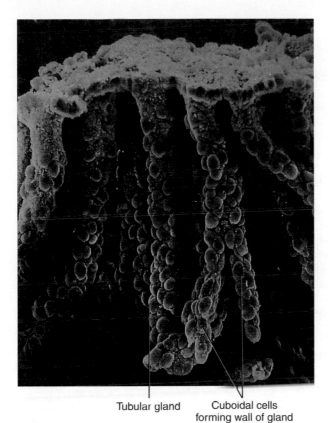

Tubular gland   Cuboidal cells
forming wall of gland

FIGURE 3-15 Simple cuboidal epithelium. This scanning electron micrograph shows how a single layer of cuboidal cells can form glands. The secreting cells arrange themselves into single or branched tubules that open onto a surface — the lining of the stomach in this case.

Connective Tissue ✳

Connective tissue is the most abundant and widely distributed tissue in the body (Table 3-7). It also exists in more varied forms than any of the other tissue types. It is found in skin, membranes, muscles, bones, nerves, and all internal organs. Connective tissue exists as delicate, paper-thin webs that hold internal organs together and give them shape. It also exists as strong and tough cords, rigid bones, and even in the form of a fluid—blood.

The functions of connective tissue are as varied as its structure and appearance. It connects tissues to each other and forms a supporting framework for the body as a whole and for its individual organs. As blood, it transports substances throughout the body. Several other kinds of connective tissue function to defend us against microbes and other invaders.

Connective tissue differs from epithelial tissue in the arrangement and variety of its cells and in the amount and kinds of intercellular material, called **matrix,** found between its cells. In addition to the relatively few cells embedded in the matrix of most types of connective tissue, varying numbers and kinds of fibers are also present. The structural quality and appearance of the matrix and fibers determine the qualities of each type of connective tissue. The matrix of blood, for example, is a liquid, but other types of connective tissue, such as cartilage, have the consistency of firm rubber. The matrix of bone is hard and rigid, although the matrix of connective tissues such as tendons and ligaments is strong and flexible.

The following list identifies a number of the major types of connective tissue in the body. Photomicrographs of several are also shown.

1. Areolar connective tissue
2. Adipose or fat tissue
3. Fibrous connective tissue
4. Bone
5. Cartilage
6. Blood
7. Hematopoietic tissue

Areolar and Adipose Connective Tissue

Areolar (ah-REE-oh-lar) **connective tissue** is the most widely distributed of all connective tissue types. It is the "glue" that helps keep the organs of the body together. Also called *loose connective tissue*, it consists of webs of fibers and of a variety of cells embedded in a loose matrix of soft, sticky gel. Some of the fibers are made of **collagen,** a strong but flexible fibrous protein. Some are stretchy fibers made of rubbery **elastin** proteins. These *elastic fibers* help tissues return to a shorter length after having been stretched, as in the loose tissue beneath the skin.

It is mainly areolar tissue that makes up the **fascia** (FAY-shah) of the body, which is the fibrous material that helps bind the skin, muscles, bones, and other organs of the body together.

When it begins to store lipids, areolar tissue can develop into **adipose** (AD-i-pohs), or **fat tissue.** In Figure 3-16, numerous vesicles have formed inside the adipose cells where large quantities of fat accumulate. Adipose tissue also secretes hormones that help regulate metabolism and fuel storage in the body. A special kind of adipose tissue called *brown fat* actually burns its fuel when the body is

TABLE 3-7

Connective Tissues

TISSUE	STRUCTURE	LOCATION(S)	FUNCTION(S)
Areolar (loose)	Loose arrangement of collagen fibers, elastic fibers, and cells	Area between other tissues and organs	Connection
Adipose (fat)	Cells contain large fat vesicles	Area under skin; padding at various points	Protection, insulation, support, nutrient reserve
Dense fibrous	Dense arrangement of collagen fiber bundles	Tendons, ligaments, fascia, scar tissue	Flexible but strong connection
Bone	Hard, calcified matrix arranged in osteons	Skeleton	Support, protection
Cartilage	Hard but somewhat flexible gel matrix with embedded chondrocytes	Part of nasal septum, area covering articular surfaces of bones, larynx, rings in trachea and bronchi	Firm but flexible support
		Disks between vertebrae	Withstands pressure
		External ear	Flexible support
Blood	Liquid matrix with flowing red and white cells	Blood vessels	Transportation
Hematopoietic	Liquid matrix with dense arrangement of blood cell–producing cells	Red bone marrow	Blood cell formation

cold to produce heat. This heat, along with shivering by muscles, helps restore homeostasis of body temperature (see Figure 1-10, p. 13).

Another type of fibrous connective tissue called **reticular tissue** has thin, delicate webs of collagen fibers call *reticular* (netlike) *fibers*. This type of tissue is found in bone marrow, for example, where it helps support blood-forming cells.

Dense Fibrous Connective Tissue

Dense fibrous connective tissue (Figure 3-17) consists mainly of thick bundles of strong, white

FIGURE 3-16 **Adipose tissue.** Photomicrograph showing the large lipid storage spaces inside the adipose cells.

FIGURE 3-17 **Dense fibrous connective tissue.** The bundles of wavy collagen fibers are roughly parallel to one another. The dark nuclei of fiber-producing cells are also visible in this photomicrograph of a tendon.

collagen fibers arranged in parallel rows. This type of connective tissue composes tendons. It provides great strength and flexibility, but it does not stretch. Such characteristics are ideal for these structures that anchor our muscles to our bones.

Bone and Cartilage

Bone is one of the most highly specialized forms of connective tissue. The matrix of bone is hard and calcified. It forms numerous structural building blocks called **osteons** (OS-tee-onz), or **Haversian** (hah-VER-shun) **systems**. When bone is viewed under a microscope, we can see these circular arrangements of calcified matrix and cells that give bone its characteristic appearance (Figure 3-18). Bones are a storage area for calcium and provide support and protection for the body.

Cartilage differs from bone in that its matrix is the consistency of a firm plastic or a gristlelike gel. Cartilage cells, which are called **chondrocytes** (KON-droh-sytes), are located in many tiny spaces distributed throughout the matrix (Figure 3-19).

Blood and Hematopoietic Tissue

Because its matrix is liquid, blood is perhaps the most unusual form of connective tissue. It has transportation and protective functions in the body. Red and white blood cells are the cell types common to blood (Figure 3-20).

Hematopoietic (hee-MAH-toh-poy-EE-tik) **tissue** is the bloodlike connective tissue found in the

FIGURE 3-19 **Cartilage.** Photomicrograph showing the chondrocytes distributed throughout the gel-like matrix.

FIGURE 3-20 **Blood.** Photomicrograph of a human blood smear. This smear shows two white blood cells surrounded by a number of smaller red blood cells. The liquid matrix of this tissue is also called *plasma.*

red marrow cavities of bones and in organs such as the spleen, tonsils, and lymph nodes. This type of tissue is responsible for the formation of blood cells and lymphatic system cells important in our defense against disease (see Table 3-7).

Muscle Tissue

Muscle cells are the movement specialists of the body. They have a higher degree of contractility (ability to shorten or contract) than any other

FIGURE 3-18 **Bone tissue.** Photomicrograph of dried, ground bone. A wheel-like structural unit of bone, known as an *osteon* (Haversian system), is apparent in this section.

3 kinds

tissue cells. Unfortunately, injured muscle cells are often slow to heal and often are replaced by scar tissue if injured. There are three kinds of muscle tissue: **skeletal, cardiac,** and **smooth** (Table 3-8).

Skeletal Muscle Tissue

Skeletal or striated muscle is called voluntary because willed or *voluntary* control of skeletal muscle contractions is possible. Note in Figure 3-21 that, when viewed under a microscope, skeletal muscle is characterized by many cross striations and many nuclei per cell. Individual cells are long and threadlike and are often called *fibers*. Skeletal muscles are attached to bones and, when contracted, produce voluntary and controlled body movements.

Cardiac Muscle Tissue

Cardiac muscle forms the walls of the heart, and the regular but involuntary contractions of cardiac muscle produce the heartbeat. Under the light microscope (Figure 3-22), cardiac muscle fibers have faint cross striations (as in skeletal muscle) and thicker dark bands called *intercalated disks*. Cardiac muscle fibers branch and connect to various other cardiac fiber branches to produce a three-dimensional, interlocking mass of contractile tissue.

Smooth Muscle Tissue

Smooth (visceral) muscle is said to be involuntary because it is not under conscious or willful control. Under a microscope (Figure 3-23), smooth muscle cells are seen as long, narrow fibers but not nearly as long as skeletal or striated fibers. Individual smooth muscle cells appear smooth (that is, without cross striations) and have only one nucleus per fiber. Smooth muscle helps form the walls of blood vessels and hollow organs such as the intestines and other tube-shaped structures in the body. Contractions of smooth (visceral) muscle propel food material through the digestive tract and help regulate the diameter of blood vessels. Contraction of smooth muscle in the tubes of the respiratory system, such as the bronchioles in the lungs, can impair breathing and result in asthma attacks and labored respiration.

Nervous Tissue

The function of nervous tissue is to provide rapid communication between body structures and control of body functions (see Table 3-8). Nervous tissue consists of two kinds of cells: nerve cells, or **neurons**

TABLE 3-8

Muscle and Nervous Tissues

TISSUE	STRUCTURE	LOCATION(S)	FUNCTION(S)
Muscle			
Skeletal (striated voluntary)	Long, threadlike cells with multiple nuclei and striations	Muscles that attach to bones	Maintenance of posture, movement of bones
		Eyeball muscles	Eye movements
		Upper third of esophagus	First part of swallowing
Cardiac (striated involuntary)	Branching, interconnected cylinders with faint striations	Wall of heart	Contraction of heart
Smooth (non-striated involuntary or visceral)	Threadlike cells with single nuclei and no striations	Walls of tubular viscera of digestive, respiratory, and genitourinary tracts	Movement of substances along respective tracts
		Walls of blood vessels and large lymphatic vessels	Changing of diameter of vessels
		Ducts of glands	Movement of substances along ducts
		Intrinsic eye muscles (iris and ciliary body)	Changing of diameter of pupils and shape of lens
		Arrector muscles of hairs	Erection of hairs (goose pimples)
Nervous			
	Nerve cells with large cell bodies and thin fiberlike extensions; supportive glial cells also present	Brain, spinal cord, nerves	Irritability, conduction

Striations

Nuclei of muscle fibers   Muscle fiber

FIGURE 3-21 Skeletal muscle. Photomicrograph showing the striations of the muscle cell fibers in longitudinal section.

Smooth muscle cells   Nuclei of smoo

FIGURE 3-23 Smooth muscle. Photomicrograph, longitudinal section. Note the central placement of nuclei in the spindle-shaped smooth muscle fibers.

Nucleus of muscle cell

Intercalated disks

FIGURE 3-22 Cardiac muscle. Photomicrograph showing the branched, lightly striated fibers. The darker bands, called *intercalated disks*, which are characteristic of cardiac muscle, are easily identified in this tissue section.

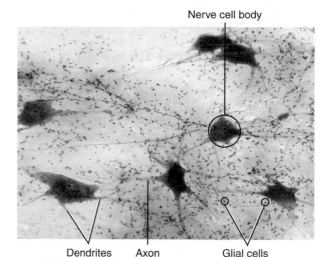

Nerve cell body

Dendrites   Axon   Glial cells

FIGURE 3-24 Nervous tissue. Photomicrograph of neurons in a smear of the spinal cord. Both neurons in this slide display characteristic cell bodies and multiple cell processes.

(NOO-ronz), which are the conducting units of the system, and special connecting and supporting cells called **glia** (GLEE-ah), or neuroglia.

All neurons are characterized by a **cell body** and two types of processes: (1) one **axon,** which transmits a nerve impulse away from the cell body, and (2) one or more **dendrites** (DEN-drytes), which carry impulses toward the cell body. Both neurons in Figure 3-24 have many dendrites extending from the cell body.

QUICK CHECK

1. What is the difference between simple and stratified epithelial tissue? Between squamous and cuboidal epithelial tissue?
2. Which main tissue type of the body is mostly matrix?
3. What are the three main types of muscle tissue?
4. What are the two main types of cell found in nervous tissue? Their functions?

Health and Well-Being

Tissues and Fitness

Achieving and maintaining an ideal body weight is a health-conscious goal. However, a better indicator of health and fitness is body composition. Exercise physiologists assess body composition to identify the percentage of the body made of lean tissue and the percentage made of fat. Body-fat percentage is often determined by using calipers to measure the thickness of skin folds at certain places on the body. A person with low body weight may still have a high ratio of fat to muscle, an unhealthy condition. In this case the individual is "underweight" but "overfat." In other words, fit-

ness depends more on the percentage and ratio of specific tissue types than the overall amount of tissue present.

Therefore one goal of a good fitness program is a desirable body-fat percentage. For men, the ideal is 12% to 18%, and for women, the ideal is 18% to 24%. Because fat contains stored energy (measured in calories), a low fat percentage means a low energy reserve. High body-fat percentages are associated with several life-threatening conditions, including cardiovascular disease, diabetes, and cancer. A balanced diet and an exercise program ensure that the ratio of fat to muscle tissue stays at a level appropriate for maintaining homeostasis.

OUTLINE SUMMARY

CELLS

A. Size and shape
  1. Human cells vary considerably in size; all are microscopic
  2. Cells differ notably in shape
B. Composition
  1. Cells contain cytoplasm, a substance found only in cells
  2. Organelles are specialized structures within the cytoplasm
  3. Cell interior is surrounded by plasma membrane
C. Structural parts
  1. Plasma membrane forms (see Figure 3-1)
    a. Forms outer boundary of cell
    b. Composed of thin, two-layered membrane of phospholipids and embedded with proteins
    c. Is selectively permeable
  2. Cytoplasm (see Figure 3-2)
    a. All cell substance from the nucleus to the plasma membrane
    b. Cytoskeleton — internal framework of cell
      (1) Made up of microfilaments and microtubules
      (2) Provides support and movement of cell and organelles
    c. Other cell parts
      (1) Ribosomes
        (a) Made of two tiny subunits of mostly ribosomal RNA (rRNA)
        (b) May attach to rough ER or lie free in cytoplasm

      (c) Manufacture enzymes and other proteins; often called *protein factories*
      (2) Endoplasmic reticulum (ER)
        (a) Network of connecting sacs and canals
        (b) Carries substances through cytoplasm
        (c) Rough ER collects, folds, and transports proteins made by ribosomes
        (d) Smooth ER synthesizes chemicals; makes new membrane
      (3) Golgi apparatus
        (a) Group of flattened sacs near nucleus
        (b) Collects chemicals into vesicles that move from the smooth ER outward to the plasma membrane
        (c) Called the *chemical processing and packaging center*
      (4) Mitochondria
        (a) Composed of inner and outer membranous sacs
        (b) Involved with energy-releasing chemical reactions (cellular respiration)
        (c) Often called *power plants* of the cell
        (d) Each mitochondrion contains one DNA molecule

(5) Lysosomes
   (a) Membrane-enclosed packets containing digestive enzymes
   (b) Have protective function (eat microbes)
   (c) Formerly thought to be responsible for apoptosis (programmed cell death)
(6) Centrosome
   (a) Microtubule-organizing region of the cytoskeleton near the nucleus
   (b) Centrioles — paired organelles that lie at right angles to each other within the centrosome and function in moving chromosomes during cell reproduction
(7) Cell extensions (see Figure 3-3)
   (a) Microvilli — short extensions of the plasma membrane that increase surface area and produce slight movements that enhance absorption by the cell
   (b) Cilia — hairlike extensions with inner microtubules found on free or exposed surfaces of all cells; serve sensory functions, but some are also capable of moving together in a wavelike fashion to propel mucus across a surface
   (c) Flagella — single projections (much longer than cilia) that act as "tails" of sperm cells
3. Nucleus
   a. Controls cell because it contains most of the genetic code (genome), instructions for making proteins, which in turn determine cell structure and function
   b. Component structures include nuclear envelope, nucleoplasm, nucleolus, and chromatin granules
   c. DNA molecules become tightly coiled chromosomes during cell division
   d. 46 nuclear chromosomes contain DNA, which contains genetic code
D. Relationship of cell structure and function
   1. Every human cell has a designated function: some help maintain the cell, and others regulate life processes
   2. Specialized functions of a cell differ depending on number and type of organelles

MOVEMENTS OF SUBSTANCES THROUGH CELL MEMBRANES

A. Passive transport processes do not require added energy and result in movement "down a concentration gradient"
   1. Diffusion (see Figure 3-4)
      a. Substances scatter themselves evenly throughout an available space, the particles moving from high to low concentration; may thus move through channels or carriers in a membrane to reach an equilibrium (equality of concentration)
      b. Passive process — it is unnecessary to add energy to the system
      c. Osmosis is diffusion of water (when some solutes cannot cross the membrane)
      d. Dialysis is diffusion of small solute particles
   2. Filtration — movement of water and solutes caused by hydrostatic pressure on one side of membrane
B. Active transport processes occur only in living cells; movement of substances is "up the concentration gradient"; requires energy from ATP
   1. Ion pumps (see Figure 3-5)
      a. An ion pump is a protein complex in the cell membrane
      b. Ion pumps use energy from ATP to move substances across cell membranes against their concentration gradients
      c. Examples: sodium-potassium pump, calcium pump
      d. Some ion pumps work with other carriers so that glucose or amino acids are transported along with ions
   2. Phagocytosis and pinocytosis
      a. Phagocytosis ("cell eating") engulfs large particles in a vesicle as a protective mechanism often used to destroy bacteria or debris from tissue damage (see Figure 3-6)
      b. Pinocytosis ("cell drinking") engulfs fluids or dissolved substances into cells
      c. Both are active transport mechanisms because they require cell energy (from ATP) to move the cytoskeleton in a way that engulfs material and pulls it into the cell

CELL REPRODUCTION AND HEREDITY
A. DNA structure
   1. Large molecule shaped like a spiral staircase; sugar (deoxyribose) and phosphate units compose sides of the molecule; base pairs (adenine-thymine or guanine-cytosine) compose "steps" (see Figure 2-14, p. 30)
   2. Base pairings always the same (complementary base pairing), but the sequence of base pairs differs in different DNA molecules
      a. A gene is a specific sequence of base pairs within a DNA molecule
      b. Genes dictate formation of enzymes and other proteins by ribosomes, thereby indirectly determining a cell's structure and functions; in short, genes are heredity determinants (see Figure 3-7)
B. Genetic code
   1. Genetic information — stored in base-pair sequences on genes and expressed through protein synthesis
   2. RNA molecules and protein synthesis
      a. DNA — contained in cell nucleus
      b. Protein synthesis — occurs in cytoplasm; thus genetic information must pass from the nucleus to the cytoplasm
      c. Process of transferring genetic information from nucleus to cytoplasm where proteins are produced requires completion of *transcription* and *translation* (see Figure 3-8)
   3. Transcription
      a. Double-stranded DNA separates to form messenger RNA (mRNA)
      b. Each strand of mRNA duplicates a particular gene (base-pair sequence) from a segment of DNA
      c. mRNA molecules pass from the nucleus to the cytoplasm where they direct protein synthesis in ribosomes and ER
   4. Translation
      a. Involves synthesis of proteins in cytoplasm by ribosomes
      b. Requires use of information contained in mRNA
      c. Codon — a series of three nucleotide bases that acts as a code for a specific amino acid

C. Cell division — reproduction of cell involving division of the nucleus (mitosis) and the cytoplasm
   1. Two daughter cells result from the division
   2. Period when the cell is not actively dividing is called *interphase*
   3. DNA replication — process by which each half of a DNA molecule becomes a whole molecule identical to the original DNA molecule; precedes mitosis
   4. Mitosis — process in cell division that distributes identical nuclear chromosomes (DNA molecules) to each new cell formed when the original cell divides; enables cells to reproduce their own kind; makes heredity possible (see Figure 3-9)
      a. Prophase — first stage
         (1) Chromatin granules become organized
         (2) Chromosomes (pairs of linked chromatids) appear
         (3) Centrioles move away from nucleus
         (4) Nuclear envelope disappears, freeing genetic material
         (5) Spindle fibers appear
      b. Metaphase — second stage
         (1) Chromosomes align across center of cell
         (2) Spindle fibers attach themselves to each chromatid
      c. Anaphase — third stage
         (1) Centromeres break apart
         (2) Separated chromatids now called *chromosomes*
         (3) Chromosomes are pulled to opposite ends of cell
         (4) Cleavage furrow develops at end of anaphase
      d. Telophase — fourth stage
         (1) Cell division is completed
         (2) Nuclei appear in daughter cells
         (3) Nuclear envelope and nucleoli appear
         (4) Cytoplasm is divided (cytokinesis)
         (5) Daughter cells become fully functional
   5. Results of cell division
      a. Two identical cells result from cell division, growing tissues or replacing old or damaged cells

    b. Differentiation — process by which daughter cells can specialize and form different kinds of tissue

    c. Abnormalities of mitotic division can produce benign or malignant neoplasms (tumors)

TISSUES (See Tables 3-5 through 3-7)

A. Epithelial tissue
1. Covers body and lines body cavities
2. Cells packed closely together with little matrix
3. Classified by shape of cells (see Figure 3-10)
   a. Squamous
   b. Cuboidal
   c. Columnar
   d. Transitional
4. Also classified by arrangement of cells into one or more layers: simple or stratified
5. Simple squamous epithelium — single layer of scalelike cells adapted for transport (e.g., absorption) (see Figure 3-11)
6. Stratified squamous epithelium — several layers of closely packed cells specializing in protection (see Figure 3-12)
7. Simple columnar epithelium — tall, column-like cells arranged in a single layer; contain mucus-producing goblet cells; specialized for absorption (Figure 3-13)
8. Stratified transitional epithelium — up to 10 layers of roughly cuboidal cells that distort to squamous shape when stretched; found in body areas that stretch, such as urinary bladder (see Figure 3-14)
9. Pseudostratified epithelium — single layer of distorted columnar cells; each cell touches basement membrane
10. Simple cuboidal epithelium — single layer of cubelike cells often specialized for secretory activity; may secrete into ducts, directly into blood, and on body surface (see Figure 3-15)

B. Connective tissue
1. Most abundant and widely distributed tissue in body, with many different types, appearances, and functions
2. Relatively few cells in intercellular matrix

3. Types
   a. Areolar (loose connective) tissue — fibrous glue (fascia) that holds organs together; collagenous and elastic fibers, plus a variety of cell types
   b. Adipose (fat) tissue — lipid storage, metabolism regulation; brown fat produces heat (see Figure 3-16)
   c. Reticular tissue — delicate net of collagen fibers, as in bone marrow
   d. Dense fibrous tissue — bundles of strong collagen fibers; example is tendon (see Figure 3-17)
   e. Bone tissue — matrix is calcified; functions as support and protection (see Figure 3-18)
   f. Cartilage tissue — matrix is consistency of gristlelike gel; chondrocyte is cell type (see Figure 3-19)
   g. Blood tissue — matrix is fluid; functions are transportation and protection (see Figure 3-20)

C. Muscle tissue (see Figures 3-21 to 3-23)
1. Types
   a. Skeletal muscle tissue — attaches to bones; also called *striated* or *voluntary*; control is voluntary; striations apparent when viewed under a microscope (see Figure 3-21)
   b. Cardiac muscle tissue — also called *striated involuntary*; composes heart wall; ordinarily cannot control contractions (see Figure 3-22)
   c. Smooth muscle tissue — also called *nonstriated (visceral)* or *involuntary*; no cross striations; found in blood vessels and other tube-shaped organs (Figure 3-23)

D. Nervous tissue (see Figure 3-24)
1. Function — rapid communication between body structures and control of body functions
2. Neurons
   a. Conduction cells
   b. All neurons have cell body and two types of processes: axon and dendrite
      (1) Axon (one) carries nerve impulse away from cell body
      (2) Dendrites (one or more) carry nerve impulse toward the cell body
3. Glia (neuroglia) — supportive and connecting cells

NEW WORDS

adenosine triphosphate
   (ATP)
apoptosis
centromere
chondrocytes
chromatid
chromatin
chromosome
cleavage furrow
collagen
crenation
cytoplasm
cytoskeleton
deoxyribonucleic acid
   (DNA)
differentiate
elastin
endocrine
exocrine
gene
genome
gland
glia

goblet cell
hypertonic
hypotonic
interphase
interstitial fluid
lyse
matrix
messenger RNA
   (mRNA)
mitosis
   prophase
   metaphase
   anaphase
   telophase
neoplasm
neuron
   axon
   dendrite
nucleoplasm
organelle
   centriole
   centrosome
   cilia

endoplasmic reticu-
   lum (ER)
flagellum
Golgi apparatus
lysosome
microvillus (pl.,
   microvilli)
mitochondrion (pl.,
   mitochondria)
nuclear envelope
nucleolus
nucleus
plasma membrane
ribosome
vesicle
osteon (Haversian
   system)
ribonucleic acid (RNA)
sodium-potassium
   pump
solute
spindle fiber

tissue
   adipose
   areolar (loose)
   columnar
   connective
   cuboidal
   dense fibrous
   epithelial
   hematopoietic
   nervous
   reticular
   squamous
   transitional
transcription
translation
transport processes
   (active and passive)
dialysis
diffusion
filtration
osmosis
phagocytosis
pinocytosis

REVIEW QUESTIONS

1. Describe the structure of the plasma membrane.
2. List three functions of the plasma membrane.
3. Give the function of the following orga-nelles: *ribosome, Golgi apparatus, mitochondria, lysosomes,* and *centrioles.*
4. Give the function of the *nucleus* and *nucleolus.*
5. Explain the difference between *chromatin* and *chromosomes.*
6. Describe the processes of *diffusion* and *filtration.*
7. Describe the functioning of the *ion pump* and explain the process of *phagocytosis.*
8. Define *gene* and *genome.*
9. Describe the process of transcription.
10. Describe the process of translation.
11. List the four stages in active cell division (mitosis) and briefly describe what occurs in each stage.
12. What important event in mitosis occurs during interphase?

13. Name and describe three epithelial tissues.
14. Name and describe three connective tissues.
15. Name and describe two muscle tissues.
16. Name the two types of nervous tissue cells. Which is the conductive cell type, and which is the support cell type?

CRITICAL THINKING

17. Explain what is meant by tissue typing. Why has this become so important in recent years?
18. Explain what would happen if a cell con-taining 97% water were placed in a 10% salt solution.
19. If one side of a DNA molecule had a base sequence of adenine-adenine-guanine-cytosine-thymine-cytosine-thymine, what would the sequence of bases on the opposite side of the molecule be?
20. If a molecule of mRNA were made from the base sequence in Question 19, what would be the sequence of bases in the RNA?

CHAPTER TEST

1. _____ and _____ are two fat-based molecules that make up part of the structure of the plasma membrane.
2. _____ is a term that refers to small structures inside the cell. It means "little organs."
3. _____ is the movement of substances across a cell membrane using cell energy, whereas _____ is the movement of substances across the cell membrane without using cell energy.
4. _____ refers to the movement of fluids or dissolved molecules into the cell by trapping them in the plasma membrane.
5. _____ and _____ are the two nucleic acids that are involved in transcription.
6. _____ is the process in protein synthesis that uses the information in mRNA to build a protein molecule.
7. _____ is the process that forms the mRNA molecule.
8. _____ is a segment of base pairs in a chromosome.
9. _____ is the total genetic information package in a cell.
10. _____, _____, _____, and _____ are the four main types of tissues in the body.
11. Which of the following is not a specialized form of diffusion?
    a. filtration
    b. dialysis
    c. osmosis
    d. all of these are specialized forms of diffusion
12. During this stage of mitosis, the chromosomes move away from the center of the cell:
    a. interphase
    b. metaphase
    c. anaphase
    d. telophase
13. During this stage, the DNA replicates:
    a. interphase
    b. metaphase
    c. prophase
    d. telophase
14. During this stage of mitosis, the chromosomes align in the center of the cell:
    a. interphase
    b. metaphase
    c. prophase
    d. telophase
15. During this stage of mitosis, the chromatin condenses into chromosomes:
    a. interphase
    b. metaphase
    c. prophase
    d. telophase
16. During this stage of mitosis, the nuclear envelope and nuclei reappear:
    a. interphase
    b. prophase
    c. anaphase
    d. telophase

Match each function in Column B with the proper cell structure in Column A.

COLUMN A

17. _____ Ribosome
18. _____ Endoplasmic reticulum
19. _____ Golgi apparatus
20. _____ Mitochondria
21. _____ Lysosomes
22. _____ Flagella
23. _____ Cilia
24. _____ Nucleus
25. _____ Nucleoli

COLUMN B

a. A long cell projection used to propel sperm cells
b. Bags of digestive enzymes in the cell
c. Tubelike passages that carry substances through the cytoplasm
d. Short hairlike structures on the free surface of some cells
e. Chemically process and package substances from the endoplasmic reticulum
f. Directs protein synthesis; the brain of the cell
g. "Protein factories" in the cell, made of RNA
h. Small structure in the nucleus; helps in the formation of ribosomes
i. "Powerhouse" of the cell; most of the cell's ATP is formed here

OBJECTIVES

AFTER YOU HAVE COMPLETED THIS CHAPTER, YOU SHOULD BE ABLE TO:

1. Define and contrast the terms *organ* and *organ system*.
2. List the 11 major organ systems of the body.
3. Identify and locate the major organs of each major organ system.
4. Briefly describe the major functions of each major organ system.
5. Identify and discuss the major subdivisions of the reproductive system.

Organ Systems of the Body

4

The words *organ* and *system* were discussed in Chapter 1 as having special meanings when applied to the body. An organ is a structure made up of two or more kinds of tissues organized in such a way that the tissues can together perform a more complex function than can any tissue alone. A system is a group of organs arranged in such a way that they can together perform a more complex function than can any organ alone. This chapter gives an overview of the 11 major organ systems of the body.

In the chapters that follow, the presentation of information on individual organs and an explanation of how they work together to accomplish complex body functions will form the basis for the discussion of each organ system. For example, a detailed description of the skin as the primary organ of the integumentary system will be covered in Chapter 5, and information on the bones of the body as organs of the skeletal system will be presented in Chapter 6. Knowledge of individual organs and how they are organized into groups makes much more meaningful the understanding of how a particular organ system functions as a unit in the body.

When you have completed your study of the major organ systems in the chapters that follow, it will be possible to view the body not as an assembly of individual parts but as an integrated and functioning whole. This chapter names the systems of the body and the major organs that compose them, and it briefly describes the functions of each system. It is intended to provide a basic "road map" to help you anticipate and prepare for the more detailed information that follows in the remainder of the text.

STUDY TIPS

Chapter 4 is the perfect "big picture" chapter. It is a preview for most of the remaining chapters in the text.

1. Put the name of the system on one side of a flash card and the function of that system and its organs on the other side. Notice how each organ contributes to the function of the system.
2. In your study groups, go over the flash cards. Discuss how several systems need to be involved in accomplishing one function in the body, such as getting nutrients or oxygen to the cells.
3. Go over the questions in the back of the chapter and discuss possible test questions.
4. Before you begin the chapter dealing with a particular system, it would be helpful to get an overview of that system by reviewing the synopsis of that system in this chapter.

ORGAN SYSTEMS OF THE BODY

In contrast to cells, which are the smallest structural units of the body, organ systems are the body's largest and most complex structural units. The 11 major organ systems that compose the human body are listed here.

1. Integumentary
2. Skeletal
3. Muscular
4. Nervous
5. Endocrine
6. Cardiovascular (circulatory)
7. Lymphatic
8. Respiratory
9. Digestive
10. Urinary
11. Reproductive
    a. Male subdivision
    b. Female subdivision

Clinical Application

Stem Cells

Scientists all over the world are currently engaged in intensive research efforts to unravel the biological secrets of a special kind of undifferentiated cell called a **stem cell.**

Embryonic stem cells, which are obtained from a developing embryo, can be isolated and cultured in the laboratory. Using complex research methods, these primitive cells can then be stimulated to produce additional stem cells or be "directed" to produce many different kinds of differentiated daughter cell types including nerve, blood, muscle, and various types of glandular tissue.

Adult stem cells, are undifferentiated cells found scattered within differentiated mature tissues throughout the body. Current research suggests that all adult tissues have some of these undifferentiated cells that are capable of producing any of the specialized cell types within its particular tissue (see Research, Issues, & Trends box, p. 213). For example, infu-

sion of adult bone marrow stem cells is a therapy now being used to treat patients with leukemia or bone marrow damaged by toxins or high-dose x-ray treatment (see Clinical Application: Bone Marrow Transplants box, p. 253). Exciting new discoveries now suggest that some adult stem cells, like embryonic stem cells, can be coaxed into producing a variety of different types of cells.

Stem cell research has produced exciting and complex advances in biology that will have a profound impact on human health. Already, stem cell therapies for treating Parkinson disease, stroke, diabetes, and spinal cord injury, to name only a few, are being proposed by medical scientists. Although many scientific and ethical questions remain unanswered, the potential now exists for cell, tissue, and organ "engineering" that may well permit repair or total replacement of diseased or damaged organs in a functioning organ system.

Examine Figure 4-1 to find a diagrammatic listing of the body systems and the major organs in each. In addition to the information contained in Figure 4-1, each system is presented in visual form in Figures 4-2 through 4-13. Visual presentation of material is often useful in gaining an understanding of the interrelationships that are so important in anatomy and physiology.

For a brief 3D tour of each of the body's organ systems, go to AnimationDirect on your CD-ROM.

Integumentary System

Note in Figure 4-2 that the *skin* is the largest and most important organ in the *integumentary* (in-teg-yoo-MEN-tar-ee) *system.* Its weight in most adults is 20 pounds or more, accounting for about 16% of total body weight and making it the body's heaviest organ. The integumentary system includes the skin and its *accessory structures,* which include the *hair, nails,* and specialized *sweat-* and *oil-producing glands.* In addition, a number of microscopic and highly specialized *sense organs* are embedded in the skin. They permit the body to respond to various stimuli such as pain, pressure, touch, and changes in temperature.

The integumentary system is crucial to survival. Its primary function is *protection.* The skin protects underlying tissue against invasion by harmful bacte-

ria, bars entry of most chemicals, and minimizes the chances of mechanical injury to underlying structures. In addition, the skin regulates body temperature by sweating and by controlling blood flow and therefore heat loss at the body surface. The skin also synthesizes important chemicals, such as vitamin D, and functions as a sophisticated sense organ.

Skeletal System

The sternum or breastbone, the humerus, and the femur shown in Figure 4-3 are examples of the 206 individual organs (bones) found in the *skeletal system.* The system includes not only **bones** but also related tissues such as *cartilage* and *ligaments* that together provide the body with a rigid framework for support and protection. In addition, the skeletal system, through the existence of **joints** between bones, makes possible the movements of body parts. Without joints, we could make no movements. Our bodies would be rigid, immobile hulks. Bones also serve as storage areas for important minerals such as calcium and phosphorus. The formation of blood cells in the red marrow of certain bones is another crucial function of the skeletal system.

Muscular System

Individual skeletal muscles are the organs of the *muscular system.* Muscles not only produce movement and maintain body posture but also generate

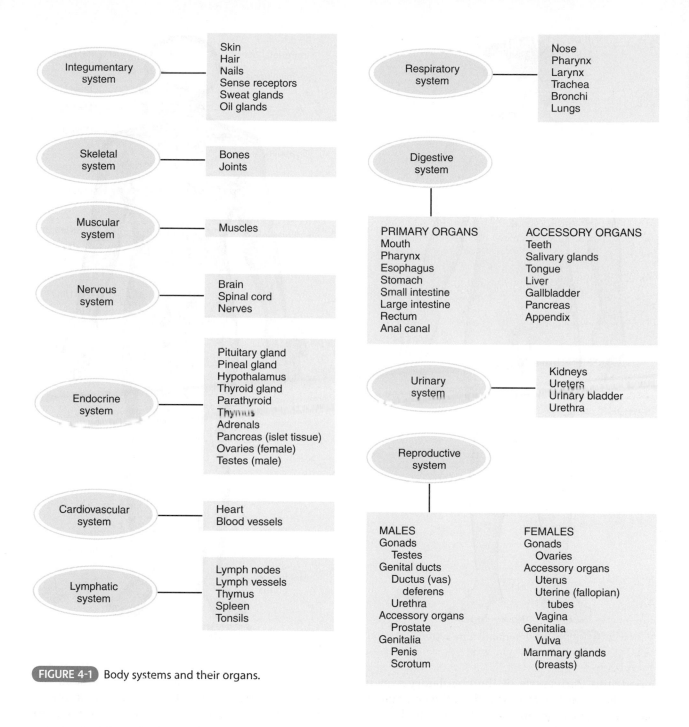

FIGURE 4-1 Body systems and their organs.

the heat required for maintaining a constant core body temperature. The skeletal muscles are called **voluntary,** or **striated, muscles** because their contractions are under conscious control and their individual cells appear striated when viewed with a microscope. In addition to the skeletal or voluntary muscles that constitute the muscular system, two other important types of muscle tissue are found in the body. **Involuntary,** or **smooth, muscle** tissue is found in blood vessel walls, other tubular structures, and in the lining of hollow organs such as the stomach and small intestine. **Cardiac muscle** is the specialized type of involuntary muscle tissue of the heart. By contracting, it pumps

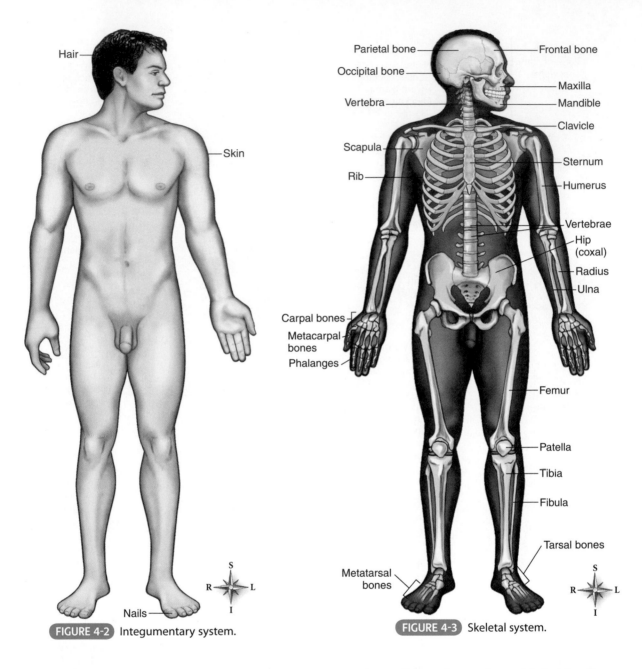

FIGURE 4-2 Integumentary system.

FIGURE 4-3 Skeletal system.

blood into the vessels of the circulatory system. Specialized cardiac muscle cells in the heart generate the electrical impulses that cause the heart to beat in a controlled and rhythmic way.

The tendon labeled in Figure 4-4 represents how tendons attach muscles to bones. When stimulated by a nervous impulse, muscle tissue shortens or contracts. Voluntary movement occurs when skeletal muscles contract because of the way muscles are attached to bones and the way bones articulate or join together with one another in

joints. Contraction of smooth muscle in blood vessel walls helps maintain blood pressure. In the digestive tube, contraction of smooth muscle propels food through the system and then moves undigested residue from the body.

Nervous System

The *brain, spinal cord,* and *nerves* are the organs of the *nervous system.* As you can see in Figure 4-5, nerves extend from the brain and spinal cord to

Sternocleidomastoid

Deltoid

Pectoralis
major

Biceps
brachii

External
abdominal
oblique

Rectus
abdominis

Sartorius

Rectus femoris

Patellar tendon

Tibialis anterior

S
R ——★—— L
I

FIGURE 4-4 Muscular system.

Brain

Eye
(sense organ)

Cranial nerves

Spinal cord

Spinal
nerves

☐ Central nervous
system (CNS)

☐ Peripheral nervous
system (PNS)

S
R ——★—— L
I

FIGURE 4-5 Nervous system.

every area of the body. The extensive networking of the components of the nervous system makes it possible for this complex system to perform its primary functions. These include the following:

1. Communication between body functions
2. Integration of body functions
3. Control of body functions
4. Recognition of sensory stimuli

These functions are accomplished by specialized signals called **nerve impulses.** In general, the functions of the nervous system result in rapid activity that lasts usually for a short duration. For example, we can chew our food normally, walk, and perform coordinated muscular movements only if our nervous system functions properly. The nerve impulse permits the rapid and precise control of diverse body functions. Other types of nerve impulses cause glands to secrete fluids. In addition, elements of the nervous system can recognize certain **stimuli**

(STIM-yoo-lye), such as heat, light, pressure, or temperature, that affect the body. When stimulated, these specialized components of the nervous system, called *sense organs* (discussed in Chapter 9), generate nervous impulses that travel to the brain or spinal cord where analysis or relay occurs and, if needed, appropriate action is initiated.

Endocrine System

The *endocrine system* is composed of specialized glands and cells that secrete chemicals known as **hormones** directly into the blood. Sometimes called *ductless glands*, the organs of the endocrine system perform the same general functions as the nervous system: communication, integration, and control. The nervous system provides rapid, brief control by way of fast-traveling nerve impulses. The endocrine system provides slower but longer-lasting control by hormone secretion. For example, secretion of growth hormone controls the rate of development over long periods of gradual growth.

In addition to controlling growth, hormones are the main regulators of metabolism, reproduction, and other body activities. They play important roles in fluid and electrolyte balance, acid-base balance, and energy metabolism.

As you can see in Figure 4-6, the endocrine glands are widely distributed throughout the body. The **pituitary** (pi-TOO-i-tair-ee) **gland, pineal** (PIN-ee-al) **gland,** and **hypothalamus** (hye-poh-THAL-ah-muss) are located in the skull. The **thyroid** (THY-royd) and **parathyroid** (PAIR-ah-THY-royd) **glands** are in the neck, and the **thymus** (THY-muss) **gland** is in the thoracic cavity, specifically in the mediastinum (see Figure 1-4, p. 6). The **adrenal** (ah-DREE-nal) **glands** and **pancreas** (PAN-kree-as), which also serves as an accessory organ of digestion, are found in the abdominal cavity. Note in Figure 4-6 that the ovaries in the female and the testes in the male also function as endocrine glands. They secrete the sex hormones that stimulate the development of the *secondary sexual characteristics,* including the beard in men and maturation of breasts in adolescent girls.

Cardiovascular (Circulatory) System

The *cardiovascular,* or *circulatory, system* consists of the *heart,* which is a muscular pumping device as shown in Figure 4-7, and a closed system of

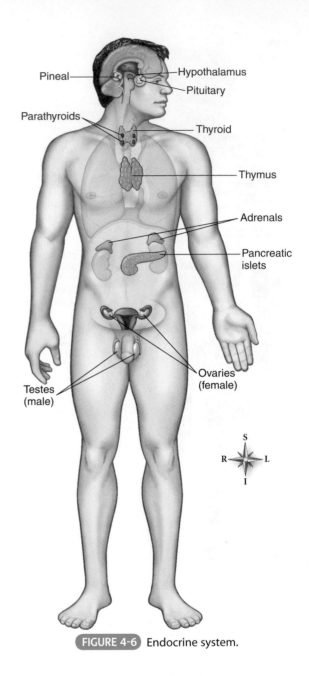

FIGURE 4-6 Endocrine system.

blood vessels made up of **arteries, veins,** and **capillaries.** As the name implies, blood contained in this system is pumped by the heart around a closed circle or circuit of vessels as it passes through the body.

The primary function of the circulatory system is *transportation.* The need for an efficient transportation system in the body is critical. Transportation needs include continuous movement of oxygen and carbon dioxide, nutrients, hormones, and

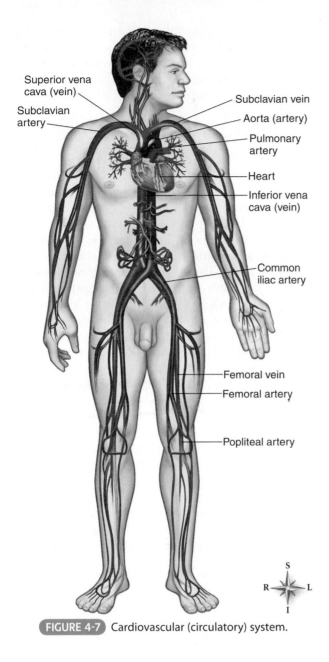

Superior vena cava (vein)

Subclavian artery

Subclavian vein

Aorta (artery)

Pulmonary artery

Heart

Inferior vena cava (vein)

Common iliac artery

Femoral vein

Femoral artery

Popliteal artery

S

R — L

I

FIGURE 4-7 Cardiovascular (circulatory) system.

other important substances. Wastes produced by the cells are released into the bloodstream on an ongoing basis and are transported by the blood to the excretory organs. The circulatory system also helps regulate body temperature by distributing heat throughout the body and by assisting in retaining or releasing heat from the body by regulating blood flow near the body surface. Certain cells of the circulatory system also are involved in the defense of the body or immunity.

Lymphatic System

The *lymphatic system* is composed of **lymph nodes, lymphatic vessels,** and specialized lymphatic organs such as the **tonsils, thymus,** and **spleen.** Note that the thymus in Figure 4-8 functions as an endocrine gland and as a lymphatic gland. Instead of containing blood, the lymphatic vessels are filled with *lymph,* a whitish, watery fluid that contains lymphocytes, proteins, and some fatty molecules. No red blood cells are present. The lymph is formed from the fluid around the body cells and diffuses into the lymph vessels. However, unlike blood, lymph does not circulate repeatedly through a closed circuit or loop of vessels. Instead, lymph flowing through lymphatic vessels eventually enters the circulatory system by passing through large ducts, including the **thoracic duct** shown in Figure 4-8, which in turn connect with veins in the upper area of the thoracic cavity. Collections of lymph nodes can be seen in the axillary (armpit) and in the inguinal (groin) areas of the body in Figure 4-8. The formation and movement of lymph are discussed in Chapter 13.

The functions of the lymphatic system include movement of fluids and certain large molecules from the tissue spaces around the cells and movement of fat-related nutrients from the digestive tract back to the blood. The lymphatic system is also involved in the functioning of the immune system, which plays a critical role in the defense mechanism of the body against disease.

Respiratory System

The organs of the *respiratory system* include the **nose, pharynx** (FAIR-inks), **larynx** (LAIR-inks), **trachea** (TRAY-kee-ah), **bronchi** (BRONG-kye), and **lungs** (Figure 4-9). Together these organs permit the movement of air into the tiny, thin-walled sacs of the lungs called *alveoli* (al-VEE-oh-lye). In the alveoli, oxygen from the air is exchanged for the waste product carbon dioxide, which is car-

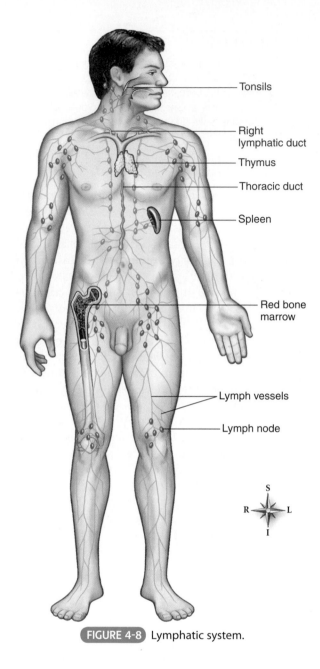

Tonsils

Right
lymphatic duct

Thymus

Thoracic duct

Spleen

Red bone
marrow

Lymph vessels

Lymph node

S
R — L
I

FIGURE 4-8 Lymphatic system.

cus that covers the lining of many respiratory passages and then eliminated from the body. The respiratory system is also involved in regulating the acid-base balance of the body—a function that is discussed in Chapter 19.

Digestive System

The organs of the *digestive system* (Figure 4-10) are often separated into two groups: the *primary organs* and the *secondary* or *accessory organs* (see Figure 4-1). They work together to ensure proper digestion and absorption of nutrients. The primary organs include the **mouth, pharynx, esophagus, stomach, small intestine, large intestine, rectum,** and **anal canal.** The accessory organs of digestion include the **teeth, salivary glands, tongue, liver, gallbladder, pancreas,** and **appendix.**

The primary organs of the digestive system form a tube, open at both ends, called the **gastrointestinal** (GAS-troh-in-TESS-tih-nul) or **GI tract.** Food that enters the tract is digested, its nutrients are absorbed, and the undigested residue is eliminated from the body as waste material called *feces* (FEE-seez). The accessory organs assist in the mechanical or chemical breakdown of ingested food. The appendix, although classified as an accessory organ of digestion and physically attached to the digestive tube, is not functionally important in the digestive process. However, inflammation of the appendix, called **appendicitis** (ah-pen-di-SYE-tis) is a very serious clinical condition and often requires surgery.

Urinary System

The organs of the *urinary system* include the **kidneys, ureters** (YOOR-eh-terz), **bladder,** and **urethra** (yoo-REE-thrah).

The kidneys (Figure 4-11) "clear" or clean the blood of the waste products continually produced by the metabolism of nutrients in the body cells. The kidneys also play an important role in maintaining the electrolyte, water, and acid-base balances in the body.

The waste product produced by the kidneys is called *urine* (YOOR-in). After it is produced by the kidneys, it flows out of the kidneys through the ureters into the urinary bladder, where it is stored. Urine passes from the bladder to the outside of the

ried to the lungs by the blood so that it can be eliminated from the body. The organs of the respiratory system perform a number of functions in addition to permitting movement of air into the alveoli. For example, if you live in a cold or dry environment, incoming air can be warmed and humidified as it passes over the lining of the respiratory air passages. In addition, inhaled irritants such as pollen or dust passing through the respiratory tubes can be trapped in the sticky mu-

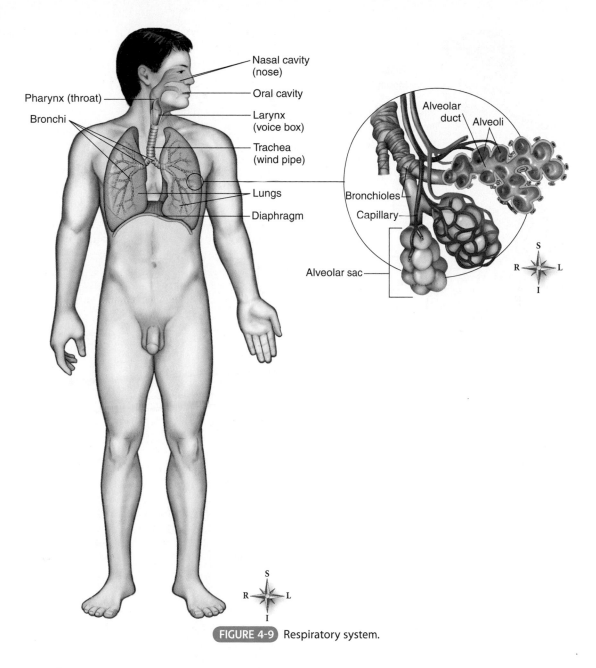

FIGURE 4-9 Respiratory system.

body through the urethra. In the male the urethra passes through the penis, which has a double function: it transports urine and also semen or seminal fluid. Therefore it has urinary and reproductive purposes. In the female the urinary and reproductive passages are completely separate, so the urethra performs only a urinary function.

Organs other than those of the urinary system are also involved in the elimination of body wastes. Undigested food residues and metabolic wastes are eliminated from the intestinal tract as feces, and the lungs rid the body of carbon dioxide. The skin also serves an excretory function by eliminating water and some salts in sweat.

Reproductive Systems

The normal function of the *reproductive system* is different from the normal function of other organ systems of the body. The proper functioning of the

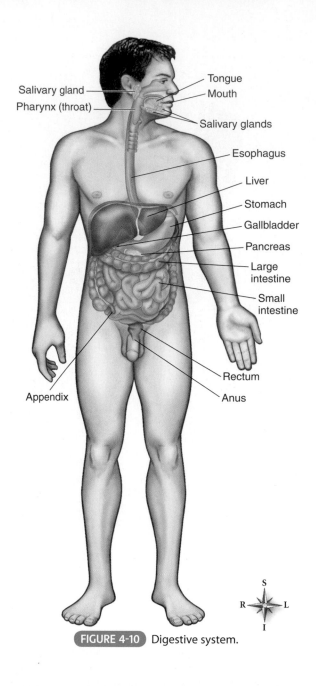

Salivary gland
Pharynx (throat)
Tongue
Mouth
Salivary glands
Esophagus
Liver
Stomach
Gallbladder
Pancreas
Large intestine
Small intestine
Rectum
Anus
Appendix

S
R — L
I

FIGURE 4-10 Digestive system.

Kidney
Ureter
Urinary bladder
Urethra

S
R — L
I

FIGURE 4-11 Urinary system.

Radiography
Wilhelm Röntgen (1845-1923)

In 1895, the German physicist Wilhelm Röntgen (RENT-gen) made one of the most important medical discoveries of the modern age: radiographic imaging of the body. **Radiography,** or x-ray photography, is the oldest and still the most widely used method of noninvasive imaging of internal body structures and earned Röntgen a Nobel Prize. While studying the effects of electricity passing through gas under low pressures, Röntgen accidentally discovered x rays when they caused a plate coated with special chemicals to glow. Not long after that, he showed that they could produce shadows of internal organs such as bones on photographic film. His first, and most famous, radiograph was of his wife Bertha's hand. Although a little fuzzy, it clearly showed Bertha's finger bones and the outline of her ring. When this radiograph was published by a Vienna newspaper, the entire world became instantly aware of his breakthrough discovery.

The figure at right shows how radiography works. A source of waves in the x band of the radiation spectrum beams the x rays through a body and to a piece of photographic film or phosphorescent screen. The resulting image shows the outlines of bones and other dense structures that absorb the x rays. As the figure shows, one way to make soft, hollow structures such as digestive organs more visible is to use radiopaque contrast material. For example, barium sulfate (which absorbs x rays) can be introduced into the colon to make it more visible in a radiograph.

Today, many variations of Röntgen's invention are used to study internal organs without having to cut into the body. For example, computed tomography (CT) scanning is a modern, computerized type of x-ray photography. Radiographic technicians are health professionals whose chief responsibility is to make radiographs, and radiologists are responsible for interpreting these images. Many medical, veterinary, and dental professionals rely on these images and interpretations in their diagnosis, assessment, and treatment of patients. In addition, radiography is used in many industrial and investigative settings—even by archaeologists studying mummies.

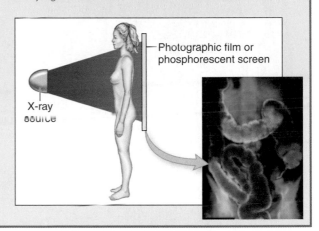

Photographic film or phosphorescent screen

X-ray source

---

reproductive systems ensures survival, not of the individual but of the species, that is, the human race. In addition, production of the hormones that permit the development of sexual characteristics occurs as a result of normal reproductive system activity.

Male Reproductive System

The male reproductive structures shown in Figure 4-12 include the **gonads** (GO-nadz), called **testes** (TES-teez), which produce the sex cells or **sperm;** one of the important *genital ducts*, called the **vas deferens** (vas DEF-er-enz); and the **prostate** (PROSS-tayt), which is classified as an *accessory organ* in the male. The **penis** (PEE-nis) and **scrotum** (SKROH-tum) are supporting structures and together are known as the **genitalia** (jen-i-TAIL-yah). The *urethra*, which is identified in Figure 4-11 as part of the urinary system, passes through the pe-

nis. It serves as a genital duct that carries sperm to the exterior and also as a passageway for the elimination of urine. Functioning together, these structures produce, transfer, and ultimately introduce sperm into the female reproductive tract, where fertilization can occur. Sperm produced by the testes travel through a number of genital ducts, including the vas deferens, to exit the body. The prostate and other accessory organs add fluid and nutrients to the sex cells as they pass through the ducts and the penis, thus permitting transfer of sex cells and seminal fluid into the female reproductive tract.

Female Reproductive System

The female **gonads** are the **ovaries.** The *accessory organs* shown in Figure 4-13 include the **uterus** (YOO-ter-us); **uterine** (YOO-ter-in), or **fallopian, tubes;** and the **vagina** (vah-JYE-nah). In the female

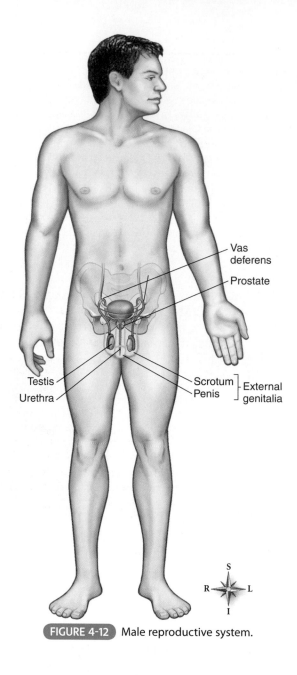

FIGURE 4-12 Male reproductive system.

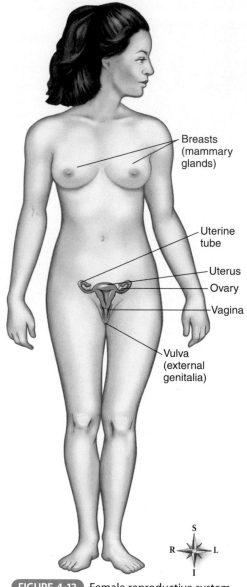

FIGURE 4-13 Female reproductive system.

the term **vulva** (VUL-vah) is used to describe the external genitalia. The breasts, or **mammary glands,** are also classified as external accessory sex organs in the female.

The reproductive organs in the female produce the sex cells, known as **ova;** receive the male sex cells (sperm); transfer the sex cells to the uterus; permit fertilization; and allow for the development, birth, and nourishment of offspring.

QUICK CHECK

1. What are the functions of the lymphatic system?
2. What functions besides gas exchange are performed by the respiratory system?
3. What are some of the accessory organs of the digestive system?
4. What organ in males is shared by both the urinary system and the reproductive system?

Health and Well-Being

Cancer Screening Tests

A knowledge of the structure and function of the body organ systems is a critically important "first step" in understanding and using information that empowers us to become more sophisticated guardians of our own health and well-being. For example, a better understanding of the reproductive system helps individuals participate in a more direct and personal way in cancer prevention screening techniques.

Breast and testicular self-examinations to detect cancer are two important ways that women and men can participate directly in protecting their own health. In addition, regular examination of the skin surface to detect changes in moles or the appearance, or change in appearance, of other growths or pigmented areas can help in the early detection of skin cancer. Indeed, many other "danger signs of cancer," such as changes in bowel habits, persistent cough, or difficulty in swallowing, can be better understood and appropriate action steps can be initiated earlier with an understanding of the structure and function of the organ systems of the body. Information and specific instructions concerning cancer screening tests are available from the American Cancer Society and from most hospitals, clinics, and health care providers.

THE BODY AS A WHOLE

As you study the more detailed structure and function of the organ systems in the chapters that follow, always relate the system and its component organs to the body as a whole. No one body system functions entirely independently of other systems. Instead, you will find that they are structurally and functionally interrelated and interdependent.

 Health and Well-Being

Paired Organs

Have you ever wondered what advantage there might be in having two kidneys, two lungs, two eyes, and two of many other organs? Although the body could function well with only one of each, most of us are born with a pair of these organs. For paired organs that are vital to survival, such as the kidneys, this arrangement allows for the accidental loss of one organ without immediate threat to the survival of the individual. Athletes who have lost one vital organ through injury or disease are often counseled against participating in contact sports that carry the risk of damaging the remaining organ. If the second organ is damaged, total loss of a vital function, such as sight, or even death, may result.

OUTLINE SUMMARY

DEFINITIONS AND CONCEPTS
A. Organ — a structure made up of two or more kinds of tissues organized in such a way that they can together perform a more complex function than can any tissue alone
B. Organ system — a group of organs arranged in such a way that they can together perform a more complex function than can any organ alone
C. Knowledge of individual organs and how they are organized into groups makes the understanding of how a particular organ system functions as a whole more meaningful

ORGAN SYSTEMS
A. Integumentary system (see Figure 4-2)
   1. Structure — organs
      a. Skin
      b. Hair
      c. Nails
      d. Sense receptors
      e. Sweat glands
      f. Oil glands
   2. Functions
      a. Protection
      b. Regulation of body temperature
      c. Synthesis of chemicals
      d. Sense organ

B. Skeletal system (see Figure 4-3)
  1. Structure
    a. Bones
    b. Joints
  2. Functions
    a. Support
    b. Movement (with joints and muscles)
    c. Storage of minerals
    d. Blood cell formation
C. Muscular system (see Figure 4-4)
  1. Structure
    a. Muscles
      (1) Voluntary, or striated
      (2) Involuntary, or smooth
      (3) Cardiac
  2. Functions
    a. Movement
    b. Maintenance of body posture
    c. Production of heat
    d. Contraction of heart
    e. Blood pressure maintenance
    f. Intestinal movement to eliminate feces
D. Nervous system (see Figure 4-5)
  1. Structure
    a. Brain
    b. Spinal cord
    c. Nerves
    d. Sense organs
  2. Functions
    a. Communication
    b. Integration
    c. Control
    d. Recognition of sensory stimuli
  3. System functions by production of nerve impulses caused by stimuli of various types
  4. Control is fast-acting and of short duration
E. Endocrine system (see Figure 4-6)
  1. Structure
    a. Pituitary gland
    b. Pineal gland
    c. Hypothalamus
    d. Thyroid gland
    e. Parathyroid glands
    f. Thymus gland
    g. Adrenal glands
    h. Pancreas
    i. Ovaries (female)
    j. Testes (male)
  2. Functions
    a. Secretion of special substances called *hormones* directly into the blood
    b. Same as nervous system — communication, integration, control
    c. Control is slow and of long duration
    d. Examples of hormone regulation:
      (1) Growth
      (2) Metabolism
      (3) Reproduction
      (4) Fluid and electrolyte balance
F. Cardiovascular (circulatory) system (see Figure 4-7)
  1. Structure
    a. Heart
    b. Blood vessels
      (1) Arteries
      (2) Veins
      (3) Capillaries
  2. Functions
    a. Transportation
    b. Regulation of body temperature
    c. Immunity (body defense)
G. Lymphatic system (see Figure 4-8)
  1. Structure
    a. Lymph nodes
    b. Lymphatic vessels
    c. Tonsils
    d. Thymus
    e. Spleen
  2. Functions
    a. Transportation
    b. Immunity (body defense)
H. Respiratory system (see Figure 4-9)
  1. Structure
    a. Nose
    b. Pharynx
    c. Larynx
    d. Trachea
    e. Bronchi
    f. Lungs
  2. Functions
    a. Exchange of waste gas (carbon dioxide) for oxygen occurs in the *alveoli* of the lungs
    b. Warm and humidify incoming air
    c. Filtration of irritants from inspired air
    d. Regulation of acid-base balance

I. Digestive system (see Figure 4 10)
   1. Structure
      a. Primary organs
         (1) Mouth
         (2) Pharynx
         (3) Esophagus
         (4) Stomach
         (5) Small intestine
         (6) Large intestine
         (7) Rectum
         (8) Anal canal
      b. Accessory organs
         (1) Teeth
         (2) Salivary glands
         (3) Tongue
         (4) Liver
         (5) Gallbladder
         (6) Pancreas
         (7) Appendix
   2. Functions
      a. Mechanical and chemical breakdown (digestion) of food
      b. Absorption of nutrients
      c. Undigested waste product that is eliminated is called *feces*
   3. Appendix
      a. Structural but not a functional part of digestive system
      b. Inflammation of appendix is called *appendicitis*

J. Urinary system (see Figure 4-11)
   1. Structure
      a. Kidneys
      b. Ureters
      c. Urinary bladder
      d. Urethra
   2. Functions
      a. "Clearing" or cleaning blood of waste products — waste product excreted from body is called *urine*
      b. Electrolyte balance
      c. Water balance
      d. Acid-base balance
      e. In males, urethra has urinary and reproductive functions

K. Reproductive system (see Figures 4-12 and 4-13)
   1. Structure
      a. Male
         (1) Gonads — testes
         (2) Genital ducts — vas deferens, urethra
         (3) Accessory gland — prostate
         (4) Supporting structures — genitalia (penis and scrotum)
      b. Female
         (1) Gonads — ovaries
         (2) Accessory organs — uterus, uterine (fallopian) tubes, vagina
         (3) Supporting structures — genitalia (vulva), mammary glands (breasts)
   2. Functions
      a. Survival of genes
      b. Production of sex cells (male: sperm; female: ova)
      c. Transfer and fertilization of sex cells
      d. Development and birth of offspring
      e. Nourishment of offspring
      f. Production of sex hormones

NEW WORDS

radiography
    See the individual chapters for each of the body systems for more detailed explanations of the new words highlighted in this chapter.

REVIEW QUESTIONS

Review the names of organ systems and individual organs in Figures 4-1 through 4-13.

1. Define *organ* and *organ system*.
2. Give examples of the stimuli to which the skin sense organs can respond.
3. How is the skin able to assist in the body's ability to regulate temperature?
4. What is the function of tendons?
5. What are some of the differences between the lymphatic and cardiovascular systems?
6. Name the organs that help rid the body of waste. What type of waste does each organ remove?
7. Besides bone, what other types of tissues are included in the skeletal system?
8. List the 11 organ systems discussed in this chapter.
9. Most of the organ systems have more than one function. List two functions for the following systems: integumentary system, skeletal system, muscular system, lymphatic system, respiratory system, and urinary system.
10. What is unique about the reproductive system?

CRITICAL THINKING

11. Explain the differences between the nervous and endocrine systems. Include what types of functions are regulated and the "message carriers" for each system.
12. The term *balance* is used in this chapter. This is another term for *homeostasis*. Review the functions of the systems and list those functions that are homeostatic.

CHAPTER TEST

1. The primary organs of the digestive system make a long tube called the _____.
2. _____ is another term for voluntary muscle.
3. _____ is another term for involuntary muscle.
4. The nervous system can generate special electrochemical signals called _____.
5. The _____, _____, _____, and _____ are called the accessory structures of the skin.
6. The _____ is part of both the lymphatic and endocrine systems.
7. The _____ is part of both the male reproductive and urinary systems.
8. The gonads for the male reproductive system are the _____. For the female reproductive system, the gonads are the _____.
9. The skeletal system is composed of bone tissue and these two related tissues: _____ and _____.

Match each function in Column B with the proper cell structure in Column A.

COLUMN A

10. _____ Integumentary
11. _____ Skeletal
12. _____ Muscular
13. _____ Nervous
14. _____ Endocrine
15. _____ Cardiovascular
16. _____ Lymphatic
17. _____ Respiratory
18. _____ Digestive
19. _____ Urinary
20. _____ Reproductive

COLUMN B

a. Provides movement, body posture, and heat
b. Uses hormones to regulate body functions
c. Transports fatty nutrients from the digestive system to the blood
d. Physical and chemical change in nutrients and absorption of them
e. Cleans the blood of metabolic wastes and regulates electrolyte balance
f. Protects underlying structures, sensory reception, and regulation of body temperature
g. Transports substances from one part of the body to another
h. Ensures the survival of the species rather than the individual
i. Uses electrochemical signals to integrate and control body functions
j. Exchanges oxygen and carbon dioxide and regulates acid-base balance
k. Provides a rigid framework for the body and stores minerals

OBJECTIVES

AFTER YOU HAVE COMPLETED THIS CHAPTER, YOU SHOULD BE ABLE TO:

1. Classify, compare the structure of, and give examples of each type of body membrane.
2. Describe the structure and function of the epidermis and dermis.
3. List and briefly describe each accessory organ of the skin.
4. List and discuss the three primary functions of the integumentary system.
5. Classify burns and describe how to estimate the extent of a burn injury.

The Integumentary System and Body Membranes

5

In Chapter 1 the concept of progressive organization of body structures from simple to complex was established. Complexity in body structure and function progresses from cells to tissues and then to organs and organ systems. This chapter discusses the skin and its accessory *structures*—the hair, the nails, and the skin glands—as an organ system. This system is called the **integumentary system. Integument** (in-TEG-yoo-ment) is another name for the skin, and the skin itself is the principal organ of the integumentary system. The skin is one of a group of anatomically simple but functionally important sheetlike structures called *membranes*. This chapter begins with classification and discussion of the important body membranes. Study of the structure and function of the integument follows. Ideally, you should study the skin and its accessory structures before proceeding to the more traditional organ systems in the chapters that follow to improve your understanding of how structure is related to function.

CLASSIFICATION OF BODY MEMBRANES

The term **membrane** refers to a thin, sheetlike structure that may have many important functions in the body. Membranes cover and protect the body surface, line body cavities, and cover the inner surfaces of the hollow organs such as the digestive, reproductive, and respiratory passageways. Some membranes anchor organs to each other or to bones, and others cover the internal organs. In certain areas of the body, membranes secrete lubricating fluids that reduce friction during organ movements such as the beating of the heart or lung expansion and contraction. Membrane lubricants also decrease friction be-

tween bones in joints. There are two major categories or types of body membranes:

1. **Epithelial membranes,** composed of epithelial tissue and an underlying layer of specialized connective tissue

2. **Connective tissue membranes,** composed exclusively of various types of connective tissue. No epithelial cells are present in this type of membrane

Epithelial Membranes

There are three types of epithelial tissue membranes in the body:

1. Cutaneous membrane
2. Serous membranes
3. Mucous membranes

Cutaneous Membrane

The **cutaneous** (kyoo-TAYN-ee-us) **membrane,** or skin, is the primary organ of the integumentary system. It is one of the most important and certainly one of the largest and most visible organs. In most individuals the skin composes some 16% of the body weight. It fulfills the requirements necessary for an epithelial tissue membrane in that it has a superficial layer of epithelial cells and an underlying layer of supportive connective tissue. Its structure is uniquely suited to its many functions. The skin is discussed in depth later in the chapter.

Serous Membranes

As with all epithelial membranes, a **serous** (SEER-us) **membrane** is composed of two distinct layers of tissue. The epithelial sheet is a thin layer of simple squamous epithelium. The connective tissue layer forms a very thin, gluelike **basement membrane** that holds and supports the epithelial cells.

The serous membrane that lines body cavities and covers the surfaces of organs in those cavities is in reality a single, continuous sheet of tissue covering two different surfaces. The name of the serous membrane is determined by its location. Using this criterion results in two types of serous membranes. The first type lines body cavities, and the second type covers the organs in those cavities. The serous membrane, which lines the walls of a body cavity much like wallpaper covers the walls of a room, is called the **parietal** (pah-RYE-i-tal) **portion.** The other type of serous membrane, which covers the surface of organs found in body cavities, is called the **visceral** (VIS-er-al) **portion.**

The serous membranes of the thoracic and abdominal cavities are identified in Figure 5-1. In the thoracic cavity the serous membranes are called

FIGURE 5-1 Types of body membranes. **A,** Epithelial membranes, including cutaneous membrane (skin), serous membranes (parietal and visceral pleura and peritoneum), and mucous membranes. **B,** Connective tissue membranes, including synovial membranes. See text for explanation.

pleura (PLOOR-ah). In the abdominal cavity, they are called **peritoneum** (pair-i-toh-NEE-um). Look again at Figure 5-1 to note the placement of the *parietal* and *visceral pleura* and the *parietal* and *visceral peritoneum.* In both cases the parietal layer forms the lining of the body cavity, and the visceral layer covers the organs found in that cavity.

Serous membranes secrete a thin, watery fluid that helps reduce friction and serves as a lubricant when organs rub against one another and against the walls of the cavities that contain them. **Pleurisy** (PLOOR-i-see) is a very painful pathological condition characterized by inflammation of the serous membranes (pleura) that line the chest cavity and cover the lungs. Pain is caused by irritation and friction as the lungs rub against the walls of the chest cavity. In severe cases the inflamed surfaces of the pleura fuse, and permanent damage may develop. The term **peritonitis** (pair-i-toh-NYE-tis) is used to describe inflammation of the serous membranes in the abdominal cavity. Peritonitis is sometimes a serious complication of an infected appendix.

> To learn more about serous membranes, go to AnimationDirect on your CD-ROM.

Mucous Membranes

Mucous (MYOO-kus) **membranes** are epithelial membranes containing both an epithelial cell and a fibrous or connective tissue layer. These membranes line body surfaces opening directly to the exterior. Examples of mucous membranes include those lining the respiratory, digestive, urinary, and reproductive tracts. The epithelial component of a mucous membrane varies, depending on its location and function. In most cases the cell composition is either stratified squamous or simple columnar epithelia. In the esophagus, for example, a tough, abrasion-resistant stratified squamous epithelium is found. This is a good example of the "form follows function" principle. Without the protection of a tough epithelial lining, ingested food that is coarse, like popcorn, might cause injury to the esophageal wall when swallowed and may result in irritation or even infection and hemorrhage. A thin layer of simple columnar epithelium lines the walls of the lower segments of the digestive tract. In the stomach and small intestine, ingested food undergoes digestion and is changed into a smooth, liquefied material that is no longer abrasive. The single layer of lining epithelial cells in these segments of the intestinal tract is well suited to a primary function: nutrient absorption.

The epithelial cells of most mucous membranes secrete a thick, slimy material called **mucus** that keeps the membranes moist and soft. The fibrous connective tissue underlying the epithelium in mucous membranes is called the **lamina propria** (LAM-min-uh PRO-pre-uh). Note that the term

mucous identifies the type of membrane, whereas *mucus* refers to the secretion produced by that membrane.

The term **mucocutaneous junction** (myoo-koh-kyoo-TAY-nee-us JUNK-shun) is used to describe the transitional area that serves as a point of "fusion" where skin and mucous membranes meet. Such junctions lack accessory organs such as hair or sweat glands that characterize skin. These transitional areas are generally moistened by mucous glands within the body orifices or openings where these junctions are located. The eyelids, lips, nasal openings, vulva, and anus have mucocutaneous junctions that may become sites of infection or irritation.

> To learn more about mucous membranes, go to AnimationDirect on your CD-ROM.

Connective Tissue Membranes

Unlike cutaneous, serous, and mucous membranes, connective tissue membranes do not contain epithelial components. The **synovial** (si-NO-vee-al) **membranes** lining the joint capsules that surround and attach the ends of articulating bones in movable joints are classified as connective tissue membranes (see Figure 5-1, *B* and Figure 6-20 on p. 127). These membranes are smooth and slick and secrete a thick, colorless lubricating fluid called **synovial fluid.** The membrane itself, with its specialized fluid, helps reduce friction between the opposing surfaces of bones in movable joints. Synovial membranes also line the small, cushion-like sacs called **bursae** (BER-see) found between many moving body parts.

> To learn more about connective tissue and synovial membrane, go to AnimationDirect on your CD-ROM.

✓ QUICK CHECK

1. What are the four main types of membranes in the body?
2. Which of the body's membranes are types of epithelial membranes?
3. What fluid(s) is/are produced by each of the four main membrane types? What is the function of each fluid?

THE SKIN

The brief description of the skin in Chapter 4 (see p. 72) identified it not only as the primary organ of the integumentary system but also as the largest and one of the most important organs of the body. The skin is an architectural marvel. Consider the incredible number of structures fitting into 1 square inch of skin: 500 sweat glands; more than 1,000 nerve endings; yards of tiny blood vessels; nearly 100 oil or **sebaceous** (seh-BAY-shus) **glands;** 150 sensors for pressure, 75 for heat, and 10 for cold; and millions of cells.

Structure of the Skin

The skin, or cutaneous membrane, is a sheetlike organ composed of the following layers of distinct tissue (Figure 5-2):

1. The **epidermis** is the outermost layer of the skin. It is a relatively thin sheet of stratified squamous epithelium.

FIGURE 5-2 **Microscopic view of the skin.** The epidermis, shown in longitudinal section, is raised at one corner to reveal the ridges in the dermis.

2. The **dermis** is the deeper of the two layers. It is thicker than the epidermis and is made up largely of connective tissue.

As you can see in Figure 5-2, the layers of the skin are supported by a thick layer of loose connective tissue and fat called **subcutaneous** (sub-kyoo-TAY-nee-us) **tissue,** or the **hypodermis** (hye-poh-DER-mis). Fat in the subcutaneous layer insulates the body from extremes of heat and cold. It also serves as a stored source of energy for the body and can be used as a food source if required. In addition, the subcutaneous tissue acts as a shock-absorbing pad and helps protect underlying tissues from injury caused by bumps and blows to the body surface.

Epidermis

The tightly packed epithelial cells of the epidermis are arranged in five distinct layers. The cells of the innermost layer, called the **stratum germinativum** (STRAH-tum jer-mi-na-TE-vum), undergo mitosis and reproduce themselves (see Figure 5-2). As they move toward the surface of the skin, these new cells "specialize" in ways that increase their ability to provide protection for the body tissues that lie below them. This ability is of critical clinical significance. It enables the skin to repair itself if it is injured. The self-repairing characteristic of normal skin makes it possible for the body to maintain an effective barrier against infection, even when it is subjected to injury and normal wear and tear. As new cells are produced in the deep layer of the epidermis, they move upward through additional layers, or "strata" of cells. As they approach the surface, the cytoplasm is replaced by one of nature's most unique proteins, a substance called **keratin** (KER-ah-tin). Keratin is a tough, waterproof material that provides cells in the outer layer of the skin with a horny, abrasion-resistant, and protective quality. The tough outer layer of the epidermis is called the **stratum corneum** (STRAH-tum KOR-nee-um). Cells filled with keratin are continually pushed to the surface of the epidermis. In the photomicrograph of the skin shown in Figure 5-3, many of the outermost cells of the stratum corneum have been dislodged. These dry, dead cells filled with keratin "flake off" by the thousands onto our clothes, into our bath water, and onto things we handle. Millions of epithelial cells reproduce daily to replace the millions shed. This is just one example of the work our

"Flaked" cells from stratum corneum · Epidermis · Dermis

FIGURE 5-3 Photomicrograph of the skin. New cells of the epidermis are produced in stratum germinativum, where they are pushed upward and eventually die and flatten out to form stratum corneum (*arrow* shows dead cell falling away from skin). The deep region of the skin is the dermis, made up of connective tissue having few cells.

bodies do without our knowledge, continuing even when we seem to be resting.

Skin Pigment

The deepest cell layer of the epidermis identified in Figure 5-2 is responsible for the production of a specialized **pigment** substance that gives color to the skin. The term *pigment* comes from a Latin word meaning "paint." It is this epidermal layer that gives color to the skin. The brown pigment **melanin** (MEL-ah-nin) is produced by specialized cells in this layer. These cells are called **melanocytes** (MEL-ah-no-sytes). The higher the concentration of melanin, the deeper is the color of skin. The primary function of melanin is to absorb harmful ultraviolet (UV) radiation from sunlight before it reaches tissues below the outer layers of the epidermis. The amount and type of melanin in your skin depends first on the skin color genes you have inherited. That is, heredity determines how dark or light your basic skin color is. However, other factors such as sunlight exposure can modify this hereditary effect. Prolonged exposure to sunlight in light-skinned people darkens the exposed area because it leads to increased melanin deposits in the epidermis—a protective mechanism that keeps deeper tissues safe from UV radiation. If the skin contains little melanin, as under the nails where there is no melanin at all, a change in color can occur if the volume of blood in the skin changes significantly or if the amount of oxygen in the blood is increased or decreased. In these individuals, increased blood flow to the skin or increased blood oxygen levels can cause a pink flush to appear. However, if blood oxygen levels decrease or if actual blood flow is reduced dramatically, the skin turns a blue-gray color—a condition called **cyanosis** (SYE-ah-NO-sis). In general, the less abundant the melanin deposits in the skin are, the more visible will be the changes in color caused by the change in skin blood volume or oxygen level. Conversely, the richer the skin's pigmentation is, the less noticeable such changes will be.

Dermal-Epidermal Junction

The junction that exists between the thin epidermal layer of skin above and the dermal layer below forms a specialized type of basement membrane called the **dermal-epidermal junction.** The deeper cells of the epidermis are packed tightly together. They are held firmly to one another and to the dermis below by specialized junctions between the membranes of adjacent cells, sometimes described as "spot welds," and by a unique type of gel that serves to "glue" the two layers of the skin together and provide support for the epidermis attached to its upper surface. Small nipplelike bumps that project upward from the dermis into the epidermis, called **dermal papillae** (DER-mal pah-PIL-ee)—which are discussed below—also play an important role in stabilizing the dermal-epidermal junction (see Figure 5-2). If the junction is weakened or destroyed, the skin falls apart. When this occurs over a limited area because of burns, friction injuries, or exposure to irritants, **blisters** may result. Any widespread detachment of a large area of epidermis from the dermis is an extremely serious condition that may result in overwhelming infection and death.

Dermis

The dermis is the deeper of the two primary skin layers and is much thicker than the epidermis. The mechanical strength of the skin is in the dermis. It is composed largely of connective tissue. Instead of cells being crowded close together like the epithelial cells of the epidermis, they are scattered far apart, with many fibers in between. Some of the fibers are tough and strong (collagen or white fibers), and others are stretchable and elastic (elastic or yellow fibers).

Papillary Layer. The upper region, or *papillary layer,* of the dermis is characterized by parallel rows of tiny bumps called *dermal papillae,* which are visible in Figure 5-2. The papillary layer takes its name from the papillae on its surface. These upward projections are interesting and useful features. As noted above, they form an important part of the dermal-epidermal junction that helps bind the skin layers together. In addition, they form the ridges and grooves that make up your fingerprints and footprints.

You can observe these ridges on the tips of the fingers and on the skin covering the palms of your hands. Observe in Figure 5-2 how the epidermis follows the contours of the dermal papillae. These ridges develop sometime before birth. Not only is their pattern unique in each individual but also the pattern never changes except to grow larger— two facts that explain why our fingerprints or footprints can provide positive identification of who we are. The biological function of skin ridges is to improve our grip when making or using tools, for example, or walking barefooted on smooth surfaces. The papillary layer and its papillae are composed essentially of loose connective tissue elements and a fine network of thin collagenous and elastic fibers (see Chapter 3, p. 55).

Reticular Layer. The deeper area, or *reticular layer,* of the dermis is filled with a dense network of interlacing fibers. Most of the fibers in this area are collagen that gives toughness to the skin. However, elastic fibers are also present. These make the skin stretchable and elastic (able to rebound). As we age, the number of elastic fibers in the dermis decreases, and the amount of fat stored in the subcutaneous tissue is reduced. Wrinkles develop as the skin loses elasticity. The skin sags and becomes less soft and pliant (Figure 5-4).

In addition to connective tissue elements, the dermis contains a specialized network of nerves and nerve endings to process sensory information such as pain, pressure, touch, and temperature. At various levels of the dermis, there are muscle fibers, hair follicles, sweat and sebaceous glands, and many blood vessels.

Subcutaneous Tissue

The **subcutaneous tissue** is often called the *superficial fascia* by anatomists. It is not a part or layer of the skin. Instead, it lies deep to the dermis and forms a connection between the skin and underlying structures of the body such as muscle and

FIGURE 5-4 **Aged skin.** In late adulthood, wrinkles in the skin often develop, especially in areas of frequent movement such as on the hands, around the mouth, and around the eyelids.

bone. If you ever skin a piece of chicken before cooking, separation of the skin will occur in the "cleavage plane" that exists between the superficial fascia and the underlying structures. The spongy nature of subcutaneous tissue determines the relative mobility of the skin. Liquid medicines such as insulin are often administered by *subcutaneous injection* into this area. Loose fibrous and adipose tissue are prominent in subcutaneous tissue, and in obese individuals fat content in this layer may exceed 10 cm or more in thickness.

Clinical Application

Weight Loss Surgery and Liposuction

In individuals who are significantly overweight or **obese,** much of the excess fat accumulates in the subcutaneous tissue. Because the skin stretches to accommodate the excess fat, loose, sagging skin folds will remain after massive weight loss, especially in areas such as the abdomen, arms, and thighs. Removal of excess skin is often required following gastric bypass procedures or surgical "banding" of the stomach (see Clinical Application: Gallstones and Weight Loss box, p. 363) that result in massive weight loss.

Liposuction is a surgical procedure that involves insertion of hollow cannulas into the subcutaneous tissue to remove fat using a vacuum aspirator. It is not intended as a weight loss procedure. Instead, it is used in individuals who may not be overweight but have an inability to lose subcutaneous fatty deposits in problem areas such as the hips, lower abdomen, inner thighs, and knees. Unfortunately the process, sometimes called *body contouring*, may result in hanging skin folds that require additional surgery to remove.

Accessory Structures of the Skin

Hair

The human body is covered with millions of hairs. Indeed, at the time of birth most of the specialized structures called **follicles** (FOL-li-kulz) that are required for hair growth are already present. They develop early in fetal life and by birth are present in most parts of the skin. The hair of a newborn infant is extremely fine and soft. It is called **lanugo** (lah-NOO-go) from the Latin word meaning "down." In premature infants, lanugo may be noticeable over most of the body, but soon after birth the lanugo is lost and replaced by new hair that is stronger and more pigmented. Although only a few areas of the skin are hairless—notably the lips, the palms of the hands, and the soles of the feet—most body hair remains almost invisible. Hair is most visible on the scalp, eyelids, and eyebrows. The coarse hair that first appears in the pubic and axillary regions at the time of puberty develops in response to the secretion of hormones.

Hair growth begins when cells of the epidermal layer of the skin grow down into the dermis, forming a small tube called the *hair follicle.* The relationship of a hair follicle and its related structures to the epidermal and dermal layers of the skin is shown in Figure 5-5. Hair growth begins from a small, cap-shaped cluster of cells called the **hair papilla** (pah-PIL-ah), which is located at the base of the follicle. The papilla is nourished by a dermal blood vessel. Note in Figure 5-5 that part of the hair, namely the *root,* lies hidden in the follicle. The visible part of a hair is called the *shaft.*

As long as cells in the papilla of the hair follicle remain alive, new hair will replace any that is cut or plucked. Contrary to popular belief, frequent cutting or shaving does not make hair grow faster or become coarser. Why? Because neither process affects the epithelial cells that form the hairs, because they are embedded in the dermis.

A tiny, smooth (involuntary) muscle can be seen in Figure 5-5. It is called an **arrector pili** (ah-REK-tor PYE-lye) muscle. It is attached to the base of a dermal papilla above and to the side of a hair follicle below. Generally, these muscles contract only when we are frightened or cold. When contraction occurs, each muscle simultaneously pulls on its two points of attachment (that is, up on a hair follicle but down on a part of the skin). This produces little raised places, commonly known as *goose bumps,* between the depressed points of the skin

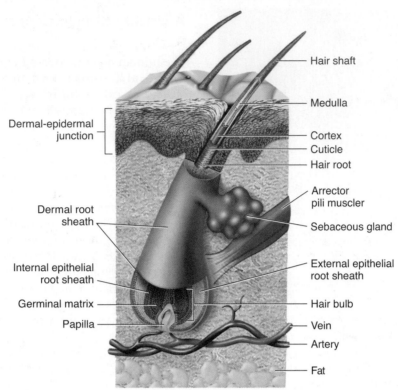

Dermal-epidermal junction

Hair shaft

Medulla

Cortex

Cuticle

Hair root

Arrector pili muscler

Sebaceous gland

External epithelial root sheath

Dermal root sheath

Internal epithelial root sheath

Germinal matrix

Papilla

Hair bulb

Vein

Artery

Fat

FIGURE 5-5   **Hair follicle.** Relationship of a hair follicle and related structures to the epidermal and dermal layers of the skin.

and at the same time pulls the hairs up until they are more or less straight. The name *arrector pili* describes the function of these muscles. It is Latin for "erectors of the hair." We unconsciously recognize these facts in expressions such as "I was so frightened my hair stood on end."

Receptors

Receptors in the skin make it possible for the body surface to act as a sense organ, relaying messages to the brain concerning sensations such as touch, pain, temperature, and pressure. Receptors differ in structure from the highly complex to the very simple. Look again at Figure 5-2 and identify both a **tactile (Meissner)** (MYZ-ner) **corpuscle** and a **lamellar (Pacini)** (pah-SIN-ee) **corpuscle.** The lamellar corpuscle is deep in the dermis. It is capable of detecting *deep pressure* on the skin surface. The tactile corpuscle is generally located close to the skin surface. It is capable of detecting sensations of *light touch.* Both specialized receptors are widely distributed in skin. Additional receptors in the skin respond to other types of stimuli. For example, **free nerve endings** respond to pain, and receptors called **bulboid corpuscles (Krause end**

bulbs) detect low-frequency vibration. Other receptors mediate sensations such as crude touch and vibration. The various sense organs found in the skin are discussed in detail in Chapter 9.

Nails

Nails are classified as accessory organs of the skin and are produced by cells in the epidermis. They form when epidermal cells over the terminal ends of the fingers and toes fill with keratin and become hard and platelike. The components of a typical fingernail and its associated structures are shown in Figure 5-6. In this illustration the fingernail of the index finger is viewed from above and in sagittal section. (Recall that a sagittal section divides a body part into right and left portions.) Look first at the nail as seen from above. The visible part of the nail is called the **nail body.** The rest of the nail, namely the **root,** lies in a groove and is hidden by a fold of skin called the **cuticle** (KYOO-ti-kul). In the sagittal section you can see the nail root from the side and note its relationship to the cuticle, which is folded back over its upper surface. The nail body nearest the root has a crescent-shaped white area known as the **lunula** (LOO-nyoo-lah),

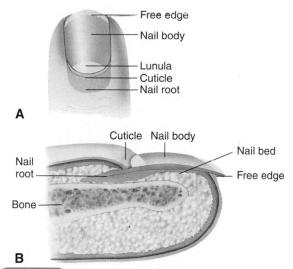

A

B

FIGURE 5-6 Structure of nails. **A,** Fingernail viewed from above. **B,** Sagittal section of fingernail and associated structures.

or "little moon." You should be able to identify this area easily on your own nails. It is most noticeable on the thumbnail. Under the nail lies a layer of epithelium called the *nail bed*, which is labeled on the sagittal section in Figure 5-6. Because it contains abundant blood vessels, it appears pink in color through the translucent nail bodies. If blood oxygen levels drop and cyanosis develops, the nail bed will turn blue.

Skin Glands

The skin glands include the two varieties of **sweat,** or **sudoriferous** (soo-doh-RIF-er-us), **glands** and the microscopic **sebaceous glands** (see Figure 5-2).

Sweat (Sudoriferous) Glands. Sweat glands are the most numerous of the skin glands. They can be classified into two groups—**eccrine** (EK-rin) and **apocrine** (AP-oh-krin)—based on type of secretion and location. **Eccrine sweat glands** are by far the more numerous, important, and widespread sweat glands in the body. They are quite small and, with few exceptions, are distributed over the total body surface. Throughout life they produce a transparent, watery liquid called **perspiration,** or *sweat.* Sweat assists in the elimination of waste products such as ammonia and uric acid. In addition to elimination of waste, sweat plays a critical role in helping the body maintain a constant temperature. Anatomists estimate that a single square inch of skin on the palms of the hands contains about 3,000

eccrine sweat glands. With a magnifying glass you can locate the pinpoint-size openings on the skin that you probably call **pores.** The pores are outlets of small ducts from the eccrine sweat glands.

Apocrine sweat glands are found primarily in the skin in the armpit (axilla) and in the pigmented skin areas around the genitals. They are larger than the eccrine glands, and instead of watery sweat, they secrete a thicker secretion. The odor associated with apocrine gland secretion is not caused by the secretion itself. Instead, it is caused by the contamination and decomposition of the secretion by skin bacteria. Apocrine glands enlarge and begin to function at puberty.

Sebaceous Glands. Sebaceous glands secrete oil for the hair and skin. Oil or sebaceous glands grow where hairs grow. Their tiny ducts open into hair follicles (see Figure 5-5) so that their secretion, called **sebum** (SEE-bum), lubricates the hair and skin. Someone aptly described sebum as "nature's skin cream" because it prevents drying and cracking of the skin. Sebum secretion increases during adolescence, stimulated by the increased blood levels of the sex hormones. Frequently sebum accumulates in and enlarges some of the ducts of the sebaceous glands, forming white pimples. This sebum often darkens when exposed to air, forming a **blackhead.** Sebum secretion decreases in late

---

Health and Well-Being

Exercise and the Skin

Excess heat produced by the skeletal muscles during exercise increases the core body temperature far beyond the normal range. Because blood in vessels near the skin's surface dissipates heat well, the body's control centers adjust blood flow so that more warm blood from the body's core is sent to the skin for cooling. During exercise, blood flow in the skin can be so high that the skin takes on a redder coloration.

To help dissipate even more heat, sweat production increases to as high as 3 liters per hour during exercise. Although each sweat gland produces very little of this total, more than 3 million individual sweat glands are found throughout the skin. Sweat evaporation is essential to keeping body temperature in balance, but excessive sweating can lead to a dangerous loss of fluid. Because normal amounts of drinking may not replace the water lost through sweating, it is important to increase fluid consumption during and after any type of exercise to avoid **dehydration.**

adulthood, contributing to increased wrinkling and cracking of the skin.

Skin Cancer

The three most common types of skin cancer are **squamous** (SKWAY-muss) **cell carcinoma, basal cell carcinoma,** and **malignant** (mah-LIG-nant) **melanoma** (mel-ah-NO-mah). Although genetic predisposition plays a role, pathophysiologists believe that exposure to the sun's ultraviolet (UV) radiation is the most important factor in causing the common skin cancers. UV radiation damages the deoxyribonucleic acid (DNA) in skin cells, causing the mistakes in mitosis that produce cancer. Skin cells have a natural ability to repair UV damage to the DNA, but in some people, this inherent mechanism may not be able to deal with a massive amount of damage. **Kaposi** (KAH-pohsee) **sarcoma** is a rare form of skin cancer (Figure 5-7, *D*) frequently associated with AIDS and other immune deficiencies.

Squamous Cell Carcinoma

A common type of skin cancer, squamous cell carcinoma, is a slow-growing malignant tumor of the epidermis. Lesions typical of this form of skin can-

FIGURE 5-7 Examples of skin cancer lesions. **A,** Squamous cell carcinoma. **B,** Basal cell carcinoma. **C,** Malignant melanoma. **D,** Kaposi sarcoma.

ccr begin as hard, raised nodules that are usually painless (Figure 5-7, *A*). If not treated, squamous cell carcinomas will grow in size and eventually *metastasize* (meh-TAS-tah-syze), or spread, invading other organs and areas of the body.

Basal Cell Carcinoma

Basal cell carcinoma, the most common type of skin cancer, usually appears on the upper face. Originating in cells at the base of the epidermis, this type of skin cancer is much less likely to metastasize than other types. It often appears first as a small, raised lesion that erodes in the center to form a bleeding, crusted crater (Figure 5-7, *B*).

Melanoma

Malignant melanoma is the most serious form of skin cancer. This type of cancer sometimes develops from a *benign* (bee-NYNE) or noncancerous pigmented mole, and then transforms into a dark, spreading cancerous lesion (Figure 5-7, *C*). Benign moles should be checked regularly for warning signs of melanoma because early detection and removal are essential for successful treatment. The "ABCD" rule of self-examination of moles is summarized in Table 5-1. Unfortunately, the incidence of melanoma in the U.S. population is increasing. Epidemiological studies now show that adults who had more than two blistering sunburns before the age of 20 have a much greater risk of developing melanoma than someone who experi-

enced no such burns. Those who grew up in the 1970s and 1980s are now, as older adults, exhibiting melanoma at a much higher rate than those in previous generations.

Functions of the Skin

The skin, or cutaneous membrane, serves a number of important functions that contribute to survival. The most important functions are:

1. Protection
2. Temperature regulation
3. Sense organ activity
4. Excretion
5. Synthesis of vitamin D

 To learn more about pressure ulcers, go to AnimationDirect on your CD-ROM.

Protection

The skin as a whole is often described as our "first line of defense" against a multitude of hazards. It protects us against the daily invasion of deadly microbes. The tough, keratin-filled cells of the stra-

TABLE 5-1	
Warning Signs of Malignant Melanoma	
ABCD	**RULE**
Asymmetry	Benign moles are usually symmetrical. Their halves are mirror images of each other. Melanoma lesions are asymmetrical or lopsided.
Border	Benign moles are outlined by a distinct border, but malignant melanomal lesions are often irregular or indistinct in shape.
Color	Benign moles may be any shade of brown but are relatively evenly colored. Melanoma lesions tend to be unevenly colored, exhibiting a mixture of shades or colors.
Diameter	By the time a melanoma lesion exhibits characteristics A, B, and C, it also is probably larger than 6 mm (¼ inch).

 Clinical Application

Pressure Ulcers

Family members, nurses, or other professionals who provide health care services for bedridden or otherwise immobilized individuals need to be aware of the causes and nature of **pressure ulcers.** Also called *bedsores,* these lesions appear after blood flow to a local area of skin slows because of pressure on the skin covering a bony prominence such as the heel (see figure). Ulcers form and infections develop as lack of blood flow causes tissue damage. Frequent changes in body position and soft support cushions help prevent pressure ulcers.

tum corneum also resist the entry of harmful chemicals and protect against physical tears and cuts. Because it is waterproof, keratin also protects the body from excessive fluid loss. Melanin in the pigment layer of the skin prevents the sun's harmful UV rays from penetrating the interior of the body.

Temperature Regulation

The skin plays a key role in regulating the body's temperature. Incredible as it seems, on a hot and humid day the skin can serve as a means for releasing almost 3,000 calories of body heat—enough heat energy to boil more than 20 liters of water! It accomplishes this feat by regulating sweat secretion and by regulating the flow of blood close to the body surface. When sweat evaporates from the body surface, heat is also lost. The principle of heat loss through evaporation is basic to many cooling systems. When increased quantities of blood are allowed to fill the vessels close to the skin, heat is also lost by radiation. Blood supply to the skin far exceeds the amount needed by the skin. Such an abundant blood supply primarily enables the regulation of body temperature.

Changes in skin color noted in a hot or cold environment are related to the change in skin blood flow that helps regulate either heat loss or preservation of core body temperature. In addition, changes in skin blood flow, especially to the skin of the face and neck, can occur as a result of certain skin diseases or sudden emotion. When blood supply increases, the skin reddens—a condition called *flushing* or *blushing*. Contraction of skin blood vessels causes the skin to take on a bluish color referred to as *cyanosis* (sye-ah-NO-sis).

Sense Organ Activity

The skin functions as an enormous sense organ. Its millions of nerve endings serve as antennas or receivers for the body, keeping it informed of changes in its environment. The two specialized receptors shown in Figure 5-2 make it possible for the body to detect sensations of light touch (tactile corpuscles) and deep pressure (lamellar corpuscles). Other receptors make it possible for us to respond to sensations such as pain, heat, and cold.

Excretion

By regulating the volume and chemical content of sweat, the body, through a function of the skin, can influence both its total fluid volume and the

amounts of certain waste products (such as uric acid, ammonia, and urea) that are excreted. This excretory function can become more important in certain disease states or pathological conditions.

Synthesis of Vitamin D

Synthesis of vitamin D is another important function of the skin. It occurs when the skin is exposed to UV light. When this occurs, a precursor substance in skin cells is transported to the liver and kidneys where it is converted into an active form of vitamin D. Recent research has shown that vitamin D is critically important for good health, thus underscoring the importance of this skin function.

Burns

Burns constitute one of the most serious and frequent problems that affect the skin. Typically, we think of a burn as an injury caused by fire or by contact of the skin with a hot surface. However, overexposure to UV light (sunburn) or contact of the skin with an electric current or a harmful chemical such as an acid can also cause burns.

Estimating Body Surface Area

When burns involve large areas of the skin, treatment and the possibility for recovery depend in large part on the *total area involved* and the *severity of the burn*. The severity of a burn is determined by the depth of the injury, as well as by the amount of body surface area affected.

The **"rule of nines"** is one of the most commonly used methods of determining the extent of a burn injury. With this technique (Figure 5-8), the body is divided into 11 areas of 9% each, with the area around the genitals representing the additional 1% of body surface area. As you can see in Figure 5-8, in the adult 9% of the skin covers the head and each upper extremity, including front and back surfaces. Twice as much, or 18%, of the total skin area covers the front and back of the trunk and each lower extremity, including front and back surfaces.

Classification of Burns

The classification system used to describe the severity of burns is based on the number of tissue layers involved (Figure 5-9). The most severe burns destroy not only layers of the skin and subcutaneous tissue but underlying tissues as well.

FIGURE 5-8 The "rule of nines." Dividing the body into 11 areas of 9% each helps to estimate the amount of skin surface burned in an adult.

First-Degree Burns. A **first-degree burn** (e.g., a typical sunburn) causes minor discomfort and some reddening of the skin. Although the surface layers of the epidermis may peel in 1 to 3 days, no blistering occurs, and actual tissue destruction is minimal.

Second-Degree Burns. A **second-degree burn** involves the deep epidermal layers and always causes injury to the upper layers of the dermis. Although deep second-degree burns damage sweat glands, hair follicles, and sebaceous glands, complete destruction of the dermis does not occur. Blisters, severe pain, generalized swelling, and fluid loss characterize this type of burn. Scarring is common. First- and second-degree burns are called **partial-thickness burns.**

Third-Degree Burns. A **third-degree,** or **full-thickness, burn** is characterized by complete destruction of the epidermis and dermis. In addition, tissue death extends below the primary skin layers into the subcutaneous tissue. Third-degree burns often involve underlying muscles and even bone. One distinction between second- and third-degree burns is that third-degree lesions are insensitive to pain immediately after injury because of the destruction of nerve endings. The fluid loss that results from third-degree burns is a very serious problem. Another serious problem with third-degree burns is the great risk of infection.

FIGURE 5-9 Classification of burns. Thickness of the damaged skin is one way to classify burns. **A,** First-degree, or partial-thickness, burn. **B,** Second-degree, or partial-thickness, burn. **C,** Third-degree, or full-thickness, burn.

To learn more about burns, go to AnimationDirect on your CD-ROM.

QUICK CHECK

1. What are the five most important functions of the skin?
2. Can you list some of the sensory stimuli that can be detected by the skin?
3. How can the amount of skin surface area covered by a burn be estimated?

Science Application

Secrets of the Skin
Dr. Joseph E. Murray (b. 1919)

The skin is our most visible organ, so it is no wonder that observing the structure and function of skin has generated sparks that have lit the fires of scientific discovery through the ages. The ancient Romans outlined the process of inflammation in detail after observing it first in the skin. In the twentieth century, Joseph Murray (see figure) noticed that skin he grafted onto burned soldiers he treated during World War II would eventually be rejected by the body. After the war, Murray tried to understand the body's immune reactions to transplanted tissues.

His work led to the first successful kidney transplants. His breakthroughs in transplanting kidneys not only earned him a Nobel Prize in 1990, it also paved the way for all the different types of tissue and organ transplantation that we see today.

Many scientists continue to study the secrets of the skin, and many physicians and other health care professionals also pioneer new methods of skin care and treatment in the fields of dermatology, allergy, burn medicine, and reconstructive and cosmetic surgery. Additional practical applications of some of this skin science are practiced by people working with cosmetics and other skin treatments, nail treatments, and hair treatments. For example, industrial researchers, product developers, cosmeticians, spa specialists, and hair stylists all require some knowledge of current skin science to do their jobs effectively.

OUTLINE SUMMARY

CLASSIFICATION OF BODY MEMBRANES

A. Classification of body membranes (see Figure 5-1)
   1. Epithelial membranes — composed of epithelial tissue and an underlying layer of connective tissue
   2. Connective tissue membranes — composed largely of various types of connective tissue
B. Epithelial membranes
   1. Cutaneous membrane — the skin
   2. Serous membranes — simple squamous epithelium on a connective tissue basement membrane
      a. Types
         (1) Parietal — line walls of body cavities
         (2) Visceral — cover organs found in body cavities
      b. Examples
         (1) Pleura — parietal and visceral layers line walls of thoracic cavity and cover the lungs
         (2) Peritoneum — parietal and visceral layers line walls of abdominal cavity and cover the organs in that cavity
      c. Diseases
         (1) Pleurisy — inflammation of the serous membranes that line the chest cavity and cover the lungs

         (2) Peritonitis — inflammation of the serous membranes in the abdominal cavity that line the walls and cover the abdominal organs
   3. Mucous membranes
      a. Line body surfaces that open directly to the exterior
      b. Produce mucus, a thick secretion that keeps the membranes soft and moist
C. Connective tissue membranes
   1. Do not contain epithelial components
   2. Produce a lubricant called *synovial fluid*
   3. Examples are the synovial membranes lining the joint capsules that surround and attach the ends of articulating bones in movable joints and in the lining of bursal sacs

THE SKIN

A. Structure (see Figure 5-2) — two primary layers called *epidermis* and *dermis*
   1. Epidermis
      a. Outermost and thinnest primary layer of skin
      b. Composed of several layers of stratified squamous epithelium
      c. Stratum germinativum — innermost layer of cells that continually reproduce, and new cells move toward the surface (see Figure 5-3)

   d. As cells approach the surface, they are filled with a tough, waterproof protein called *keratin* and eventually flake off
   e. Stratum corneum — outermost layer of keratin-filled cells
2. Skin pigment — deepest epidermal layer is responsible for production of pigment, which gives color to the skin
   a. The brown pigment melanin is produced by specialized cells in this layer
   b. Blisters — caused by breakdown of union between cells or primary layers of skin
3. Dermal-epidermal junction — specialized area between two primary skin layers
4. Dermis
   a. Deeper and thicker of the two primary skin layers and composed largely of connective tissue
   b. Upper papillary layer of dermis characterized by parallel rows of tiny bumps called *dermal papillae*
   c. Ridges and grooves in dermis form pattern unique to each individual
      (1) Basis of fingerprinting
      (2) Improves grip for tool use and walking
   d. Deeper reticular layer of dermis filled with network of tough, interlacing, collagenous, and stretchable elastic fibers
      (1) Number of elastic fibers decreases with age and contributes to wrinkle formation (see Figure 5-4)
      (2) Dermis also contains nerve endings, muscle fibers, hair follicles, sweat and sebaceous glands, and many blood vessels
B. Accessory structures of the skin
   1. Hair (see Figure 5-5)
      a. Soft hair of fetus and newborn is called *lanugo*
      b. Hair growth requires epidermal tube-like structure called *hair follicle*
      c. Hair growth begins from hair papilla
      d. Hair root lies hidden in follicle and visible part of hair called *shaft*
      e. Arrector pili — specialized smooth muscle that produces "goose bumps" and causes hair to stand up straight

2. Receptors (see Figure 5-2)
   a. Specialized nerve endings — make it possible for skin to act as a sense organ
   b. Tactile (Meissner) corpuscle — capable of detecting light touch
   c. Lamellar (Pacini) corpuscle — capable of detecting pressure
3. Nails (see Figure 5-6)
   a. Produced by epidermal cells over terminal ends of fingers and toes
   b. Visible part is called *nail body*
   c. Root lies in a groove and is hidden by cuticle
   d. Crescent-shaped area nearest root is called *lunula*
   e. Nail bed may change color with change in blood flow
4. Skin glands
   a. Sweat, or sudoriferous, glands
      (1) Eccrine sweat glands
         • Most numerous, important, and widespread of the sweat glands
         • Produce perspiration or sweat, which flows out through pores on skin surface
         • Function throughout life and assist in body heat regulation
      (2) Apocrine glands
         • Found primarily in axilla and around genitalia
         • Secrete a thicker secretion quite different from eccrine perspiration
         • Breakdown of secretion by skin bacteria produces odor
   b. Sebaceous glands
      (1) Secrete oil or sebum for hair and skin
      (2) Level of secretion increases during adolescence
      (3) Amount of secretion is regulated by sex hormones
      (4) Sebum in sebaceous gland ducts may darken to form a blackhead
C. Skin cancer (see Figure 5-7)
   1. Types
      a. Squamous cell carcinoma
      b. Basal cell carcinoma
      c. Malignant melanoma
      d. Kaposi sarcoma

2. Causes
   a. Genetic predisposition
   b. Sun's UV radiation damages skin cell DNA, causing mistakes during mitosis
3. Squamous cell carcinoma
   a. Common type of skin cancer
   b. Slow growing
   c. Lesions begin as painless, hard, raised nodules
   d. Will metastasize
4. Basal cell carcinoma (most common type of skin cancer)
   a. Originates in cells at base of epidermis — often on upper face
   b. Lesions begin as small raised areas that erode in center, bleed, and crust over
   c. Less likely to metastasize than other skin cancer types
5. Malignant melanoma
   a. Most serious form of skin cancer
   b. May develop from benign, pigmented moles or excess UV radiation
   c. Incidence in the United States is increasing
   d. ABCD rule of self-examination (see Table 5-1)

B. Functions of the skin
1. Protection — first line of defense against
   a. Infection by microbes
   b. UV rays from sun
   c. Harmful chemicals
   d. Cuts and tears
2. Temperature regulation
   a. Skin can release almost 3,000 calories of body heat per day
      (1) Mechanisms of temperature regulation
         (a) Regulation of sweat secretion
         (b) Regulation of flow of blood close to the body surface
3. Sense organ activity
   a. Skin functions as an enormous sense organ
   b. Receptors serve as receivers for the body, keeping it informed of changes in its environment

C. Burns
1. Treatment and recovery or survival depend on total area involved and severity or depth of the burn
2. Body surface area is estimated using the "rule of nines" (see Figure 5-8) in adults
   a. Body is divided into 11 areas of 9% each
   b. Additional 1% of body surface area is around the genitals
3. Classification of burns (see Figure 5-9)
   a. First-degree (partial-thickness) burns — only the surface layers of epidermis involved
   b. Second-degree (partial-thickness) burns — involve the deep epidermal layers and always cause injury to the upper layers of the dermis
   c. Third-degree (full-thickness) burns — characterized by complete destruction of the epidermis and dermis
      (1) May involve underlying muscle and bone
      (2) Lesion is insensitive to pain because of destruction of nerve endings immediately after injury — intense pain is soon experienced
      (3) Risk of infection is increased

NEW WORDS

apocrine sweat gland	bulboid corpuscles	cutaneous membrane	dermis
arrector pili	(Krause end bulbs)	cuticle	eccrine sweat gland
basal cell carcinoma	burns	cyanosis	epidermis
basement membrane	bursae	dehydration	epithelial membrane
blackhead	connective tissue	dermal-epidermal	first-degree burn
blister	membranes	junction	follicle

NEW WORDS—cont'd

free nerve endings
hair papilla
hypodermis (subcutaneous tissue)
integument
integumentary system
Kaposi sarcoma
keratin
lamellar (Pacini) corpuscle
lanugo
lunula
malignant melanoma

melanin
melanocyte
membrane
mucocutaneous junction
mucous membrane
mucus
papilla
parietal portion
partial-thickness burn
peritoneum
peritonitis
perspiration

pigment
pleura
pleurisy
pores
pressure ulcer
rule of nines
sebaceous gland
sebum
second-degree burn
serous membrane
squamous cell carcinoma
stratum corneum

stratum germinativum
subcutaneous tissue (superficial fascia)
sudoriferous gland
sweat
synovial fluid
synovial membrane
tactile (Meissner) corpuscle
third-degree, or full-thickness, burn
visceral portion

REVIEW QUESTIONS

1. Define *membrane*.
2. Explain the structure of a serous membrane. Include the difference between the parietal and visceral membranes.
3. Explain the structure of a mucous membrane. Include an explanation of the mucocutaneous junction.
4. Explain the structure of a synovial membrane. What is the function of synovial fluid?
5. Name and briefly describe the layers of the epidermis.
6. Explain the structure of the dermis.
7. Differentiate between the *hair papilla*, the *hair root*, and the *hair shaft*.
8. Explain what occurs when the arrector pili contract.
9. Name the four receptors of the skin. To what type of stimuli does each respond?
10. Give the location of the eccrine glands and their function, and describe the type of fluid they produce.
11. Give the location of the apocrine glands and their function, and describe the type of fluid they produce.
12. Give the location of the sebaceous glands and their function, and describe the type of fluid they produce.
13. Explain the difference between second-degree and third-degree burns. Which is considered a "full-thickness" burn?

CRITICAL THINKING

14. Explain the protective function of melanin.
15. Explain fully the role of the skin in temperature regulation.
16. If a person burned all of his back, the back of his right arm, and the back of his right thigh, approximately what percent of his body surface area would be involved? How did you determine this?

CHAPTER TEST

1. The _____, _____, and _____ are the three types of epithelial membranes.
2. Epithelial membranes are usually composed of two distinct layers: the epithelial layer and a supportive connective tissue layer called the _____.
3. The membrane lining the interior of the chest wall is called the _____.
4. The membrane covering the organs of the abdomen is called the _____.
5. The connective tissue membrane that lines the space between the bone and joints is called the _____.
6. The two main layers of the epidermis of the skin are the _____ and the _____.
7. As new skin cells approach the surface of the skin, their cytoplasm is replaced by a unique waterproof protein called _____.

8. The upper region of the dermis forms projections called _____ that form unique fingerprints.
9. The _____ are sweat glands that can be found all over the body and produce a transparent watery liquid.
10. The _____ are sweat glands that can be found in the armpits and produce a thicker secretion.
11. The sebaceous glands secrete an oil called _____.
12. _____, _____, and _____ are the three functions of the skin.
13. The receptors in the skin that respond to pain are the:
    a. tactile (Meissner) corpuscle
    b. lamellar (Pacini) corpuscle
    c. free nerve endings
    d. bulboid (Krause end bulbs)

CHAPTER TEST—cont'd

14. The receptors in the skin that respond to low-frequency vibration are the:
    a. tactile (Meissner) corpuscles
    b. lamellar (Pacini) corpuscles
    c. free nerve endings
    d. bulboid (Krause end bulbs)

15. The receptors in the skin that respond to light touch are the:
    a. tactile (Meissner) corpuscles
    b. lamellar (Pacini) corpuscles
    c. free nerve endings
    d. bulboid (Krause end bulbs)

16. The receptors in the skin that respond to deep pressure are the:
    a. tactile (Meissner) corpuscles
    b. lamellar (Pacini) corpuscles
    c. free nerve endings
    d. bulboid (Krause end bulbs)

Match each description of a part of the hair in Column B with the name of the structure in Column A.

COLUMN A

17. _____ Hair follicle
18. _____ Hair papilla
19. _____ Hair root
20. _____ Hair shaft

COLUMN B

a. The part of the hair hidden in the follicle
b. The growth of the epidermal cells into the dermis forming a small tube
c. The part of the hair that is visible and extends from the follicle
d. A cuplike cluster of cells where hair growth begins

OBJECTIVES

AFTER YOU HAVE COMPLETED THIS CHAPTER, YOU SHOULD BE ABLE TO:

1. List and discuss the generalized functions of the skeletal system.
2. Identify the major anatomical structures found in a typical long bone.
3. Discuss the microscopic structure of bone and cartilage, including the identification of specific cell types and structural features.
4. Explain how bones are formed, how they grow, and how they are remodeled.
5. Identify the two major subdivisions of the skeleton and list the bones found in each area.
6. List and compare the major types of joints in the body and give an example of each.

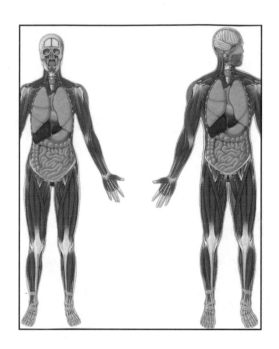

Clear View of the Human Body

Developed by: **Kevin Patton** and **Paul Krieger**

Illustrated by: **Dragonfly Media Group**

INTRODUCTION

A complete understanding of human anatomy and physiology requires an appreciation for how structures within the body relate to one another. Such appreciation for anatomical structure has become especially important in the 21st century with the explosion in the use of diverse methods of medical imaging that rely on the ability to interpret sectional views of the human body.

The best way to develop your understanding of overall anatomical structure is to carefully dissect a large number of male and female human cadavers—then have those dissected specimens handy while reading and learning about each system of the body. Obviously, such multiple dissections and constant access to specimens are impractical for nearly everyone. However, the experience of a simple dissection can be approximated by layering several partially transparent, two-dimensional anatomical diagrams in a way that allows a student to "virtually" dissect the human body simply by paging through the layers.

This Clear View of the Human Body provides a handy tool for dissecting simulated male and female bodies. It also provides views of several different parts of the human body in a variety of cross sections. The many different anterior and posterior views also give you a perspective on body structure that is not available with ordinary anatomical diagrams. This Clear View is an always-available tool to help you learn the three-dimensional structure of the body in a way that allows you to see how they relate to each other in a complete body. It will always be right here in your textbook,

so place a bookmark here and refer to the Clear View frequently as you study each of the systems of the human body.

HINTS FOR USING THE CLEAR VIEW OF THE BODY

1. Starting at the first page of the Clear View, slowly lift the page as you look at the anterior view of the male and female bodies. You will see deeper structures appear, as if you had dissected the body. As you lift each successive layer of images, you will be looking at deeper and deeper body structures. A key to the labels is found in the gray sidebar.

2. Starting with the second section of the Clear View, notice that you are looking at the posterior aspect of the male and female body. Lift each layer from the left edge to reveal body structures in successive layers from the back to the front. This very unique view will help you understand structural relationships even better.

3. On each page of the Clear View, look at the horizontal section represented in the sidebar. The section you are looking at on any one page is from the location shown in the larger diagram as a red line. In other words, if you cut the body at the red line and tilted the upper part of the body toward you, you would see what is shown in the section diagram. Notice that each section has its own labeling system that is separate from the labels used in the larger images.

KEY

1. Epicranius m.
2. Temporalis m.
3. Orbicularis oculi m.
4. Masseter m.
5. Orbicularis oris m.
6. Pectoralis major m.
7. Serratus anterior m.
8. Basilic vein
9. Brachial fascia
10. Cephalic vein
11. Rectus sheath
12. Linea alba
13. Rectus abdominis m.
14. Umbilicus
15. Abdominal oblique m., external
16. Abdominal oblique m., internal
17. Transverse abdominis m.
18. Inguinal ring, external
19. Fossa ovalis
20. Fascia of the thigh
21. Great saphenous vein
22. Parietal bone
23. Frontal bone
24. Temporal bone
25. Zygomatic bone
26. Maxilla
27. Mandible
28. Sternocleidomastoid m.
29. Sternohyoid muscle
30. Omohyoid muscle
31. Deltoid m.
32. Pectoralis minor m.
33. Sternum
34. Rib (costal) cartilage
35. Rib
36. Greater omentum
37. Frontal lobe
38. Parietal lobe
39. Temporal lobe
40. Cerebellum
41. Nasal septum
42. Brachiocephalic vein
43. Superior vena cava
44. Thymus gland
45. Right lung
46. Left lung
47. Pericardium
48. Liver
49. Gall bladder
50. Stomach
51. Transverse colon
52. Small intestines
53. Biceps brachii m.
54. Brachioradialis m.
55. Adductor longus m.
56. Sartorius m.
57. Quadriceps femoris m.
58. Patellar ligament
59. Tibialis anterior m.
60. Sup. extensor retinaculum
61. Inf. extensor retinaculum
62. Cerebrum of brain
63. Cerebellum
64. Brain stem
65. Maxillary sinus
66. Nasal cavity
67. Tongue
68. Thyroid gland
69. Heart
70. Hepatic veins
71. Esophagus
72. Spleen
73. Celiac artery
74. Portal vein
75. Duodenum
76. Pancreas
77. Mesenteric artery
78. Ascending colon
79. Transverse colon
80. Descending colon
81. Sigmoid colon
82. Mesentery
83. Appendix
84. Inguinal ligament
85. Pubic symphysis
86. Extensor carpi radialis m.
87. Pronator teres m.
88. Flexor carpi radialis m.
89. Flexor digitorum profundus m.
90. Quadriceps femoris m.
91. Extensor digitorum longus m.
92. Thyroid cartilage
93. Trachea
94. Aortic arch
95. Right lung
96. Left lung
97. Pulmonary artery
98. Right atrium
99. Right ventricle
100. Left atrium
101. Left ventricle
102. Coracobrachialis m.
103. Inferior vena cava
104. Descending aorta
105. Right kidney
106. Left kidney
107. Right ureter
108. Rectum
109. Urinary bladder
110. Prostate gland
111. Iliac artery and vein
112. Uterus
113. Parietal bone
114. Frontal sinus
115. Sphenoidal sinus
116. Occipital bone
117. Palatine process
118. Cervical vertebrae
119. Corpus callosum
120. Thalamus
121. Trapezius m.
122. Acromion process
123. Coracoid process
124. Humerus
125. Subscapularis m.
126. Deltoid m. (cut)
127. Triceps m.
128. Brachialis m.
129. Brachioradialis m.
130. Radius
131. Ulna
132. Diaphragm
133. Thoracic duct
134. Quadratus lumborum m.
135. Psoas m.
136. Lumbar vertebrae
137. Iliacus m.
138. Gluteus medius m.
139. Iliofemoral ligament
140. Sacral nerves
141. Sacrum
142. Coccyx
143. Femur
144. Vastus lateralis m.
145. Femoral artery and vein
146. Adductor magnus m.
147. Patella
148. Fibula
149. Tibia
150. Fibularis longus m.
151. Spinal cord
152. Nerve root
153. Platysma m.
154. Splenius capitis m.
155. Levator scapulae m.
156. Rhomboideus m.
157. Infraspinatis m.
158. Teres major m.
159. Lumbodorsal fascia
160. Erector spinae m.
161. Serratus post. inf. m.
162. Latissimus dorsi m.
163. Gluteus medius m.
164. Gluteus maximus m.
165. Iliotibial tract
166. Flexor carpi ulnaris m.
167. Extensor carpi ulnaris m.
168. Extensor digitorum m.
169. Carpal ligament, dorsal
170. Interosseus m.
171. Gluteus minimus m.
172. Piriformis m.
173. Gemellus sup. m.
174. Obturator internus m.
175. Gemellus inf. m.
176. Quadratus femoris m.
177. Biceps femoris m.
178. Gastrocnemius m.
179. Calcaneal (Achilles) tendon
180. Calcaneus bone
181. Subcutaneous fat
182. Corpus spongiosum
183. Corpora cavernosa
184. Umbilical ligaments
185. Epigastric artery and vein
186. Right testis
187. Transverse thoracic m.
188. Parietal pleura
189. Common bile duct
190. Lesser omentum
191. Flexor digitorum profundus
192. Epiglottis

Head - Cross Section

A. Vitreous body of eye
B. Ethmoidal cells
C. Temporalis m.
D. Optic nerve
E. Sphenoidal sinus
F. Brain

Lungs/Heart - Cross Section

Abdomen - Cross Section

A. Esophagus
B. Descending aorta
C. Azygos vein
D. Right lung
E. Left lung
F. Right atrium
G. Right ventricle
H. Left atrium
I. Left ventricle
J. Liver
K. Stomach
L. Pancreas
M. Intervertebral disc
N. Left kidney
O. Spleen

Anterior View

1. Epicranius m.
2. Temporalis m.
3. Orbicularis oculi m.
4. Masseter m.
5. Orbicularis oris m.
6. Pectoralis major m.
7. Serratus anterior m.
8. Basilic vein
9. Brachial fascia
10. Cephalic vein
11. Rectus sheath
12. Linea alba
13. Rectus abdominis m.
14. Umbilicus
15. Abdominal oblique m., external
16. Abdominal oblique m., internal
17. Transverse abdominis m.
18. Inguinal ring, external
19. Fossa ovalis
20. Fascia of the thigh
21. Great saphenous vein

Lungs/Heart - Cross Section

Abdomen - Cross Section

A. Esophagus
B. Descending aorta
C. Azygos vein
D. Right lung
E. Left lung
F. Right atrium
G. Right ventricle
H. Left atrium
I. Left ventricle
J. Liver
K. Stomach
L. Pancreas
M. Intervertebral disc
N. Left kidney
O. Spleen

Anterior View

1. Epicranius m.
2. Temporalis m.
3. Orbicularis oculi m.
4. Masseter m.
5. Orbicularis oris m.
6. Pectoralis major m.
7. Serratus anterior m.
8. Basilic vein
9. Brachial fascia
10. Cephalic vein
11. Rectus sheath
12. Linea alba
13. Rectus abdominis m.
14. Umbilicus
15. Abdominal oblique m., external
16. Abdominal oblique m., internal
17. Transverse abdominis m.
18. Inguinal ring, external
19. Fossa ovalis
20. Fascia of the thigh
21. Great saphenous vein

Upper Arm - Cross Section

A. Biceps brachii m.
B. Brachialis m.
C. Humerus
D. Triceps brachii m., medial
E. Triceps brachii m., lateral

Posterior View

1. Epicranius m.
2. Temporalis m.
4. Masseter m.
15. Abdominal oblique m., external
31. Deltoid m.
121. Trapezius m.
127. Triceps m.
153. Platysma m.
154. Splenius capitis m.
155. Levator scapulae m.
156. Rhomboideus m.
157. Infraspinatus m.
158. Teres major m.
159. Lumbodorsal fascia
160. Erector spinae m.
161. Serratus post. inf. m.
162. Latissimus dorsi m.
162a. Latissimus dorsi m. (cut)
163. Gluteus medius m.
164. Gluteus maximus m.
165. Iliotibial tract
166. Flexor carpi ulnaris m.
167. Extensor carpi ulnaris m.
168. Extensor digitorum m.
169. Carpal ligament, dorsal
170. Interosseus m.
171. Gluteus minimus m.
172. Piriformis m.
173. Gemellus sup. m.
174. Obturator internus m.
175. Gemellus inf. m.
176. Quadratus femoris m.
177. Biceps femoris m.
178. Gastrocnemius m.
179. Calcaneal (Achilles) tendon
180. Calcaneus bone

Posterior View

1. Epicranius m.
2. Temporalis m.
3. Orbicularis oculi m.
4. Masseter m.
5. Orbicularis oris m.
6. Pectoralis major m.
7. Serratus anterior m.
8. Basilic vein
11. Rectus sheath
12. Linea alba
13. Rectus abdominis m.
14. Umbilicus
15. Abdominal oblique m., external
17. Transverse abdominis m.
19. Fossa ovalis
21. Great saphenous vein
153. Platysma m.
181. Subcutaneous fat
182. Corpus spongiosum
183. Corpora cavernosa
184. Umbilical ligaments
185. Epigastric artery and vein
186. Right testis

The Skeletal System

The primary organs of the skeletal system—bones—lie buried beneath the muscles and other soft tissues, providing a rigid framework and support structure for the whole body. In this respect the skeletal system functions like steel girders in a building. However, unlike steel girders, bones can be moved. Bones are also living organs. They can remodel themselves and help the body respond to a changing environment. This ability of bones to change allows our bodies to grow and adapt to new situations.

Our study of the skeletal system begins with an overview of its function. We then classify bones by their structure and describe the characteristics of a typical bone. After discussing the microscopic structure of skeletal tissues, we briefly outline bone growth and formation. Having this information, the study of specific bones and the way they are assembled in the skeleton will be more meaningful. The chapter ends with a discussion of skeletal functions and an overview of joints, or **articulations** (ar-tik-yoo-LAY-shunz).

An understanding of how bones articulate with one another in joints and how they relate to other body structures provides a basis for understanding the functions of many other organ systems. Coordinated movement, for example, is possible only because of the way bones are joined to one another and because of the way muscles are attached to those bones. In addition, knowing where specific bones are in the body will assist you in locating other body structures that are discussed later.

STUDY TIPS

To make the study of the skeletal system more efficient, we suggest these tips:

1. Before starting your study of Chapter 6, go back to Chapter 4 and review the synopsis of the skeletal system.
2. A number of terms in this chapter have prefixes or suffixes that help explain their meanings. The prefixes *epi-* and *endo-* were discussed earlier. *Peri-* means "around," *osteo-* or *os-* refers to bone, and *chondro-* refers to cartilage. The suffix *-cyte* means "cell," *-blast* means "young cell," and *-clast* means "to destroy." Knowing the meanings of these prefixes and suffixes will make some of the terms self-explanatory.
3. When studying the microscopic structures of bone, remember that bone tissue, which has living cells throughout, heals fairly easily, whereas cartilage, a more static tissue, does not. Bone tissue cells must have food and oxygen and a way to get rid of waste products. The structure of the osteon allows this to occur.
4. Most of the names of the bones should be somewhat familiar to you. Studying the figures of the full skeletons and the figure of the skull may be the best way to learn them.
5. The joints are named based on the amount of movement they allow (*arthro-* means "joint"). The joint capsule is an example of a synovial membrane, which was discussed in Chapter 5.
6. In your study groups you can use flash cards to study the terms related to bone structure and joints.
7. Discuss bone formation and the structure of the osteon.
8. A photocopy of each of the skeleton figures, with the labels blacked out, will help you learn the names of the bones. There is no real shortcut to learning the names and locations of the bones, but quizzing each other will help.
9. Go over the questions at the end of the chapter and discuss possible test questions.

FUNCTIONS OF THE SKELETAL SYSTEM

Support

Bones form the body's supporting framework. All the softer tissues of the body literally hang from the skeletal framework.

Protection

Hard, bony "boxes" protect delicate structures enclosed within them. For example, the skull protects the brain. The breastbone and ribs protect vital organs (heart and lungs). Many bones also protect a vital tissue: red bone marrow, the blood cell–forming tissue.

Movement

Muscles are anchored firmly to bones. As muscles contract and shorten, they pull on bones and thereby move them. Movable joints in the skeleton make such movement possible.

Storage

Bones play an important part in maintaining homeostasis of blood calcium, a vital substance required for normal nerve and muscle function. They serve as a safety deposit box for calcium. When the amount of calcium in blood increases to an above-normal level, calcium moves out of the blood and into the bones for storage. Conversely, when blood calcium decreases to a below-normal level, calcium moves in the opposite direction. It comes out of storage in bones and enters the blood.

The balance of calcium deposits and withdrawals to and from the skeleton is regulated by a balance of hormones. For example, **calcitonin** (kal-si-TOH-nin) **(CT)** from the *thyroid gland* increases mineralization of bone and thus reduces blood calcium. **Parathyroid hormone (PTH)** from the *parathyroid glands* counterbalances the effects of calcitonin by decreasing calcium in the bone and thus increasing blood calcium.

Hematopoiesis

The term **hematopoiesis** (hee-MA-toh-poy-EE-sis) is used to describe the process of blood cell forma-

tion. It is a combination of two Greek word parts: *hemato* (hee-MA-toh) meaning "blood" and *poiesis* (poy-EE-sis) meaning "to make." Blood cell formation is a vital process carried on in **red bone marrow.** Red bone marrow is soft connective tissue inside the hard walls of some bones.

TYPES OF BONES

There are four major types of bones, classified according to overall structure. Their names suggest their shapes: *long* (for example, humerus or arm bone), *short* (for example, carpals or wrist bones), *flat* (for example, frontal or skull bone), and *irregular* (for example, vertebrae or spinal bones). Some scientists recognize an additional category called *sesamoid* ("like a sesame seed") or *round,* which may develop within a tendon. An example of sesamoid bone is the kneecap (patella), which develops within the patellar tendon.

Many important bones in the skeleton are classified as long bones, and all bones of the body have several common characteristics. By studying a typical long bone, you can become familiar with the structural features of the entire group of human bones.

Structure of Long Bones

Figure 6-1 will help you learn the names of the main parts of a long bone. Identify each of the following:

1. **Diaphysis** (dye-AF-i-sis), or shaft—a hollow tube made of hard, compact bone, hence a rigid and strong structure light enough in weight to permit easy movement
2. **Medullary cavity**—the hollow area inside the diaphysis of a bone; contains soft **yellow bone marrow,** an inactive, fatty form of marrow found in the adult skeleton
3. **Epiphyses** (eh-PIF-i-seez), or the ends of the bone—red bone marrow fills in small spaces in the spongy bone composing the epiphyses
4. **Articular cartilage**—a thin layer of cartilage covering each epiphysis; functions like a small rubber cushion would if it were placed over the ends of bones where they form a joint
5. **Periosteum**—a strong fibrous membrane covering a long bone everywhere except at

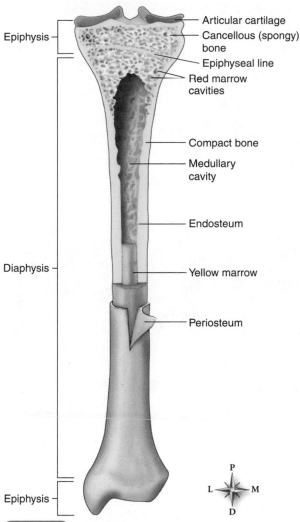

FIGURE 6-1 Long bone. Frontal section of the right humerus (long bone of the arm) showing the typical structures of a long bone.

FIGURE 6-2 Flat bone. The diploe is a spongy bone layer sandwiched between two compact bone layers.

✓ QUICK CHECK

1. Name some of the organs of the skeletal system.
2. What are the five major functions of the skeletal system?
3. What are the four categories of bones in the skeleton?
4. Describe the major features of a long bone. How does the typical flat bone differ?

---

joint surfaces, where it is covered by articular cartilage

6. **Endosteum**—a thin membrane that lines the medullary cavity

Structure of Flat Bones

Flat bones, such as the sternum (breastbone), the ribs, and many of the skull bones have a simpler structure than most long bones. As Figure 6-2 shows, flat bones have a layer of spongy bone sandwiched between outer layers of compact bone. The spongy bone layer is called the **diploe** (DIP-lo-EE).

MICROSCOPIC STRUCTURE OF BONE AND CARTILAGE

The skeletal system contains two major types of connective tissue: *bone* and *cartilage*. Bone has different appearances and textures, depending on its location. In Figure 6-3, *A*, the outer layer of bone is hard and dense. Bone of this type is called **compact bone.** Compact bone appears solid to the naked eye. The porous bone in the end of the long bone is called **spongy bone** or **cancellous bone.** As the name implies, spongy bone contains many spaces that may be filled with marrow. The needlelike threads of spongy bone that surround this network of spaces are called **trabeculae** (trah-BEK-yoo-lee). Figure 6-3, *B*, shows the microscopic appearance of spongy and compact bone.

As you can see in Figures 6-3 and 6-4, compact bone does not contain a network of open spaces. Instead, the matrix is organized into numerous structural units called **osteons** or *haversian systems*. Each circular and tubelike osteon is composed of calcified matrix arranged in multiple layers that resemble the rings of an onion. Each ring is called a **concentric lamella** (lah-MEL-ah). The circular rings, or lamellae, surround the *central canal*, which contains a blood vessel.

FIGURE 6-3 Microscopic structure of bone. **A,** Longitudinal section of a long bone shows the location of the microscopic section illustrated in **B.** Note that the compact bone forming the hard shell of the bone is constructed of cylindrical units called *osteons.* Spongy bone is constructed of bony projections called *trabeculae.*

Bones are not lifeless structures. Within their hard, seemingly lifeless matrix are many living bone cells called **osteocytes** (OS-tee-oh-sytes). Osteocytes are mature bone cells that lie between the hard layers of the lamellae in little spaces called **lacunae** (lah-KOO-nee). In Figures 6-3, *B,* and 6-4, note that tiny passageways, or canals, called **canaliculi** (kan-ah-LIK-yoo-lye) connect the lacunae with one another and with the central canal in each osteon. Nutrients pass from the blood vessel in the central canal through the canaliculi to the osteocytes. Note also in Figure 6-3, *B,* that numerous blood vessels from the outer **periosteum**

(pair-ee-OS-tee-um) enter the bone and eventually pass through the central canals.

Cartilage both resembles and differs from bone. As with bone, it consists more of intercellular substance than of cells. Innumerable collagenous fibers reinforce the matrix of both tissues. However, in cartilage the fibers are embedded in a firm gel instead of in a calcified cement substance like they are in bone. As a result, cartilage has the flexibility of a firm plastic rather than the rigidity of bone. Note in Figure 6-5 that cartilage cells, called **chondrocytes** (KON-droh-sytes), as with the osteocytes of bone, are located in lacunae. In cartilage,

FIGURE 6-4 **Compact bone.** Photomicrograph shows osteon system of organization. (The letter C shows the central canal.)

Matrix   Chondrocyte   Perichondrium
               in lacuna

FIGURE 6-5 **Cartilage tissue.** Photomicrograph shows chondrocytes scattered around the tissue matrix in spaces called lacunae.

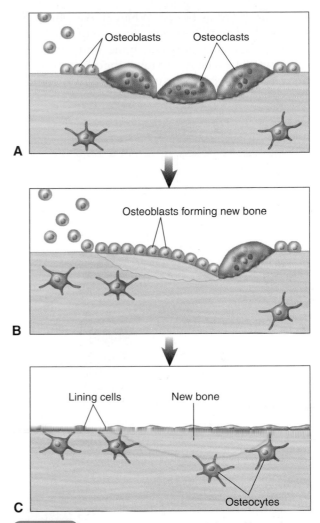

FIGURE 6-6 **Bone cells.** During remodeling of bone, bone-dissolving osteoclasts remove the hard calcium salts in bone matrix (**A**). Osteoblasts then form new bone matrix in the area (**B**) until they eventually become surrounded and "trapped" by hard bone and are then called osteocytes (**C**).

lacunae are suspended in the cartilage matrix much like air bubbles in a block of firm gelatin. Because there are no blood vessels in cartilage, nutrients must diffuse through the matrix to reach the cells. Because of this lack of blood vessels, cartilage rebuilds itself very slowly after an injury.

BONE FORMATION AND GROWTH

When the skeleton begins to form in a baby before its birth, it consists not of bones but of cartilage and fibrous structures shaped like bones.

Gradually these cartilage "models" become transformed into real bones when the cartilage is replaced with calcified bone matrix. This process of constantly "remodeling" a growing bone as it changes from a small cartilage model to the characteristic shape and proportion of the adult bone requires continuous activity by bone-forming cells called **osteoblasts** (OS-tee-oh-blasts) and bone-reabsorbing cells called **osteoclasts** (OS-tee-oh-klasts), both seen in Figure 6-6. The laying down of calcium salts by osteoblasts in the gel-like matrix of the forming bones is an ongoing process. This calcification process is what makes bones as "hard as bone." When an osteoblast becomes "trapped" between lamellae of hard bone matrix, they stop forming bone and are called osteocytes. Osteocytes resume their bone-making activity when osteoclasts (or an injury) remove the surrounding bone.

The combined action of the osteoblasts and osteoclasts sculpts bones into their adult shapes (Figure 6-7). The process of "sculpting" by the bone-forming and bone-reabsorbing cells allows bones to respond to stress or injury by changing size, shape, and density. The stresses placed on

FIGURE 6-7 Endochondral ossification. **A,** Bone formation begins with a cartilage model. **B** and **C,** Invasion of the diaphysis (shaft) by blood vessels and the combined action of osteoblast and osteoclast cells result in cavity formation, calcification, and the appearance of bone tissue. **D** and **E,** Centers of ossification also appear in the epiphyses (ends) of the bone. **F,** Note the epiphyseal plate, which indicates that this bone is not yet mature and that additional growth is possible. **G,** In a mature bone, only a faint epiphyseal line marks where the cartilage once was and indicates the centers of ossification have fused together.

certain bones during exercise increase the rate of bone deposition. For this reason, athletes or dancers may have denser, stronger bones than less active people.

Most bones of the body are formed from cartilage models, as illustrated in Figures 6-7 and 6-8. This process is called **endochondral** (en-doh-KON-dral) **ossification** (os-i-fi-KAY-shun), meaning "formed in cartilage." A few flat bones, such as the skull bones illustrated in Figure 6-8, are formed by another process in connective tissue membranes.

As you can see in Figure 6-7, a long bone grows and ultimately becomes "ossified" from small centers located in both ends of the bone, called **epiphyses,** and from a larger center located in the shaft, or the **diaphysis,** of the bone. As long as any cartilage, called an **epiphyseal plate,** remains between the epiphyses and the diaphysis, growth continues. Growth ceases when all epiphyseal cartilage is transformed into bone. All that remains is an *epiphyseal line* that marks the location where the two centers of ossification have fused

Health and Well-Being

Osteoporosis

Osteoporosis (os-tee-oh-poh-ROH-sis) is one of the most common and serious of all bone diseases. It is characterized by excessive loss of calcified matrix and collagenous fibers from bone. Osteoporosis occurs most often in elderly white females. Although white and black males are also susceptible, black women are seldom affected by it.

Because sex hormones play important roles in stimulating osteoblast activity after puberty, decreasing levels of these hormones in the blood of elderly persons reduce new bone growth and the maintenance of existing bone mass. Therefore some reabsorption of bone and subsequent loss of bone mass are accepted consequences of advancing years. However, bone loss in osteoporosis goes far beyond the modest decrease normally seen in old age. The result is a dangerous pathological condition resulting in bone degeneration, increased susceptibility to "spontaneous fractures," and pathological curvature of the spine. Treatment may include drug therapy and dietary supplements of calcium and vitamin D to replace deficiencies or to offset intestinal malabsorption. Some of the effects of osteoporosis can be prevented by starting exercise while still a young adult, which strengthens bone, and maintaining a diet sufficient in calcium throughout life.

together. Physicians sometimes use this knowledge to determine whether a child is going to grow any more. They have an x-ray study performed on the child's wrist. If it shows a layer of epiphyseal cartilage, they know that additional growth will occur. However, if it shows no epiphyseal cartilage, they know that growth has stopped and that the individual has attained adult height.

To learn more about bone formation and growth, go to AnimationDirect on your CD-ROM.

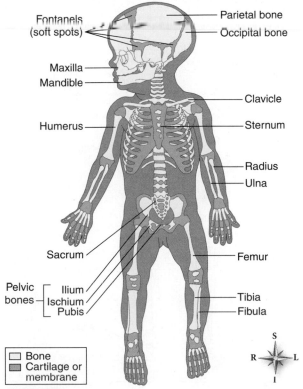

Fontanels (soft spots)
Parietal bone
Occipital bone
Maxilla
Mandible
Clavicle
Humerus
Sternum
Radius
Ulna
Sacrum
Femur
Pelvic bones — Ilium, Ischium, Pubis
Tibia
Fibula

□ Bone
■ Cartilage or membrane

FIGURE 6-8 Bone development in a newborn. An infant's skeleton has many bones that are not yet completely ossified.

✓ QUICK CHECK

1. What is the basic structural unit of compact bone tissue called?
2. What are osteocytes? Where would you find them in bone tissue?
3. How does cartilage differ from bone?
4. What is ossification? What is the role of the osteoblast?

DIVISIONS OF SKELETON

The human skeleton has two divisions: the **axial skeleton** and the **appendicular skeleton.** Bones of the center, or axis, of the body make up the axial skeleton. The bones of the skull, spine, and chest and the hyoid bone in the neck are all in the axial skeleton. The bones of the upper and lower extremities or appendages make up the appendicular skeleton. The appendicular skeleton consists of the bones of the upper extremities (shoulder, pectoral girdles, arms, wrists, and hands) and the

FIGURE 6-9 **Human skeleton.** The axial skeleton is distinguished by a blue tint in this illustration. **A,** Anterior view. The axial skeleton is distinguished by a blue tint in this illustration. **B,** Posterior view.

lower extremities (hip, pelvic girdles, legs, ankles, and feet) (Table 6-1). Locate the various parts of the axial skeleton and the appendicular skeleton in Figure 6-9.

Axial Skeleton

Skull

The skull consists of 8 bones that form the **cranium,** 14 bones that form the **face,** and 6 tiny bones in the **middle ear.** You can learn the names and locations of these bones by studying Table 6-2. Find as many of them as you can on Figure 6-10. Feel their outlines in your own body where possible. Examine them on a skeleton if you have access to one.

TABLE 6-1

Main Parts of the Skeleton*

AXIAL SKELETON†	APPENDICULAR SKELETON‡
Skull	Upper extremities
Cranial bones	Pectoral (shoulder) girdle
Ear bones	Arm and forearm bones
Face bones	Wrist bones
Spine	Hand bones
Vertebrae	Lower extremities
Thorax	Pelvic (hip) girdle
Ribs	Thigh and leg bones
Sternum	Ankle bones
Hyoid bone	Foot bones

*Total bones = 206.
†Total = 80 bones.
‡Total = 126 bones.

TABLE 6-2

Bones of the Skull

NAME	NUMBER	DESCRIPTION
Cranial Bones		
Frontal	1	Forehead bone; also forms front part of floor of cranium and most of upper part of eye sockets; cavity inside bone above upper margins of eye sockets (orbits) called *frontal sinus*; lined with mucous membrane
Parietal	2	Form bulging topsides of cranium
Temporal	2	Form lower sides of cranium; contain middle and inner ear structures; *mastoid sinuses* are mucosa-lined spaces in *mastoid process*, the protuberance behind ear; *external auditory canal* is tube leading into temporal bone; muscles attach to *styloid process*
Occipital	1	Forms back of skull; spinal cord enters cranium through large hole *(foramen magnum)* in occipital bone
Sphenoid	1	Forms central part of floor of cranium; pituitary gland located in small depression in sphenoid called *sella turcica (Turkish saddle);* muscles attach to *pterygoid process*
Ethmoid	1	Uniquely shaped bone that helps form floor of cranium; side walls, roof of nose, and part of its middle partition (nasal septum—made up of the *vomer* bone and the *perpendicular plate* of the ethmoid bone); and part of orbit. Contains honeycomb-like spaces, the *ethmoid sinuses; superior* and *middle conchae* are projections of ethmoid bone that form "ledges" along side wall of each nasal cavity
Face Bones		
Nasal	2	Small bones that form upper part of bridge of nose
Maxilla	2	Upper jawbones; also help form roof of mouth, floor, and side walls of nose and floor of orbit; large cavity in maxillary bone is *maxillary sinus*
Zygomatic	2	Cheek bones; also help form orbit
Mandible	1	Lower jawbone articulates with temporal bone at *condyloid process;* only bone of skull that moves freely; *mental foramen* is hole for blood vessels and nerves
Lacrimal	2	Small bones; help form medial wall of eye socket and side wall of nasal cavity
Palatine	2	Form back part of roof of mouth and floor and side walls of nose and part of floor of orbit
Inferior nasal concha	2	Form curved "ledge" along inside of side wall of nose, below middle concha
Vomer	1	Forms lower, back part of nasal septum
Ear Bones		
Malleus	2	Malleus, incus, and stapes are tiny bones in middle ear cavity in temporal bone; *malleus* means "hammer"—shape of bone
Incus	2	*Incus* means "anvil"—shape of bone
Stapes	2	*Stapes* means "stirrup"—shape of bone

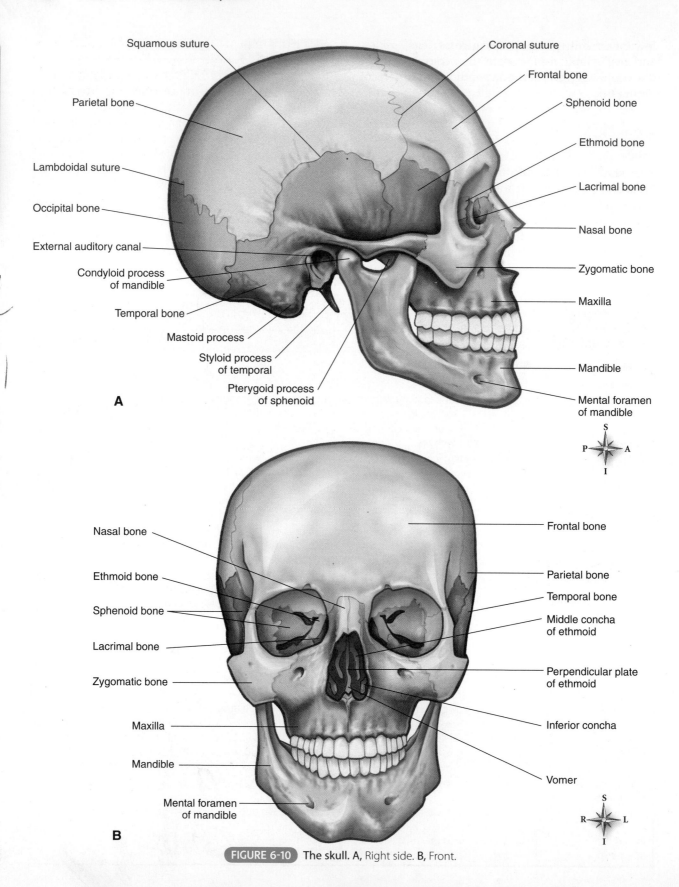

Squamous suture

Coronal suture

Frontal bone

Parietal bone

Sphenoid bone

Ethmoid bone

Lambdoidal suture

Lacrimal bone

Occipital bone

Nasal bone

External auditory canal

Condyloid process
of mandible

Zygomatic bone

Temporal bone

Maxilla

Mastoid process

Styloid process
of temporal

Mandible

Pterygoid process
of sphenoid

Mental foramen
of mandible

A

Nasal bone

Frontal bone

Ethmoid bone

Parietal bone

Sphenoid bone

Temporal bone

Middle concha
of ethmoid

Lacrimal bone

Zygomatic bone

Perpendicular plate
of ethmoid

Maxilla

Inferior concha

Mandible

Vomer

Mental foramen
of mandible

B

FIGURE 6-10 **The skull. A,** Right side. **B,** Front.

"My sinuses give me so much trouble." Have you ever heard this complaint or perhaps uttered it yourself? **Sinuses** are spaces or cavities within some of the cranial bones (Figure 6-11). Four pairs of them (those within the frontal, maxillary, sphenoid, and ethmoid bones) have openings into the nose and thus are referred to as **paranasal sinuses.** Air-filled sinuses are necessary to make the skull light enough for the neck to hold the head upright. But sinuses can give trouble when the mucous membrane that lines them becomes inflamed, swollen, and painful. For example, inflammation in the frontal sinus *(frontal sinusitis)* often starts from a common cold. (The suffix *-itis* added to a word means "inflammation of.")

Note in Figure 6-10 that the two parietal bones, which give shape to the bulging topside of the skull, form immovable joints called **sutures** with several bones: the *lambdoidal suture* with the occipital bone, the *squamous suture* with the temporal bone and part of the sphenoid, and the *coronal suture* with the frontal bone.

You may be familiar with the "soft spots" on a baby's skull. These are six **fontanels,** or areas where ossification is incomplete at birth. You can see them in Figure 6-8. Fontanels allow some compression of

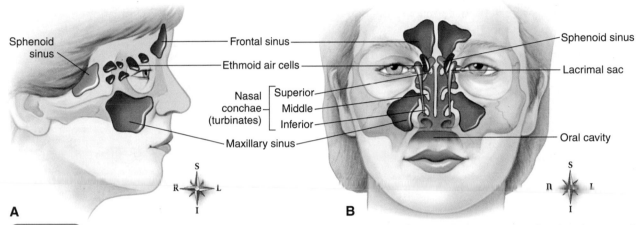

FIGURE 6-11   **Paranasal sinuses. A,** Lateral view of the head, showing location of sinuses. **B,** Anterior view, showing sinuses and their relationship to the nasal cavity.

Clinical Application

Epiphyseal Fracture

The point of articulation between the epiphysis and diaphysis of a growing long bone is susceptible to injury if overstressed, especially in the young child or preadolescent athlete. In these individuals the epiphyseal plate can be separated from the diaphysis or epiphysis, causing an epiphyseal fracture. This x-ray study shows such a fracture in a young boy. Without successful treatment, an epiphyseal fracture may inhibit normal growth. Stunted bone growth, in turn, may cause the affected limb to be shorter than the normal limb.

the skull during birth without much risk of breaking the skull bones. They may also be important in determining the position of the baby's head before delivery. The soft membranes of the fontanels also allow additional bone to form around the margins of the skull bones, thus permitting early rapid growth of an infant's skull. The fontanels eventually fuse to form the immovable joints called *sutures* before a baby is 2 years old.

Spine (Vertebral Column)

The term *vertebral column* may conjure up a mental picture of the spine as a single long bone shaped like a column in a building, but this is far from true. The vertebral column consists of a series of separate bones, or **vertebrae,** connected in such a

way that they form a flexible curved rod (Figure 6-12). Different sections of the spine have different names: cervical region, thoracic region, lumbar region, sacrum, and coccyx. They are illustrated in Figure 6-12 and described in Table 6-3.

Although individual vertebrae are small bones that are irregular in shape, they have several well-defined parts. Note, for example, in Figure 6-13, the body of the lumbar vertebra, its spinous process (or spine), its two transverse processes, and the hole in its center, called the *vertebral foramen.* The superior and inferior articular processes permit limited and controlled movement between adjacent vertebrae. To feel the tip of the spinous process of one of your vertebrae, simply bend your head forward and run your fingers down the

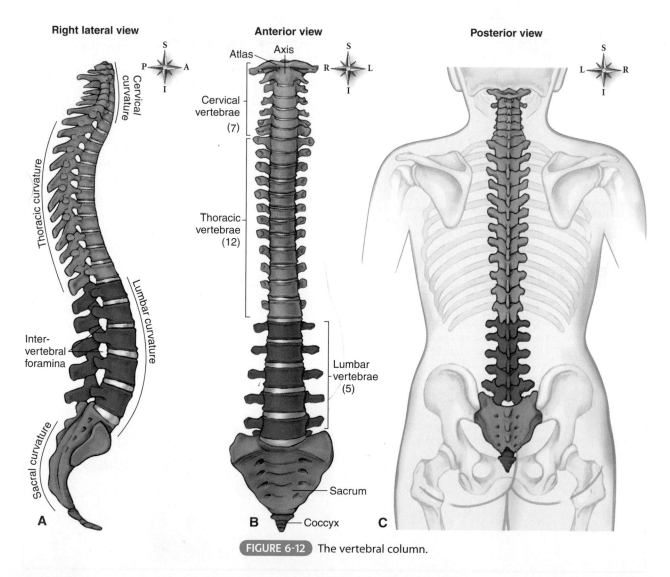

FIGURE 6-12 The vertebral column.

TABLE 6-3

Bones of the Vertebral Column

NAME	NUMBER	DESCRIPTION
Cervical	7	Upper seven vertebrae, in neck region; first cervical vertebra called *atlas*; second, *axis*
Thoracic vertebrae	12	Next 12 vertebrae; ribs attach to these
Lumbar vertebrae	5	Next five vertebrae; located in small of back
Sacrum	1	In child, five separate vertebrae; in adult, fused into one
Coccyx	1	In child, three to five separate vertebrae; in adult, fused into one

back of your neck until you feel a projection of bone at shoulder level. This is the tip of the seventh cervical vertebra's long, forked spinous process. The seven cervical vertebrae form the supporting framework of the neck.

Have you ever noticed the four curves in your spine? Your neck and the small of your back curve slightly inward or forward, whereas the chest region of the spine and the lowermost portion curve in the opposite direction (see Figure 6-12). When you look at the spine from the rear, you will see the cervical and lumbar curves of the spine, called *concave curves*, and the thoracic and sacral curves, called *convex curves*. This is not true, however, of a newborn baby's spine. It forms a continuous convex curve from top to bottom (Figure 6-14). Gradually, as the baby learns to hold up his or her head, a reverse or concave curve develops in the neck (cervical region). Later, as the baby learns to stand, the lumbar region of his or her spine also becomes concave.

The normal curves of the spine have important functions. They give it enough strength to support the weight of the rest of the body. These curves also make it possible to balance the weight of the body, which is necessary for us to stand and walk on two feet instead of having to crawl on all fours. A curved structure has more strength than a straight one of the same size and materials. (The next time you pass a bridge, look to see whether or not its supports form a curve.) Clearly the spine needs to be a strong structure. It supports the head that is balanced on top of it, the ribs and internal organs that are suspended from it in front, and the hips and legs that are attached to it below.

Thorax

Twelve pairs of ribs, the sternum (breastbone), and the thoracic vertebrae form the bony cage known as the **thorax** or **chest.** Each of the 12 pairs of ribs is attached posteriorly to a vertebra. Also, all of the ribs, except the lower two pairs, are attached to the sternum and so have anterior and posterior anchors. Look closely at Figure 6-15 and you can see that the first seven pairs of ribs (sometimes referred to as the *true ribs*) are attached to the sternum by costal cartilage. The eighth, ninth, and

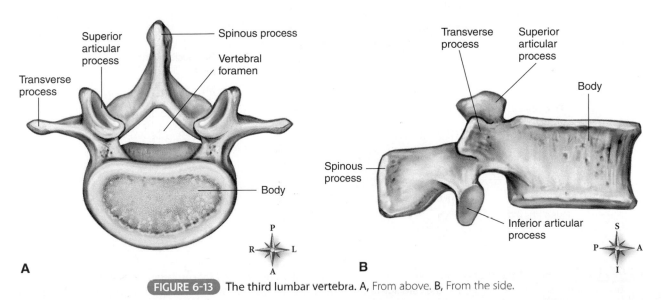

FIGURE 6-13   The third lumbar vertebra. **A,** From above. **B,** From the side.

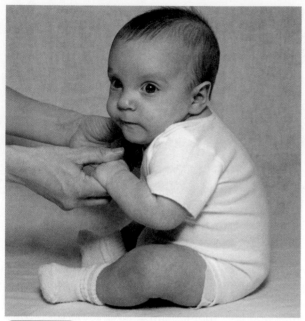

FIGURE 6-14 **Spinal curvature of an infant.** The spine of the newborn baby forms a continuous convex curve.

TABLE 6-4

Bones of the Thorax

NAME	NUMBER	DESCRIPTION
True ribs	14	Upper seven pairs; attached to sternum by *costal cartilages*
False ribs	10	Lower five pairs; first three pairs attached to sternum by costal cartilage of seventh ribs; lowest two pairs do not attach to sternum, therefore called *floating ribs*
Sternum	1	Breastbone; shaped like a dagger; piece of cartilage at lower end of bone called *xiphoid process*; superior portion called the *manubrium*

tenth pairs of ribs are attached to the cartilage of the seventh ribs and are sometimes called *false ribs.* The last two pairs of ribs, in contrast, are not attached to any costal cartilage and consequently seem to float free in front, hence their descriptive name, *floating ribs* (Table 6-4).

QUICK CHECK

1. What is the difference between the axial skeleton and the appendicular skeleton?
2. What is a suture? A fontanel? A sinus?
3. What are the three major categories of vertebrae? How many bones in each?
4. How is a false rib different from a True rib?

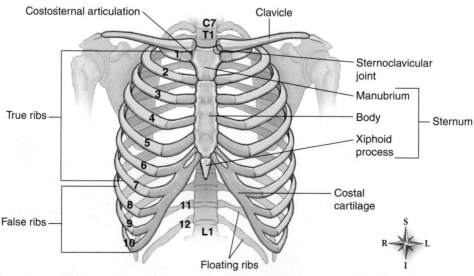

FIGURE 6-15 **Bones of the thorax.** Rib pairs 1 through 7, the true ribs, are attached by cartilage to the sternum. Rib pairs 8 through 10, the false ribs, are attached to the cartilage of the seventh pair. Rib pairs 11 and 12 are called floating ribs because they have no anterior cartilage attachments.

Appendicular Skeleton

Of the 206 bones that form the skeleton as a whole, 126 are contained in the appendicular subdivision. Look again at Figure 6-9 to identify the appendicular components of the skeleton. Note that the bones in the shoulder or pectoral girdle connect the bones of the arm, forearm, wrist, and hands to the axial skeleton of the thorax, and the hip or pelvic girdle connects the bones of the thigh, leg, ankle, and foot to the axial skeleton of the pelvis.

Upper Extremity

The **scapula** (SKAP-yoo-lah), or shoulder blade, and the **clavicle** (KLAV-i-kul), or collarbone, compose the *shoulder,* or **pectoral girdle.** This connects the upper extremity to the axial skeleton. The only direct point of attachment between these bones occurs at the **sternoclavicular** (ster-no-klah-VIK-yoo-lar) **joint** between the clavicle and the sternum or breastbone. As you can see in Figures 6-9 and 6-15, this joint is very small. Because the upper extremity is capable of a wide range of motion, great pressures can occur at or near the joint. As a result, fractures of the clavicle are very common.

The **humerus** (HYOO-mer-us) is the long bone of the arm and the second longest bone in the body.

It is attached at the concave *glenoid cavity* of the scapula at its proximal end, where it is held in place and permitted to move by a group of muscles that are together called the *rotator cuff*. The distal end of the humerus articulates with the two bones of the forearm at the elbow joint. The bones of the forearm are the **radius** and the **ulna.** The anatomy of the elbow is a good example of how structure is related to function. Note in Figure 6-16 that the large bony process of the ulna, called the **olecranon** (oh-LEK-rah-nahn), fits nicely into a large depression on the posterior surface of the humerus, called the **olecranon fossa.** This structural relationship makes possible movement at the joint.

The radius and the ulna of the forearm articulate with each other and with the distal end of the humerus at the elbow joint. In addition, they also touch each another distally where they articulate with the bones of the wrist. In the anatomical position, with the arm at the side and the palm facing forward, the radius runs along the lateral side of the forearm, and the ulna is located along the medial border.

The wrist and the hand have more bones in them for their size than any other part of the body—8 **carpal** (KAR-pal) or wrist bones, 5 **metacarpal** (met-ah-KAR-pal) bones that form the

FIGURE 6-16 Bones of the right arm, elbow, and forearm. A, B, and C are anterior views. D is posterior view.

support structure for the palm of the hand, and 14 **phalanges** (fah-LAN-jeez), or finger, bones—27 bones in all (Table 6-5). This composition is very important structurally. The presence of many small bones in the hand and wrist and the many movable joints between them makes the human hand highly maneuverable—allowing us to easily make and use tools. Figure 6-17 shows the relationships between the bones of the wrist and hand.

Lower Extremity

The *hip,* or **pelvic girdle,** connects the legs to the trunk. The pelvic girdle as a whole consists of two large **coxal bones,** one located on each side of the pelvis, attached inferiorly to the *sacrum* of the vertebral column. This ringlike arrangement of bones provide a strong base of support for the torso and connects the lower extremities to the axial skeleton. In an infant's body, each coxal bone consists of three separate bones—the **ilium** (IL-ee-um), the **ischium** (IS-kee-um), and the **pubis** (PYOO-bis) (see Figure 6-8). These bones grow together to become one bone in an adult (see Figures 6-9 and 6-21).

Just as the humerus is the only bone in the arm, the **femur** (FEE-mur) is the only bone in the thigh (Figure 6-18). It is the longest bone in the body and articulates proximally at the hip with the coxal bone in a deep, cup-shaped socket called the

---

TABLE 6-5

Bones of the Upper Extremities

NAME	NUMBER	DESCRIPTION
Clavicle	2	Collarbones; only joints between pectoral (shoulder) and axial skeleton are those between each clavicle and sternum *(sternoclavicular joints)*
Scapula	2	Shoulder blades; scapula plus clavicle forms *pectoral (shoulder)*; *acromion process*—tip of shoulder that forms joint with clavicle; *glenoid cavity*—arm socket
Humerus	2	Arm bone (Muscles are attached to the *greater tubercle* and to the *medial* and *lateral epicondyles*; the *trochlea* articulates with the ulna; the *surgical neck* is a common fracture site.)
Radius	2	Bone on thumb (lateral) side of forearm (Muscles are attached to the *radial tuberosity* and to the *styloid process.*)
Ulna	2	Bone on little finger (medial) side of forearm; *olecranon*—process of ulna known as *elbow* or "funny bone" (Muscles are attached to the *coronoid process* and to the *styloid process.*)
Carpal bones	16	Short bones at upper end of hand; anatomical wrist
Metacarpals	10	Form framework of palm of hand
Phalanges	28	Finger bones; three in each finger, two in each thumb

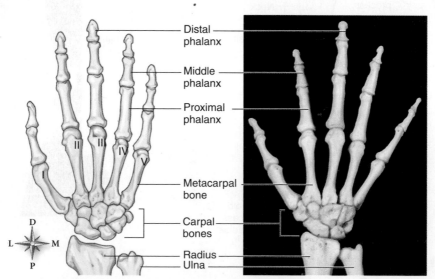

FIGURE 6-17 Bones of the right hand and wrist. There are 14 phalanges in each hand. Each of these bones is called a *phalanx* (dorsal view).

FIGURE 6-18 Bones of the right thigh, knee joint, and leg. A, B, and C are anterior views. D is a posterior view.

Phalanges

Distal phalanx

Middle phalanx

Proximal phalanx

Metatarsals

Cuneiform bones

Cuboid bone

Navicular bone

Tarsals

Talus

Calcaneus bone

FIGURE 6-19 **Bones of the right foot.** Compare the names and numbers of foot bones (viewed here from above) with those of the hand bones shown in Figure 6-17.

acetabulum (ass-eh-TAB-yoo-lum). The articulation of the head of the femur in the acetabulum is more stable than the articulation of the head of the humerus with the scapula in the upper extremity. As a result, dislocation of the hip occurs less often than does disarticulation of the shoulder. Distally, the femur articulates with the knee cap, or **patella** (pah-TEL-ah), and the **tibia,** or "shinbone." The tibia forms a rather sharp edge or crest along the front of your leg. A slender, non–weight-bearing, and rather fragile bone named the **fibula** lies along the outer or lateral border of the leg.

Toe bones have the same name as finger bones—**phalanges.** There is the same number of toe bones as finger bones, a fact that might surprise you because toes are shorter than fingers. Foot bones comparable to the metacarpals and carpals of the hand have slightly different names. They are called **metatarsals** and **tarsals** in the foot (Figure 6-19). Just as each hand contains five metacarpal bones, each foot contains five metatarsal bones. However, the foot has only seven tarsal bones, in contrast to the hand's eight carpals. The largest tarsal bone is the **calcaneus,** or heel bone. The bones of the lower extremities are summarized in Table 6-6.

You stand on your feet, so certain features of their structure make them able to support the body's weight. The great toe, for example, is considerably more solid and less mobile than the

TABLE 6-6

Bones of the Lower Extremities

NAME	NUMBER	DESCRIPTION
Coxal bone	2	Hip bone; *ilium*—upper flaring part of pelvic bone; *ischium*—lower back part; *pubic bone*—lower front part; *acetabulum*—hip socket; *symphysis pubis*—cartilaginous joint in midline between two pubic bones; *pelvic inlet*—opening into *true pelvis* or pelvic cavity; if pelvic inlet is misshapen or too small, infant skull cannot enter true pelvis for natural birth
Femur	2	Thigh bones; *head of femur*—ball-shaped upper end of bone; fits into acetabulum (Muscles are attached to the *greater* and *lesser trochanters* and to the *lateral* and *medial epicondyles*; the *lateral* and *medial condyles* form articulations at the knee.)
Patella	2	Kneecap
Tibia	2	Shinbone; *medial malleolus*—rounded projection at lower end of tibia commonly called *inner anklebone*; muscles are attached to the *tibial tuberosity*
Fibula	2	Long slender bone of lateral side of leg; *lateral malleolus*—rounded projection at lower end of fibula commonly called *outer anklebone*
Tarsal bones	14	Form heel and back part of foot; anatomical ankle; largest is the *calcaneus*
Metatarsals	10	Form part of foot to which toes are attached; tarsal and metatarsal bones arranged so that they form three arches in foot; *inner longitudinal arch* and *outer longitudinal arch*, which extend from front to back of foot, and *transverse* or *metatarsal arch*, which extends across foot
Phalanges	28	Toe bones; three in each of the smaller toes, two in each great toe

FIGURE 6-20   Arches of the foot. **A,** Medial and lateral longitudinal arches. (Arrows show direction of force.) **B,** "Flatfoot" occurs when tendons and ligaments weaken and the arches fall. **C,** Transverse arch.

thumb. The foot bones are held together in such a way as to form springy lengthwise and crosswise arches. These provide great supporting strength and a highly stable base. Strong ligaments and leg muscle tendons normally hold the foot bones firmly in their arched positions. Frequently, however, the foot ligaments and tendons weaken. The arches then flatten, a condition appropriately called *fallen arches* or *flatfeet* (Figure 6-20, *B*).

Two arches extend in a lengthwise direction in the foot (Figure 6-20, *A*). One lies on the inside part of the foot and is called the **medial longitudinal arch.** The other lies along the outer edge of the foot and is named the **lateral longitudinal arch.** Another arch extends across the ball of the foot. This arch is called the **transverse,** or **metatarsal, arch** (Figure 6-20, *C*).

DIFFERENCES BETWEEN A MAN'S AND A WOMAN'S SKELETON

A man's skeleton and a woman's skeleton differ in several ways. If you were to examine a male skeleton and a female skeleton placed side by side, you would probably first notice the difference in their sizes. Most male skeletons have bones that are larger, with more distinct bumps and other markings, than most female skeletons. This difference results partly from the difference in muscle tension on bones—the more tension on bone, the

bigger and denser the bone gets at the points of muscle attachment. These male-female distinctions are visible in nearly every bone of the body, so it is no wonder that forensic scientists can often accurately determine the sex of human remains using just a few bones.

Perhaps the most obvious of the many structural differences between the male and female skeletons are in the *pelvic girdle* or **pelvis**—the ring formed by the two pelvic (coxal) bones and sacrum. The word *pelvis* means "basin." The wide structure of the female pelvis allows the body of a fetus to be cradled in it before birth, and its wide opening allows the baby to pass through it during birth. Although the individual male coxal bones are generally larger than the individual female coxal bones, together the male coxal bones form a narrower structure than do the female coxal bones. A man's pelvis is shaped more like a funnel than the broad, shallow basin of the female pelvis (Figure 6-21).

You can also see in Figure 6-21 that the openings from the abdomen into and through the pelvis—the pelvic inlet and pelvic outlet—are both normally much wider in the female than in the male. This effect is partly because the angle at the front of the female pelvis where the two pubic bones join is wider than in the male. Such an arrangement allows more room for a fetus's head to move through during childbirth.

Male

Female

FIGURE 6-21 Comparison of the male pelvis and female pelvis. Notice the narrower width of the male pelvis, giving it a more funnel-like shape than the female pelvis. The insets show how the hand can be used to show how the pubic angles differ.

QUICK CHECK

1. Name some of the bones of the upper extremity. Name some of the lower extremity.
2. What are the phalanges? Why are there two different sets of phalanges?
3. What are metacarpal bones? How do they differ from metatarsal bones?
4. How does the female pelvis differ from the male pelvis?

JOINTS (ARTICULATIONS)

Every bone in the body, except one, connects to at least one other bone. In other words, every bone but one forms a joint with some other bone. (The excep-

tion is the hyoid bone in the neck, to which the tongue anchors.) Most of us probably never think much about our joints unless something goes wrong with them and they do not function properly. Then their tremendous importance becomes painfully clear. Joints hold our bones together securely and at the same time make it possible for movement to occur between the bones—between most of them, that is. Without joints we could not move our arms, legs, or many other of our body parts. Our bodies would, in short, be rigid, immobile hulks. Try, for example, to move your arm at your shoulder joint in as many directions as you can. Try to do the same thing at your elbow joint. Now examine the shape of the bones at each of these joints on a skeleton or in Figure 6-9. Do you see why you cannot move your arm at your elbow in nearly as many directions as you can at your shoulder?

Kinds of Joints

One method classifies joints into three types according to the degree of movement they allow:

1. Synarthroses (sin-ar-THROH-seez) — no movement
2. Amphiarthroses (am-fee-ar-THROH-seez) — slight movement
3. Diarthroses (dye-ar-THROH-seez) — free movement

Differences in joint structure account for differences in the degree of movement that is possible.

Synarthroses

A **synarthrosis** is a joint in which fibrous connective tissue grows between the articulating (joining) bones holding them close together. The joints between cranial bones are synarthroses, commonly called *sutures* (Figure 6-22, *A*).

Amphiarthroses

An **amphiarthrosis** is a joint in which cartilage connects the articulating bones. The symphysis pubis, the joint between the two pubic bones, is an amphiarthrosis (Figure 6-22, *B*).

Joints between the bodies of the vertebrae are also amphiarthroses. These joints make it possible to flex the trunk forward or sideways and even to circumduct and rotate it. Strong ligaments connect the bodies of the vertebrae, and fibrous disks lie between them. The central core of these intervertebral disks consists of a pulpy, elastic substance that loses some of its resiliency with age.

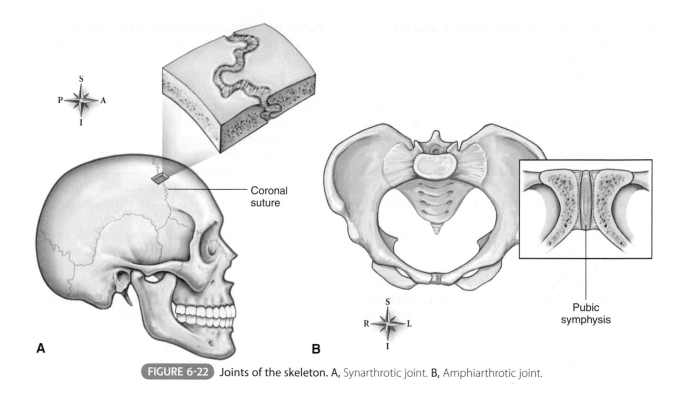

FIGURE 6-22 Joints of the skeleton. **A,** Synarthrotic joint. **B,** Amphiarthrotic joint.

Diarthroses

Fortunately most of our joints are diarthroses. Such joints allow considerable movement, sometimes in many directions and sometimes in only one or two directions.

Structure. **Diarthroses** (freely movable joints) are made alike in certain ways. All have a joint capsule, a joint cavity, and a layer of cartilage over the ends of two joining bones (Figure 6-23). The *joint capsule* is made of the body's strongest and toughest material—fibrous connective tissue—and is lined with a smooth, slippery synovial membrane. The capsule fits over the ends of the two bones somewhat like a sleeve. Because it attaches firmly to the shaft of each bone to form its covering (called the *periosteum, peri* means "around," and *osteum* means "bone"), the joint capsule holds the bones securely together but at the same time permits movement at the joint. The structure of the joint capsule, in other words, helps make possible the joint's function.

Ligaments (cords or bands made of the same strong fibrous connective tissue as the joint capsule) also grow out of the periosteum and lash the two bones together even more firmly.

The layer of **articular cartilage** over the joint ends of bones acts like a rubber heel on a shoe—it

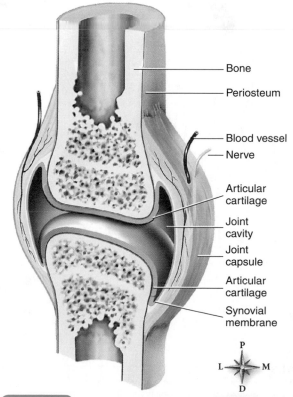

FIGURE 6-23 **Structure of a diarthrotic joint.** Each diarthrosis has a joint capsule, a joint cavity, and a layer of cartilage over the ends of the joined bones.

absorbs jolts. The articular cartilage also provides a smooth surface so the bones of the joint can move with little friction.

A joint cavity where the bones join together is lined with **synovial membrane,** which secretes a lubricating fluid (synovial fluid) that allows easier movement with less friction. In some joints, the synovial membrane forms a pocketlike extension or a pouch filled alongside a joint. Called a **bursa,** this pocket of fluid acts as a shock-absorbing cushion around the bones of the joint. Irritation, injury, or infection of a bursa can cause inflammation—a condition called *bursitis.*

Function. There are several types of diarthroses: ball-and-socket, hinge, pivot, saddle, gliding, and condyloid (Figure 6-24). Because they differ in structure, they differ also in their possible range of movement. In a ball-and-socket joint, a ball-shaped head of one bone fits into a concave socket of another bone. Shoulder and hip joints, for example, are ball-and-socket joints. Of all the joints in our bodies, these permit the widest range of move-

ments. Think for a moment about how many ways you can move your arms. You can move them forward, you can move them backward, you can move them away from the sides of your body, and you can move them back down to your sides. You can also move them around so as to visually describe a circle with your hands.

Hinge joints, like the hinges on a door, allow movements in only two directions, namely, *flexion* and *extension.* **Flexion** is bending a joint, and **extension** is straightening it out (Table 6-7). Elbow and knee joints and the joints in the fingers are hinge joints.

Pivot joints are those in which a small projection of one bone pivots in an arch of another bone. For example, a projection of the *axis* (second cervical vertebra) is a point around which an arch of the *atlas* (first cervical vertebra) can pivot. This permits **rotation** of the head, which rests on the atlas.

Only one pair of saddle joints exists in the body—between the metacarpal bone of each thumb

FIGURE 6-24 **Types of diarthrotic joints.** Notice that the structure of each type dictates its function (movement). The mechanical diagrams represent the type of action at the highlighted anatomical joints.

TABLE 6-7

Types of Joint Movements

MOVEMENT	EXAMPLE	DESCRIPTION
Flexion (to flex a joint)	Flexion	Reduces the angle of the joint, as in bending the elbow
Extension (to extend a joint)	Extension	Increases the angle of a joint, as in straightening a bent elbow
Rotation (to rotate a joint)	Rotation	Spins one bone relative to another, as in rotating the head at the neck joint

Continued

TABLE 6-7

Types of Joint Movements—cont'd

MOVEMENT	EXAMPLE	DESCRIPTION
Circumduction (to circumduct a joint)	Circumduction	Moves the distal end of a bone in a circle, while circumducting a joint, keeping the proximal end relatively stable, as in moving the arm in a circle and thus circumducting the shoulder joint
Abduction (to abduct a joint)	Abduction	Increases the angle of a joint to move a part away from the midline, as in moving the arm to the side and away from the body
Adduction (to adduct a joint)	Adduction	Decreases the angle of a joint to move a part toward the midline, as in moving the arm in and down from the side

Your study of these movements continues in Chapter 7, beginning on p. 151.

and a carpal bone of the wrist (the name of this carpal bone is the *trapezium*). Because the articulating surfaces of these bones are saddle-shaped, they make possible the human thumb's great mobility, a mobility no animal's thumb possesses. We can **flex, extend, abduct, adduct,** and **circumduct** our thumbs, and most important of all, we can move our thumbs to touch the tip of any one of our fingers. (This movement is called *opposing the thumb to the fingers.*) Without the saddle joints at the base of

Clinical Application

Palpable Bony Landmarks

Health professionals often identify externally palpable bony landmarks when dealing with the sick and injured. **Palpable bony landmarks** are bones that can be touched and identified through the skin. They serve as reference points in identifying other body structures.

There are externally palpable bony landmarks throughout the body. Many skull bones, such as the zygomatic bone, can be palpated. The medial and lateral epicondyles of the humerus, the olecranon of the ulna, and the styloid process of the ulna and the radius at the wrist can be palpated on the upper extremity. The highest corner of the shoulder is the acromion process of the scapula.

When you put your hands on your hips, you can feel the superior edge of the ilium called the *iliac crest*. The anterior end of the crest, called the *anterior superior iliac spine,* is a prominent landmark used often as a clinical reference. The medial malleolus of the tibia and the lateral malleolus of the fibula are prominent at the ankle. The calcaneus or heel bone is easily palpated on the posterior aspect of the foot. On the anterior aspect of the lower extremity, examples of palpable bony landmarks include the patella, or knee cap; the anterior border of the tibia, or shinbone; and the metatarsals and phalanges of the toes. Try to identify as many of the externally palpable bones of the skeleton as possible on your own body. Using these as points of reference will make it easier for you to visualize the placement of other bones that cannot be touched or palpated through the skin.

- Zygomatic bone
- Acromion process of scapula
- Medial epicondyle of humerus
- Lateral epicondyle of humerus
- Iliac crest
- Styloid process of radius
- Styloid process of ulna
- Patella
- Anterior border of tibia
- Lateral malleolus of fibula
- Medial malleolus of tibia
- Calcaneus

each of our thumbs, we could not do such a simple act as picking up a pin or grasping a pencil between thumb and forefinger.

Gliding joints are the least movable diarthrotic joints. Their flat articulating surfaces allow limited gliding movements, such as that at the superior and inferior articulating processes between successive vertebrae.

Condyloid (KON-di-loyd) joints are those in which a condyle (an oval projection) fits into an elliptical socket. An example is the fit of the distal end of the radius into depressions in the carpal bones.

 To learn more about types of joint movement, go to AnimationDirect on your CD-ROM.

✓ QUICK CHECK

1. What are the three major types of joints in the skeleton? Give an example of each.
2. What membrane in a diarthrotic joint provides lubrication for movement?
3. What is a ligament?
4. What is meant by "flexing" the elbow? Extending the elbow?

Clinical Application

Total Hip Replacement

Because total hip replacement (THR) is the most common orthopedic operation performed on older persons (more than 300,000 procedures per year in the United States), home health care professionals often work with patients recovering from THR surgery.

The THR procedure involves replacement of the femoral head by a metal prosthesis and the acetabular socket by a polyethylene cup. The prostheses are usually coated with a porous material that allows natural growth of bone to mesh with the artificial material. Such meshing of tissue and prostheses ensures stability of the parts without the loosening that the use of glues in the past often allowed. First introduced in 1953, THR technique has advanced to the state that the procedure has a success rate of about 85% in older adults.

Patients at home after THR surgery should progress through proper surgical healing and recovery, including stabilization of the prostheses as new tissue grows into their porous surfaces. THR patients should also expect some improvement in regained use of the affected hip, including weight-bearing and walking movements.

Science Application

Bones and Joints
Hippocrates (ca. 460-377 B.C.E.)

Ever since 400 B.C.E., when Hippocrates (the Greek physician often regarded as a founder of the medical profession) first described treatments of human bone and joint disorders and injuries, many approaches to treating the human skeleton have been taken. For example, physical and occupational therapists help patients regain movement in joints through physical exercises, and orthopedic surgeons help their patients by means of surgical operations. Because the skeleton, with its many bones and joints, is the framework of the entire body, it is not surprising to learn that many different health professionals deal directly with the skeleton. For example, podiatrists work with the bones and joints of the foot and ankle, sports trainers and physicians work with many parts of the skeleton, and chiropractic physicians often work to align the vertebral column. Of course, radiographic technicians and radiologists are often called upon to make medical images of the bones and joints and interpret the meaning of the images.

Health and Well-Being

The Knee Joint

The knee is the largest and most vulnerable joint. Because the knee is often subjected to sudden, strong forces during athletic activity, knee injuries are among the most common type of athletic injury. Sometimes, the concave disks of articular cartilage called **menisci** (meh-NIS-kye) on the tibia tear when the knee twists while bearing weight. The ligaments holding the tibia and femur together can also be injured in this way. The figure shows tears in the lateral and medial ligaments outside the joint cavity as well as tears in the crossed **cruciate** (KRU-shee-ayt) **ligaments** inside the joint. Knee injuries may also occur when a weight-bearing knee is hit by another person or a moving object.

OUTLINE SUMMARY

FUNCTIONS OF THE SKELETAL SYSTEM
A. Supports and gives shape to the body
B. Protects internal organs
C. Helps make movements possible when bones at moveable joints are pulled by muscles
D. Stores calcium — hormones regulate calcium storage: calcitonin (CT) increases storage and parathyroid hormone (PTH) reduces stores of calcium
E. Hematopoiesis — blood cell formation in red bone marrow

TYPES OF BONES
A. Four major types, according to overall shape of the bone
   1. Long — Example: humerus (arm)
   2. Short — Example: carpals (wrist)
   3. Flat — Example: frontal (skull)
   4. Irregular — Example: vertebrae (spinal cord)
   5. Some also recognize a sesamoid (round) bone category — Example: patella (kneecap)
B. Structure of long bones (see Figure 6-1)
   1. Diaphysis or shaft — hollow tube of hard compact bone
   2. Medullary cavity — hollow area inside diaphysis that contains yellow marrow
   3. Epiphyses, or ends of the bone — spongy bone that contains red bone marrow
   4. Articular cartilage — covers epiphyses and functions as a cushion
   5. Periosteum — strong membrane covering bone everywhere except at joint surfaces
   6. Endosteum — thin membrane lining medullary cavity
C. Structure of flat bones (see Figure 6-2)
   1. Spongy bone layer sandwiched between two compact bone layers
   2. Diploe — spongy bone layer of a flat bone

MICROSCOPIC STRUCTURE OF BONE AND CARTILAGE
A. Bone types (see Figure 6-3)
   1. Spongy
      a. Texture results from needlelike threads of bone called *trabeculae* surrounded by a network of open spaces

b. Found in epiphyses of bones
      c. Spaces contain red bone marrow
   2. Compact
      a. Structural unit is an osteon — calcified matrix arranged in multiple layers or rings called concentric lamella (see Figure 6-4)
      b. Bone cells are called *osteocytes* and are found inside spaces called *lacunae,* which are connected by tiny tubes called *canaliculi*
B. Cartilage (see Figure 6-5)
   1. Cell type called *chondrocyte*
   2. Matrix is gel-like and lacks blood vessels

BONE FORMATION AND GROWTH
A. Early bone development (before birth) consists of cartilage and fibrous structures
B. Osteoblasts form new bone, and osteoclasts reabsorb bone; osteocytes are inactive osteoblasts (see Figure 6-6)
C. Cartilage models gradually replaced by calcified bone matrix — process called *endochondral ossification* (see Figures 6-7 and 6-8)

DIVISIONS OF SKELETON
Skeleton is composed of the following divisions and their subdivisions:
A. Axial skeleton
   1. Skull
   2. Spine (vertebral column)
   3. Thorax
   4. Hyoid bone
B. Appendicular skeleton
   1. Upper extremities, including shoulder (pectoral) girdle
   2. Lower extremities, including hip (pelvic) girdle
C. Location and description of bones — see Figures 6-9 to 6-20 and Tables 6-2 to 6-6

DIFFERENCES BETWEEN A MAN'S AND A WOMAN'S SKELETON
A. Size — male skeleton generally larger
B. Shape of pelvis — male pelvis deep and narrow, female pelvis shallow and broad
C. Size of pelvic inlet — female pelvic inlet generally wider, normally large enough for

baby's head to pass through it (see Figure 6-21)

D. Pubic angle — angle between pubic bones of female generally wider

JOINT (ARTICULATIONS)

A. Every bone except the hyoid (which anchors the tongue) connects to at least one other bone.

B. Kinds of joints (see Figures 6-22 to 6-24)

  1. Synarthroses (no movement) — fibrous connective tissue grows between articulating bones; for example, sutures of skull

  2. Amphiarthroses (slight movement) — cartilage connects articulating bones; for example, symphysis pubis

  3. Diarthroses (free movement) — most joints belong to this class

    a. Structure

      (1) Structures of freely movable joints — joint capsule and ligaments hold adjoining bones together but permit movement at joint

      (2) Articular cartilage — covers joint ends of bones where they form joints with other bones

      (3) Synovial membrane — lines joint capsule and secretes lubricating fluid

      (4) Joint cavity — space between joint ends of bones

      (5) Bursa — fluid-filled pouch that absorbs shock; inflammation of bursa is called *bursitis*

    b. Functions of freely movable joints — ball-and-socket, hinge, pivot, saddle, gliding, and condyloid — allow different kinds of movements determined by the structure of each joint (see Table 6-7)

NEW WORDS

abduct, abduction	cruciate ligament	ligament	phalanx (pl. phalanges)
acetabulum	diaphysis (pl. diaphyses)	medial longitudinal arch	pubic
adduct, adduction			radius
amphiarthrosis (pl. amphiarthroses)	diarthrosis (pl. diarthroses)	medullary cavity	red bone marrow
		meniscus (pl. menisci)	rotation
appendicular skeleton	diploe	metacarpal	scapula
articular cartilage	endochondral ossification	metatarsal	sinus
articulation		middle ear	spongy bone (cancellous bone)
axial skeleton	endosteum	olecranon	
bursa (pl. bursae)	epiphyseal plate	olecranon fossa	sternoclavicular joint
calcaneus	epiphysis (pl. epiphyses)	osteoblast	suture
calcitonin (CT)		osteoclast	synarthrosis (pl. synarthroses)
canaliculus (pl. canaliculi)	extend, extension	osteocyte	
	face	osteon	synovial membrane
carpal	femur	osteoporosis	tarsal
cartilage	fibula	palpable	thorax
chest	flex, flexion	paranasal sinus	tibia
chondrocyte	fontanel	parathyroid hormone (PTH)	trabecula (pl. trabeculae)
circumduct, circumduction	hematopoiesis		
	humerus	patella (pl. patellae)	transverse (metatarsal) arch
clavicle	ilium	pectoral girdle	
compact bone	ischium	pelvic girdle	ulna
concentric lamella (pl. lamellae)	lacuna (pl. lacunae)	pelvis (pl. pelves or pelvises)	vertebrae
coxal bone	lateral longitudinal arch	periosteum	yellow bone marrow
cranium			

REVIEW QUESTIONS

1. List and briefly explain the five functions of the skeletal system.
2. Describe the structure of the osteon.
3. Describe the structure of cartilage.
4. Explain briefly the process of endochondral ossification. Include the function of osteoblasts and osteoclasts.
5. Explain the importance of the epiphyseal plate.
6. In general, what bones are included in the axial skeleton and the appendicular skeleton?
7. The vertebral column is divided into five sections based on location. Name the sections and give the number of vertebrae in each section.
8. Distinguish between true, false, and floating ribs. How many of each are there?
9. Describe and give an example of a synarthrotic joint.
10. Describe and give an example of an amphiarthrotic joint.
11. Describe and give an example of two types of diarthrotic joints.
12. Briefly describe a joint capsule.

CRITICAL THINKING

13. When a patient receives a bone marrow transplant, what vital process is being restored?
14. Explain how the canaliculi allow bone to heal more efficiently than cartilage.
15. What effect does the task of childbearing have on the differences between the male and female skeleton?

CHAPTER TEST

1. The thin layer of cartilage on the end of bones where they form joints is called the _____.
2. The hollow area in the shaft of long bones where marrow is located is called the _____.
3. The needlelike threads of spongy bone are called _____.
4. The structural units of compact bone are called _____.
5. Osteocytes and chondrocytes live in small spaces in the matrix called _____.
6. Bone-reabsorbing cells are called _____.
7. Bone-forming cells are called _____.
8. The process of forming bone from cartilage is called _____.
9. If a(n) _____ remains between the epiphysis and diaphysis, bone growth can continue.
10. The two major divisions of the human skeleton are the _____ skeleton and the _____ skeleton.
11. The three types of joints named based on the amount of movement they allow are _____, _____, and _____.
12. The _____ are cords or bands made of strong connective tissue that holds two bones together.

CHAPTER TEST—cont'd

13. Which of the following is not a function of the skeletal system?
    a. mineral storage
    b. blood formation
    c. heat regulation
    d. protection
14. The strong fibrous membrane covering a long bone everywhere except for the joint is called the:
    a. endosteum
    b. periosteum
    c. diaphysis
    d. epiphysis
15. The fibrous inner lining of the hollow tube in a long bone is called the:
    a. endosteum
    b. periosteum
    c. diaphysis
    d. epiphysis
16. The end of a long bone is called the:
    a. endosteum
    b. periosteum
    c. diaphysis
    d. epiphysis
17. The shaft of a long bone is called the:
    a. endosteum
    b. periosteum
    c. diaphysis
    d. epiphysis

Match the bones in Column A with their locations in Column B.

COLUMN A

18. _____ ulna
19. _____ mandible
20. _____ humerus
21. _____ metatarsals
22. _____ tibia
23. _____ rib
24. _____ fibula
25. _____ sternum
26. _____ scapula
27. _____ femur
28. _____ metacarpals
29. _____ frontal bone
30. _____ patella
31. _____ zygomatic bone
32. _____ clavicle
33. _____ occipital bone
34. _____ carpals
35. _____ maxilla

COLUMN B

a. skull
b. upper extremity
c. trunk
d. lower extremity

OBJECTIVES

AFTER YOU HAVE COMPLETED THIS CHAPTER, YOU
SHOULD BE ABLE TO:

1. List, locate in the body, and compare the structure
   and function of the three major types of muscle
   tissue.
2. Discuss the microscopic structure of a skeletal muscle sarcomere and motor unit.
3. Discuss how a muscle is stimulated and compare
   the major types of skeletal muscle contractions.
4. List and explain the most common types of movement produced by skeletal muscles.
5. Name, identify on a model or diagram, and give
   the function of the major muscles of the body discussed in this chapter.

The Muscular System

Although we will initially review the three types of muscle tissue introduced earlier (see Chapter 4), the plan for this chapter is to focus on skeletal or voluntary muscle—those muscle masses that attach to bones and actually move them about when contraction or shortening of muscle cells, or muscle fibers, occurs. If you weigh 120 pounds, about 50 pounds of your weight comes from your skeletal muscles, the "red meat" of the body that is attached to your bones.

Muscular movement occurs when chemical energy from nutrient molecules is transferred to protein filaments in each muscle fiber and then converted to mechanical energy that attempts to shorten (contract) the muscle. As the muscle fibers in a muscle contract they pull on the bones to which they are attached and thus produce movement of the body.

Movements caused by skeletal muscle contraction vary in complexity from blinking an eye to the coordinated and fluid movements of a gifted athlete. Not many of our body structures can claim as great an importance for happy, useful living as can our voluntary muscles, and only a few can boast of greater importance for life itself. Our ability to survive often depends on our ability to adjust to the changing conditions of our environment. Movements frequently constitute a major part of this adjustment.

MUSCLE TISSUE

Under the microscope, threadlike and cylindrical **skeletal muscle** cells appear in bundles. They are characterized by many crosswise stripes and multiple nuclei (Figure 7-1, *A*). Each fine thread is a muscle cell—usually called a **muscle fiber.** This type of muscle tissue

STUDY TIPS

To make the study of the muscular system more efficient, we suggest these tips:

1. Before starting Chapter 7, go back to Chapter 4 and review the synopsis of the muscular system. Also review the three types of muscle tissue covered in Chapter 3.
2. There are two prefixes that refer to muscle: *myo-* and *sarco-*. Several terms in the chapter have one of these prefixes.
3. Make sure you understand the terms *origin* and *insertion* when they are first presented. They will come up repeatedly later in the chapter.
4. Movement is one of the functions of the muscle system. To create movement, muscle cells (muscle fibers) must get shorter. Watch for the mechanisms that make muscle fibers shorter and supply the energy to do so.
5. The names of the muscles are probably less familiar to you than the names of the bones. However, you will find that muscle names can give you some information about the muscles themselves, such as their shape and other characteristics. These "hints" may make the terms easier to recall once you learn them.
6. To create movement, muscle fibers usually get shorter. The sarcomere is the structure in the muscle that actually shortens or pulls. The sliding filament model explains how this shortening occurs. The shortening of the sarcomere requires energy. ATP supplies this energy and is most efficiently formed when oxygen is supplied to the muscle. When you can't supply the muscle with enough oxygen, your muscle "borrows" energy, using a process that creates lactic acid and develops an "oxygen debt."
7. Muscle names give you some information about the muscles that help you remember them. Muscles are named for their shape: *deltoid*, *trapezius*. They are named for a bone they are near: rectus *femoris*, *tibialis anterior*. They are named for their number of origins: *triceps* brachii; their points of attachments: *sternocleidomastoid*; their size: gluteus *maximus*; and the direction of the muscle fibers: *rectus* abdominis (*rectus* means having fibers running parallel to the midline of the body). When you are learning the muscles, try to look for meaning in the muscle names.

Continued on page 142.

STUDY TIPS—cont'd

8. Most of the terms for muscle movement are fairly straightforward. One way to remember the difference between supination and pronation is that when your hand is supinated, you can hold a bowl of soup. And in *adduction*, you *add* to your body; you pull the appendage into the trunk (silly, but effective).

9. In your study group you should make use of flash cards to help you learn the terms in the chapter.

10. Discuss the processes of contraction and fatigue, and be sure you understand the movement terms.

11. If you are asked to learn just the names and locations of the muscles, photocopies of each of the muscle figures with the labels blackened out can be used to quiz each other. If you are asked to learn the functions, origins, and insertions, you need to also use flash cards.

12. Go over the questions at the end of the chapter and discuss possible test questions.

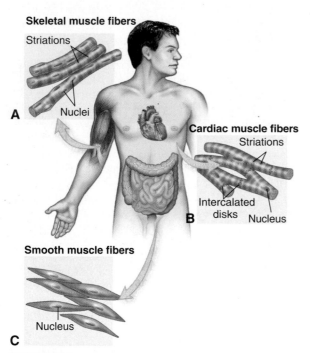

FIGURE 7-1 Muscle tissue. **A,** Skeletal muscle. **B,** Cardiac muscle. **C,** Smooth muscle.

has three names: *skeletal muscle,* because it attaches to bone; *striated muscle,* because of its cross stripes or striations; and *voluntary muscle,* because its contractions can be controlled voluntarily.

In addition to **skeletal muscle,** the body also contains two other types of muscle tissue: cardiac muscle and smooth muscle. **Cardiac muscle** com-

poses the bulk of the heart. Fibers in this type of muscle tissue are also cylindrical, branch frequently (Figure 7-1, *B*), and then recombine into a continuous mass of interconnected tissue. As with skeletal muscle fibers, the cardiac muscle fibers have cross striations. They also have unique dark bands called *intercalated disks,* where the plasma membranes of adjacent cardiac fibers come in contact with each other. Cardiac muscle tissue demonstrates the principle that "form follows function." The interconnected nature of cardiac muscle fibers helps the tissue to contract as a unit and increases the efficiency of the heart muscle in pumping blood.

Smooth muscle fibers are tapered at each end and have a single nucleus (Figure 7-1, *C*). Because they lack cross stripes or striations, they are sometimes called *nonstriated* muscle fibers. They have a smooth, even appearance when viewed through a microscope. They are called *involuntary* because we normally do not have control over their contractions. Smooth or involuntary muscle forms an important part of blood vessel walls and of many hollow internal organs (viscera) such as the gut, urethra, and ureters. Because of its location in many visceral structures, it is sometimes also called *visceral muscle.* Although we cannot willfully control the action of smooth muscle, its contractions are highly regulated, which promotes efficient food passage through the digestive tract or urine through the ureters into the bladder.

All three muscle fiber types—skeletal, cardiac, and smooth—specialize in contraction or shortening. Every movement we make is produced by contractions of skeletal muscle fibers. Contractions of cardiac muscle fibers pump the blood through the heart, and smooth muscle contractions help pump blood through our other hollow organs.

STRUCTURE OF SKELETAL MUSCLE

Muscle Organs

A skeletal muscle is an organ composed mainly of skeletal muscle fibers and connective tissue. Fibrous connective tissue wraps around each individual muscle fiber, then continues as it wraps around groups of muscle fibers called *fascicles,* and then forms a "wrapper" around the entire muscle organ. *Fascia* is the loose connective tissue outside the muscle organs that forms a flexible, sticky "packing material" between muscles, bones, and the skin.

Most skeletal muscles attach to two bones that have a movable joint between them. In other words, most muscles extend from one bone across a joint to another bone. Also, one of the two bones is usually more stationary during a given movement than the other. The muscle's attachment to this more stationary bone is called its **origin.** Its attachment to the more movable bone is called the muscle's **insertion.** The rest of the muscle (all of it except its two ends) is called the *body* of the muscle (Figure 7-2).

Tendons anchor muscles firmly to bones and are made of dense, fibrous connective tissue that extends from the muscle "wrappers" described earlier. In the shape of heavy cords or broad sheets, tendons have great strength. They do not tear or pull away from bone easily. Yet any emergency room nurse or physician sees many tendon injuries—severed tendons and tendons torn loose from bones.

Small fluid-filled sacs called **bursae** (BER-see) lie between some tendons and the bones beneath them. Recall from Chapter 6 that these small connective tissue sacs are lined with **synovial membrane.** The synovial membrane secretes a slippery lubricating fluid *(synovial fluid)* that fills the bursa. Like a small, flexible cushion, a bursa makes it easier for a tendon to slide over a bone when the tendon's muscle shortens.

Tendon sheaths enclose some tendons. Because these tube-shaped structures are also lined with synovial membrane and are moistened with synovial fluid, they, like the bursae, facilitate body movement.

Microscopic Structure and Function

Skeletal muscle tissue consists of elongated contractile cells, or *muscle fibers,* that look like long, tapered cylinders. Their flexible connective tissue wrappings hold them together in parallel groups, allowing the muscle fibers to all pull together in the same direction—as a team.

Each skeletal muscle fiber has a unique cytoskeleton structure. The fiber's internal framework is organized into many long cylinders, each made up of two kinds of threadlike microfilaments called **thick** and **thin myofilaments** (my-oh-FIL-ah-ments). The thick myofilaments are formed from a protein called **myosin,** and the thin myofilaments are composed mainly of the protein **actin.**

Each shaftlike myosin molecule has a "head" that sticks out toward the actin molecules. At rest, the actin is blocked from connecting with the myosin heads by small proteins attached to the actin. During contraction, however, the blocking proteins release actin and the myosin heads connect to form *cross bridges* between the thick and thin filaments.

Find the label **sarcomere** (SAR-koh-meer) in Figure 7-3. Think of the sarcomere as the basic functional or *contractile unit* of skeletal muscle. The submicroscopic structure of a sarcomere consists of numerous thick and thin myofilaments arranged so that, when viewed under a microscope, dark and light stripes, or cross striations, are seen. The repeating units, or sarcomeres, are separated from each other by dark bands called *Z lines* or *Z disks.*

Although the sarcomeres in the upper portion (Figure 7-3, *A*) and in the electron photomicrograph (EM) of Figure 7-3, *B,* are in a relaxed state, the thick and thin myofilaments, which are lying parallel to each other, still overlap. Now look at the diagrams in the lower portion of Figure 7-3, *A.* Note that contraction of the muscle causes the two types of myofilaments to slide toward each other

FIGURE 7-2 Attachments of a skeletal muscle. A muscle originates at a relatively stable part of the skeleton (origin) and inserts at the skeletal part that is moved when the muscle contracts (insertion).

Labels: Origin, Tendons, Muscle body, Tendon, Insertion

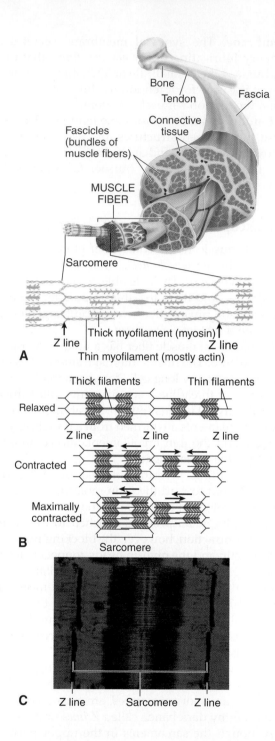

A

B

C

FIGURE 7-3 Structure of skeletal muscle. **A,** Each muscle organ has many muscle fibers, each containing many bundles of thick and thin filaments. The expanded diagram shows the overlapping thick and thin filaments arranged to form adjacent segments called *sarcomeres.* **B,** During contraction, the thin filaments are pulled toward the center of each sarcomere, shortening the whole muscle. **C,** This electron micrograph shows that the overlapping thick and thin filaments within each sarcomere create a pattern of dark striations in the muscle. The extreme magnification allowed by electron microscopy has revolutionized our concept of the structure and function of skeletal muscle and other tissues.

According to this model, during contraction, the thick and thin myofilaments in a muscle fiber first attach to one another by forming cross bridges that then act as levers to ratchet or pull the myofilaments past each other.

The connecting bridges between the myofilaments form only if calcium is present. During the relaxed state, calcium ions (Ca^{++}) are stored within the smooth endoplasmic reticulum (ER) in the muscle cell. When a nerve signal stimulates the muscle fiber, the ER releases Ca^{++} into the cytoplasm. There, the Ca^{++} ions bind to the blocking proteins in thin filaments and permit actin to react with myosin. The myosin heads connect to actin, pull, release, and then pull again. This ratcheting of myosin heads thus pulls the thin filaments toward the center of the sarcomere—producing the muscle contraction (Figure 7-4).

The contraction process of a muscle cell also requires energy. This energy is supplied by glucose and other nutrients. The energy must be transferred to myosin heads by adenosine triphosphate (ATP) molecules, the energy-transfer molecules of the cell. Oxygen is required to transfer energy to ATP and make it available to the myosin heads, so it is not surprising that many muscles have high oxygen requirements. To supplement the oxygen carried to muscle fibers by the hemoglobin of blood, muscle fibers contain **myoglobin** (MY-oh-GLO-bin)—a red, oxygen-storing pigment similar to hemoglobin. We discuss the processes of transferring energy to ATP to cellular processes in Chapter 16.

and shorten the sarcomere and thus the entire muscle. When the muscle relaxes, the sarcomeres can return to resting length, and the filaments resume their resting positions.

An explanation of how a skeletal muscle contracts is provided by the **sliding filament model.**

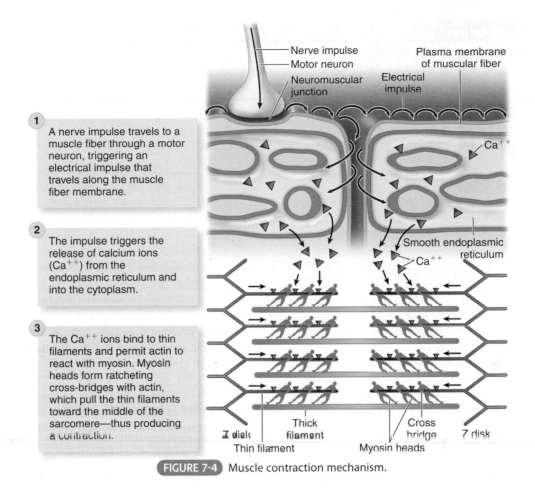

1 A nerve impulse travels to a muscle fiber through a motor neuron, triggering an electrical impulse that travels along the muscle fiber membrane.

2 The impulse triggers the release of calcium ions (Ca^{++}) from the endoplasmic reticulum and into the cytoplasm.

3 The Ca^{++} ions bind to thin filaments and permit actin to react with myosin. Myosin heads form ratcheting cross-bridges with actin, which pull the thin filaments toward the middle of the sarcomere—thus producing a contraction.

Nerve impulse
Motor neuron
Neuromuscular junction
Plasma membrane of muscular fiber
Electrical impulse
Ca^{++}
Smooth endoplasmic reticulum
Ca^{++}
Z disk
Thick filament
Thin filament
Cross bridge
Z disk
Myosin heads

FIGURE 7-4 Muscle contraction mechanism.

QUICK CHECK

1. What are the three main types of muscle tissue? How do they differ?
2. What is a muscle's origin? Its insertion?
3. How do a muscle's myofilaments provide the mechanism for movement?

FUNCTIONS OF SKELETAL MUSCLE

The three primary functions of the muscular system are:

1. Movement
2. Posture or muscle tone
3. Heat production

Movement

Muscles move bones by pulling on them. Because the length of a skeletal muscle becomes shorter as its fibers contract, the bones to which the muscle attaches move closer together. As a rule, only the insertion bone moves. Look again at Figure 7-2. As the ball is lifted, the shortening of the muscle body pulls the insertion bone toward the origin bone. The origin bone stays put, holding firm, while the insertion bone moves toward it. One tremendously important function of skeletal muscle contractions therefore is to produce body movements. Remember this simple rule: a muscle's insertion bone moves toward its origin bone. It can help you understand muscle actions.

Although we will use the shortening of a muscle as our primary example of muscle action in this chapter, it is important to remember that muscles can also produce tension as they extend. This occurs when muscles lengthen under tension, as the muscle insertion is pulled by a load away from the origin. For example, when you lower a heavy bowling ball from your shoulder the muscles in your arm produce tension as they lengthen and allow you to gently lower it—otherwise the ball would suddenly

Muscle Function
Andrew F. Huxley (b. 1917)

The British physiologist Andrew F. Huxley is largely responsible for explaining how muscle fibers contract. After making pioneering discoveries in how nerves conduct impulses, a feat for which he shared the 1963 Nobel Prize in Medicine or Physiology, Huxley turned his attention to muscle fibers. It was he who, in the 1950s, proposed the sliding filament model along with its mechanical explanation of muscle contraction.

Today, research physiologists continue to find out more about how muscle fibers work. These discoveries are being applied in many different professions. For example, nutritionists use this information in advising athletes and others concerning what and when to eat to maximize muscular strength and endurance. Athletes themselves, along with their coaches and trainers, use current concepts of muscle science in helping them improve their performance. Of course, health professionals such as physicians, nurses, and physical therapists use information about muscular problems such as myasthenia gravis and muscular dystrophy to help treat patients. Many other professions, such as massage therapy, occupational therapy, ergonomics, physical education and fitness, dance, art, and biomechanical engineering also rely on up-to-date information on muscle structure and function.

fall and possibly cause injury. Tension during muscle lengthening is often called *eccentric contraction.*

Voluntary muscular movement is normally smooth and free of jerks and tremors because skeletal muscles generally work in coordinated teams, not singly. Several muscles contract while others relax to produce almost any movement that you can imagine. Of all the muscles contracting simultaneously, the one that is mainly responsible for producing a particular movement is called the **prime mover** for that movement. The other muscles that help in producing the movement are called **synergist** (SIN-er-jists) **muscles.** As prime movers and synergist muscles at a joint contract, other muscles, called **antagonist** (an-TAG-oh-nist) **muscles,** relax. When antagonist muscles contract, they produce a movement opposite to that of the prime movers and their synergist muscles.

Locate the biceps brachii, brachialis, and triceps brachii muscles in Figure 7-7. All of these muscles are involved in bending and straightening the forearm at the elbow joint. The biceps brachii is the prime mover during bending, and the brachialis is its helper or synergist muscle. When the biceps brachii and brachialis muscles bend the forearm, the triceps brachii relaxes. Therefore while the forearm bends, the triceps brachii is the antagonistic muscle. While the forearm straightens, these three muscles continue to work as a team. However, during straightening, the triceps brachii becomes the prime mover and the biceps brachii and brachialis become the antagonistic muscles. This combined and coordinated activity is what makes our muscular movements smooth and graceful.

Posture

We are able to maintain our body position because of a continuous, low-strength muscle contraction called *muscle tone* or **tonic contraction.** Because relatively few of a muscle's fibers shorten at one time in a tonic contraction, the muscle as a whole does not shorten, and no movement occurs. Consequently, tonic contractions do not move any body parts. They do hold muscles in position, however. In other words, muscle tone maintains **posture.** Good posture means that body parts are held in the positions that favor best function. These positions balance the distribution of weight and therefore put the least strain on muscles, tendons, ligaments, and bones.

Skeletal muscle tone maintains posture by counteracting the pull of gravity. Gravity tends to pull the head and trunk down and forward, but the tone in certain back and neck muscles pulls just hard enough in the opposite direction to overcome the force of gravity and hold the head and trunk erect.

Heat Production

Healthy survival depends on our ability to maintain a constant body temperature. A fever or elevation in body temperature of only a degree or two above 37° C (98.6° F) is almost always a sign of illness. Just as serious is a fall in body temperature. Any decrease below normal, a condition called **hypothermia** (hye-poh-THER-mee-ah), drastically affects cellular activity and normal body function. The contraction of muscle fibers produces most of the heat required to maintain body temperature.

Energy required to produce a muscle contraction is obtained from ATP. Some of the energy transferred to ATP and released during a muscular contraction is used to shorten the muscle fibers. However, much of the energy is lost as heat during its transfer to ATP. This heat helps us to maintain our body temperature at a constant level. But sometimes the heat from generating ATP during heavy muscle use can produce too much heat, and we have to sweat or shed layers of clothing to cool back down to our set point temperature.

Fatigue

If muscle fibers are stimulated repeatedly without adequate periods of rest, the strength of the muscle contraction decreases, resulting in **fatigue.** If repeated stimulation occurs, the strength of the contraction continues to decrease, and eventually the muscle loses its ability to contract.

During exercise, the stored ATP required for muscle contraction becomes depleted. Formation of more ATP results in a rapid consumption of oxygen and nutrients, often outstripping the ability of the muscle's blood supply to replenish them. When oxygen supplies run low, the muscle fibers switch to a type of energy conversion that does not require oxygen. This process produces lactic acid that may contribute to a burning sensation in muscle during exercise. The simple term **oxygen debt** describes the continued increased metabolism that must occur in a cell to remove excess lactic acid that accumulates during prolonged exercise. Thus the depleted energy reserves are replaced. Labored breathing after the cessation of exercise is required to "pay the debt" of oxygen required for the metabolic effort. The technical name for oxygen debt used by exercise physiologists is *excess post-exercise oxygen consumption (EPOC),* a term that more directly describes what happens after exercise.

The oxygen debt mechanism is a good example of homeostasis at work. The body returns the cells' energy and oxygen reserves to normal, resting levels.

ROLE OF OTHER BODY SYSTEMS IN MOVEMENT

Remember that muscles do not function alone. Other structures, such as bones and joints, must function along with them. Most skeletal muscles

---

 Health and Well-Being

Slow and Fast Muscle Fibers

Sports physiologists know there are three basic skeletal muscle fiber types in the body: slow, fast, and intermediate fibers. Each type is best suited to a particular style of muscular contraction—a fact that is useful when considering how different muscles are used in various athletic activities.

Slow fibers are also called "red fibers" because they have a high content of oxygen-storing myoglobin (a red pigment similar to hemoglobin). Slow fibers are best suited to endurance activities such as long-distance running (pictured) because they do not fatigue easily. Muscles that maintain body position—posture—have a proportion of slow fibers.

Fast fibers are also called "white fibers" because they have a low red myoglobin content. Fast fibers are best suited for quick, powerful contractions because even though they fatigue quickly, they can produce a great amount of ATP very quickly. Fast fibers are well suited to sprinting and weightlifting events. Muscles that move the fingers have a high proportion of fast fibers—a big help when playing computer games or musical instruments.

Intermediate fibers have characteristics between the extremes of slow and fast fibers. This muscle type is found in muscles such as the calf muscle (gastrocnemius), which is used both for posture and occasional brief, powerful contractions such as jumping.

Each muscle of the body is a mixture of varying proportions of slow, fast, and intermediate fibers.

cause movements by pulling on bones across movable joints.

However, the respiratory, circulatory, nervous, muscular, and skeletal systems all play essential roles in producing normal movements. This fact has great practical importance. For example, a person might have perfectly normal muscles and still not be able to move normally. He or she might have a nervous system disorder that shuts off impulses to certain skeletal muscles, which results in **paralysis.** *Multiple sclerosis (MS)* acts in this way, but so do some other conditions such as a brain hemorrhage, a brain tumor, or a spinal cord injury. Skeletal system disorders, especially arthritis, have disabling effects on body movement. Muscle functioning, then, depends on the functioning of many other parts of the body. This fact illustrates a principle that is repeated often in this book. It can be simply stated: Each part of the body is one of many components in a large, interactive system. The normal function of one part depends on the normal function of the other parts.

> **✓ QUICK CHECK**
>
> 1. What are the three primary functions of the muscular system?
> 2. When a prime mover muscle contracts, what does its antagonist do?
> 3. How would you define the term *posture*?
> 4. How does muscle function affect body temperature?
> 5. What is *oxygen debt*?

MOTOR UNIT

Before a skeletal muscle can contract and pull on a bone to move it, the muscle must first be stimulated by nerve impulses. Muscle fibers are stimulated by a nerve fiber called a **motor neuron** (Figure 7-5). The point of contact between the nerve ending and the muscle fiber is called a **neuromuscular junction (NMJ).** Signal chemicals called *neurotransmitters* are released by the motor neuron in response to a nervous impulse. These chemicals then generate events within the muscle

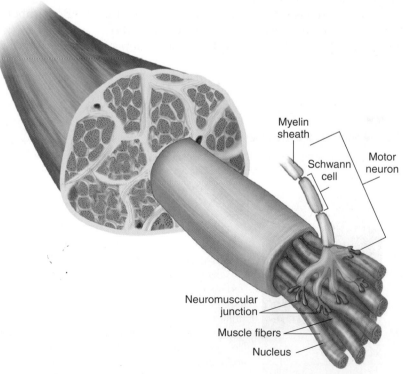

Myelin sheath
Schwann cell
Motor neuron
Neuromuscular junction
Muscle fibers
Nucleus

FIGURE 7-5 **Motor neuron.** A motor unit consists of one motor neuron and the muscle fibers supplied by its branches.

fiber that result in contraction or shortening of the muscle fiber. A single motor neuron, with the muscle fibers it innervates, is called a **motor unit** (see Figure 7-5).

MUSCLE STIMULUS

In a laboratory setting a single muscle fiber can be isolated and subjected to stimuli of varying intensities so that it can be studied. Such experiments show that a muscle fiber does not contract until an applied stimulus reaches a certain level of intensity. The minimal level of stimulation required to cause a fiber to contract is called the **threshold stimulus.**

When a muscle fiber is subjected to a threshold stimulus, it contracts completely. Because of this, muscle fibers are said to respond **"all or none."** However, a muscle is composed of many muscle fibers that are controlled by different motor units and that have different threshold-stimulus levels. Although each fiber in a muscle such as the biceps brachii responds all or none when subjected to a threshold stimulus, the muscle as a whole does not. This fact has tremendous importance in everyday life. It allows you to pick up a 2-liter bottle of soda or a 20-kg weight because different numbers of motor units can be activated for different loads. Once activated, however, each fiber always responds all or none.

TYPES OF SKELETAL MUSCLE CONTRACTION

In addition to the specialized tonic contraction of muscle that maintains muscle tone and posture, other types of contraction also occur. These additional types of muscle contraction include the following:

1. Twitch contraction
2. Tetanic contraction
3. **Isotonic contraction**
4. Isometric contraction

Twitch and Tetanic Contractions

A **twitch** is a quick, jerky response to a stimulus. Twitch contractions can be seen in isolated muscles during research, but they play a minimal role in normal muscle activity. To accomplish the coordinated and fluid muscular movements needed for most daily tasks, muscles must contract not in a jerky but in a smooth and sustained way.

A **tetanic contraction** is a more sustained and steady response than a twitch. It is produced by a series of stimuli bombarding the muscle in rapid succession. Contractions "melt" together to produce a sustained contraction, or **tetanus.** About 30 stimuli per second, for example, evoke a tetanic contraction in certain types of skeletal muscle. Tetanic contraction is not necessarily a maximal contraction in which each muscle fiber responds at the same time. In most cases, only a few groups of muscle fibers undergo contractions at any one time.

Isotonic Contraction

In most cases, **isotonic contraction** of muscle produces movement at a joint. With this type of contraction, the muscle changes length, and the insertion end moves relative to the point of origin (Figure 7-6, *A*).

There are two types of isotonic contraction. One is **concentric contraction,** in which the muscle shortens. The other is **eccentric contraction,** in which the muscle lengthens but still provides work. For example lifting this book requires concentric contraction of the biceps muscle that flexes your elbow. Lowering the book slowly and safely requires eccentric contraction of the biceps muscle. Thus what we call muscle "contraction" really means any pulling of the muscle whether it shortens or not.

Walking, running, breathing, lifting, twisting, and most body movements are examples of isotonic contraction.

Isometric Contraction

Contraction of a skeletal muscle does not always produce movement. Sometimes it increases the tension within a muscle but does not change the length of the muscle. When the muscle contracts and no movement results, it is called an **isometric contraction.** The word *isometric* comes from Greek words that mean "equal measure." In other words, a muscle's length during an isometric contraction and during relaxation is about equal. Although muscles do not shorten (and thus produce no movement) during isometric contractions, tension

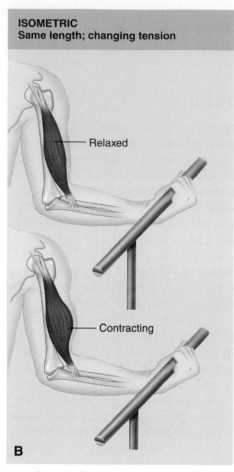

FIGURE 7-6 Types of muscle contraction. **A,** In isotonic contraction the muscle changes length, producing movement. **B,** In isometric contraction the muscle pulls forcefully against a load but does not shorten.

within them increases (Figure 7-6, *B*). Because of this, repeated isometric contractions make muscles grow larger and stronger. Pushing against a wall or other immovable object is a good example of isometric exercise. Although no movement occurs and the muscle does not shorten, its internal tension increases dramatically.

EFFECTS OF EXERCISE ON SKELETAL MUSCLES

We know that exercise is good for us. Some of the benefits of regular, properly practiced exercise are greatly improved muscle tone, better posture,

To learn more about types of skeletal muscle contractions, go to AnimationDirect on your CD-ROM.

more efficient heart and lung function, less fatigue, and looking and feeling better.

Skeletal muscles undergo changes that correspond to the amount of work that they normally do. During prolonged inactivity, muscles usually shrink in mass, a condition called **disuse atrophy.** Exercise, on the other hand, may cause an increase in muscle size called **hypertrophy.**

Muscle hypertrophy can be enhanced by **strength training,** which involves contracting muscles against heavy resistance. Isometric exercises and weight lifting are common strength-training activities. This type of training results in increased numbers of myofilaments in each muscle fiber. Although the number of muscle fibers stays the same, the increased number of myofilaments greatly increases the mass of the muscle.

Endurance training, often called **aerobic training,** does not usually result in muscle

Clinical Application

Carpal Tunnel Syndrome

Some physicians specialize in the field of occupational health, the study of health matters related to work or the workplace. Many problems seen by occupational health experts are caused by repetitive motions of the wrists or other joints. Word processors (typists) and meat cutters, for example, are at risk of developing conditions caused by repetitive motion injuries.

One common problem often caused by such repetitive motion is **tenosynovitis** (ten-oh-sin-oh-VYE-tis)—inflammation of the tendon sheath. Tenosynovitis can be painful, and the swelling characteristic of this condition can limit movement in affected parts of the body. For example, swelling of the tendon sheath around tendons in an area of the wrist known as the *carpal tunnel* can limit movement of the wrist, hand, and fingers. The figure shows the relative positions of the tendon sheath and medial nerve within the carpal tunnel. If this swelling, or any other lesion in the carpal tunnel, presses on the *median nerve*, a condition called **carpal tunnel syndrome** may result. Because the median nerve connects to the palm and radial side (thumb side) of the hand, carpal tunnel syndrome is characterized by weakness, pain, and tingling in this part of the hand. The pain and tingling may also radiate to the forearm and shoulder. Prolonged and severe cases of carpal tunnel syndrome may be relieved by injection of anti-inflammatory agents. A permanent cure is sometimes

accomplished by surgical cutting or removal of the swollen tissue pressing on the median nerve.

hypertrophy. Instead, this type of exercise program increases a muscle's ability to sustain moderate exercise over a long period. Aerobic activities such as running, bicycling, or other primarily isotonic movements increase the number of blood vessels in a muscle without significantly increasing its size. The increased blood flow allows a more efficient delivery of oxygen and glucose to muscle fibers during exercise. Aerobic training also causes an increase in the number of mitochondria in muscle fibers. This allows production of more ATP as a rapid energy source.

QUICK CHECK

1. What is a *motor unit?*
2. How does a muscle produce different levels of strength?
3. What is the difference between *isotonic* and *isometric* muscle contractions?
4. How does strength training affect a person's muscles?

MOVEMENTS PRODUCED BY SKELETAL MUSCLE CONTRACTIONS

The particular type of movement that at any joint depends on the muscle acting at that joint, on their origin and insertion points, on the shapes of the bones involved, and the joint type (see Chapter 6). Muscles acting on some joints produce movement in several directions, whereas only limited movement is possible at other joints. The terms most often used to describe body movements are as follows:

1. Flexion
2. Extension
3. Abduction
4. Adduction
5. Rotation
6. Supination and pronation
7. Dorsiflexion and plantar flexion
8. Inversion and eversion

Flexion is a movement that makes the angle between two bones at their joint smaller than it was at the beginning of the movement. Most flexions are movements commonly described as bending. If you bend your elbow or your knee, you flex it. **Extension** movements are the opposite of flexions. They make the angle between two bones at their joint larger than it was at the beginning of the movement. Therefore, extensions are straightening or stretching movements rather than bending movements. Figures 7-7 and 7-8 illustrate flexion and extension of the elbow and knee.

Abduction means moving a part away from the midline of the body, such as moving your arm out to the side. **Adduction** means moving a part toward the midline, such as bringing your arms down to your sides from an elevated position. Figure 7-9, *A*, shows abduction and adduction.

Rotation is movement around a longitudinal axis. You rotate your head and neck by moving your skull from side to side as in shaking your head "no" (Figure 7-9, *B*). **Circumduction** moves a part so that its distal end moves in a circle. When a pitcher winds up to throw a ball, she circumducts her arm.

Supination and **pronation** refer to hand positions that result from rotation of the forearm. (The term *prone* refers to the body as a whole lying face down. *Supine* means lying face up.) Supination results in a hand position with the palm turned to the anterior position (as in the anatomical position), and pronation occurs when you turn the palm of your hand so that it faces posteriorly (Figure 7-9, *C*).

Dorsiflexion and **plantar flexion** refer to ankle movements. In dorsiflexion the dorsum, or top, of the foot is elevated with the toes pointing upward. In plantar flexion the bottom of the foot is directed downward so that you are in effect standing on your toes (Figure 7-9, *D*).

Inversion and **eversion** are also ankle movements. Inversion moves turn the ankle so that the bottom of the foot faces toward the midline of the body (Figure 7-9, *E*). Eversion turns the ankle in the opposite direction, so that the bottom of the foot faces toward the side of the body (Figure 7-9, *F*).

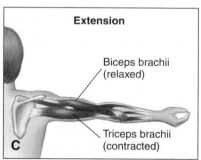

FIGURE 7-7 Flexion and extension of the elbow. **A** and **B,** When the elbow is flexed, the biceps brachii contracts while its antagonist, the triceps brachii, relaxes. **B** and **C,** When the elbow is extended, the biceps brachii relaxes while the triceps brachii contracts.

FIGURE 7-8 Flexion and extension of the knee. **A** and **B,** When the knee flexes, muscles of the hamstring group contract while their antagonists in the quadriceps femoris group relax. **B** and **C,** When the knee extends, the hamstring muscles relax while the quadriceps femoris muscle contracts.

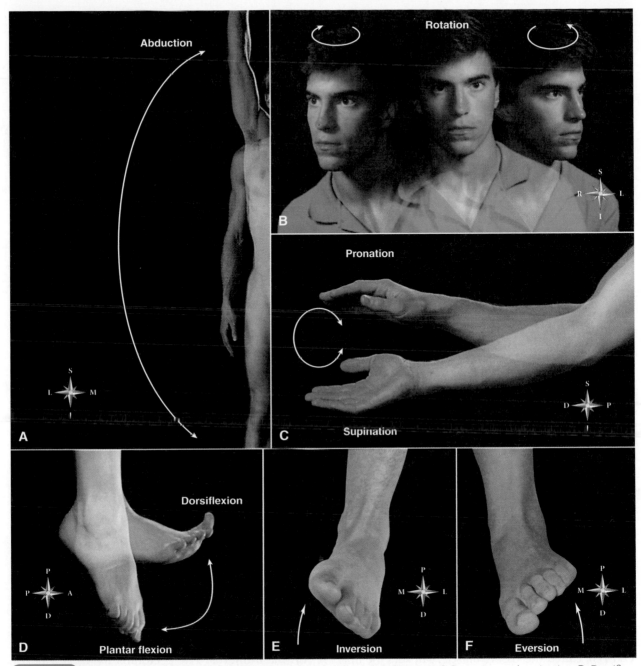

FIGURE 7-9 Examples of body movements. **A,** Adduction and abduction. **B,** Rotation. **C,** Pronation and supination. **D,** Dorsiflex-ion and plantar flexion. **E,** Inversion. **F,** Eversion.

As you study the illustrations and learn to rec-ognize the muscles discussed in this chapter, you should attempt to group them according to func-tion, as in Table 7-1. You will note, for example, that flexors produce many of the movements used for walking, sitting, swimming, typing, and many other activities. Extensors also function in these activities but perhaps play their most important role in maintaining an upright posture.

To learn more about movement produced by skeletal muscle contractions, go to AnimationDirect on your CD-ROM.

TABLE 7-1

Muscles Grouped According to Function

PART MOVED	FLEXORS	EXTENSORS	ABDUCTORS	ADDUCTORS
Upper arm	Pectoralis major	Latissimus dorsi	Deltoid	Pectoralis major and latissimus dorsi contracting together
Lower arm	Biceps brachii	Triceps brachii	None	None
Thigh	Iliopsoas and sartorius	Gluteus maximus	Gluteus medius	Adductor group
Lower leg	Hamstrings	Quadriceps group	None	None
Foot	Tibialis anterior	Gastrocnemius and soleus	Fibularis longus	Tibialis anterior

---

✓ QUICK CHECK

1. When a person flexes the knee, what movement is this?
2. What happens when a person abducts his or her arm?
3. How is dorsiflexion of the foot performed?

SKELETAL MUSCLE GROUPS

In the paragraphs that follow, representative muscles from the most important skeletal muscle groups are discussed. Refer to Figure 7-10 often so that you will be able to see a muscle as you read about its placement on the body and its function. Table 7-2 identifies and groups muscles according to function and provides information about muscle action and points of origin and insertion. Keep in mind that muscles move bones, and the bones that they move are their insertion bones.

Muscles of the Head and Neck

The *muscles of facial expression* (Figure 7-11) allow us to communicate many different emotions nonverbally. Contraction of the **frontal muscle,** for example, allows you to raise your eyebrows in surprise and furrow the skin of your forehead into a frown. The **orbicularis oris** (or-bik-yoo-LAIR-is OH-ris), called the *kissing muscle,* puckers the lips. The **zygomaticus** (zye-goh-MAT-i-kus) elevates the corners of the mouth and lips and has been called the *smiling muscle.*

The *muscles of mastication* are responsible for closing the mouth and producing chewing movements. The term **mastication** refers to chewing. As a group, they are among the strongest muscles in the body. The two largest muscles of the group, identified in Figure 7-11, are the **masseter** (mas-EET-er), which elevates the mandible, and the **temporal** (TEM-poh-ral), which assists the masseter in closing the jaw.

The **sternocleidomastoid** (stern-oh-klye-doh-MAS-toyd) and **trapezius** (trah-PEE-zee-us) muscles are easily identified in Figures 7-10 and 7-11. The two sternocleidomastoid muscles are located on the anterior surface of the neck. They originate on the sternum and then pass up and cross the neck to insert on the mastoid process of the skull. Working together, they flex the head on the chest. If only one contracts, the head is both flexed and tilted to the opposite side. The triangular-shaped trapezius muscles form the line from each shoulder to the neck on its posterior surface. They have a wide line of origin extending from the base of the skull down the spinal column to the last thoracic vertebra. When contracted, the trapezius muscles help elevate the shoulders and extend the head backward.

Muscles That Move the Upper Extremities

The upper extremity is attached to the thorax by the fan-shaped **pectoralis** (pek-teh-RAH-liss) **major** muscle, which covers the upper chest, and by the **latissimus** (lah-TIS-i-muss) **dorsi** muscle, which originates from structures over the lower back (Figures 7-10 and 7-12). Both muscles insert on the humerus. The pectoralis major is a flexor, and the latissimus dorsi is an extensor of the upper arm.

The **deltoid** muscle forms the thick, rounded prominence over the shoulder and upper arm (see Figure 7-10). The muscle takes its origin from the scapula and clavicle and inserts on the humerus. It is a powerful abductor of the upper arm.

As the name implies, the **biceps brachii** (bye-seps BRAY-kee-eye) is a two-headed muscle that serves as a primary flexor of the forearm (see

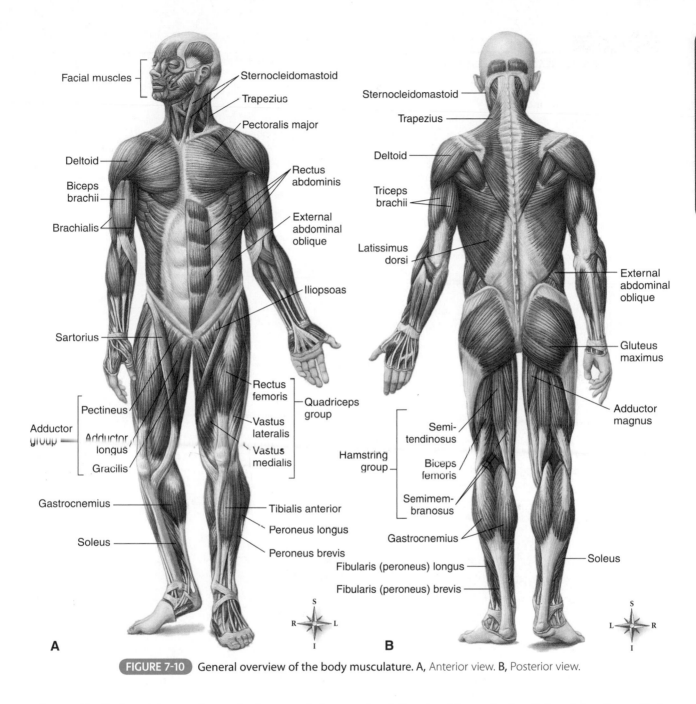

Facial muscles
Sternocleidomastoid
Trapezius
Pectoralis major
Deltoid
Biceps brachii
Brachialis
Rectus abdominis
External abdominal oblique
Iliopsoas
Sartorius
Rectus femoris
Vastus lateralis
Vastus medialis
Quadriceps group
Pectineus
Adductor group
Adductor longus
Gracilis
Gastrocnemius
Soleus
Tibialis anterior
Peroneus longus
Peroneus brevis

Sternocleidomastoid
Trapezius
Deltoid
Triceps brachii
Latissimus dorsi
External abdominal oblique
Gluteus maximus
Adductor magnus
Hamstring group
Semitendinosus
Biceps femoris
Semimembranosus
Gastrocnemius
Soleus
Fibularis (peroneus) longus
Fibularis (peroneus) brevis

A

B

FIGURE 7-10   General overview of the body musculature. **A,** Anterior view. **B,** Posterior view.

Figure 7-10). It originates from the bones of the shoulder girdle and inserts on the radius in the forearm.

The **triceps brachii** is on the posterior or back surface of the upper arm. It has three heads of origin from the shoulder girdle and inserts into the olecranon process of the ulna. The triceps is an extensor of the elbow and thus performs a straightening function. Because this muscle is responsible for delivering blows during fights, it is often called the *boxer's muscle*.

Muscles of the Trunk ✴

The muscles of the anterior or front side of the abdomen are arranged in three layers, with the fibers in each layer running in different directions much like the layers of wood in a sheet of plywood

TABLE 7-2

Principal Muscles of the Body

MUSCLE	FUNCTION	INSERTION	ORIGIN
Muscles of the Head and Neck			
Frontal	Raises eyebrow	Skin of eyebrow	Occipital bone
Orbicularis oculi	Closes eye	Maxilla and frontal bone	Maxilla and frontal bone (encircles eye)
Orbicularis oris	Draws lips together	Encircles lips	Encircles lips
Zygomaticus	Elevates corners of mouth and lips	Angle of mouth and upper lip	Zygomatic
Masseter	Closes jaw	Mandible	Zygomatic arch
Temporal	Closes jaw	Mandible	Temporal region of the skull
Sternocleidomastoid	Rotates and flexes head and neck	Mastoid process	Sternum and clavicle
Trapezius	Extends head and neck	Scapula	Skull and upper vertebrae
Muscles That Move the Upper Extremities			
Pectoralis major	Flexes and helps adduct upper arm	Humerus	Sternum, clavicle, and upper rib cartilages
Latissimus dorsi	Extends and helps adduct upper arm	Humerus	Vertebrae and ilium
Deltoid	Abducts upper arm	Humerus	Clavicle and scapula
Biceps brachii	Flexes elbow	Radius	Scapula
Triceps brachii	Extends elbow	Ulna	Scapula and humerus
Muscles of the Trunk			
External oblique	Compresses abdomen	Midline of abdomen	Lower thoracic cage
Internal oblique	Compresses abdomen	Midline of abdomen	Pelvis
Transversus abdominis	Compresses abdomen	Midline of abdomen	Ribs, vertebrae, and pelvis
Rectus abdominis	Flexes trunk	Lower rib cage	Pubis
Muscles That Move the Lower Extremities			
Iliopsoas	Flexes thigh or trunk	Femur	Ilium and vertebrae
Sartorius	Flexes thigh and rotates lower leg	Tibia	Ilium
Gluteus maximus	Extends thigh	Femur	Ilium, sacrum, coccyx
Adductor Group			
Adductor longus	Adducts thigh	Femur	Pubis
Gracilis	Adducts thigh	Tibia	Pubis
Pectineus	Adducts thigh	Femur	Pubis
Hamstring Group			
Semimembranosus	Flexes knee	Tibia	Ischium
Semitendinosus	Flexes knee	Tibia	Ischium
Biceps femoris	Flexes knee	Fibula	Ischium and femur
Quadriceps Group			
Rectus femoris	Extends knee	Tibia	Ilium
Vastus lateralis, intermedius, and medialis	Extend knee	Tibia	Femur
Fibularis Group			
Fibularis longus and brevis	Evert and plantar flex ankle	Tarsal and metatarsals (ankle and foot)	Tibia and fibula
Tibialis Anterior	Dorsiflexes ankle	Metatarsals (foot)	Tibia
Gastrocnemius	Plantar flexes ankle	Calcaneus (heel)	Femur
Soleus	Plantar flexes ankle	Calcaneus (heel)	Tibia and fibula

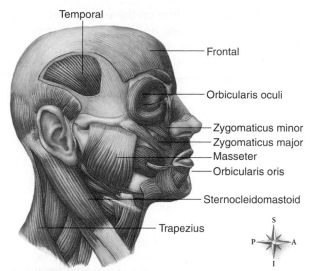

FIGURE 7-11 Muscles of the head and neck. Muscles that produce most facial expressions surround the eyes, nose, and mouth. Large muscles of mastication stretch from the upper skull to the lower jaw. These powerful muscles produce chewing movements. The neck muscles connect the skull to the trunk of the body, rotating the head or bending the neck.

(see Figure 7-12). The result is a very strong "girdle" of muscle that covers and supports the abdominal cavity and its internal organs.

The three layers of muscle in the anterolateral (side) abdominal walls are arranged as follows: the outermost layer or **external oblique;** a middle layer or **internal oblique;** and the innermost layer or **transversus abdominis.** In addition to these sheetlike muscles, the band- or strap-shaped **rectus abdominis** muscle runs down the midline of the abdomen from the thorax to the pubis. The rectus abdominis and external oblique muscles can be seen in Figure 7-12. In addition to protecting the abdominal viscera, the rectus abdominis flexes the spinal column.

The *respiratory muscles* are discussed in Chapter 14. **Intercostal muscles,** located between the ribs, and the sheetlike **diaphragm** separating the thoracic and abdominal cavities change the size and shape of the chest during breathing. As a result, air is moved into or out of the lungs.

Muscles That Move the Lower Extremities

The **iliopsoas** (il-ee-op-SO-us) originates from deep within the pelvis and the lower vertebrae to insert on the lesser trochanter of the femur and capsule of the hip joint. It is generally classified as a flexor of the thigh and an important postural muscle that stabilizes and keeps the trunk from falling over backward when you stand. However, if the thigh is fixed so that it cannot move, the iliopsoas flexes the *trunk.* An example would be doing sit-ups.

The **gluteus maximus** (GLOO-tee-us MAX-i-mus) forms the outer contour and much of the

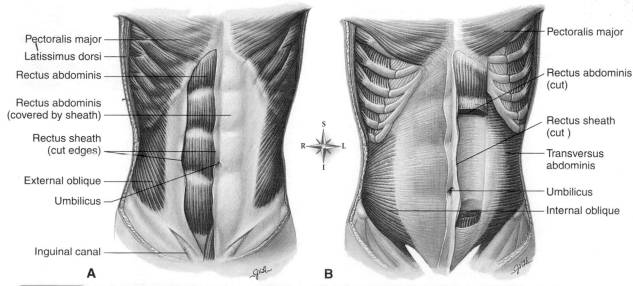

FIGURE 7-12 Muscles of the trunk. **A,** Anterior view showing superficial muscles. **B,** Anterior view showing deeper muscles.

substance of the buttock. It is an important extensor of the thigh (see Figure 7-10) and supports the torso in the erect position.

The **adductor muscles** originate on the bony pelvis and insert on the femur. They are located on the inner or medial side of the thighs. These muscles adduct, or press, the thighs together.

The three **hamstring muscles** are called the *semimembranosus, semitendinosus,* and *biceps femoris.* Acting together, they serve as powerful flexors of the lower leg (see Figure 7-10). They originate on the ischium and insert on the tibia or fibula.

The **quadriceps femoris** (KWOD-reh-seps feh-MOR-is) muscle group covers the upper thigh. The four thigh muscles—the *rectus femoris* and three *vastus* muscles—extend the lower leg (see Figure 7-10 and Table 7-2). One component of the quadri-

ceps group has its origin on the pelvis, and the remaining three originate on the femur. All four insert on the tibia. Only two of the vastus muscles are visible in Figure 7-10. The vastus intermedius is covered by the rectus femoris and is not visible.

The **tibialis** (tib-ee-AL-is) **anterior** muscle (see Figure 7-10) is located on the anterior or front surface of the leg. It dorsiflexes the foot. The **gastrocnemius** (gas-trok-NEE-mee-us) is the primary calf muscle. Note in Figure 7-10 that it has two fleshy components arising from both sides of the femur. It inserts through the calcaneal (Achilles) tendon into the heel bone or calcaneus. The gastrocnemius is responsible for plantar flexion of the foot. Since it is used to stand on tiptoe, it is sometimes called the *toe dancer's muscle.* A group of three muscles called the **fibularis group** or

Clinical Application

Muscle Injury

Injuries to skeletal muscles resulting from overexertion or trauma usually result in a *muscle strain.* Muscle strains are characterized by muscle pain, or *myalgia* (my-AL-jee-ah), and involve overstretching or tearing of muscle fibers. If an injury occurs in the area of a joint and a ligament is damaged, the injury may be called a *sprain.*

Any muscle inflammation, including that caused by a muscle strain, is termed *myositis* (my-oh-SYE-tis). If tendon inflammation occurs with myositis, as when one experiences a *charley horse,* the condition is termed *fibromyositis* (fye-broh-my-oh-SYE-tis). Although inflammation may subside in a few hours or days, it usually takes several weeks for damaged muscle fibers to repair themselves. Some damaged muscle cells may be replaced by fibrous tissue, forming scars. Occasionally, hard calcium is deposited in the scar tissue.

Cramps are painful muscle spasms (involuntary twitches). Cramps often result from mild myositis or fibromyositis, but they also can be a symptom of any irritation or of an ion and water imbalance.

Minor trauma to the body, especially a limb, may cause a muscle *bruise* or *contusion* (kon-TOO-zhun). Muscle contusions involve local internal bleeding and inflammation. Severe trauma to a skeletal muscle may cause a *crush injury.* Crush injuries not only greatly damage the affected muscle tissue but also cause the release of muscle fiber contents into the bloodstream, which can be life threatening. For example, the reddish muscle pigment *myoglobin* can accumulate in the blood and cause kidney failure.

Stress-induced muscle tension can result in myalgia and stiffness in the neck and back and is thought to be one

cause of "stress headaches." Headache and back pain clinics use a variety of strategies to treat stress-induced muscle tension. These treatments include massage, biofeedback, and relaxation training.

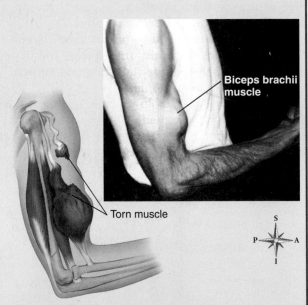

Muscle strain. Severe strain of the biceps brachii muscle. When a muscle is severely strained, it may break in two pieces, causing a visible gap in muscle tissue under the skin. Notice how the broken ends of the muscle reflexively contract (spasm) to form a knot of tissue.

Research, Issues, & Trends

Enhancing Muscle Strength

The most obvious and effective way of increasing skeletal muscle strength is by strength training; that is, regularly pulling against heavy resistance. The maximal amount of muscular strength one can achieve is determined mainly by genetics. However, there are a number of chemical enhancements athletes have tried over the centuries to improve strength. An early fad among athletes in the twentieth century was the overuse of vitamin supplements. Although moderate vitamin supplementation will ensure adequate intake of vitamins necessary for good muscle function, overuse may lead to *hypervitaminosis* and possibly serious consequences.

Another type of chemical often abused by athletes is *anabolic steroids*. Anabolic steroids are usually synthetic de-

rivatives of the male hormone *testosterone*. As with naturally produced testosterone, they do in fact stimulate an increase in muscle size and strength, making them attractive to coaches and athletes wanting to win their events. However, prolonged use of these hormones can cause serious, even life-threatening, hormonal imbalances. For this reason, anabolic steroids are banned from most organized sports.

Sports physiologists are now investigating a whole variety of chemicals, such as creatine phosphate and various coenzymes that are reported to enhance strength or endurance. Always carefully review the latest research findings on these substances with the help of a health or exercise professional before using them yourself, or you may suffer serious health consequences.

---

peroneus group (see Figure 7-10) is found along the sides of the lower leg. As a group, these muscles evert and plantar flex the foot. A long tendon from one component of the group—the *fibularis longus* muscle tendon—forms a support arch for the foot (see Figure 6-20).

QUICK CHECK

1. What do the *muscles of mastication* do for a person?
2. Why is the triceps brachii muscle sometimes called the "boxer's muscle"?
3. What action does the hamstring muscle perform?

OUTLINE SUMMARY

INTRODUCTION
A. Muscular tissue enables the body and its parts to move
  1. Three types of muscle tissue exist in body (see Chapter 3)
  2. Movement caused by muscle cells (called *fibers*) either shortening or contracting
  3. Muscle movement occurs when chemical energy (obtained from food) is converted into mechanical energy

MUSCLE TISSUE
A. Types of muscle tissue (see Figure 7-1)
  1. Skeletal muscle — also called *striated* or *voluntary muscle*
    a. Microscope reveals crosswise stripes or striations
    b. Contractions can be voluntarily controlled
  2. Cardiac muscle — composes bulk of heart
    a. Cardiac muscle fibers are branched
    b. Has dark bands called *intercalated disks*

    c. Cardiac muscle fiber interconnections allow heart to contract efficiently as a unit
  3. Nonstriated muscle, or involuntary muscle — also called *smooth* or *visceral muscle*
    a. Lacks striations when seen under a microscope; appears smooth
    b. Found in walls of hollow structures such as digestive tract, blood vessels, etc.
    c. Contractions not under voluntary control
B. Function — all muscle fibers specialize in contraction (shortening)

STRUCTURE OF SKELETAL MUSCLE
A. Muscle organs — mainly striated muscle fibers and connective tissue
  1. Connective tissue forms "wrappers" around each muscle fiber, around fascicles (groups) of muscle fibers, and around the

entire muscle; fascia surrounds muscle organs and nearby structures
2. Most skeletal muscles extend from one bone across a joint to another bone
3. Regions of a skeletal muscle (see Figure 7-2)
   a. Origin — attachment to the bone that remains relatively stationary or fixed when movement at the joint occurs
   b. Insertion — point of attachment to the bone that moves when a muscle contracts
   c. Body — main part of the muscle
4. Muscles attach to bone by tendons — strong cords or sheets of fibrous connective tissue that extend from the muscle organ; some tendons enclosed in synovial-lined tubes (tendon sheaths) and lubricated by synovial fluid
5. Bursae — small synovial-lined sacs containing a small amount of synovial fluid; located between some tendons and underlying bones

B. Microscopic structure and function (see Figure 7-3)
1. Contractile cells are called *muscle fibers*; connective tissue holds muscle fibers in parallel groupings
2. Fibers of the cytoskeleton form cylinders that contain thick myofilaments (containing myosin) and thin myofilaments (containing mainly actin)
3. Basic functional (contractile) unit called *sarcomere*
   a. Sarcomeres separated from each other by dark bands called *Z lines*
   b. Sliding filament model explains mechanism of contraction
      (1) Thick and thin myofilaments slide past each other to contract
      (2) Contraction requires calcium and energy-rich ATP molecules (see Figure 7-4)

FUNCTIONS OF SKELETAL MUSCLE

A. Movement
1. Muscles produce movement by pulling on bones as a muscle contracts
   a. The insertion bone is pulled closer to the origin bone
   b. Movement occurs at the joint between the origin and the insertion

2. Groups of muscles usually contract to produce a single movement
   a. Prime mover — mainly responsible for producing a given movement
   b. Synergist — helps the prime mover produce a given movement
   c. Antagonist — opposes the action of a prime mover in any given movement

B. Posture
1. A continuous, low-strength muscle contraction called *tonic contraction* (muscle tone) enables us to maintain body position
   a. Only a few of a muscle's fibers shorten at one time
   b. Produces no movement of body parts
   c. Maintains muscle tone called *posture*
2. Good posture favors best body functioning
3. Skeletal muscle tone maintains good posture by counteracting the pull of gravity

C. Heat production
1. Survival depends on the body's ability to maintain a constant body temperature
   a. Fever — an elevated body temperature — often a sign of illness
   b. Hypothermia — a reduced body temperature
2. Contraction of muscle fibers produces most of the heat required to maintain normal body temperature

D. Fatigue
1. Reduced strength of muscle contraction
2. Caused by repeated muscle stimulation without adequate periods of rest
3. Repeated muscular contraction depletes cellular ATP stores and outstrips the ability of the blood supply to replenish oxygen and nutrients
4. Contraction in the absence of adequate oxygen produces lactic acid, which contributes to muscle soreness
5. *Oxygen debt* — term used to describe the metabolic effort required to burn excess lactic acid that may accumulate during prolonged periods of exercise
   a. Labored breathing after strenuous exercise is required to "pay the debt"
   b. This increased metabolism helps restore energy and oxygen reserves to pre-exercise levels

ROLE OF OTHER BODY SYSTEMS IN MOVEMENT

A. Muscle functioning depends on the functioning of many other parts of the body
B. Most muscles cause movements by pulling on bones across movable joints
C. Respiratory, circulatory, nervous, muscular, and skeletal systems play essential roles in producing normal movements
D. Multiple sclerosis, brain hemorrhage, and spinal cord injury are examples of how pathological conditions in other body organ systems can dramatically affect movement

MOTOR UNIT

A. Stimulation of a muscle by a nerve impulse is required before a muscle can shorten and produce movement
B. Motor neuron — nerve cell that transmits an impulse to a muscle, causing contraction
C. Neuromuscular junction (NMJ) — point of contact between a nerve ending and a muscle fiber
D. Motor unit — combination of a motor neuron with the muscle fibers it controls (see Figure 7-5)

MUSCLE STIMULUS

A. A muscle will contract only if an applied stimulus reaches a certain level of intensity
   1. Threshold stimulus — minimal level of stimulation required to cause a muscle fiber to contract
B. Once stimulated by a threshold stimulus, a muscle fiber will contract completely, a response called *all or none*
C. Different muscle fibers in a muscle are controlled by different motor units having different threshold-stimulus levels
   1. Although individual muscle fibers always respond all or none to a threshold stimulus, the muscle as a whole does not
   2. Different motor units responding to different threshold stimuli permit a muscle as a whole to execute contractions of graded force

TYPES OF SKELETAL MUSCLE CONTRACTION

A. Twitch and tetanic contractions
   1. Twitch contractions are laboratory phenomena, not normal muscle activity; they are a single contraction of muscle fibers caused by a single threshold stimulus
   2. Tetanic contractions are sustained muscular contractions caused by stimuli hitting a muscle in rapid succession
B. Isotonic contractions (see Figure 7-6)
   1. Contractions that produce movement at a joint because the muscle changes length
   2. Concentric contractions — the muscle shortens insertion end of the muscle to move toward to the point of origin
   3. Eccentric contractions — the muscle lengthens under tension, thus moving the insertion away from the origin
   4. Most types of body movements (walking, running, etc.) are produced by isotonic contractions
C. Isometric contractions (see Figure 7-6)
   1. Contractions that do not produce movement; the muscle as a whole does not shorten
   2. Although no movement occurs, tension within the muscle increases

EFFECTS OF EXERCISE ON SKELETAL MUSCLES

A. Exercise, if regular and properly practiced, improves muscle tone and posture, results in more efficient heart and lung functioning, and reduces fatigue
B. Muscles change in relation to the amount of work they normally do
   1. Prolonged inactivity causes disuse atrophy
   2. Regular exercise increases muscle size, called *hypertrophy*
C. Strength training is exercise involving contraction of muscles against heavy resistance
   1. Strength training increases the numbers of myofilaments in each muscle fiber, and as a result, the total mass of the muscle increases
   2. Strength training does not increase the number of muscle fibers
D. Endurance training is exercise that increases a muscle's ability to sustain moderate exercise over a long period; it is sometimes called *aerobic training*
   1. Endurance training allows more efficient delivery of oxygen and nutrients to a muscle via increased blood flow
   2. Endurance training does not usually result in muscle hypertrophy

MOVEMENTS PRODUCED BY SKELETAL MUSCLE CONTRACTIONS (See Figures 7-7 through 7-9)
A. Flexion — decreases an angle
B. Extension — increases an angle
C. Abduction — away from the midline
D. Adduction — toward the midline
E. Rotation — around an axis
F. Circumduction — move distal end of a part in a circle
F. Supination and pronation — hand positions that result from twisting of the forearm
G. Dorsiflexion and plantar flexion — foot movements (upward and downward ankle movement)
H. Inversion and eversion — foot movements (sideways)

SKELETAL MUSCLE GROUPS (See Table 7-2)
A. Muscles of the head and neck (see Figures 7-10 and 7-11)
  1. Facial muscles
    a. Orbicularis oculi
    b. Orbicularis oris
    c. Zygomaticus
  2. Muscles of mastication
    a. Masseter
    b. Temporal
  3. Sternocleidomastoid — flexes head
  4. Trapezius — elevates shoulders and extends head

B. Muscles that move the upper extremities
  1. Pectoralis major — flexes upper arm
  2. Latissimus dorsi — extends upper arm
  3. Deltoid — abducts upper arm
  4. Biceps brachii — flexes forearm
  5. Triceps brachii — extends forearm
C. Muscles of the trunk (See Figure 7-12)
  1. Abdominal muscles
    a. Rectus abdominis
    b. External oblique
    c. Internal oblique
    d. Transversus abdominis
  2. Respiratory muscles
    a. Intercostal muscles
    b. Diaphragm
D. Muscles that move the lower extremities
  1. Iliopsoas — flexes thigh
  2. Gluteus maximus — extends thigh
  3. Adductor muscles — adduct thighs
  4. Hamstring muscles — flex lower leg
    a. Semimembranosus
    b. Semitendinosus
    c. Biceps femoris
  5. Quadriceps femoris group — extends lower leg
    a. Rectus femoris
    b. Vastus muscles
  6. Tibialis anterior — dorsiflexes foot
  7. Gastrocnemius — plantar flexes foot
  8. Peroneus group — flexes foot

NEW WORDS

abduct, abduction
actin
adduct, adduction
adductor muscle
aerobic training
all or none
antagonist muscle
biceps brachii
bursa (pl. bursae)
cardiac muscle
carpal tunnel syndrome
circumduct,
  circumduction
concentric contraction
deltoid
diaphragm
disuse atrophy
dorsiflex, dorsiflexion
eccentric contraction
endurance training
evert, eversion
extend, extension

external oblique
fatigue
fibularis group
flex, flexion
frontal muscle
gastrocnemius
gluteus maximus
hamstring muscle
hypertrophy
hypothermia
iliopsoas
insertion
intercostal muscle
internal oblique
invert, inversion
isometric contraction
isotonic contraction
latissimus dorsi
masseter
mastication
motor neuron
motor unit

muscle fiber
myofilament
myoglobin
myosin
neuromuscular junction (NMJ)
orbicularis oris
origin
oxygen debt
paralysis
pectoralis major
peroneus group
plantar flex, plantar flexion
posture
prime mover
pronate, pronation
quadriceps femoris
rectus abdominis
rotate, rotation
sarcomere
skeletal muscle

sliding filament model
smooth muscle
sternocleidomastoid
strength training
supinate, supination
synergist muscle
synovial membrane
temporal
tendon
tendon sheath
tenosynovitis
tetanic contraction, tetanus
threshold stimulus
tibialis anterior
tone, tonic contraction
transversus abdominis
trapezius
triceps brachii
twitch
zygomaticus

REVIEW QUESTIONS

1. Briefly describe the structure of cardiac muscle.
2. Briefly describe the structure of smooth muscle.
3. Briefly describe the structure and give the functions of tendons, bursae, and synovial membranes.
4. Explain how tonic contractions help maintain posture.
5. Give an example of how two body systems other than the muscular system contribute to the movement of the body.
6. Explain twitch and tetanic contractions.
7. Explain isotonic contractions.
8. Explain isometric contractions.
9. What is strength training and what are its results?
10. What is endurance training and what are its results?
11. Describe the following movements: flexion, extension, abduction, adduction, and rotation.
12. Name two muscles of the trunk and give their origin, insertion, and function.
13. Name two muscles of the head or neck and give their origin, insertion, and function.
14. Name two muscles that move the upper extremity and give their origin, insertion, and function.
15. Name three muscles that move the lower extremity and give their origin, insertion, and function.

CRITICAL THINKING

16. Draw and label a relaxed sarcomere, and include actin, myosin, and Z lines. Explain the process that causes the sarcomere to contract.
17. Explain the interaction of the prime mover, the synergist, and the antagonist in efficient movement.
18. Describe the conditions that cause a muscle to develop an "oxygen debt." How is the oxygen debt "paid off"?

CHAPTER TEST

1. _____ is another name for muscle cell.
2. Cardiac muscle makes up the bulk of the tissue of the _____.
3. The muscle attachment to the more movable bone is called the _____.
4. The muscle attachment to the more stationary bone is called the _____.
5. _____ is the protein that makes up the thin myofilaments.
6. _____ is the protein that makes up the thick myofilaments.
7. The _____ is the basic functional unit of contraction in a skeletal muscle.
8. The three functions of the skeletal system are _____, _____, and _____.
9. The molecule _____ supplies energy for muscle contraction.
10. _____ is the waste product produced when the muscle must switch to an energy supplying process that does not require oxygen.
11. A single motor neuron with all the muscle fibers it innervates is called a _____.
12. _____ is the minimal level of stimulation required to cause a muscle fiber to contract.

13. _____ is a type of muscle contraction that produces movement in a joint and allows the muscle to shorten.
14. _____ is a type of muscle contraction that does not produce movement and does not allow the muscle to shorten but does increase muscle tension.
15. _____ is a term describing movement of a body part away from the midline of the body.
16. _____ is a term used to describe the movement that is the opposite of flexion.
17. _____ describes the hand position when the body is in anatomical position.
18. Skeletal muscles can also be called:
    a. visceral muscles
    b. voluntary muscles
    c. cardiac muscles
    d. all of the above
19. Smooth muscles can also be called:
    a. visceral muscles
    b. involuntary muscles
    c. nonstriated muscles
    d. all of the above

Match the muscles in Column A with the locations in Column B.

COLUMN A

20. _____ temporal muscle
21. _____ biceps brachii
22. _____ sartorius
23. _____ gastrocnemius
24. _____ masseter
25. _____ pectoralis major
26. _____ external oblique
27. _____ gluteus maximus
28. _____ sternocleidomastoid
29. _____ rectus abdominis
30. _____ rectus femoris
31. _____ triceps brachii

COLUMN B

a. muscles of the head or neck
b. muscles that move the upper extremity
c. muscles of the trunk
d. muscles that move the lower extremity

OBJECTIVES

AFTER YOU HAVE COMPLETED THIS CHAPTER, YOU SHOULD BE ABLE TO:

1. List the organs and divisions of the nervous system and describe the generalized functions of the system as a whole.
2. Identify the major types of cells in the nervous system and discuss the functions of each.
3. Identify the anatomical and functional components of a three-neuron reflex arc. Compare and contrast the propagation of a nerve impulse along a nerve fiber and across a synaptic cleft.
4. Identify the major anatomical components of the brain and spinal cord and briefly comment on the functions of each.
5. Compare and contrast spinal and cranial nerves.
6. Discuss the anatomical and functional characteristics of the two divisions of the autonomic nervous system.

The Nervous System

8

The normal body must accomplish a gigantic and enormously complex job—keeping itself alive and healthy. Each one of its billions of cells performs some activity that is a part of this function. Control of the body's billions of cells is accomplished in part by two body-wide communication systems: the nervous system and the endocrine system. Both systems transmit information from one part of the body to another, but they do it in different ways. The nervous system transmits information very rapidly by nerve impulses conducted from one body area to another. The endocrine system transmits information more slowly by chemicals secreted by ductless glands into the bloodstream and then circulated from the glands to other parts of the body. Nerve impulses and hormones communicate information to body structures, increasing or decreasing their activities as needed for healthy survival. In other words, the communication systems of the body are also its control and integrating systems. They combine the body's hundreds of functions into its one overall function of keeping itself alive and healthy.

Recall that homeostasis is the balanced and controlled internal environment of the body that is basic to life itself. Homeostasis is possible only if our physiological control and integration systems function properly. Our plan for this chapter is to name the cells, organs, and divisions of the nervous system; discuss the generation of nervous impulses; and then explain how these impulses move between one area of the body and another. We will not only study the major components of the nervous system, such as the brain, spinal cord, and nerves but also learn how they function to maintain and regulate homeostasis. In Chapter 9, we consider the senses.

STUDY TIPS

To make the study of the nervous system more efficient, we suggest these tips:

1. Before starting Chapter 8, review the synopsis of the nervous system in Chapter 4.
2. There is a great deal of material in Chapter 8. It can be made somewhat easier if you divide the chapter into three parts: the microscopic structure and function of the nervous system, the central nervous system, and the peripheral nervous system. However, keep in mind that the nervous system functions as one organized system. The divisions in the system are merely a way to simplify the system; they are not separate entities.
3. It may help to learn the terminology if you remember that neuro- refers to nerves, dendro- means "branch," and oligo- means "few" or "little." So oligodendrocyte, a glia cell, means "a cell with few branches."
4. The function of the nervous system is accomplished by two processes: the conduction of nerve impulses and the passing of the nerve impulses across a synapse. Nerve impulses are an exchange of ions between the interior and exterior of the neuron. The synapse requires the production, release, and deactivation of neurotransmitters. Neurotransmitters function by stimulating receptors in the neuron on the other side of the synapse.
5. When studying the autonomic nervous system, remember the basic function of each part. The parasympathetic nervous system tries to maintain a quiet homeostasis. The sympathetic nervous system prepares the body for emergency situations—the "fight-or-flight" response.
6. The material on the central nervous system can best be learned by using flash cards to match the structure and the function.
7. In your study groups, you should (a) go over the terms from the first part of the chapter; (b) discuss the processes of nerve impulse transmission and what occurs at the synapse; (c) go over the flash cards with the names and functions of the parts of the central nervous system; and (d) review the questions at the end of the chapter and discuss possible test questions.
8. Remember that most of the structures in the central nervous system have more than one function.
9. If you remember the general functions of the sympathetic and parasympathetic nervous system, the specific effects of the systems will be easier to remember.

ORGANS AND DIVISIONS OF THE NERVOUS SYSTEM

The organs of the nervous system as a whole include the brain and spinal cord, the numerous nerves of the body, the special sense organs such as the eyes and ears, and the microscopic sense organs such as those found in the skin. The system as a whole consists of two principal divisions called the *central nervous system* and the *peripheral nervous system* (Figure 8-1). Because the brain and spinal cord occupy a midline or central location in the body, together they are called the **central nervous system,** or **CNS.** Similarly, the usual designation for the nerves of the body is the **peripheral nervous system,** or **PNS.** The term *peripheral* is appropriate because nerves extend to outlying or peripheral parts of the body. A subdivision of the peripheral nervous system, called the **autonomic nervous system,** or **ANS,** consists of structures that regulate the body's automatic or involuntary functions (for example, the heart rate, the contractions of the stomach and intestines, and the secretion of chemical compounds by glands).

 To learn more about the divisions of the nervous system, go to AnimationDirect on your CD-ROM.

CELLS OF THE NERVOUS SYSTEM

The two types of cells found in the nervous system are called **neurons** (NOO-ronz) or nerve cells and **glia** (GLEE-ah), which are support cells. Neurons conduct impulses, whereas glia support neurons.

Neurons

Each neuron consists of three parts: a main part called the neuron **cell body,** one or more branching projections called **dendrites** (DEN-drytes), and one elongated projection known as an **axon.** Identify each part on the neuron shown in Figure 8-2. Dendrites are the processes or projections that transmit impulses to the neuron cell bodies, and axons are the processes that transmit impulses away from the neuron cell bodies.

The three types of neurons are classified according to the direction in which they transmit impulses:

1. Sensory neurons
2. Motor neurons
3. Interneurons

Sensory neurons transmit impulses to the spinal cord and brain from all parts of the body. Sensory neurons are also called **afferent neurons.**

Motor neurons transmit impulses in the opposite direction—away from the brain and spinal cord. They do not conduct impulses to all parts of the body—only to two kinds of tissue—muscle and glandular epithelial tissue. Motor neurons are called **efferent neurons.**

Interneurons conduct impulses from sensory neurons to motor neurons. They also often connect with each other to form complex, central networks of nerve fibers. Interneurons are sometimes called *central* or *connecting* neurons.

The axon shown in Figure 8-2, *B*, is surrounded by a segmented wrapping of a material called **myelin** (MY-eh-lin). Myelin is a white, fatty substance formed by *Schwann cells* that wrap around some axons outside the central nervous system. Such fibers are called **myelinated fibers.** In Figure 8-2, *B*, one such axon has been enlarged to show

FIGURE 8-1 Divisions of the nervous system.

FIGURE 8-2 Neuron. **A,** Diagram of a typical neuron showing dendrites, a cell body, and an axon. **B,** Photomicrograph of a neuron. **C,** Segment of a myelinated axon cut to show detail of the concentric layers of the Schwann cell filled with myelin.

additional detail. **Nodes of Ranvier** (rahn-vee-AY) are indentations between adjacent Schwann cells.

The outer cell membrane of a Schwann cell is called the **neurilemma** (noo ri LEM mah). It is clinically significant that axons in the brain and spinal cord have no neurilemma, because neurilemma plays an essential part in the regeneration of cut and injured axons. Therefore the potential for regeneration in the brain and spinal cord is far less than it is in the peripheral nervous system.

Glia

Glia—or *neuroglia* (noo-ROG-lee-ah)—do not specialize in transmitting impulses. Instead, they are special types of supporting cells. Their name is appropriate because it is derived from the Greek word *glia* meaning "glue." One function of glia cells is to hold the functioning neurons together and protect them. An important reason for discussing glia is that one of the most common types of brain tumor—called **glioma** (glee-OH-mah)—develops from them. We now know that glia perform many different functions, including the regulation of neuron function. Therefore, they not only act as "glue" in the physical sense but also help bring the various functions of nervous tissue together into a coordinated whole.

Glia vary in size and shape (Figure 8-3). Some are relatively large cells that look somewhat like stars because of the threadlike extensions that jut out from their surfaces. These glia cells are called **astrocytes** (ASS-troh-sytes), a word that means "star cells" (see Figure 8-3, *A*). Their threadlike branches attach to neurons and to small blood vessels, holding these structures close to each other. Along with the walls of the blood vessels, astrocyte branches form a two-layer structure called the **blood-brain barrier (BBB).** As its name implies, the BBB separates the blood tissue and nervous tissue to protect vital brain tissue from harmful chemicals that might be in the blood.

Microglia (my-KROG-lee-ah) are smaller than astrocytes. They usually remain stationary, but in inflamed or degenerating brain tissue, they enlarge, move about, and act as microbe-eating scavengers. They surround the microbes, draw them into their cytoplasm, and digest them. They likewise help clean up cell damage resulting from injury or disease. Recall from Chapter 3 that phagocytosis is the scientific name for this important cellular process.

The **oligodendrocytes** (ohl-i-go-DEN-droh-sytes) help to hold nerve fibers together and also serve another and probably more important function: they produce the fatty myelin sheath that envelops nerve fibers located in the brain and spinal cord. **Schwann cells** are glial cells that also form myelin sheaths but do so only in the peripheral nervous system. Notice in Figure 8-3, *C*, that each oligodendrocyte can form part of the myelin sheath around several axons but Schwann cells wrap entirely around only one axon.

> ### ✓ QUICK CHECK
> 1. What is the difference between the central nervous system and the peripheral nervous system?
> 2. What are the major features of a neuron?
> 3. How are glia different from neurons?

NERVES AND TRACTS

A **nerve** is a group of peripheral nerve fibers (axons) bundled together like the strands of a cable. Peripheral nerve fibers usually have a myelin sheath. Because myelin is white, peripheral nerves often look white.

CENTRAL NERVOUS SYSTEM NEUROGLIA

Foot processes

Capillary

Astrocytes

A

Microglia

B

Oligodendrocyte

Nerve fiber

Myelin sheath

C

FIGURE 8-3 Glia. **A,** Astrocytes have extensions attached to blood vessels in the brain. **B,** Microglia within the central nervous system can enlarge and consume microbes by phagocytosis. **C,** Oligodendrocytes have extensions that form myelin sheaths around axons in the central nervous system.

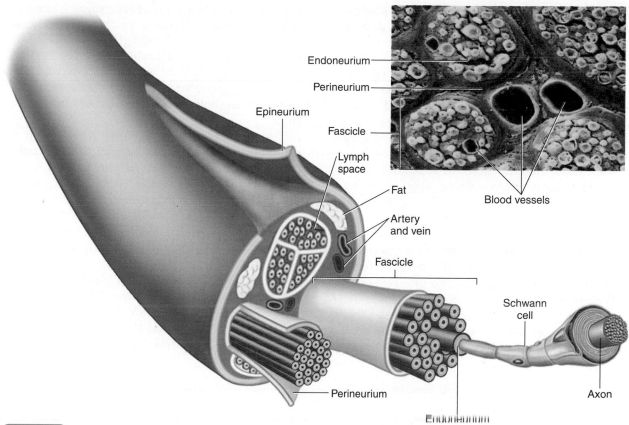

Endoneurium
Perineurium
Epineurium
Fascicle
Lymph space
Fat
Artery and vein
Blood vessels
Fascicle
Schwann cell
Perineurium
Axon
Endoneurium

FIGURE 8-4   **The nerve.** Each nerve contains axons bundled into fascicles. A connective tissue called *epineurium* wraps the entire nerve. Perineurium surrounds each fascicle. Inset shows a scanning electron micrograph of a cross section of a nerve.

Bundles of axons in the CNS, called **tracts,** also are myelinated and thus form the **white matter** of the brain and cord. Brain and cord tissue composed of cell bodies and unmyelinated axons and dendrites is called **gray matter** because of its characteristic gray appearance.

Figure 8-4 shows that each axon in a nerve is surrounded by a thin wrapping of fibrous connective tissue called the **endoneurium** (en-doh-NOO-ree-um). Groups of these wrapped axons are called **fascicles.** Each fascicle is surrounded by a thin, fibrous **perineurium** (pair-i-NOO-ree-um). A tough, fibrous sheath called the **epineurium** (ep-i-NOO-ree-um) covers the whole nerve.

REFLEX ARCS

During every moment of our lives, nerve impulses speed over neurons to and from our spinal cords and brains. If all impulse conduction ceases, life itself ceases. Only neurons can provide the rapid communication between cells that is necessary for maintaining life. Hormonal messages are the only other kind of communications the body can send, and they travel much more slowly than impulses. They can move from one part of the body to another only via circulating blood. Compared with impulse conduction, circulation is a very slow process.

Nerve impulses, also called **action potentials,** can travel over trillions of routes—routes made up of neurons because they are the cells that conduct impulses. Hence the routes traveled by nerve impulses are sometimes spoken of as *neuron pathways.* A basic type of neuron pathway, called a **reflex arc,** is important to nervous system functioning. The simplest kind of reflex arc is a two-neuron arc, so-called because it consists of only two types of neurons: sensory neurons and motor neurons. Three-neuron arcs are the next simplest kind. They, of course, consist of all three kinds of neurons: sensory neurons, interneurons, and motor neurons.

Reflex arcs are like one-way streets: they allow impulse conduction in only one direction. The next paragraph describes this direction in detail. Look frequently at Figure 8-5 as you read it.

Impulse conduction normally starts in receptors. **Receptors** are the beginnings of dendrites of sensory neurons. They are often located at some distance from the spinal cord (in tendons, skin, or mucous membranes, for example). In Figure 8-5 the sensory receptors are located in the quadriceps muscle group. In the reflex that is illustrated there, stretch receptors are stimulated when muscles are stretched as a result of a tap on the patellar ligament from a rubber hammer used by a physician to elicit a reflex during a physical examination. The nerve impulse that is generated, its neurological pathway, and its ultimate "knee-jerk" effect are an example of the simplest form of a two-neuron reflex arc.

In the knee-jerk reflex, only sensory and motor neurons are involved. The nerve impulse that is generated by stimulation of the stretch receptors travels along the length of the sensory neuron's dendrite to its cell body located in the *dorsal (posterior) root ganglion*. A **ganglion** (GANG-lee-un) is a group of nerve-cell bodies located in the PNS. This ganglion is located near the spinal cord. Each spinal ganglion contains not one sensory neuron cell body, as shown in Figure 8-5, but hundreds of them.

The axon of the sensory neuron travels from the cell body in the dorsal root ganglion and ends near the dendrites of another neuron located in the gray matter of the spinal cord. A microscopic space separates the axon ending of one neuron from the dendrites of another neuron. This space is called a **synapse.** The nerve impulse stops at the synapse, chemical signals are sent across the gap, and the impulse then continues along the dendrites, cell body, and axon of the motor neuron.

The motor neuron axon forms a synapse with a structure called an **effector,** an organ that puts nerve signals "into effect." Effectors are muscles or glands, and muscle contractions and gland

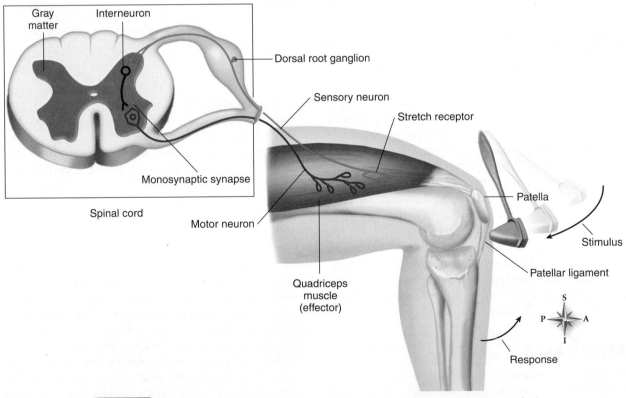

FIGURE 8-5 **Knee-jerk reflex.** The neural pathway involved in the knee-jerk (patellar) reflex.

secretion are the only kinds of reflexes operated by these effectors.

The response to impulse conduction over a reflex arc is called a **reflex.** In short, impulse conduction by a reflex arc causes a reflex to occur. In our example reflex, the nerve impulses that reach the quadriceps muscle (the effector) result in the "knee-jerk" response.

Now turn your attention to the *interneuron* shown in Figure 8-5. Some reflexes involve three rather than two neurons. In these more complex types of responses, an interneuron, in addition to a sensory and a motor neuron, is involved. In three-neuron reflexes, the end of the sensory neuron's axon synapses first with an interneuron before chemical signals are sent across a second synapse, resulting in conduction through the motor neuron. For example, application of an irritating stimulus to the skin of the thigh initiates a three-neuron reflex response that causes contraction of muscles to pull the leg away from the irritant—a three-neuron arc reaction called the **withdrawal reflex**.

All interneurons lie entirely within the gray matter of the brain or spinal cord. Gray matter forms the H-shaped inner core of the spinal cord. Because of the presence of an interneuron, three-neuron reflex arcs have two synapses. A two-neuron reflex arc, however, has only a sensory neuron and a motor neuron with one synapse between them.

Identify the motor neuron in Figure 8-5. Observe that its dendrites and cell body, like those of an interneuron, are located in the spinal cord's gray matter. The axon of this motor neuron, however, runs through the ventral (anterior) root of the spinal nerve and terminates in a muscle.

Clinical Application

Multiple Sclerosis (MS)

Many diseases are associated with disorders of the oligodendrocytes. Because these glia cells are involved in myelin formation, these diseases are called **myelin disorders.** The most common primary disease of the CNS is a myelin disorder called **multiple sclerosis,** or **MS.** It is characterized by myelin loss and destruction accompanied by varying degrees of oligodendrocyte cell injury and death. The result is demyelination of the white matter of the CNS. Hard, plaque-like lesions replace the destroyed myelin, and affected areas are invaded by inflammatory cells. As the myelin around axons is lost, nerve conduction is impaired, and weakness, incoordination, visual impairment, and speech disturbances occur. Although the disease occurs in both sexes and all age groups, it is most common in women between 20 and 40 years.

The cause may be related to autoimmunity and viral infections in some individuals. It is relapsing and chronic in nature, but some cases of acute and unremitting disease have been reported. In most cases, MS is prolonged, with remissions and relapses occurring over many years. Television personality and author Montel Williams reports that he lived with recurring episodes of MS for 20 years before he realized that he has the condition. Although there is not yet a cure for MS, early diagnosis and treatment can slow or stop its progression.

Effects of multiple sclerosis (MS). A, A normal myelin sheath allows rapid conduction. **B,** In MS, the myelin sheath is damaged, disrupting nerve conduction.

NERVE IMPULSES

What are nerve impulses? Here is one widely accepted definition: a nerve impulse is a self-propagating wave of electrical disturbance that travels along the surface of a neuron's plasma membrane. You might visualize this as a tiny spark sizzling its way along a fuse.

Nerve impulses do not continually race along every nerve cell's surface. First they have to be initiated by a stimulus, a change in the neuron's environment. Pressure, temperature, and chemical changes are the usual stimuli.

The membrane of each resting neuron has a slight positive charge on the outside and a negative charge on the inside, a state called *polarization*, as shown in Figure 8-6. This occurs because there is normally an excess of sodium ions (Na^+) on the outside of the membrane. When a section of the membrane is stimulated, its Na^+ channels suddenly open, and Na^+ rushes inward. The inside of the membrane temporarily becomes positive, and the outside becomes negative—a process called *depolarization*. This section of the membrane then immediately recovers—a process called *repolarization*. However, the depolarization has already stimulated Na^+ channels in the next section of the membrane to open. The impulse—or *action potential*—cannot go backwards during the brief moment of repolarization and recovery of the previous section of membrane. Thus a self-propagating wave of electrical disturbance—a nerve impulse—travels in one direction across the neuron's surface (see Figure 8-6, *A*).

Nerve impulses are also called *action potentials* because each one is a difference in charge (called "electrical potential") that usually triggers an action by the cell—in this case, transmission of the impulse itself.

If the traveling impulse encounters a section of membrane covered with insulating myelin, it simply "jumps" around the gaps in the myelin sheath.

Called **saltatory conduction,** this type of impulse travel is much faster than is possible in nonmyelinated sections. Saltatory conduction is illustrated in Figure 8-6, *B*.

> To learn more about nerve impulses, go to AnimationDirect on your CD-ROM.

THE SYNAPSE

Transmission of signals from one neuron to the next—across the synapse—is an important part of the nerve conduction process. By definition, a synapse is the place where impulses are transmitted from one neuron, called the **presynaptic neuron,** to another neuron, called the **postsynaptic neuron.**

Three structures make up a synapse: a synaptic knob, a synaptic cleft, and the plasma membrane of a postsynaptic neuron.

A **synaptic knob** is a tiny bulge at the end of a terminal branch of a presynaptic neuron's axon (Figure 8-7). Each synaptic knob contains many small sacs or vesicles. Each vesicle contains a very small quantity of a chemical compound called a *neurotransmitter.* When a nerve impulse arrives at the synaptic knob, neurotransmitter molecules are released from the vesicles into the **synaptic cleft.**

The synaptic cleft is the space between a synaptic knob and the plasma membrane of a *postsynaptic neuron*. It is an incredibly narrow space—only about two millionths of a centimeter in width. Identify the synaptic cleft in Figure 8-7.

The plasma membrane of a postsynaptic neuron has protein molecules embedded in it opposite each synaptic knob. These serve as receptors to which neurotransmitter molecules bind. This binding can initiate an impulse in the postsynaptic neuron by opening ion channels in the postsynaptic membrane.

After impulse conduction by postsynaptic neurons is initiated, neurotransmitter activity is rapidly terminated. Either one or both of two mechanisms cause this. Some neurotransmitter molecules are transported out of the synaptic cleft back into synaptic knobs. Other neurotransmitter molecules are metabolized into inactive compounds by specific enzymes.

Neurotransmitters are chemicals by which neurons communicate. As previously noted, at trillions of synapses in the CNS, presynaptic neurons

FIGURE 8-6 **Conduction of nerve impulses. A,** In an unmyelinated fiber, a nerve impulse (action potential) is a self-propagating wave of electrical disturbance. **B,** In a myelinated fiber, the action potential "jumps" around the insulating myelin in a rapid type of conduction called *saltatory conduction.*

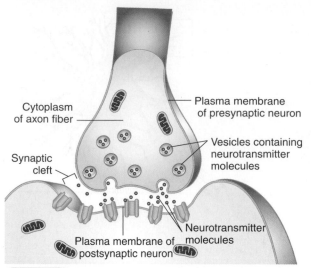

FIGURE 8-7 **Components of a synapse.** Diagram shows synaptic knob or axon terminal of presynaptic neuron, the plasma membrane of a postsynaptic neuron, and a synaptic cleft. On the arrival of an action potential at a synaptic knob, neurotransmitter molecules are released from vesicles in the knob into the synaptic cleft. The combining of neurotransmitter and receptor molecules in the plasma membrane of the postsynaptic neuron opens ion channels and thereby initiates impulse conduction in the postsynaptic neuron.

release neurotransmitters that assist, stimulate, or inhibit postsynaptic neurons. At least 30 different compounds have been identified as neurotransmitters. They are not distributed randomly through the spinal cord and brain. Instead, specific neurotransmitters are localized in discrete groups of neurons and released in specific pathways.

For example, the substance named **acetylcholine** (ass-ee-til-KOH-leen) is released at some of the synapses in the spinal cord and at neuromuscular (nerve-muscle) junctions. Other well-known neurotransmitters include **norepinephrine** (nor-ep-i-NEF-rin), **dopamine** (DOH-pah-meen), and **serotonin** (sair-oh-TOH-nin). They belong to a group of compounds called **catecholamines** (kat-eh-KOHL-ah-meenz), which may play a role in sleep, motor function, mood, and pleasure recognition.

Two morphinelike neurotransmitters called **endorphins** (en-DOR-finz) and **enkephalins** (en-KEF-ah-linz) are released at various spinal cord and brain synapses in the pain conduction pathway. These neurotransmitters inhibit conduction of pain impulses. They are natural pain killers.

Very small molecules such as **nitric oxide (NO)** have an important role as neurotransmitters. Un-

Health and Well-Being

Suppressing Pain During Exercise

Research shows that the release of endorphins increases during heavy exercise. Endorphins inhibit pain, so it is no wonder that pain associated with muscle fatigue decreases when endorphins are present. Normally, pain is a warning signal that calls attention to injuries or dangerous circumstances. However, it is better to inhibit severe pain if it would stop us from continuing an activity that may be necessary for survival. Athletes and others who exercise heavily have even reported a unique feeling of well-being or euphoria associated with elevated endorphin levels.

like most other neurotransmitters, NO diffuses directly across the plasma membrane of neurons rather than being released from vesicles.

QUICK CHECK

1. How does myelin increase the speed of nerve impulse conduction?
2. What is a synapse?
3. How do neurotransmitters transmit signals across the synapse?
4. What is a postsynaptic neuron?

CENTRAL NERVOUS SYSTEM

The central nervous system (CNS), as its name implies, is centrally located. Its two major structures, the brain and spinal cord, are found along the midline of the body (Figure 8-8). The brain is protected in the cranial cavity of the skull, and the spinal cord is surrounded in the spinal cavity by the vertebral column. In addition, the brain and spinal cord are also covered by protective membranes called *meninges*, which are discussed in a later section of this chapter.

Divisions of the Brain

The brain, one of our largest organs, consists of the following major divisions, named in ascending order, beginning with most inferior part:

I. Brainstem
  A. Medulla oblongata
  B. Pons
  C. Midbrain
II. Cerebellum

III. Diencephalon
   A. Hypothalamus
   B. Thalamus
IV. Cerebrum

Observe in Figure 8-9 the location and relative sizes of the medulla, pons, cerebellum, and cerebrum. Also identify the midbrain.

Brainstem

The lowest part of the brainstem is the medulla oblongata. Immediately above the medulla lies the pons and above that the midbrain. Together these three structures are called the *brainstem* (see Figure 8-9).

The **medulla oblongata** (meh-DUL-ah ob-long-GAH-tah) is an enlarged, upward extension of the spinal cord. It lies just inside the cranial cavity above the large hole in the occipital bone called the *foramen magnum*. As with the spinal cord, the medulla consists of gray and white matter, but the arrangement differs in the two organs. In the medulla, bits of gray matter mix closely and intricately with white matter to form the **reticular formation** (*reticular* means "netlike"). In the spinal cord, gray and white matter do not intermingle. Gray matter forms the interior core of the cord, and white matter surrounds it. The pons and **midbrain,** like the medulla, consist of white matter and scattered bits of gray matter.

All three parts of the brainstem function as two-way conduction paths. Sensory fibers conduct impulses up from the cord to other parts of the brain, and motor fibers conduct impulses down from the brain to the cord. In addition, many important reflex centers lie in the brainstem. The cardiac, respiratory, and vasomotor centers (collectively called the *vital centers*), for example, are located in the medulla. Impulses from these centers control heartbeat, respiration, and blood vessel diameter (which is important in regulating blood pressure).

Cerebellum

Structure. Look at Figure 8-9 to find the location, appearance, and size of the cerebellum. The **cerebellum** is the second largest part of the human brain. It lies under the occipital lobe of the cerebrum. In the cerebellum, folded gray matter composes the thin outer layer and forms a large surface area of nervous connections that allow for a huge amount of information processing. White matter tracts form most of the interior. Notice that

Brain

Spinal cord

Nerves

☐ Central nervous system (CNS)
☐ Peripheral nervous system (PNS)

S
R · L
I

FIGURE 8-8 **The nervous system.** The brain and spinal cord (highlighted green) constitute the central nervous system (CNS) shown in orange, and the nerves make up the peripheral nervous system (PNS) shown in yellow.

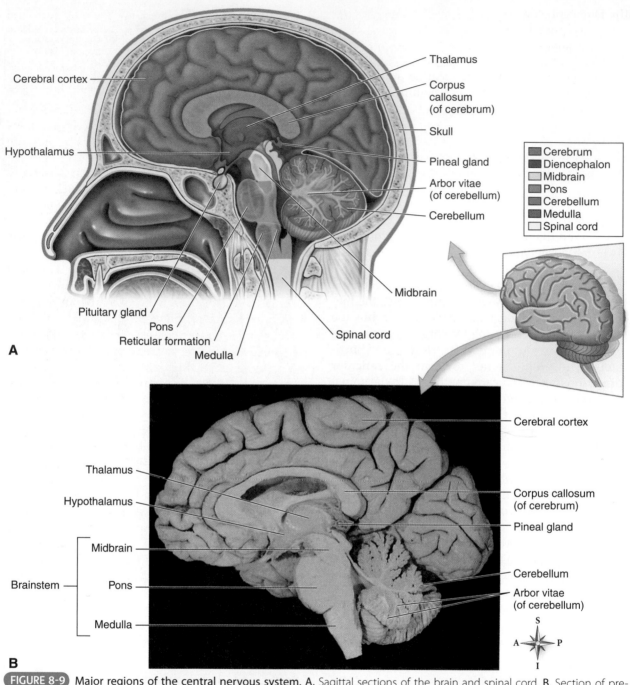

FIGURE 8-9 Major regions of the central nervous system. **A,** Sagittal sections of the brain and spinal cord. **B,** Section of preserved brain.

these tracts branch in a treelike pattern called the *arbor vitae* (literally, "living tree").

Function. Most of our previous knowledge about cerebellar functions has come from observing patients who have some sort of disease of the cerebellum and from animals that have had the cerebellum removed. From such observations, we know that the cerebellum plays an essential part in the production of normal movements.

Perhaps a few examples will make this clear. A patient who has a tumor of the cerebellum frequently loses his balance and topples over; he may feel like a drunken man when he walks. He cannot coordinate his muscles normally. He may complain, for instance, that he is clumsy about everything he does—that he cannot even drive a nail or draw a straight line. With the loss of normal cerebellar functioning, he has lost the ability to make precise movements. The most obvious functions of the cerebellum, then, are to produce smooth coordinated movements, maintain equilibrium, and sustain normal postures.

Recent studies using new brain imaging methods show that the cerebellum may have far more functions than earlier observed. The cerebellum may assist the cerebrum and other parts of the brain, perhaps having an overall coordinating function for the whole brain.

Diencephalon

The **diencephalon** (dye-en-SEF-ah-lon) is a small but important part of the brain located between the midbrain below and the cerebrum above. It consists of three major structures: hypothalamus, thalamus, and pineal gland. Find these structures in Figure 8-9 before reading further.

Hypothalamus. The **hypothalamus** (hye-poh-THAL-ah-muss), as its name suggests, is located below the thalamus. The posterior pituitary gland, the stalk that attaches it to the undersurface of the brain, and areas of gray matter located in the side walls of a fluid-filled space called the *third ventricle* are extensions of the hypothalamus. Identify the pituitary gland and the hypothalamus in Figure 8-9.

The old adage, "Don't judge by appearances," applies well to appraising the importance of the hypothalamus. Measured by size, it is one of the least significant parts of the brain, but measured by its contribution to healthy survival, it is one of the most important brain structures. Impulses from neurons whose dendrites and cell bodies lie in the hypothalamus are conducted by their axons to neurons located in the spinal cord, and many of these impulses are then relayed to muscles and glands all over the body. Thus the hypothalamus exerts major control over virtually all internal organs. Among the vital functions that it helps control are the heartbeat, constriction and dilation of blood vessels, and contractions of the stomach and intestines.

Some neurons in the hypothalamus function in a surprising way; they make the hormones that the posterior pituitary gland secretes into the blood. Because one of these hormones (called **antidiuretic hormone,** or **ADH**) affects the volume of urine excreted, the hypothalamus plays an essential role in maintaining the body's water balance.

Some of the neurons in the hypothalamus function as endocrine (ductless) glands. Their axons secrete chemicals called *releasing hormones* into the blood, which then carries them to the anterior pituitary gland. Releasing hormones, as their name suggests, control the release of certain anterior pituitary hormones. These in turn influence the hormone secretion of other endocrine glands. Thus the hypothalamus indirectly helps control the functioning of every cell in the body.

The hypothalamus is a crucial part of the mechanism for maintaining body temperature. Therefore marked elevation in body temperature in the absence of disease frequently characterizes injuries or other abnormalities of the hypothalamus. In addition, this important center is involved in functions such as the regulation of water balance, sleep cycles, and the control of appetite and many emotions involved in pleasure, fear, anger, sexual arousal, and pain.

Thalamus. Just above the hypothalamus is a dumbbell-shaped section of gray matter called the **thalamus** (THAL-ah-muss). Each enlarged end of the dumbbell lies in a lateral wall of a fluid-filled chamber called the *third ventricle*. The thin center section of the thalamus passes from left to right through this ventricle, which is discussed in more detail later in this chapter. The thalamus is composed chiefly of dendrites and cell bodies of neurons that have axons extending up toward the sensory areas of the cerebrum. The thalamus performs the following functions:

1. It helps produce sensations. Its neurons relay impulses to the cerebral cortex from the sense organs of the body.
2. It associates sensations with emotions. Almost all sensations are accompanied by a feeling of some degree of pleasantness or unpleasantness. The way that these pleasant and unpleasant feelings are produced is unknown except that they seem to be associated with the arrival of sensory impulses in the thalamus.
3. It plays a part in the so-called *arousal* or alerting mechanism.

Pineal Body. Posterior to the thalamus is a tiny mass protruding from the back of the diencephalon called the **pineal gland** or *pineal body*. It resembles a small pine nut or kernel of corn. The pineal gland receives sensory information about the strength of light seen by the eyes and adjusts its output of the hormone *melatonin*. Melatonin is known as "the timekeeping hormone" because it helps keep the body's clock "on time" with the daily, monthly, and seasonal cycles of sunlight and moonlight. We will return to this amazing little organ in Chapter 10 (p. 243).

Cerebrum

The **cerebrum** (seh-REE-brum) is the largest and uppermost part of the brain. If you were to look at the outer surface of the cerebrum, the first features you might notice is its many ridges and grooves. The ridges are called *convolutions* or **gyri** (JYE-rye), and the grooves are called **sulci** (SUL-kye). The deepest sulci are called *fissures;* the longitudinal fissure divides the cerebrum into right and left halves or hemispheres. These halves are almost separate structures except for their lower midportions, which are connected by a structure called the **corpus callosum** (KOHR-pus kah-LOH-sum) (see Figure 8-9). Two deep sulci subdivide each cerebral hemisphere into four major lobes and each lobe into numerous convolutions. The lobes are named for the bones that lie over them: the frontal lobe, the parietal lobe, the temporal lobe, and the occipital lobe. Identify these in Figure 8-10, *A.*

A thin layer of gray matter called the **cerebral cortex,** made up of neuron dendrites and cell bodies, forms the surface of the cerebrum. White matter, made up of bundles of nerve fibers (tracts), composes most of the interior of the cerebrum. Within this white matter, however, are a few islands of gray matter known as the **basal nuclei** or *basal ganglia,* whose functioning is essential for producing automatic movements and postures.

 ## Research, Issues, & Trends

Parkinson Disease

Parkinson disease (PD) is a chronic nervous disorder resulting from a deficiency of the neurotransmitter *dopamine* in the basal nuclei of the cerebrum. The group of signs associated with this disorder is a syndrome called *parkinsonism.* Parkinsonism is characterized by rigidity and trembling of the head and extremities, a forward tilt of the trunk, and shuffling manner of walking, as you can see in the figure. You may have noticed these characteristics in former boxing champion Muhammad Ali, the actor Michael J. Fox, or others you may know with PD. All of these characteristics result from a lack of dopamine, leading to misinformation in the part of the brain that normally prevents the skeletal muscles from being overstimulated.

Dopamine injection into the blood and dopamine pills are not effective treatments because dopamine cannot cross the blood-brain barrier. A breakthrough in the treatment of Parkinson disease came when the drug *levodopa* or L-*dopa* was found to increase the dopamine levels in afflicted patients. Neurons use L-dopa, which can cross the blood-brain barrier, to make dopamine. For some reason, L-dopa does not always have the desired effects in individual patients, so a number of alternatives have been developed. One option that has had some success is the surgical grafting of normal dopamine-secreting cells into the brains of individuals with PD. Another experimental option is an artificial implant that gives electrical stimulation to the basal nuclei, causing them to produce more dopamine.

Forward tilt of trunk

Rigidity and trembling of head

Reduced arm swinging

Rigidity and trembling of extremities

Shuffling gait with short steps

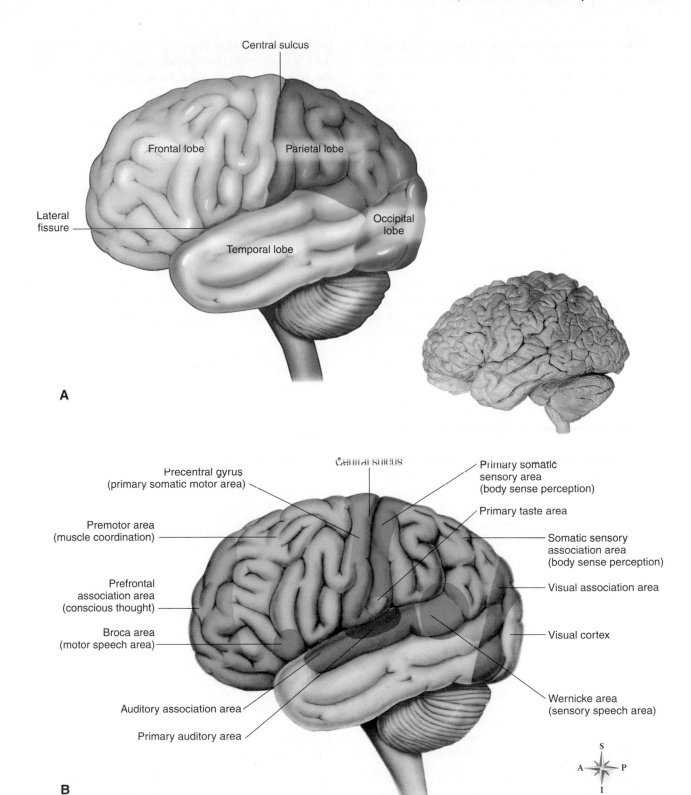

Central sulcus

Frontal lobe

Parietal lobe

Lateral fissure

Occipital lobe

Temporal lobe

A

Central sulcus

Precentral gyrus (primary somatic motor area)

Premotor area (muscle coordination)

Prefrontal association area (conscious thought)

Broca area (motor speech area)

Auditory association area

Primary auditory area

Primary somatic sensory area (body sense perception)

Primary taste area

Somatic sensory association area (body sense perception)

Visual association area

Visual cortex

Wernicke area (sensory speech area)

S
A   P
I

B

FIGURE 8-10 **The cerebrum. A,** The lobes of the cerebrum. **B,** Functional regions of the cerebral cortex. Association areas are so named because they put together (associate) information from many different parts of the brain.

What functions does the cerebrum perform? This is a hard question to answer briefly because the neurons of the cerebrum do not function alone. They function with many other neurons in many other parts of the brain and in the spinal cord. Neurons of these various structures continually bring impulses to cerebral neurons and also continually transmit impulses away from them. If all other neurons were functioning normally and only cerebral neurons were not functioning, here are some of the things that you could not do. You could not think or use your will. You could not remember anything that has ever happened to you. You could not decide to make the smallest movement, nor could you make it. You would neither see nor hear. You could not experience any of the sensations that make life so rich and varied. Nothing would anger or frighten you, and nothing would bring you joy or sorrow. You would, in short, be unconscious. These terms sum up cerebral functions: consciousness, thinking, memory, sensations, emotions, and willed movements. Figure 8-10, *B*, shows the areas of the cerebral cortex essential for willed movements, general sensations, vision, hearing, and normal speech.

Injury or disease can destroy neurons. A common example is the destruction of neurons of the motor area of the cerebrum that results from a **cerebrovascular accident (CVA),** which is a hemorrhage from or cessation of blood flow through cerebral blood vessels. When this happens, the victim can no longer voluntarily move the parts of the body on the side opposite to the side on which the CVA occurred. In nontechnical language, he or she has suffered a stroke. Note in Figure 8-10, *B*, the location of the motor area in the frontal lobe of the cerebrum.

It is important to understand that specific areas of the cortex have specific functions. For example, the temporal lobe's auditory areas interpret incoming nervous signals from the ear as very specific sounds. The visual area of the cortex in the occipital lobe helps you identify and understand specific images. Localized areas of the cortex are directly related to specific functions, as shown in Figure 8-10, *B*. This explains the specific symptoms associated with an injury to localized areas of the cerebral cortex after a stroke or traumatic injury to the head. Table 8-1 summarizes the major components of the brain and their main functions.

 To learn more about areas of the brain that control body functions, go to AnimationDirect on your CD-ROM.

✓ QUICK CHECK

1. What are the four main divisions of the brain? Where is each division?
2. What regions make up the brainstem?
3. Why is the hypothalamus said to be a link between the nervous system and endocrine system?
4. In which part of your brain do you do your thinking?

TABLE 8-1

Functions of Major Divisions of the Brain

BRAIN AREA	FUNCTION
Brainstem	
Medulla oblongata	Two-way conduction pathway between the spinal cord and higher brain centers; cardiac, respiratory, and vasomotor control center
Pons	Two-way conduction pathway between areas of the brain and other regions of the body; influences respiration
Midbrain	Two-way conduction pathway; relay for visual and auditory impulses
Cerebellum	Muscle coordination; maintenance of equilibrium and posture
Diencephalon	
Hypothalamus	Regulation of body temperature, water balance, sleep-cycle control, appetite, and sexual arousal
Thalamus	Sensory relay station from various body areas to cerebral cortex; emotions and alerting or arousal mechanisms
Pineal gland	Adjusts output of melatonin in response to changes in external light, to keep the body's internal clock on time
Cerebrum	Sensory perception, emotions, willed movements, consciousness, and memory

Spinal Cord

Structure

If you are of average height, your spinal cord is about 17 or 18 inches long (Figure 8-11). It lies inside the spinal column in the spinal cavity and extends from the occipital bone down to the bottom of the first lumbar vertebra. Place your hands on your hips, and they will line up with your fourth lumbar vertebra. Your spinal cord ends just above this level.

Look now at Figure 8-12. Notice the H-shaped core of the spinal cord. It consists of gray matter and so is composed mainly of dendrites and cell bodies of neurons. Columns of white matter form the outer portion of the spinal cord, and bundles

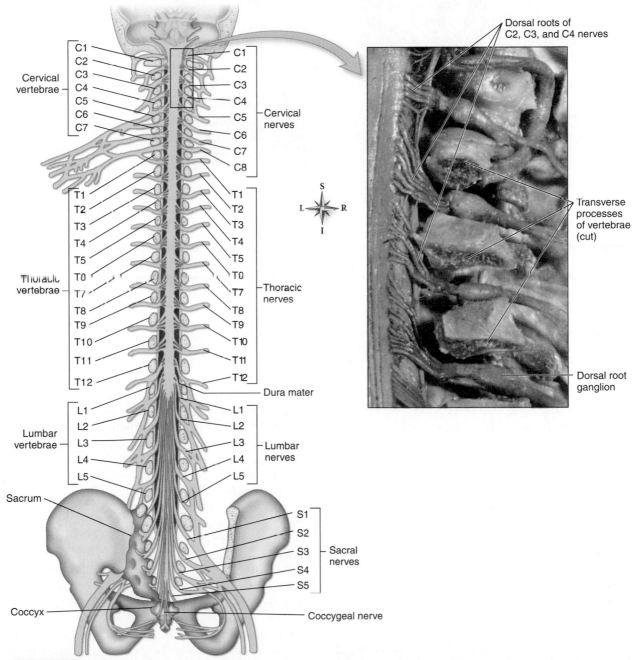

FIGURE 8-11   **Spinal cord and spinal nerves.** Inset is a dissection of the cervical segment of the spinal cord showing emerging cervical nerves. The spinal cord is viewed from behind (posterior aspect).

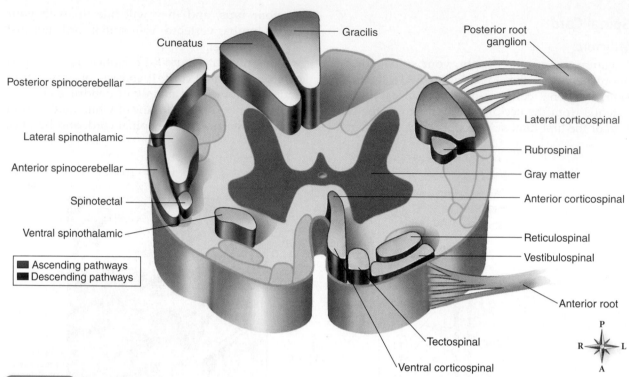

FIGURE 8-12 **Spinal cord cross section.** Cross section of the spinal cord showing some of the major ascending and descending pathways (nerve tracts) highlighted in color. You can also see the gray matter in the center of the cord and the nerve roots attached to the cord.

of myelinated nerve fibers—the **spinal tracts**—make up the white columns.

Spinal cord tracts provide two-way conduction paths to and from the brain. *Ascending tracts* conduct impulses up the cord to the brain. *Descending tracts* conduct impulses down the cord from the brain. Tracts are functional organizations in that all axons composing one tract serve one general function. For instance, fibers of the spinothalamic tracts serve a sensory function. They transmit impulses that produce sensations of crude touch, pain, and temperature. Other ascending tracts shown in Figure 8-12 include the gracilis and cuneatus tracts, which transmit sensations of touch and pressure up to the brain, and the anterior and posterior spinocerebellar tracts, which transmit information about muscle length to the cerebellum. Descending tracts include the lateral and ventral corticospinal tracts, which transmit impulses controlling many voluntary movements.

Functions

To try to understand spinal cord functions, think about a hotel telephone switching system. Suppose a guest in Room 108 calls the switching sys-

tem and keys in the extension number for Room 520, and in a second or so, someone in that room answers. Very briefly, three events took place: a message traveled into the switching system, the system routed the message along the proper path, and the message traveled out from the switching system toward Room 520. The telephone switching system provided the network of connections that made possible the completion of the call. We might say that the switching system transferred the incoming call to an outgoing line.

The spinal cord functions similarly. It contains the centers for thousands and thousands of reflex arcs. Look back at Figure 8-5. The interneuron shown there is an example of a spinal cord reflex center. It switches or transfers incoming sensory impulses to outgoing motor impulses, thereby making it possible for a reflex to occur. Reflexes that result from conduction over arcs whose centers lie in the spinal cord are called *spinal cord reflexes*. Two common kinds of spinal cord reflexes are withdrawal and jerk reflexes. An example of a withdrawal reflex is pulling one's hand away from a hot surface. The familiar knee jerk is an example of a jerk reflex.

In addition to functioning as the primary reflex center of the body, the spinal cord tracts, as previously noted, carry impulses to and from the brain. Sensory impulses travel up to the brain in ascending tracts, and motor impulses travel down from the brain in descending tracts. Therefore if an injury cuts the cord all the way across, impulses can no longer travel to the brain from any part of the body located below the injury, nor can they travel from the brain down to these parts. In short, this kind of spinal cord injury produces a loss of sensation, which is called **anesthesia** (an-es-THEE-zhah), and a loss of the ability to make voluntary movements, which is called **paralysis** (pah-RAL-i-sis).

Coverings and Fluid Spaces of the Brain and Spinal Cord

Nervous tissue is not a sturdy tissue. Even moderate pressure can kill nerve cells, so nature safeguards the chief organs made of this tissue—the spinal cord and the brain—by surrounding them with a tough, fluid-containing membrane called the **meninges** (meh-NIN-jeez). The meninges are then surrounded by bone.

The spinal meninges form a tubelike covering around the spinal cord and line the bony vertebral foramen of the vertebrae that surround the cord. Look at Figure 8-13, and you can identify the three layers of the spinal meninges. They are the **dura mater** (DOO-rah MAH-ter), which is the tough outer layer that lines the vertebral canal, the **pia** (PEE-ah) **mater,** which is the innermost membrane covering the spinal cord itself, and the **arachnoid** (ah-RAK-noyd) **mater,** which is the membrane between the dura and the pia mater. The arachnoid mater resembles a cobweb with fluid in its spaces. The word *arachnoid* means "like a spider web." It comes from *arachne,* the Greek word for spider.

The meninges that form the protective covering around the spinal cord also extend up and around the brain to enclose it completely. Fluid fills the subarachnoid spaces between the pia mater and arachnoid in the brain and spinal cord. This fluid is called **cerebrospinal** (seh-ree-broh-SPY-nal) **fluid (CSF).**

CSF also fills spaces in the brain called cerebral **ventricles.** In Figure 8-14, you can see the irregular shapes of the ventricles of the brain. These illustrations can also help you visualize the location of the ventricles if you remember that these large spaces

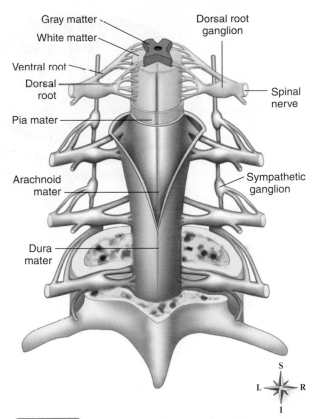

Gray matter
White matter
Ventral root
Dorsal root
Pia mater
Arachnoid mater
Dura mater
Dorsal root ganglion
Spinal nerve
Sympathetic ganglion

FIGURE 8-13 Spinal cord and its coverings. The meninges, spinal nerves, and sympathetic trunk are visible.

lie deep inside the brain and that there are two lateral ventricles. One lies inside the right half of the cerebrum (the largest part of the human brain), and the other lies inside the left half.

CSF is one of the body's circulating fluids. It forms continually from fluid filtering out of the blood in a network of brain capillaries known as the **choroid plexus** (KOH-royd PLEK-sus) and into the ventricles. CSF seeps from the lateral ventricles into the third ventricle and flows down through the cerebral aqueduct (find this in Figures 8-14 and 8-15) into the fourth ventricle. Most of the CSF moves through tiny openings from the fourth ventricle into the subarachnoid space near the cerebellum. Some of it moves into the small, tubelike central canal of the cord and then out into the subarachnoid spaces. Then it moves leisurely down and around the cord and up and around the brain (in the subarachnoid spaces of their meninges) and returns to the blood (in the veins of the brain).

Remembering that this fluid forms continually from blood, circulates, and is resorbed into blood can be useful. It can help you understand certain

FIGURE 8-14 **Fluid spaces of the brain. A,** The ventricles highlighted within the brain in a left lateral view. **B,** The ventricles as seen from above.

FIGURE 8-15 **Flow of cerebrospinal fluid (CSF).** The fluid produced by filtration of blood by the choroid plexus of each ventricle flows inferiorly through the lateral ventricles, interventricular foramen, third ventricle, cerebral aqueduct, fourth ventricle, and subarachnoid space and to the blood.

Clinical Application

Lumbar Puncture

The meninges, the fluid-containing membranes surrounding the brain and spinal cord, extend beyond the spinal cord, an anatomical fact that is most convenient in regard to being able to perform lumbar punctures without putting the spinal cord at risk of injury. A **lumbar puncture,** or "spinal tap," is the withdrawal of some cerebrospinal fluid (CSF) from the subarachnoid space in the lumbar region of the spinal cord. The physician inserts a needle just above or below the fourth lumbar vertebra, knowing that the spinal cord ends an inch or more above this level. The fourth lumbar vertebra can be easily located because it lies on a line with the iliac crest. Placing an adult patient on his side and having him arch his back by drawing the knees and chest together separates the vertebrae sufficiently to introduce the needle. Lumbar punctures are often performed when CSF is needed for analysis or when it is necessary to reduce pressure caused by swelling of the brain or spinal cord after injury or disease. The normal sample of CSF from a lumbar puncture shown here is slightly yellowish and clear, but the red color in the abnormal sample indicates bleeding (in this case, a hemorrhage in the subarachnoid space).

Lumbar puncture

abnormalities. Suppose a person has a brain tumor that presses on the cerebral aqueduct. This blocks the way for the return of CSF to the blood. Because the fluid continues to form but cannot drain away, it accumulates in the ventricles or in the meninges. Other conditions can cause an accumulation of CSF in the ventricles. An example is **hydrocephalus** (hye-droh-SEF-ah-lus) or "water on the brain." One form of treatment involves surgical placement of a hollow tube or catheter through the blocked channel so that CSF can drain into another location in the body.

QUICK CHECK

1. What are the major functions of the spinal cord?
2. What are spinal tracts?
3. Name the three meninges that cover the brain and spinal cord.
4. What is cerebrospinal fluid?

PERIPHERAL NERVOUS SYSTEM

The nerves connecting the brain and spinal cord to other parts of the body constitute the peripheral nervous system (PNS). This system includes **cranial** and **spinal nerves** that connect the brain and spinal cord, respectively, to peripheral structures such as the skin surface and the skeletal muscles. In addition, other structures in the autonomic nervous system (ANS) are considered part of the PNS. These connect the brain and spinal cord to various glands in the body and to the cardiac and smooth muscles in the thorax and abdomen.

Cranial Nerves

Twelve pairs of cranial nerves are attached to the undersurface of the brain, extending from the brainstem. Figure 8-16 shows the attachments of these nerves. Their fibers conduct impulses between the brain and structures in the head and neck and in the thoracic and abdominal cavities. For instance, the second cranial nerve (optic nerve) conducts impulses from the eye to the brain, where these impulses produce vision. The third cranial nerve (oculomotor nerve) conducts impulses from the brain to muscles in the eye, where they cause contractions that move the eye. The tenth cranial nerve (vagus nerve) conducts impulses between the medulla oblongata and structures in the neck and thoracic and abdominal cavities. The names of each cranial nerve and a brief description of their functions are listed in Table 8-2.

FIGURE 8-16 **Cranial nerves.** View of the undersurface of the brain shows attachments of the cranial nerves.

 To learn more about cranial nerves, go to AnimationDirect on your CD-ROM.

Spinal Nerves

Structure

Thirty-one pairs of nerves are attached to the spinal cord in the following order: 8 pairs are attached to the cervical segments, 12 pairs are attached to the thoracic segments, 5 pairs are attached to the lumbar segments, 5 pairs are attached to the sacrospinal segments, and 1 pair is attached to the coccygeal segment (see Figure 8-11).

Unlike cranial nerves, spinal nerves have no special names; instead, a letter and number identify each one. C1, for example, indicates the pair of spinal nerves attached to the first segment of the cervical part of the cord, and T8 indicates nerves attached to the eighth segment of the thoracic part of the spinal cord.

In Figure 8-11 the cervical area of the spine has been dissected to show the emerging spinal nerves in that area. After spinal nerves exit from the spinal cord, they branch to form the many peripheral nerves of the trunk and limbs. Sometimes, nerve fibers from several spinal nerves are reorganized to form a single peripheral nerve. This reorganization

TABLE 8-2

Cranial Nerves

NERVE*		CONDUCT IMPULSES	MAIN FUNCTIONS
I	Olfactory	From nose to brain	Sense of smell
II	Optic	From eye to brain	Vision
III	Oculomotor	From brain to eye muscles	Eye movements
IV	Trochlear	From brain to external eye muscles	Eye movements
V	Trigeminal	From skin and mucous membrane of head and from teeth to brain; also from brain to chewing muscles	Sensations of face, scalp, and teeth; chewing movements
VI	Abducens	From brain to external eye muscles	Eye movements
VII	Facial	From taste buds of tongue to brain; from brain to face muscles	Sense of taste; contraction of muscles of facial expression
VIII	Vestibulocochlear	From ear to brain	Hearing; sense of balance
IX	Glossopharyngeal	From throat and taste buds of tongue to brain; also from brain to throat muscles and salivary glands	Sensations of throat, taste, swallowing movements, secretion of saliva
X	Vagus	From throat, larynx, and organs in thoracic and abdominal cavities to brain; also from brain to muscles of throat and to organs in thoracic and abdominal cavities	Sensations of throat and larynx and of thoracic and abdominal organs; swallowing, voice production, slowing of heartbeat, acceleration of peristalsis (gut movements)
XI	Accessory	From brain to certain shoulder and neck muscles	Shoulder movements; turning movements of head
XII	Hypoglossal	From brain to muscles of tongue	Tongue movements

*The first letters of the words in the following sentence are the first letters of the names of the cranial nerves, in the correct order. Many anatomy students find that using this sentence, or one like it, helps in memorizing the names and numbers of the cranial nerves. It is "**O**n **O**ld **O**lympus' **T**iny **T**ops, **A** **F**riendly **V**iking **G**rew **V**ines **A**nd **H**ops."

can be seen as a network of intersecting or "braided" branches called a **plexus.** Figure 8-11 shows several plexuses.

Functions

Spinal nerves conduct impulses between the spinal cord and the parts of the body not supplied by cranial nerves. The spinal nerves shown in Figure 8-11 contain, as do all spinal nerves, sensory and motor fibers. Spinal nerves therefore function to make possible sensations and movements. A disease or injury that prevents conduction by a spinal nerve thus results in a loss of feeling and a loss of movement in the part supplied by that nerve.

Detailed mapping of the skin's surface reveals a close relationship between the source on the spinal cord of each spinal nerve and the part of the body that it innervates. Knowledge of the segmental arrangement of spinal nerves is useful to physicians. For instance, a neurologist can identify the site of a spinal cord or nerve abnormality by noting the area of the body that is insensitive to a pinprick.

Skin surface areas that are supplied by a single spinal nerve are called **dermatomes** (DER-mah-tohmz). A dermatome "map" of the body is shown in Figure 8-17.

QUICK CHECK

1. How many cranial nerves does a person have? How many spinal nerves?
2. What is a spinal nerve *plexus?*
3. What are *dermatomes?*

AUTONOMIC NERVOUS SYSTEM

The autonomic nervous system (ANS) consists of certain motor neurons that conduct impulses from the spinal cord or brainstem to the following kinds of tissues:

1. Cardiac muscle tissue
2. Smooth muscle tissue
3. Glandular epithelial tissue

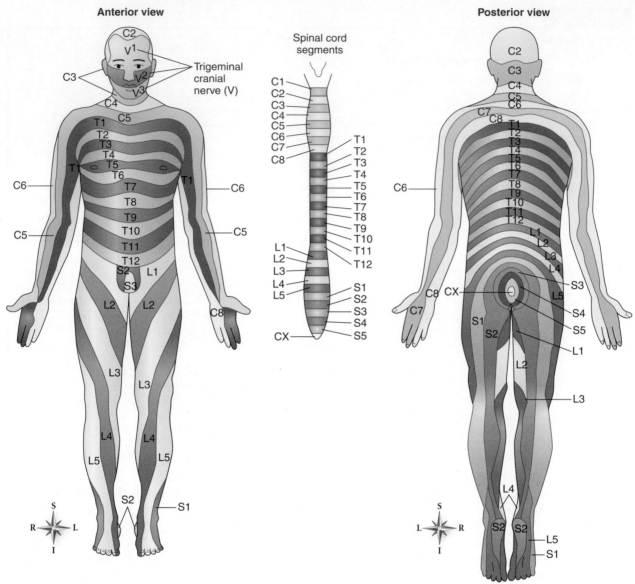

FIGURE 8-17 **Dermatomes.** Segmental dermatome distribution of spinal nerves to the front, back, and side of the body. *C,* Cervical segments; *T,* thoracic segments; *L,* lumbar segments; *S,* sacral segments; *CX,* coccygeal segment.

The ANS consists of the parts of the nervous system that regulate involuntary functions (for example, the heartbeat, contractions of the stomach and intestines, and secretions by glands). On the other hand, motor nerves that control the voluntary actions of skeletal muscles are sometimes called the *somatic nervous system.*

The ANS consists of two divisions called the **sympathetic nervous system** and the **parasympathetic nervous system** (Figure 8-18).

Functional Anatomy

Autonomic neurons are the motor neurons that make up the ANS. The dendrites and cell bodies of some autonomic neurons are located in the gray matter of the spinal cord or brainstem. Their axons extend from these structures and terminate in peripheral "junction boxes" called **ganglia.** These autonomic neurons are called **preganglionic neurons** because they conduct impulses between the spinal

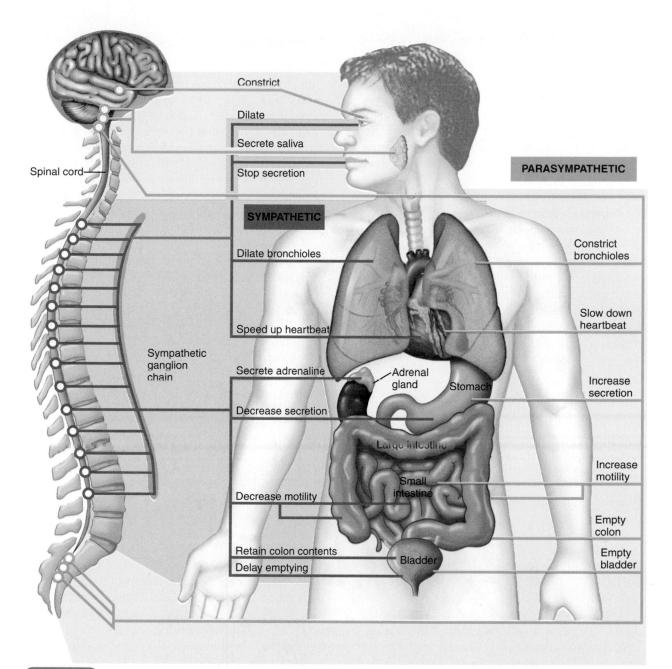

Constrict

Dilate

Secrete saliva

Stop secretion

Spinal cord

PARASYMPATHETIC

SYMPATHETIC

Dilate bronchioles

Constrict bronchioles

Speed up heartbeat

Slow down heartbeat

Sympathetic ganglion chain

Secrete adrenaline

Adrenal gland

Stomach

Increase secretion

Decrease secretion

Large intestine

Increase motility

Small intestine

Decrease motility

Empty colon

Retain colon contents

Bladder

Empty bladder

Delay emptying

FIGURE 8-18   **Innervation of the major target organs by the autonomic nervous system.** The sympathetic pathways are highlighted with orange, and the parasympathetic pathways are highlighted with green.

cord and a ganglion. In the ganglia the axon endings of preganglionic neurons synapse with the dendrites or cell bodies of postganglionic neurons. **Postganglionic neurons,** as their name suggests, conduct impulses from a ganglion to cardiac muscle, smooth muscle, or glandular epithelial tissue.

Autonomic or **visceral effectors** are the tissues to which autonomic neurons conduct impulses. Specifically, visceral effectors are cardiac muscle that makes up the wall of the heart, smooth muscle that partially makes up the walls of blood vessels and other hollow internal organs, and glandular epithelial tissue that makes up the secreting part of a gland.

Autonomic Conduction Paths

Conduction paths to visceral and somatic effectors from the CNS (spinal cord or brainstem) differ somewhat. Autonomic paths to visceral effectors, as the right side of Figure 8-19 shows, consist of two-neuron relays. Impulses travel over preganglionic neurons from the spinal cord or brainstem to autonomic ganglia. There, they are relayed across synapses to postganglionic neurons, which then conduct the impulses from the ganglia to visceral effectors.

Compare the autonomic conduction path with the somatic conduction path illustrated on the left side of Figure 8-19. Somatic motor neurons, like the ones shown here, conduct all the way from the spinal cord or brainstem to somatic effectors with no intervening synapses.

Sympathetic Nervous System

Structure

Sympathetic preganglionic neurons have dendrites and cell bodies in the gray matter of the thoracic and upper lumbar segments of the spinal cord. The sympathetic system has also been referred to as the *thoracolumbar system*. Look now at the right side of Figure 8-19. Follow the course of the axon of the sympathetic preganglionic neuron shown there. It leaves the spinal cord in the anterior (ventral) root of a spinal nerve. It next enters the spinal nerve but soon leaves it to extend to and through a sympathetic ganglion and terminate in a collateral ganglion. There, it synapses with several postganglionic neurons whose axons extend to terminate in visceral effectors. Also shown in Figure 8-19, branches of the preganglionic axon may ascend or descend to terminate in ganglia above and below their point of origin. All sympathetic preganglionic axons therefore

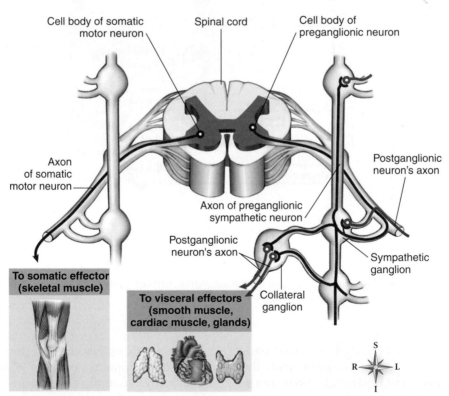

FIGURE 8-19   Autonomic conduction paths. The left side of the diagram shows that one somatic motor neuron conducts impulses all the way from the spinal cord to a somatic effector. Conduction from the spinal cord to any visceral effector, however, requires a relay of at least two autonomic motor neurons—a preganglionic and a postganglionic neuron, shown on the right side of the diagram.

synapse with many postganglionic neurons, and these frequently terminate in widely separated organs. Hence sympathetic responses are usually widespread, involving many organs rather than just one.

Sympathetic postganglionic neurons have dendrites and cell bodies in sympathetic ganglia. Sympathetic ganglia are located in front of and at each side of the spinal column. Because short fibers extend between the sympathetic ganglia, they look a little like two chains of beads and are often referred to as the *sympathetic chain ganglia.* Axons of sympathetic postganglionic neurons travel in spinal nerves to blood vessels, sweat glands, and arrector pili hair muscles all over the body. Separate autonomic nerves distribute many sympathetic postganglionic axons to various internal organs.

Functions

The sympathetic nervous system functions as an emergency system. Impulses over sympathetic fibers take control of many internal organs when we exercise strenuously and when strong emotions—anger, fear, hate, anxiety—are elicited. In short, when we must cope with stress of any kind, sympathetic impulses increase to many visceral effectors and rapidly produce widespread changes within our bodies.

The middle column of Table 8-3 indicates many sympathetic responses. The heart beats faster. Most blood vessels constrict, causing blood pressure to increase. Blood vessels in skeletal muscles dilate, supplying the muscles with more blood. Sweat glands and adrenal glands secrete more abundantly. Salivary and other digestive glands secrete more sparingly. Digestive tract contractions (peristalsis) become sluggish, hampering digestion. Together, these sympathetic responses make us ready for strenuous muscular work, or they prepare us for *fight or flight.* The group of changes induced by sympathetic control is known as the **fight-or-flight response.**

Parasympathetic Nervous System

Structure

The dendrites and cell bodies of parasympathetic preganglionic neurons are located in the gray matter of the brainstem and the sacral segments of the spinal cord. The parasympathetic system has also been referred to as the *craniosacral system.* The preganglionic parasympathetic axons extend some distance before terminating in the parasympathetic ganglia located in the head and in the thoracic and abdominal cavities close to the visceral effectors that they control. The dendrites and cell bodies of

TABLE 8-3		
Autonomic Functions		
VISCERAL EFFECTORS	**SYMPATHETIC CONTROL**	**PARASYMPATHETIC CONTROL**
Heart muscle	Accelerates heartbeat	Slows heartbeat
Smooth muscle		
Of most blood vessels	Constricts blood vessels	None
Of blood vessels in skeletal muscles	Dilates blood vessels	None
Of the digestive tract	Decreases peristalsis; inhibits defecation	Increases peristalsis
Of the anal sphincter	Stimulates—closes sphincter	Inhibits—opens sphincter for defecation
Of the urinary bladder	Inhibits—relaxes bladder	Stimulates—contracts bladder
Of the urinary sphincters	Stimulates—closes sphincter	Inhibits—opens sphincter for urination
Of the eye		
Iris	Stimulates radial fibers—dilation of pupil	Stimulates circular fibers—contraction of pupil
Ciliary	Inhibits—accommodation for far vision (flattening of lens)	Stimulates—accommodation for near vision (bulging of lens)
Of hairs (arrector pili)	Stimulates— "goose pimples"	No parasympathetic fibers
Glands		
Adrenal medulla	Increases epinephrine secretion	None
Sweat glands	Increases sweat secretion	None
Digestive glands	Decreases secretion of digestive juices	Increases secretion of digestive juices

parasympathetic postganglionic neurons lie in these outlying parasympathetic ganglia, and their short axons extend into the nearby structures. Therefore each parasympathetic preganglionic neuron synapses only with postganglionic neurons to a single effector. For this reason, parasympathetic stimulation frequently involves response by only one organ. This is not true of sympathetic responses; as noted, sympathetic stimulation usually results in responses by numerous organs.

Functions

The parasympathetic system dominates control of many visceral effectors under normal, everyday conditions. Impulses over parasympathetic fibers, for example, tend to slow heartbeat, increase peristalsis, and increase secretion of digestive juices and insulin (see Table 8-3). Thus we can think of parasympathetic function as counterbalancing sympathetic function.

Autonomic Neurotransmitters

Turn your attention now to Figure 8-20. It reveals information about autonomic neurotransmitters, the chemical compounds released from the axon terminals of autonomic neurons. Observe that three of the axons shown in Figure 8-20—the sympathetic preganglionic axon, the parasympathetic preganglionic axon, and the parasympathetic postganglionic axon—release acetylcholine. These axons are therefore classified as **cholinergic fibers.** Only one type of autonomic axon releases the neurotransmitter norepinephrine (noradrenaline). This is the axon of a sympathetic postganglionic neuron, and such neurons are classified as **adrenergic fibers.** That each division of the ANS signals its effectors with a different neurotransmitter explains how an organ can tell which division is stimulating it. The heart, for example, responds to acetylcholine from the parasympathetic division by slowing down. The presence of norepinephrine at the heart, on the other hand, is a signal from the sympathetic division, and the response is an increase in heart activity.

Autonomic Nervous System as a Whole

The function of the autonomic nervous system is to regulate the body's automatic, involuntary functions in ways that maintain or quickly restore homeostasis. Many internal organs are doubly

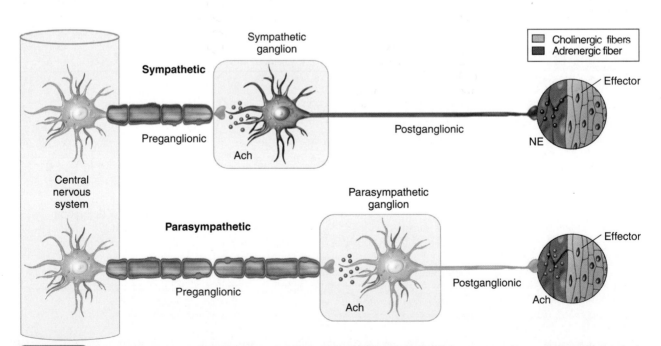

FIGURE 8-20 **Autonomic neurotransmitters.** Three of the four fiber types are cholinergic, secreting the neurotransmitter acetylcholine *(Ach)* into a synapse. Only the sympathetic postganglionic fiber is adrenergic, secreting norepinephrine *(NE)* into a synapse.

innervated by the ANS. In other words, they receive fibers from parasympathetic and sympathetic divisions. Parasympathetic and sympathetic impulses continually bombard them and, as Table 8-3 indicates, influence their function in opposite or antagonistic ways. For example, the heart continually receives sympathetic impulses that make it beat faster and parasympathetic impulses that slow it down. The ratio between these two antagonistic forces, determined by the ratio between the two different autonomic neurotransmitters, determines the actual heart rate.

The term *autonomic nervous system* is something of a misnomer. It seems to imply that this part of the nervous system is independent from other parts. But this is not true. Dendrites and cell bodies of preganglionic neurons are located, as observed in Figures 8-19 and 8-20, in the spinal cord and brainstem. They are continually influenced directly or indirectly by impulses from neurons located above them, notably by some in the hypothalamus and in the parts of the cerebral cortex called the **limbic system** or *emotional brain*. Through conduction paths from these areas, emotions can produce widespread changes in the automatic functions of our bodies, in cardiac and smooth muscle contractions, and in secretion by glands. Anger and fear, for example, lead to increased sympathetic activity and the fight-or-flight response.

According to some physiologists, the altered state of consciousness known as *meditation* leads to decreased sympathetic activity and a group of changes opposite to those of the fight-or-flight response.

QUICK CHECK

1. What kinds of tissues are controlled by the autonomic nervous system (ANS)?
2. What are the two main divisions of the ANS?
3. What division of the ANS produces the *fight-or-flight response?*
4. Which two neurotransmitters are used by autonomic nerve pathways?

Clinical Application

Herpes Zoster, or Shingles

Herpes zoster, or **shingles,** is a unique viral infection that almost always affects the skin of a single dermatome. It is caused by a varicella zoster virus (VZV) of chickenpox. Nearly 15% of the population will suffer from shingles at least once by the time they reach the age of 80. In most cases the disease results from reactivation of the varicella virus. The virus probably traveled through a cutaneous nerve and remained dormant in a dorsal root ganglion for years after an episode of chickenpox. If the body's immunological protective mechanism becomes diminished in the elderly after stress, or in individuals undergoing radiation therapy or taking immunosuppressive drugs, the virus may reactivate. If this occurs, the virus travels over the sensory nerve to the skin of a single dermatome. The result is a painful eruption of red, swollen plaques or vesicles that eventually rupture and crust before clearing in 2 to 3 weeks. In severe cases, extensive inflammation, hemorrhagic blisters, and secondary bacterial infection may lead to permanent scarring. In most cases, the eruption of vesicles is preceded by 4 to 5 days of preeruptive pain, burning, and itching in the affected dermatome. Although an attack of herpes zoster does not confer lasting immunity, only 5% of cases are recurrences.

Some health officials are concerned about a possible shingles epidemic among adults caused by widespread use of chickenpox vaccines in children. Apparently, adults who have not had occasional immune-boosting exposures to children with chickenpox have an increased risk of developing shingles. A shingles vaccine is available for use in people 60 and older who have had chickenpox.

Neuroscience
Otto Loewi (1873-1961)

The Austrian scientist Otto Loewi started his studies in the humanities, not science. When he did begin university studies in medicine, he often skipped his science classes to attend lectures in philosophy. But after Dr. Loewi turned his attention to human biology, he was brilliant. In 1921, when trying to design an experiment to find out how neurons communicate with other cells, he had a dream in which the answer came to him. He rushed to his lab and performed a famous experiment in which he discovered what we know as acetylcholine. For his work that showed that it is neurotransmitters that carry signals from neurons, Loewi shared a Nobel Prize in 1936. And, not surprisingly, Loewi later spent some of his time studying how dreams may help us understand subconscious thoughts.

Many professions depend on neuroscience researchers like Otto Loewi to provide information they need to help us improve our lives. For example, neurologists, psychiatrists, and other medical professionals use this information to treat disorders of the nervous system. Pharmacologists and pharmacy professionals use these ideas to develop drug treatments that affect the nervous system. Mental health professionals such as psychologists and counselors use concepts derived from neuroscience to better understand human emotions and behavior. Even people who specialize in business and marketing use some of the neuroscience discoveries—their focus is learning how to entice buyers to buy certain products or, perhaps, to predict the behavior of crowds.

OUTLINE SUMMARY

ORGANS AND DIVISIONS OF THE NERVOUS SYSTEM (See Figure 8-1)
A. Central nervous system (CNS) — brain and spinal cord
B. Peripheral nervous system (PNS) — all nerves
C. Autonomic nervous system (ANS)

CELLS OF THE NERVOUS SYSTEM
A. Neurons
  1. Consist of three main parts — dendrites, cell body of neuron, and axon (see Figure 8-2)
    a. Dendrites — branching projections that conduct impulses *to* cell body of neuron
    b. Axon — elongated projection that conducts impulses *away* from cell body of neuron
  2. Neurons classified according to function
    a. Sensory (afferent) neurons — conduct impulses to the spinal cord and brain
    b. Motor (efferent) neurons — conduct impulses away from brain and spinal cord to muscles and glands
    c. Interneurons — conduct impulses from sensory neurons to motor neurons or among a network of interneurons; also known as *central* or *connecting neurons*

B. Glia (neuroglia)
  1. Support cells, bringing the cells of nervous tissue together structurally and functionally
  2. Three main types of glial cells of the CNS (see Figure 8-3)
    a. Astrocytes — star-shaped cells that anchor small blood vessels to neurons
    b. Microglia — small cells that move in inflamed brain tissue carrying on phagocytosis
    c. Oligodendrocytes — form myelin sheaths on axons in the CNS
  3. Schwann cells form myelin sheaths on axons of the PNS (see Figure 8-2)

NERVES AND TRACTS (See Figure 8-4)
A. Nerve — bundle of peripheral axons
  1. Tract — bundle of central axons
  2. White matter — tissue composed primarily of myelinated axons (nerves or tracts)
  3. Gray matter — tissue composed primarily of cell bodies and unmyelinated fibers
B. Nerve coverings — fibrous connective tissue
  1. Endoneurium — surrounds individual fibers within a nerve

2. Perineurium — surrounds a group (fascicle) of nerve fibers
3. Epineurium — surrounds the entire nerve

REFLEX ARCS

A. Nerve impulses are conducted from receptors to effectors over neuron pathways or reflex arcs; conduction by a reflex arc results in a reflex (that is, contraction by a muscle or secretion by a gland)
B. The simplest reflex arcs are two-neuron arcs — consisting of sensory neurons synapsing in the spinal cord with motor neurons
C. Three-neuron arcs consist of sensory neurons synapsing in the spinal cord with interneurons that synapse with motor neurons (see Figure 8-5)

NERVE IMPULSES

A. Definition — self-propagating wave of electrical disturbance that travels along the surface of a neuron membrane (also called *action potential*)
B. Mechanism
   1. At rest, the neuron's membrane is slightly positive on the outside — polarized — from a slight excess of Na^+ on the outside
   2. A stimulus triggers the opening of Na^+ channels in the plasma membrane of the neuron
   3. Inward movement of Na^+ depolarizes the membrane by making the inside more positive than the outside at the stimulated point; this depolarization is a nerve impulse (action potential)
   4. The stimulated section of membrane immediately repolarizes, but by that time the depolarization has already triggered the next section of membrane to depolarize, thus propagating a wave of electrical disturbances (depolarizations) all the way down the membrane

THE SYNAPSE

A. Definition — the place where impulses are transmitted from one neuron to another (the postsynaptic neuron) (see Figure 8-7)
B. Synapse made of three structures — synaptic knob, synaptic cleft, and plasma membrane

C. Neurotransmitters bind to specific receptor molecules in the membrane of a postsynaptic neuron, opening ion channels and thereby stimulating impulse conduction by the membrane
D. Names of neurotransmitters — acetylcholine, catecholamines (norepinephrine, dopamine, and serotonin), endorphins, enkephalins, nitric oxide (NO), and other compounds

CENTRAL NERVOUS SYSTEM

A. Divisions of the brain (see Figure 8-9 and Table 8-1)
   1. Brainstem
      a. Consists of three parts of brain, named in ascending order: the medulla oblongata, pons, and midbrain
      b. Structure — white matter with bits of gray matter scattered through it
      c. Functions
         (1) All three parts of brainstem are two-way conduction paths
            (a) Sensory tracts in the brainstem conduct impulses to the higher parts of the brain
            (b) Motor tracts conduct from the higher parts of the brain to the spinal cord
         (2) Gray matter areas in the brainstem function as important reflex centers
   2. Cerebellum
      a. Structure
         (1) Second largest part of the human brain
         (2) Gray matter outer layer is thin but highly folded, forming a large surface area for processing information
         (3) *Arbor vitae* — internal, treelike network of white matter tracts
      b. Function
         (1) Helps control muscle contractions to produce coordinated movements so that we can maintain balance, move smoothly, and sustain normal postures
         (2) Variety of additional coordinating effects, assisting the cerebrum and other regions of the brain

3. Diencephalon
   a. Hypothalamus
      (1) Consists mainly of the posterior pituitary gland, pituitary stalk, and gray matter
      (2) Acts as the major center for controlling the ANS; therefore it helps control the functioning of most internal organs
      (3) Controls hormone secretion by anterior and posterior pituitary glands; therefore it indirectly helps control hormone secretion by most other endocrine glands
      (4) Contains centers for controlling body temperature, appetite, wakefulness, and pleasure
   b. Thalamus
      (1) Dumbbell-shaped mass of gray matter extending toward each cerebral hemisphere
      (2) Relays sensory impulses to cerebral cortex sensory areas
      (3) In some way produces the emotions of pleasantness or unpleasantness associated with sensations
   c. Pineal gland (pineal body)
      (1) Small body resembling a pine nut behind the thalamus
      (2) Adjusts output of "timekeeping hormone" melatonin in response to changing levels of external light (sunlight and moonlight)
4. Cerebrum
   a. Largest part of the human brain
   b. Outer layer of gray matter is the cerebral cortex; made up of lobes; composed mainly of dendrites and cell bodies of neurons
   c. Interior of the cerebrum composed mainly of white matter
      (1) Tracts — nerve fibers arranged in bundles
      (2) Basal nuclei — islands of gray matter regulate automatic movements and posture
   d. Functions of the cerebrum — mental processes of all types, including sensations, consciousness, memory, and voluntary control of movements

B. Spinal cord (see Figure 8-11)
   1. Columns of white matter, composed of bundles of myelinated nerve fibers, form the outer portion of the H-shaped core of the spinal cord; bundles of axons called *tracts*
   2. Interior composed of gray matter made up mainly of neuron dendrites and cell bodies
   3. Spinal cord tracts provide two-way conduction paths — ascending and descending
   4. Spinal cord functions as the primary center for all spinal cord reflexes; sensory tracts conduct impulses to the brain, and motor tracts conduct impulses from the brain
C. Coverings and fluid spaces of the brain and spinal cord
   1. Coverings (see Figure 8-13)
      a. Cranial bones and vertebrae
      b. Cerebral and spinal meninges — the dura mater, the pia mater, and the arachnoid mater
   2. Fluid spaces (see Figure 8-14)
      a. Subarachnoid spaces of meninges
      b. Central canal inside cord
      c. Ventricles in brain

PERIPHERAL NERVOUS SYSTEM
A. Cranial nerves (see Figure 8-16 and Table 8-2)
   1. Twelve pairs — attached to undersurface of the brain
   2. Connect brain with the neck and structures in the thorax and abdomen
B. Spinal nerves
   1. Thirty-one pairs — contain dendrites of sensory neurons and axons of motor neurons
   2. Conduct impulses necessary for sensations and voluntary movements
C. Dermatome — skin surface area supplied by a single cranial or spinal nerve

AUTONOMIC NERVOUS SYSTEM
A. Functional anatomy
   1. Autonomic nervous system — motor neurons that conduct impulses from the central nervous system to cardiac muscle, smooth muscle, and glandular epithelial tissue; regulates the body's automatic or involuntary functions (see Figure 8-18)

2. Autonomic neurons — preganglionic autonomic neurons conduct from spinal cord or brainstem to an autonomic ganglion; postganglionic neurons conduct from autonomic ganglia to cardiac muscle, smooth muscle, and glandular epithelial tissue

3. Autonomic or visceral effectors — tissues to which autonomic neurons conduct impulses (that is, cardiac and smooth muscle and glandular epithelial tissue)

4. Composed of two divisions — the sympathetic system and the parasympathetic system

B. Autonomic conduction paths
   1. Consist of two-neuron relays (that is, preganglionic neurons from the central nervous system to autonomic ganglia, synapses, postganglionic neurons from ganglia to visceral effectors)
   2. In contrast, somatic motor neurons conduct all the way from the CNS to somatic effectors with no intervening synapses

C. Sympathetic nervous system
   1. Dendrites and cell bodies of sympathetic preganglionic neurons are located in the gray matter of the thoracic and upper lumbar segments of the spinal cord
   2. Axons leave the spinal cord in the anterior roots of spinal nerves, extend to sympathetic or collateral ganglia, and synapse with several postganglionic neurons whose axons extend to spinal or autonomic nerves to terminate in visceral effectors
   3. A chain of sympathetic ganglia is in front of and at each side of the spinal column
   4. Functions of the sympathetic nervous system
      a. Serves as the emergency or stress system, controlling visceral effectors during strenuous exercise and when strong emotions (anger, fear, hate, or anxiety) are triggered
      b. Group of changes induced by sympathetic control is called the *fight-or-flight response*

D. Parasympathetic nervous system
   1. Structure
      a. Parasympathetic preganglionic neurons have dendrites and cell bodies in the gray matter of the brainstem and the sacral segments of the spinal cord
      b. Parasympathetic preganglionic neurons terminate in parasympathetic ganglia located in the head and the thoracic and abdominal cavities close to visceral effectors
      c. Each parasympathetic preganglionic neuron synapses with postganglionic neurons to only one effector
   2. Function—dominates control of many visceral effectors under normal, everyday conditions; counterbalances sympathetic function

E. Autonomic neurotransmitters
   1. Cholinergic fibers — preganglionic axons of parasympathetic and sympathetic systems and parasympathetic postganglionic axons release acetylcholine
   2. Adrenergic fibers — axons of sympathetic postganglionic neurons release norepinephrine (noradrenaline)

F. Autonomic nervous system as a whole
   1. Regulates the body's automatic functions in ways that maintain or quickly restore homeostasis
   2. Many visceral effectors are doubly innervated (that is, they receive fibers from parasympathetic and sympathetic divisions and are influenced in opposite ways by the two divisions)

NEW WORDS

acetylcholine
action potential
adrenergic fiber
afferent neuron
anesthesia
arachnoid mater
astrocyte
autonomic effector
autonomic nervous
  system (ANS)
autonomic neuron
axon
basal nuclei
blood-brain barrier
  (BBB)
catecholamine
cell body
central nervous system
  (CNS)
cerebral cortex
cerebrospinal fluid
cerebrovascular acci-
  dent (CVA)
cerebrum
cholinergic fiber
choroid plexus
corpus callosum
cranial nerve

dendrite
dermatome
dopamine
dura mater
effector
efferent neuron
enkephalin
endoneurium
endorphin
epineurium
fascicle
fight-or-flight response
ganglion (pl. ganglia)
glia
glioma
gray matter
gyri
herpes zoster
hydrocephalus
hypothalamus
interneuron
limbic system
lumbar puncture
medulla oblongata
meninx (pl. meninges)
microglia
midbrain
motor neuron

multiple sclerosis (MS)
myelin
myelin disorder
myelinated fiber
nerve
neurilemma
neuron
neurotransmitter
nitric oxide (NO)
node of Ranvier
norepinephrine
oligodendrocyte
paralysis
parasympathetic
  nervous system
Parkinson disease (PD)
perineurium
peripheral nervous
  system (PNS)
pia mater
pineal gland
plexus
pons
postganglionic neuron
postsynaptic neuron
preganglionic neuron
presynaptic neuron
receptor

reflex
reflex arc
reticular formation
saltatory conduction
Schwann cell
sensory neuron
serotonin
shingles
spinal nerve
spinal tract
sulcus (pl. sulci)
sympathetic nervous
  system
sympathetic postgan-
  glionic neuron
sympathetic pregangli-
  onic neuron
synapse
synaptic cleft
synaptic knob
thalamus
tract
ventricle
visceral effector
white matter
withdrawal reflex

REVIEW QUESTIONS

1. Draw and label the three parts of the neuron and explain the function of the dendrite and axon.
2. Name the three types of neurons classified according to the direction in which the impulse is transmitted. Define and explain each of them.
3. Define or explain the following terms: *myelin, node of Ranvier,* and *neurilemma.*
4. Name and give the function of the three types of glia cells.
5. Define or explain the following terms: *epineurium, perineurium,* and *endoneurium.*
6. What is the physical difference between gray matter and white matter?
7. Explain how a reflex arc functions. What are the two types of reflex arc?
8. Explain what occurs during a nerve impulse. What is *saltatory conduction*?
9. Explain fully what occurs at a synapse. Explain the two ways in which neurotransmitter activity is terminated.
10. Describe and list the functions of the medulla oblongata.
11. Describe and list the functions of the hypothalamus.
12. Describe and list the functions of the thalamus.
13. Describe and list the functions of the cerebellum.
14. Give the general functions of the cerebrum. What are the specific functions of the occipital and temporal lobes?
15. Describe and list the functions of the spinal cord.
16. Name and explain the three layers of the meninges.
17. What is the function of cerebrospinal fluid? Where and how is it produced?
18. How many nerve pairs are generated from the spinal cord? How many nerve pairs are generated from each section of the spinal cord and how are they named? What is a plexus?
19. Explain the structure and function of the sympathetic nervous system.
20. Explain the structure and function of the parasympathetic nervous system.

CRITICAL THINKING

21. Compare the functional regions of the frontal, parietal, occipital, and temporal lobes.
22. Which of the cranial nerves deals primarily with motor function? Which deal primarily with sensory function?
23. There is a type of medication that inhibits the functioning of acetylcholinesterase (the enzyme that deactivates acetylcholine). Explain the side effects the medication would have on the visceral effectors.

CHAPTER TEST

1. _____ is the name of the nervous system division that includes the nerves that extend to the outlying parts of the body.

2. _____ is the name of the nervous system division that includes the brain and spinal cord.

3. A group of peripheral axons bundled together in an epineurium is called a _____.

4. The two types of cells found in the nervous system are _____ and _____.

5. The knee jerk is of a type of neural pathway called a _____.

6. _____ is a self-propagating wave of electrical disturbance that travels along the surface of a neuron's plasma membrane.

7. The exterior of a resting neuron has a slight _____ charge, whereas the interior has a slight _____ charge.

8. During a nerve impulse, _____ is the ion that rushes into the neuron.

9. The _____ is the place where impulses are passed from one neuron to another.

10. Acetylcholine and dopamine are examples of _____, which are chemicals used by neurons to communicate.

11. _____, _____, and _____ are the three membranes that make up the meninges.

12. There are _____ pairs of cranial nerves and _____ pairs of nerves that come from the spinal cord.

13. _____ are skin surface areas supplied by a single spinal nerve.

14. _____ is the part of the autonomic nervous system that regulates effectors during nonstress conditions.

15. _____ is the part of the autonomic nervous system that regulates the "fight-or-flight" response.

16. The preganglionic axons of the sympathetic nervous system release the neurotransmitter _____. The postganglionic axons release _____.

17. The preganglionic axons of the parasympathetic nervous system release the neurotransmitter _____. The postganglionic axons release _____.

18. The autonomic nervous system consists of neurons that conduct impulses from the brain or spinal cord to _____ tissue, _____ tissue, and _____ tissue.

CHAPTER TEST—cont'd

Match each function or description in Column B with the correct term in Column A.

COLUMN A

19. _____ dendrite
20. _____ axon
21. _____ myelin
22. _____ Schwann cells
23. _____ astrocytes
24. _____ microglia
25. _____ oligodendrocyte
26. _____ medulla oblongata
27. _____ pons
28. _____ midbrain
29. _____ hypothalamus
30. _____ thalamus
31. _____ cerebellum
32. _____ cerebrum
33. _____ spinal cord

COLUMN B

a. cells that make myelin for axons outside the CNS
b. glia cells that help form the blood-brain barrier
c. a single projection that carries nerve impulses away from the cell body
d. cells that make myelin for axons inside the CNS
e. a white fatty substance that surrounds and insulates the axon
f. cells that act as microbe-eating scavengers in the CNS
g. a highly branched part of the neuron that carries impulses toward the cell body
h. part of the brainstem that is a conduction pathway between areas of the brain and body; influences respiration
i. sensory relay station from various body areas to the cerebral cortex; also involved with emotions and alerting and arousal mechanisms
j. carries messages to and from the brain to the rest of the body; also mediates reflexes
k. part of the brainstem that contains cardiac, respiratory, and vasomotor centers
l. sensory perception, willed movements, consciousness, and memory are mediated here
m. regulates body temperature, water balance, sleep-wake cycles, appetite, and sexual arousal
n. regulates muscle coordination, maintenance of equilibrium, and posture
o. part of the brainstem that contains relays for visual and auditory impulses

OBJECTIVES

AFTER YOU HAVE COMPLETED THIS CHAPTER, YOU SHOULD BE ABLE TO:

1. Classify sense organs as special or general and explain the basic differences between the two groups.
2. Discuss how a stimulus is converted into a sensation.
3. Discuss the general sense organs and their functions.
4. Describe the structure of the eye and the functions of its components.
5. Discuss the anatomy of the ear and its sensory function in hearing and equilibrium.
6. Discuss the chemical receptors and their functions.

The Senses

9

If you were asked to name the sense organs, what organs would you name? Can you think of any besides the eyes, ears, nose, and taste buds? Actually there are millions of other sense organs throughout the body in our skin, internal organs, and muscles. They constitute the many *sensory receptors* that allow us to respond to stimuli such as touch, pressure, temperature, and pain. These microscopic receptors are located at the tips of dendrites of sensory neurons.

Our ability to "sense" changes in our external and internal environments is a requirement for maintaining homeostasis and for survival itself. We can initiate protective reflexes important to homeostasis only if we can sense a change or danger. External dangers may be detected by sight or hearing. If the danger is internal, such as overstretching a muscle, detecting an increase in body temperature (fever), or sensing the pain caused by an ulcer, other receptors make us aware of the problem and permit us to take appropriate action to maintain homeostasis.

CLASSIFICATION OF SENSE ORGANS

The sense organs are often classified as either *general* sense organs or *special* sense organs. The *general sense organs* consist of microscopic receptors widely distributed throughout the body in the skin, muscles, tendons, joints, and other internal organs of the body. They are responsible for such sensations as pain, temperature, touch, and pressure. The *special sense organs* are responsible for the special senses of smell, taste, vision, hearing, and equilibrium and are grouped into localized areas such as the nasal mucosa and tongue or into such complex organs as the eye and ear.

In addition to classification as either general or special sense organs, individual receptor cells are often identified according to (1) whether they are

STUDY TIPS

Each sense must go through the following processes to perform its function: it must detect the physical stimulus to which it responds and it must convert that stimulus into a nerve impulse.

1. When you study structures and their specific functions in a sensory system, try to see how they contribute to one of the two processes. For example, the eye must let light in and focus it on a specific point; the receptors must convert that stimulus to a nerve impulse and send it to the brain.
2. Use flash cards to learn the specific structures and functions of the sensory systems.
3. In your study group, discuss how each of the sensory systems detects and responds to a stimulus.
4. Photocopy the figures of the sense organs, blacken out the labels, and quiz each other on the names, locations, and functions of the structures.
5. Review the Quick Check questions, go over the questions at the back of the chapter, and discuss possible test questions.

encapsulated or *unencapsulated*, that is, whether they are covered by some sort of capsule or are "free" or "naked" of any such covering and (2) the types of stimuli that activate them. Table 9-1 identifies the general sense organs as either free nerve endings or one of the six types of encapsulated nerve endings, whereas Table 9-2 identifies the type of receptor cells in the special sense organs that are stimulated by specific types of stimuli.

CONVERTING A STIMULUS INTO A SENSATION

All sense organs, regardless of size, type, or location, have in common some important functional characteristics. First, they must be able to sense or detect a stimulus or a change in the intensity of a particular stimulus in their environment. Of course, different sense organs detect different

TABLE 9-1

General Sense Organs

TYPE	MAIN LOCATION	GENERAL SENSES	
Free Nerve Endings (Naked Nerve Endings)			
	Skin and mucosa (epithelial layers)	Pain, crude touch, temperature, itch, tickle	
Encapsulated Nerve Endings			
Tactile (Meissner) corpuscles	Skin (in papillae of dermis) and fingertips and lips (numerous)	Fine or light touch and low-frequency vibration	
Ruffini (bulbous) corpuscles	Skin (dermal layer) and subcutaneous tissue of fingers	Persistent touch and pressure	
Lamellar (Pacini) corpuscles	Subcutaneous, submucous, and subserous tissues; around joints, in mammary glands, and external genitals of both sexes	Deep pressure and high-frequency vibration	
Bulboid corpuscles (Krause end bulbs)	Skin (dermal layer), subcutaneous tissue, mucosa of lips and eyelids, and external genitals	Touch	
Golgi tendon organs	Near junction of tendons and muscles	Proprioception (sense of muscle tension)	
Muscle spindles	Skeletal muscles	Proprioception (sense of muscle length)	Intrafusal fibers

TABLE 9-2

Special Sense Organs

SENSE ORGAN	SPECIFIC RECEPTOR	TYPE OF RECEPTOR	SENSE
Eye	Rods and cones	Photoreceptor	Vision
Ear	Organ of Corti	Mechanoreceptor	Hearing
	Cristae ampullares	Mechanoreceptor	Balance
Nose	Olfactory cells	Chemoreceptor	Smell
Taste buds	Gustatory cells	Chemoreceptor	Taste

types of stimuli. Whether it is light, sound, temperature change, mechanical pressure, or the presence of chemicals ultimately identified as taste or smell, the stimulus must be changed into an electrical signal or nerve impulse. This signal is then transmitted over a nervous system "pathway" to the brain, where the sensation is actually perceived. The sensory pathway for the general sense organs typically involves conduction of action potentials generated in the receptors through the spinal cord to the thalamus (cutaneous or skin receptors) or cerebellum (proprioceptors) where they synapse, and impulses are then relayed to specific areas of the cerebral cortex for conscious sensory interpretation.

GENERAL SENSE ORGANS

The microscopic general sense organ receptors are found in almost every part of the body but they are concentrated in the skin (Figure 9-1). However, these receptors are not evenly distributed over the body surface or in the internal organs. And they do not all respond to the same type of stimulus. To demonstrate this, try touching any point of your skin on a fingertip with the tip of a toothpick. You can hardly miss stimulating at least one receptor and almost instantaneously experiencing a sensation of touch. It is the specialized form and function of the different receptor cells that allow them to respond to different stimuli. This specialized response capability of receptor cells allows us to experience different types of sensations. For example, so-called *mechanoreceptors* are activated by mechanical stimuli that "deform" or change the position or shape of the receptor. A good example is the lamellar (Pacini) corpuscle, which senses deep pressure. Stimulation of some receptors leads to the sensation of vibration, and stimulation of still others gives the sensation of touch. The important and numerous free nerve endings respond to stimuli that permit us to sense pain, temperature, and a number of other sensations. Table 9-1 identifies the general sense receptors showing type, main location, and the sensation produced. Receptors associated with the skin are illustrated in Figure 9-1. Not listed in Table 9-1, but visible in Figure 9-1, are two additional types of free nerve endings that are associated with light touch. *Hair root plexuses* are fine basketlike nerve endings that encircle hair follicles and *tactile* (Merkel) *disks* that attach to nerve endings in the epidermis.

Some specialized receptors found near the junction between tendons and muscles and others found deep within skeletal muscle tissue are called **proprioceptors.** When stimulated, they provide us with information concerning the position or movement of the different parts of the body as well as the length and the extent of contraction and tension in our muscles. The Golgi tendon organs and muscle spindles identified in Table 9-1 are important proprioceptors.

Later in the chapter you will study about specialized photoreceptors that allow us to see, mechanoreceptors that function as the sense organs of hearing, equilibrium, and balance, and chemoreceptors that detect chemicals responsible for our senses of taste and smell.

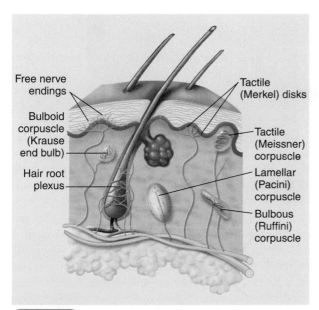

FIGURE 9-1 **General sense receptors.** This section of skin shows the placement of a number of receptors described in Table 9-1.

Labels:
Free nerve endings
Bulboid corpuscle (Krause end bulb)
Hair root plexus
Tactile (Merkel) disks
Tactile (Meissner) corpuscle
Lamellar (Pacini) corpuscle
Bulbous (Ruffini) corpuscle

✓ QUICK CHECK

1. What are different ways that sense organs can be classified into types?
2. Where is a sensation actually perceived?
3. What is the function of a *proprioceptor*?

FIGURE 9-2 Horizontal section through the left eyeball. The eye is viewed from above.

SPECIAL SENSE ORGANS

The Eye

When you look at a person's eye, you see only a small part of the whole eye. Three layers of tissue form the eyeball: the **sclera** (SKLEH-rah), the **choroid** (KOH-royd), and the **retina** (RET-i-nah) (Figure 9-2).

Sclera

The outer layer of sclera consists of tough fibrous tissue. The "white" of the eye is part of the front surface of the sclera. The other part of the front surface of the sclera is called the **cornea** (KOR-nee-ah) and is sometimes spoken of as the window of the eye because of its transparency. A lack of blood vessels and lymphatics in the cornea contributes to its transparency and to the high rate of success of corneal transplantation procedures (Figure 9-3). Inflammation of the cornea is called *keratitis.* In addition to possible loss of transparency that may result from inflammation, any change in the shape

FIGURE 9-3 Corneal transplant. Illustration shows patient with a recent corneal transplant. Note the mild swelling and sutures surrounding the transplanted cornea.

of the cornea can dramatically change the ability of the eye to focus an image on the retina. This fact explains the popularity of surgical procedures that use lasers or other specialty instruments to "sculpt" and change the shape of the cornea. The result is improvement of many visual problems without the use of eyeglasses or contact lenses (see "Refractive Eye Surgery" box on p. 209). At a casual glance, the cornea does not look transparent

Clinical Application

Refractive Eye Surgery

A surgical technique used to treat myopia (nearsightedness) that eliminated the use of eyeglasses or contact lenses became available more than 30 years ago. The procedure, called **radial keratotomy (RK),** involves surgical placement of six or more radial slits (incisions) in a spokelike pattern around the cornea. As a result, the cornea flattens and the ability to focus improves. Other incisional types of refractory eye surgery include **astigmatic keratotomy (AK),** which involves treatment of astigmatism by placement of transverse cuts across the corneal surface, and **automated lamellar keratoplasty (ALK).** The ALK technique uses a special surgical device called a *microkeratome* to cut a thin cap off the corneal surface and then shave and reshape the underlying tissue. At the end of the procedure, the corneal cap is replaced and will heal without the need for sutures. ALK is used to treat both myopia and hyperopia (farsightedness).

More recent advances in refractory eye surgery involve the use of surgical lasers. **Excimer laser surgery,** also called **photorefractive keratectomy (PRK),** uses a "cool" excimer laser beam to vaporize corneal tissue. It is used to flatten the cornea to correct mild to moderate nearsightedness. A refractive eye surgery procedure to correct myopia is called **laser-assisted in situ keratomileusis (LASIK).** This procedure employs both PRK and ALK techniques. First, a microkeratome is used to create a hinged cap of tissue, which is lifted off the corneal surface *(A).* An excimer laser is then used to vaporize and reshape the underlying tissue *(B).* At the end of the procedure, the cap is replaced *(C).* Another laser surgery approved by the U.S. Food and Drug Administration for treating hyperopia (farsightedness) is **laser thermal keratoplasty (LTK).** Ultra-short bursts of laser energy (lasting 3 seconds) are used to reshape the surface of the cornea, with no surgical cutting involved. Yet another approved treatment for correction of farsightedness is called **conductive keratoplasty (CK).** Instead of a scalpel or laser, it employs radiofrequency energy to heat hair-thin probes that are then used to change the shape of the cornea.

but appears blue, brown, gray, or green because it lies over the **iris,** a colored muscular part of the eye described below. A mucous membrane known as the **conjunctiva** (kon-junk-TI-vah) lines the eyelids and covers the sclera in front. Inflammation of this important membrane is called *conjunctivitis* (kon-junk-ti-VYE-tis) and is most often caused by bacterial or viral infection, allergy, or environmental factors. The conjunctiva is kept moist by tears formed in the **lacrimal gland.**

Choroid

The middle layer of the eyeball, the **choroid,** contains a dark pigment to prevent the scattering of incoming light rays. Two involuntary muscles make up the front part of the choroid. One is the iris, the colored structure seen through the cornea, and the other is the *ciliary muscle* (see Figure 9-2). The black center of the iris is really a hole in this doughnut-shaped muscle; it is the **pupil** of

Clinical Application

Visual Acuity

Visual acuity is the clearness or sharpness of visual perception. Acuity is affected by our focusing ability, the efficiency of the retina, and the proper function of the visual pathway and processing centers in the brain.

One common way to measure visual acuity is to use the familiar test chart on which letters or other objects of various sizes and shapes are printed. The subject is asked to identify the smallest object that he or she can see from a distance of 20 feet (6.1 m). The resulting determination of visual acuity is expressed as a double number such as "20-20." The first number represents the distance (in feet) between the subject and the test chart—the standard being 20. The second number represents the number of feet a person with normal acuity would have to stand to see the same objects clearly. Thus a finding of 20-20 is normal because the subject can see at 20 feet what a person with normal acuity can see at 20 feet. A person with 20-100 vision can see objects at 20 feet that a person with normal vision can see at 100 feet.

People whose acuity is worse than 20-200 after correction are considered to be legally blind. Legal blindness is the designation used to identify the severity of a wide variety of visual disorders so that laws that involve visual acuity can be enforced. For example, laws that govern the awarding of driving licenses require that drivers have a minimum level of visual acuity.

the eye. Some of the fibers of the iris are arranged like spokes in a wheel. When they contract, the pupils dilate, letting in more light rays. Other fibers are circular. When they contract, the pupils constrict, letting in fewer light rays. Normally, the pupils constrict in bright light and dilate in dim light.

The **lens** of the eye lies directly behind the pupil. It is held in place by a ligament attached to the ciliary muscle. When we look at distant objects, the ciliary muscle is relaxed, and the lens has only a slightly curved shape. To focus on near objects, the ciliary muscle must contract. As it contracts, it pulls the choroid coat forward toward the lens, thus causing the lens to bulge and curve even more. Most of us become more farsighted as we grow older and lose the ability to focus on close objects because our lenses lose at least some of their elasticity and can no longer bulge enough to bring near objects into focus. **Presbyopia** (pres-bee-OH-pee-ah) or "oldsightedness" is the name for this condition.

In most young people, the lens is both transparent and somewhat elastic so that it is capable of changing shape. Unfortunately, in some individuals, long-time exposure to ultraviolet (UV) radiation in sunlight may cause the lens to become hard, lose its transparency, and become "milky" in appearance. This condition is called a **cataract** (KAT-ah-rakt). Cataract formation may occur in one or both eyes. Once it begins, cataract formation tends to be progressive and may result in blindness. Cataracts can be removed surgically and the defective lens replaced with an artificial implant.

Retina

The **retina**, or innermost layer of the eyeball, contains microscopic photoreceptor cells, called *rods* and *cones* because of their shapes. Dim light can stimulate the rods, but fairly bright light is necessary to stimulate the cones. In other words, **rods** are the receptors for night vision and **cones** are the receptors for daytime vision. There are three kinds of cones; each is sensitive to a different color: red, green, or blue. Scattered throughout the central portion of the retina, these three types of cones allow us to distinguish between different colors.

There is a yellowish area near the center of the retina called the *macula lutea*. It surrounds a small depression, called the **fovea centralis,** which contains the greatest concentration of cones of any area of the retina (see Figure 9-2). In good light, greater *visual acuity*, or sharpness of visual perception, can be obtained if we look directly at an object and focus the image on the fovea. But in dim light or darkness, we see an object better if we look slightly to the side of it, thereby focusing the image nearer the periphery of the retina, where the rods are more plentiful.

Fluids fill the hollow inside of the eyeball. They maintain the normal shape of the eyeball and help refract light rays; that is, the fluids bend light rays to bring them to focus on the retina. **Aqueous humor** is the name of the watery fluid in front of the lens (in the anterior chamber of the eye), and **vitreous humor** is the name of the jellylike fluid behind the lens (in the posterior chamber). Aqueous humor is constantly being formed, drained, and replaced in the anterior chamber. If drainage is blocked for any reason, the internal pressure within the eye will increase, and damage that could lead to blindness will occur. This condition is called **glaucoma** (glaw-KOH-mah).

Visual Pathway

Light is the stimulus that results in vision (that is, our ability to see objects as they exist in our environment). Light enters the eye through the pupil and is *refracted*, or bent, so that it is focused on the retina. **Refraction** occurs as light passes through the cornea, the aqueous humor, the lens, and the vitreous humor on its way to the retina.

The innermost layer of the retina contains the rods and cones, which are the **photoreceptor cells** of the eye (Figure 9-4). They respond to a light

Clinical Application

Finding Your Blind Spot

Demonstrate the location of the blind spot in your visual field by covering your left eye and looking at the objects below. While staring at the block, begin about 35 cm (12 inches) from objects and slowly bring the figures closer to your eye. At one point, the circle will seem to disappear because its image has fallen on the blind spot.

FIGURE 9-4 Cells of the retina. Photoreceptors called *rods* and *cones* (notice their shapes) detect changes in light and relay the information to bipolar neurons. The bipolar cells, in turn, conduct the information to ganglion cells. The information eventually leaves the eye by way of the optic nerve.

Clinical Application

Macular Degeneration

A serious and widespread visual problem affecting more than 1.5 million Americans over age 65 is called *age-related macular degeneration,* or *AMD.* The most common type of AMD (about 85% of cases) is called "dry" AMD. In these individuals, as the macular area of the retina degenerates and the disease progresses over time, the central visual field is gradually lost and the ability to distinguish fine detail diminishes. Although total blindness seldom occurs and varying amounts of peripheral vision remain, AMD patients are unable to read or drive and other daily activities are severely restricted because of the loss of clear "straight-ahead" sight. A less common (10% to 15% of cases) but more severe type of AMD is called "wet" AMD. In these patients, fragile and leaking blood vessels damage the retina over the macula lutea, and rapid loss of central vision may occur.

stimulus by producing a nervous impulse. The rod and cone photoreceptor cells synapse with neurons in the bipolar and ganglionic layers of the retina. Nervous signals eventually leave the retina and exit the eye through the optic nerve on the posterior surface of the eyeball. No rods or cones are present in the area of the retina where the optic nerve fibers exit. The result is a "blind spot" known as the **optic disc** (see Figure 9-2).

After leaving the eye, the optic nerves enter the brain and travel to the visual cortex of the occipital lobe. In this area, *visual interpretation* of the nervous impulses generated by light stimuli in the rods and cones of the retina results in "seeing."

> To learn more about the process of seeing, go to AnimationDirect on your CD-ROM.

Clinical Application

Focusing Problems

Focusing a clear image on the retina is essential for good vision. In the normal eye *(A),* light rays enter the eye and are focused into a clear, upside-down image on the retina. The brain can easily right the upside-down image in our conscious perception but cannot fix an image that is not sharply focused. If our eyes are elongated *(B),* the image focuses in front of the retina rather than on it. The retina receives only a fuzzy image. This condition, called **myopia,** or *nearsightedness*, can be corrected by using contact lenses, glasses *(C),* or refractive eye surgery. If our eyes are shorter than normal *(D),* the image focuses behind the retina, also producing a fuzzy image. This condition, called **hyperopia,** or *farsightedness*, can also be corrected by lenses *(E)* or refractive surgery. *Astigmatism* is an abnormal eye condition resulting in blurred vision. It is caused by an irregular curvature of the lens.

Clinical Application

Color Blindness

Color blindness, usually an inherited condition, is caused by mistakes in producing three chemicals called **photopigments** in the cones. Each photopigment is sensitive to one of the three primary colors of light: green, blue, and red. In many cases, the green-sensitive photopigment is missing or deficient; other times, the red-sensitive photopigment is abnormal. (Deficiency of the blue-sensitive photopigment is very rare.) Color-blind individuals see colors, but they cannot distinguish between them normally.

Figures such as those shown here are often used to screen individuals for color blindness. A person with red-green blindness cannot see the 74 in Figure *A*, whereas a person with normal vision can. To determine which photopigment is deficient, a color-blind person may try a figure

similar to *B*. Persons with a deficiency of red-sensitive photopigment can distinguish only the two; those deficient in green-sensitive photopigment can only see the four.

A   **B**

Research, Issues, & Trends

Corneal Stem Cell Transplants

A new treatment for individuals who may be totally blind because of certain eye diseases, or because of scarring caused by abrasion or chemical burns to their corneas, may make it possible for them to see again. If, because of accident or disease, the clear membrane covering the cornea is permanently destroyed and cannot be regenerated, blindness results. In these cases, traditional corneal transplants are not possible because a clear membrane formed by the eye of the recipient is necessary for survival of the transplanted tissue. Research now indicates that *corneal stem cell transplants* can restore and maintain the clear covering membrane of the cornea that may have been destroyed by disease or injury.

In this procedure, adult stem cells that have the ability to develop into the clear covering membrane of the cornea are first harvested from the corneas of cadavers and then transplanted into and around the edges of the diseased or damaged corneas of the blind recipient. The new stem cells then produce the clear corneal surface membrane required for normal vision. This technique is in the research stage and has limited applications, and problems associated with rejection of the foreign stem cells and suppression of the immune system of the recipient must still be resolved. However, this exciting new development in clinical medicine can effectively treat blindness that was considered permanent in the past.

✓ QUICK CHECK

1. What are the three layers of the eyeball?
2. What are the *humors* of the eye?
3. How are rods and cones used in vision? How are they alike? How are they different?

The Ear

In addition to its role in hearing, the ear also functions as the sense organ of equilibrium and balance. As we shall later see, the stimulation or "trigger" that activates receptors involved with hearing and equilibrium is mechanical, and the receptors themselves are called **mechanoreceptors** (mek-an-oh-ree-SEP-torz). Physical forces that involve sound vibrations and fluid movements are responsible for initiating nervous impulses eventually perceived as sound and balance.

The ear is more than an appendage on the side of the head. A large part of the ear and its most important functional part lie hidden from view deep inside the temporal bone. The ear is divided into the following anatomical areas (Figure 9-5):

1. External ear
2. Middle ear
3. Inner (internal) ear

FIGURE 9-5 **The ear.** External, middle, and inner ear structures.

External Ear

The external ear has two parts: the **auricle** (AW-ri-kul), or pinna, and the **external auditory canal.** The auricle is the appendage on the side of the head surrounding the opening of the external auditory canal. The canal itself is a curving tube about 2.5 cm (1 inch) in length. It extends into the temporal bone and ends at the **tympanic** (tim-PAN-ik) **membrane,** or **eardrum,** which is a partition between the external and middle ear. The skin of the auditory canal, especially in its outer one third, contains many short hairs and **ceruminous** (seh-ROO-mi-nus) **glands** that produce a waxy substance called **cerumen** that may collect in the canal and impair hearing by absorbing or blocking the passage of sound waves. Sound waves traveling through the external auditory canal strike the tympanic membrane and cause it to vibrate.

Middle Ear

The middle ear is a tiny and very thin epithelium-lined cavity hollowed out of the temporal bone. It houses three very small bones. The names of these ear bones, called **ossicles** (OS-si-kulz), describe their shapes: **malleus** (hammer), **incus** (anvil), and **stapes** (stirrup). The "handle" of the malleus attaches to the inside of the tympanic membrane, and the "head" attaches to the incus. The incus attaches to the stapes, and the stapes presses against a membrane that covers a small opening, the *oval window.* The oval window separates the middle ear from the inner ear. When sound waves cause the eardrum to vibrate, that movement is transmitted and amplified by the ear ossicles as it passes through the middle ear. Movement of the stapes against the oval window causes movement of fluid in the inner ear.

A point worth mentioning, because it explains the frequent spread of infection from the throat to the ear, is the fact that a tube—the **auditory,** or **eustachian** (yoo-STAY-shun), **tube**—connects the throat with the middle ear. The epithelial lining of the middle ears, auditory tubes, and throat are extensions of one continuous membrane. As a consequence, a sore throat may spread to produce a middle ear infection called *otitis media* (oh-TYE-tis MEE-dee-ah).

Inner Ear

The activation of specialized mechanoreceptors in the inner ear generates nervous impulses that result in hearing and equilibrium. Anatomically, the inner ear consists of three spaces in the temporal bone, assembled in a complex maze called the **bony labyrinth** (LAB-i-rinth). This odd-shaped bony space is filled with a watery fluid called **perilymph** (PAIR-i-limf) and is divided into the following parts: **vestibule** (VES-ti-byool), **semicircular canals,** and **cochlea** (KOHK-lee-ah). The vestibule is adjacent to the oval window between the semicircular canals and the cochlea (Figure 9-6). Note in Figure 9-6 that a balloonlike membranous sac is suspended in the perilymph and follows the shape of the bony labyrinth much like a "tube within a tube." This is the **membranous labyrinth,** and it is filled with a thicker fluid called **endolymph** (EN-doh-limf).

The specialized mechanoreceptors for balance and equilibrium are located in the three semicircular canals and the vestibule. The three half-circle semicircular canals are oriented at right angles to one another (see Figure 9-6). Within each canal is a dilated area called the *ampulla* that contains a specialized receptor called a **crista ampullaris** (KRIS-tah am-pyoo-LAIR-is), which generates a nerve impulse when you move your head. The sensory cells in the cristae ampullares have hairlike extensions that are suspended in the endolymph. The sensory cells are stimulated when movement of the head causes the endolymph to move, thus causing the hairs to bend. Nerves from other receptors in the vestibule join those from the semicircular canals to form the **vestibular nerve,** which joins with the cochlear nerve to form the acoustic nerve, or cranial nerve VIII (see Figure 9-5). Eventually, nervous impulses passing through this nerve reach the cerebellum and medulla. Other connections from these areas result in impulses reaching the cerebral cortex.

The organ of hearing, which lies in the snail-shaped cochlea, is the **organ of Corti** (KOHR-tye).

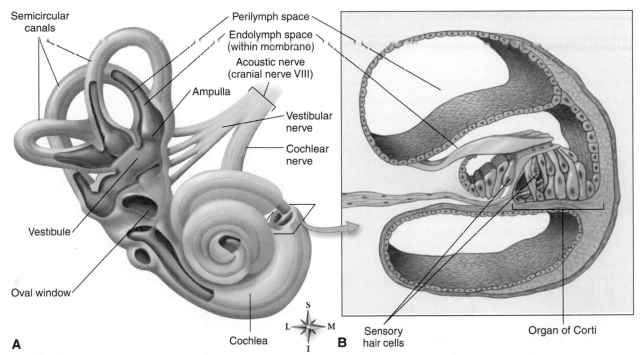

FIGURE 9-6 **The inner ear.** The bony labyrinth is the hard outer wall of the entire inner ear and includes semicircular canals, vestibule, and cochlea. Within the bony labyrinth is the membranous labyrinth *(purple),* which is surrounded by perilymph and filled with endolymph. Each ampulla in the vestibule contains a crista ampullaris that detects changes in head position and sends sensory impulses through the vestibular nerve to the brain. The inset shows a section of the membranous cochlea. Hair cells in the organ of Corti detect sound and send the information through the cochlear nerve. The vestibular and cochlear nerves join to form the acoustic nerve, or cranial nerve VIII.

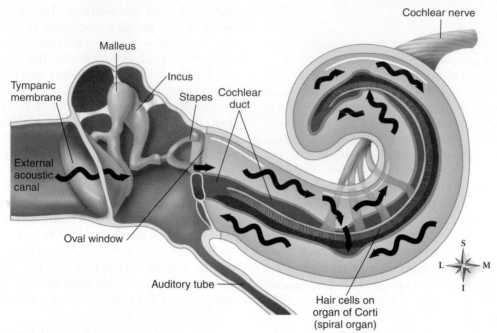

FIGURE 9-7 **Effect of sound waves on cochlear structures.** Sound waves strike the tympanic membrane and cause it to vibrate. This vibration causes the membrane of the oval window to vibrate. This vibration causes the perilymph in the bony labyrinth of the cochlea to move, which causes the endolymph in the membranous labyrinth of the cochlea or cochlear duct to move. This movement of endolymph stimulates hair cells on the organ of Corti to generate a nerve impulse. The nerve impulse travels over the cochlear nerve, which becomes a part of the eighth cranial nerve. Eventually, nerve impulses reach the auditory cortex and are interpreted as sound.

It is surrounded by endolymph, filling the membranous labyrinth, which is the membranous tube within the bony cochlea. Specialized hair cells on the organ of Corti generate nerve impulses when they are bent by the movement of endolymph set in motion by sound waves (Figures 9-6 and 9-7).

To learn more about the pathway of sound waves, go to AnimationDirect on your CD-ROM.

Health and Well-Being

Swimmer's Ear

External otitis, or *swimmer's ear*, is a common infection of the external ear in swimmers. It can be bacterial or fungal in origin and is usually associated with prolonged exposure to water. The infection generally involves, at least to some extent, the auditory canal and auricle. The ear as a whole is tender, red, and swollen. Treatment of swimmer's ear usually involves antibiotic therapy and prescription analgesics.

✓ QUICK CHECK

1. What senses are detected in the ear?
2. Can you describe the three main parts of the ear?
3. How do the ossicles work in helping a person to hear?
4. Where are the receptor cells for hearing?

The Taste Receptors

The *taste buds* are the sense organs of taste. They contain both supporting cells and the **chemoreceptors,** called **gustatory** (GUS-tah-tor-ee) **cells,** which generate the nervous impulses ultimately interpreted by the brain as taste (Figure 9-8). Although a few taste buds are located in the lining of the mouth and on the soft palate, most are located on the sides of much larger and differing shaped bumps scattered across the tongue called **papillae** (pah-PIL-ee). About 10 to 15 large *circumvallate papillae,* that form an inverted "V" pattern at the back of the tongue, contain the most taste buds. Each taste bud, as you can see in Figure 9-8, opens

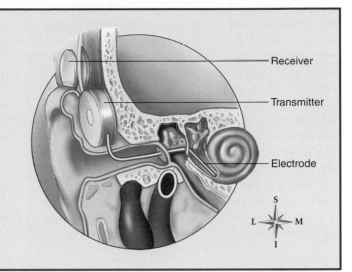

Clinical Application

Cochlear Implants

Advances in electronic circuitry are now being used to correct some forms of nerve deafness. If the hairs on the organ of Corti are damaged, nerve deafness results—even if the vestibulocochlear nerve is healthy. A surgically implanted device can improve this form of hearing loss by eliminating the need for the sensory hairs. As you can see in the figure, a transmitter just outside the scalp sends external sound information to a receiver under the scalp (behind the auricle). The receiver translates the information into an electrical code that is relayed down an electrode to the cochlea. The electrode, wired to the organ of Corti, stimulates the vestibulocochlear nerve endings directly. Thus even though the cochlear hair cells are damaged, sound can still be perceived.

FIGURE 9-8 **The tongue. A,** Dorsal surface of tongue showing circumvallate papillae. **B,** Section through a papilla with taste buds on the side. **C,** Enlarged view of a section through a taste bud.

through an opening into a trenchlike moat that surrounds the papilla and is filled with saliva. Chemicals dissolved in the saliva stimulate the chemoreceptor gustatory cells.

Scientists now emphasize that the sensation of "taste" is often a variable mixture of qualities. Physiologists who once listed only four "primary" taste sensations—sweet, sour, bitter, and salty—that result from stimulation of taste buds have now expanded the list of "primary" taste sensations to include at least two others present in most individuals. Currently, metallic taste and a meaty flavor called *umami* (oo-MOM-ee), discovered by Japanese researchers, have been added to the list of primary tastes. The list may grow. Of course, some individuals are able to sense a larger number of tastes than others. Notable examples include "experts" who, it is said, can detect literally dozens of discrete and different tastes in wine, coffee, tea, and other foods and beverages. However, most of these tastes and flavors result from a combination of taste bud and olfactory receptor stimulation. In other words, the myriad tastes we recognize are not tastes alone but tastes plus odors. For this reason, a cold virus that causes nasal congestion can interfere with the stimulation of the olfactory receptors by odors from foods in the mouth and can markedly dull taste sensations. Nervous impulses that are generated by stimulation of taste buds travel primarily through two cranial nerves (VII and IX) to end in the specialized taste area of the cerebral cortex.

The Smell Receptors

The chemoreceptors responsible for the sense of smell are located in a small area of epithelial tissue in the upper part of the nasal cavity (Figure 9-9). The location of the **olfactory receptors** is somewhat hidden, and we must often forcefully sniff the air to smell delicate odors. Each olfactory cell has a number of specialized cilia that sense different chemicals and cause the cell to respond by generating a nervous impulse. To be detected by olfactory receptors, chemicals must be dissolved in the watery mucus that lines the nasal cavity.

The olfactory receptors are extremely sensitive and respond quickly to even very slight odors. However, after a short time they develop a kind of fatigue and lose their ability to respond. This decrease in receptor sensitivity is called **adaptation** and explains why odors that are at first very noticeable are soon not sensed at all. After the olfactory cells are stimulated by odor-causing chemicals, the resulting nerve impulse travels through the olfactory nerves in the olfactory bulb and tract and then enter the thalamus for relay to the olfactory centers in the cortex of the brain, where the nervous impulses are interpreted as specific odors. The pathways taken by olfactory nerve impulses and the areas where these impulses are interpreted are closely associated with the limbic area of the brain important in memory and emotion (see Chapter 8, p. 195). For this reason, we may retain

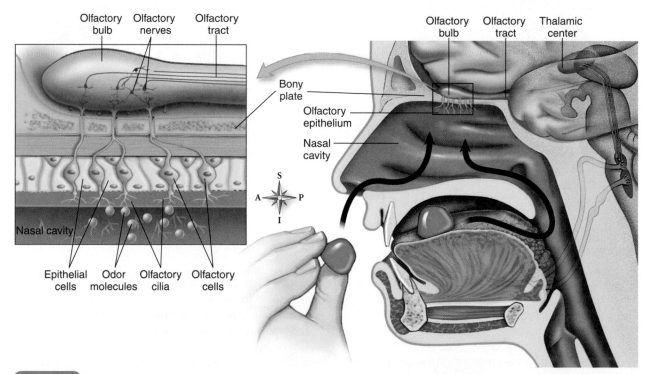

FIGURE 9-9 **Olfactory structures.** Gas molecules stimulate olfactory cells in the nasal epithelium. Sensory information is then conducted along nerves in the olfactory bulb and olfactory tract to sensory processing centers in the brain.

vivid and long-lasting memories of particular smells and odors. The pleasant smell of bread or cookies baking in a grandmother's kitchen may be part of a childhood memory that lasts a lifetime.

 To learn more about how the brain interprets odors, go to AnimationDirect on your CD-ROM.

> ✓ **QUICK CHECK**
> 1. Where are taste receptors located?
> 2. Can you name the primary tastes that humans can perceive?
> 3. What is the job of olfactory receptors?

Science Application

The Senses
Santiago Ramón y Cajal
(1852-1934)

Santiago Ramón y Cajal is considered by many to be the originator of the modern view of the nervous system's organization. He not only uncovered much about sensory centers of the cortex and the structure of the retina but also made important discoveries about nearly every part of the nervous system. Most of this Spanish researcher's ideas about the nervous system are intact today. Although Santiago wanted to be an artist, his father convinced him to follow in his footsteps and become an anatomist—a choice that led to his receiving a Nobel Prize in 1906.

The study of the sensory part of the nervous system and its relationships with the rest of the body is useful in many different fields. For example, the ideas used by optometrists and ophthalmologists, otologists and audiologists, and other professionals who assess and treat sensory disorders are based on neuroscience. Many other fields can make indirect use of neuroscience as well. For example, artists use what we know of visual perception in creating their works, musicians and architects make use of our knowledge of sound perception when performing in or designing concert halls, and aerospace professionals can use what we know of equilibrium and how it is perceived in the brain to understand motion sickness.

OUTLINE SUMMARY

CLASSIFICATION OF SENSE ORGANS
A. General sense organs (see Table 9-1)
  1. Often exist as individual cells or receptor units
  2. Widely distributed throughout the body
B. Special sense organs (see Table 9-2)
  1. Large and complex organs
  2. Localized grouping of specialized receptors
C. Classification by presence or absence of covering capsule
  1. Encapsulated
  2. Unencapsulated ("free" or "naked")
D. Classification by type of stimuli required to activate receptors
  1. Photoreceptors (light)
  2. Chemoreceptors (chemicals)
  3. Pain receptors (injury)
  4. Thermoreceptors (temperature change)
  5. Mechanoreceptors (movement or deforming of capsule)
  6. Proprioceptors (position of body parts or changes in muscle length or tension)

CONVERTING A STIMULUS INTO A SENSATION
A. All sense organs have common functional characteristics
  1. All are able to detect a particular stimulus
  2. A stimulus is converted into a nerve impulse
  3. A nerve impulse is perceived as a sensation in the central nervous system

GENERAL SENSE ORGANS (Table 9-1)
A. Distribution is widespread; single-cell receptors are common
B. Examples (see Figure 9-1, Table 9-1)
  1. Free nerve endings — pain, temperature, and crude touch
  2. Tactile (Meissner) corpuscles — fine touch and vibration

3. Bulbus (Ruffini) corpuscles — touch and pressure
4. Lamellar (Pacini) corpuscles — pressure and vibration
5. Bulboid corpuscles (Krause end bulbs) — touch
6. Golgi tendon organs — proprioception
7. Muscle spindles — proprioception

SPECIAL SENSE ORGANS

A. The eye (see Figure 9-2)
   1. Layers of eyeball
      a. Sclera — tough outer coat; "white" of eye; cornea is transparent part of sclera over iris
      b. Choroid — pigmented vascular layer prevents scattering of light; front part of this layer made of ciliary muscle and iris, the colored part of the eye; the pupil is the hole in the center of the iris; contraction of iris muscle dilates or constricts pupil
      c. Retina (see Figure 9-4) — innermost layer of the eye; contains rods (receptors for night vision) and cones (receptors for day vision and color vision)
   2. Conjunctiva — mucous membrane covering the front surface of the sclera and also lines the eyelid; kept moist by tears formed in the lacrimal gland
   3. Lens — transparent body behind the pupil; focuses or refracts light rays on the retina
   4. Eye fluids
      a. Aqueous humor — in the anterior chamber in front of the lens
      b. Vitreous humor — in the posterior chamber behind the lens
   5. Visual pathway
      a. Innermost layer of retina contains rods and cones
      b. Impulse travels from the rods and cones through the bipolar and ganglionic layers of retina (see Figure 9-4)
      c. Nerve impulse leaves the eye through the optic nerve; the point of exit is free of receptors and is therefore called a *blind spot*
      d. Visual interpretation occurs in the visual cortex of the cerebrum

B. The ear
   1. The ear functions in hearing and in equilibrium and balance—receptors called *mechanoreceptors*
   2. Divisions of the ear (see Figure 9-5)
      a. External ear
         (1) Auricle (pinna)
         (2) External auditory canal
            (a) Curving canal 2.5 cm (1 inch) in length
            (b) Contains ceruminous glands
            (c) Ends at the tympanic membrane
      b. Middle ear
         (1) Houses ear ossicles — malleus, incus, and stapes
         (2) Ends in the oval window
         (3) The auditory (eustachian) tube connects the middle ear to the throat
         (4) Inflammation called *otitis media*
      c. Inner ear (see Figure 9-6)
         (1) Bony labyrinth filled with perilymph
         (2) Subdivided into the vestibule, semicircular canals, and cochlea
         (3) Membranous labyrinth filled with endolymph
         (4) The receptors for balance in the semicircular canals are called *cristae ampullares*
         (5) Specialized hair cells on the organ of Corti respond when bent by the movement of surrounding endolymph set in motion by sound waves (see Figure 9-7)

C. The taste receptors (see Figure 9-8)
   1. Receptors are chemoreceptors called *taste buds*
   2. Cranial nerves VII and IX carry gustatory impulses
   3. Most pathologists list four kinds of "primary" taste sensations — sweet, sour, bitter, and salty
      a. Metallic and umami (meaty) tastes are also unique and are frequently added to the list of "primary" taste sensations
      b. Nasal congestion interferes with stimulation of olfactory receptors and thereby dulls taste sensations
   4. Gustatory and olfactory senses work together to permit creation of many other taste sensations

D. The smell receptors (see Figure 9-9)
  1. Receptors for fibers of olfactory or cranial nerve I lie in olfactory mucosa of nasal cavity
  2. Olfactory receptors are extremely sensitive but easily adapt (become fatigued)
  3. Odor-causing chemicals initiate a nervous signal that is interpreted as a specific odor by the brain

NEW WORDS

adaptation	endolymph	malleus	refraction
aqueous humor	eustachian tube	mechanoreceptor	retina
auricle	external auditory canal	membranous labyrinth	rod
bony labyrinth	fovea centralis	myopia	sclera
cataract	glaucoma	optic disc	semicircular canals
cerumen	gustatory cells	organ of Corti	stapes
ceruminous gland	hyperopia	ossicles	tympanic membrane
chemoreceptor	incus	papillae	(eardrum)
choroid	iris	perilymph	vestibular nerve
cochlea	lacrimal gland	photopigments	vestibule
cone	laser-assisted in situ	photoreceptor cell	vitreous humor
conjunctiva cornea	keratomileusis	presbyopia	
cornea	(LASIK)	proprioceptor	
crista ampullaris	lens	pupil	

REVIEW QUESTIONS

1. Name the general senses found in the skin or subcutaneous tissue and list the type of stimuli to which each of them respond. Which of these are unencapsulated?
2. Name the two general senses of proprioception and give the location of each.
3. With what type of information do proprioceptors provide us?
4. Explain how the iris changes the size of the pupil.
5. Explain how the ciliary muscles allow the eye to focus on near and far objects.
6. What is *presbyopia*, and what is its cause?
7. Name the two types of receptor cells in the retina. Explain the difference between these two receptors.
8. What is *glaucoma*, and what is its cause?
9. What are *cataracts*, how are they caused, and what can be done to prevent them?
10. What is meant by the visual pathway? Where is the blind spot, and what causes it?
11. Briefly explain the structure of the external ear.
12. Explain how sound waves are transmitted through the middle ear.
13. Explain how sound waves are converted to an auditory impulse.
14. Explain how the structures in the inner ear help maintain balance or equilibrium.
15. Where are gustatory cells located, and to what "primary" tastes do they respond?
16. Explain how the sense of smell is stimulated.

CRITICAL THINKING
17. Explain why food loses some of its taste when you have a bad cold with a stuffy nose.
18. Explain why the longer you are in a newly painted room, the less able you are to smell the paint.
19. Where in the eye is light sensed? Where is it perceived? (Be specific.)
20. Explain why the smell of a "doctor's office" or the smell of a turkey cooking on Thanksgiving can easily generate an emotional response.

CHAPTER TEST

1. The eye can be classified as a photoreceptor. Taste and smell can be classified as _____, and Golgi tendon organs and muscle spindles can be classified as _____.

2. The specific mechanoreceptor for hearing is the _____.

3. The specific mechanoreceptor for balance is the _____.

4. The gustatory cells are involved with the sense of _____.

5. Six "primary" kinds of taste sensations that result from the stimulation of the taste buds are _____, _____, _____, _____, _____, and _____.

6. Taste buds can be found on much larger structures on the tongue called _____.

7. The chemoreceptors responsible for the sense of smell are the _____.

Match each function or description in Column B with the corresponding structure of the eye in Column A.

COLUMN A

8. _____ sclera
9. _____ cornea
10. _____ iris
11. _____ pupil
12. _____ lacrimal
13. _____ lens
14. _____ rods
15. _____ cones
16. _____ choroid coat
17. _____ vitreous
18. _____ aqueous

COLUMN B

a. tears are formed in this gland
b. hole in the eye that lets light in
c. receptors for night or dim light vision
d. thick jellylike fluid or humor of the eye
e. tough, white outer layer of the eye
f. receptors for red, blue, and green color vision
g. ciliary muscles pull on this to help the eye focus
h. dark pigmented middle layer of the eye that prevents the scattering of incoming light
i. transparent part of the sclera, the window of the eye
j. colored part of the front of the eye
k. thin, watery humor of the eye

CHAPTER TEST—cont'd

Match each function or description in Column B with the corresponding structure of the ear in Column A.

COLUMN A

19. _____ tympanic membrane
20. _____ ossicles
21. _____ auditory tube
22. _____ perilymph
23. _____ endolymph
24. _____ cochlea
25. _____ organ of Corti

COLUMN B

a. tube connecting the middle ear and the throat
b. watery fluid that fills the bony labyrinth
c. snail-shaped structure in the inner ear
d. the organ of hearing
e. thick fluid in the membranous labyrinth
f. another term for eardrum
g. collective name for incus, malleus, and stapes

OBJECTIVES

AFTER YOU HAVE COMPLETED THIS CHAPTER, YOU SHOULD BE ABLE TO:

1. Distinguish between endocrine and exocrine glands and define the terms *hormone* and *prostaglandin*.
2. Identify and locate the primary endocrine glands and list the major hormones produced by each gland.
3. Describe the mechanisms of steroid and nonsteroid hormone action.
4. Explain how negative and positive feedback mechanisms regulate the secretion of endocrine hormones.
5. Identify the principal functions of each major endocrine hormone and describe the conditions that may result from hyposecretion or hypersecretion.
6. Define *diabetes insipidus*, *diabetes mellitus*, *gigantism*, *goiter*, *cretinism*, and *glycosuria*.

The Endocrine System 10

Have you ever known anyone with thyroid problems or diabetes? Surely you have seen the dramatic changes that happen to a person's body as he or she goes through puberty. These are all proof of the importance of the endocrine system in normal development and health.

The **endocrine system** performs the same general functions as the nervous system: communication and control. The nervous system provides rapid, brief control by way of fast-traveling nerve impulses. The endocrine system provides slower but longer-lasting control by way of hormones (chemicals) secreted into and circulated by the blood.

The organs of the endocrine system are located in widely separated parts of the body—in the neck; the cranial, thoracic, abdominal, and pelvic cavities; and also outside of the body cavities. Note the names and locations of the endocrine glands shown in Figure 10-1.

All organs of the endocrine system are glands, but not all glands are organs of the endocrine system. Of the two types of glands in the body—**exocrine glands** and **endocrine glands**—only endocrine glands belong to this system. Exocrine glands secrete their products into ducts that empty onto a surface or into a cavity. For example, sweat glands produce a watery secretion that empties onto the surface of the skin. Salivary glands are also exocrine glands, secreting saliva that flows into the mouth. Endocrine glands are ductless glands. They secrete chemicals known as **hormones** into intercellular spaces. From there, the hormones diffuse directly into the blood and are carried throughout the body. Each hormone molecule may then bind to a cell that has specific receptors for that hormone, triggering a reaction in the cell. Such a cell is called a **target cell.** The list of endocrine glands and the organs in which their target cells are found *(target organs)* contin-

STUDY TIPS

To make the study of the endocrine system more efficient, we suggest these tips:

1. Before studying Chapter 10, review the synopsis of the endocrine system in Chapter 4.
2. The function of the endocrine system is similar to that of the nervous system. The differences are in the methods used to produce an effect and the extent of the effect. The endocrine system uses chemicals in the blood (hormones) rather than nerve impulses. Hormones can have a direct effect on almost every cell in the body, an impossible task for the nervous system. Steroid hormones can act directly because they can enter the cell; protein hormones cannot enter the cell so they need a second messenger system.
3. Material from earlier chapters regarding topics such as receptor proteins in the cell membrane, adenosine triphosphate (ATP), homeostasis, and negative feedback loops will help you understand the material in this chapter.
4. Use flash cards to learn the names of the hormones, what they do, and the names and locations of the glands that produce them. Remember that hormones released by the posterior pituitary gland are made in the hypothalamus.
5. In your study group, discuss the hormone mechanisms and the negative feedback loops involved in hormone regulation.
6. Review the hormone flash cards in your study group. A photocopy of Figure 10-1 (showing the endocrine glands) may be helpful for reviewing the location of glands. Quiz each other on which gland produces what hormone.
7. Go over the questions at the end of the chapter and discuss possible test questions.

ues to grow. The names, locations, and functions of the well-known endocrine glands are given in Figure 10-1 and Table 10-1.

In this chapter you will read about the functions of the main endocrine glands and discover why

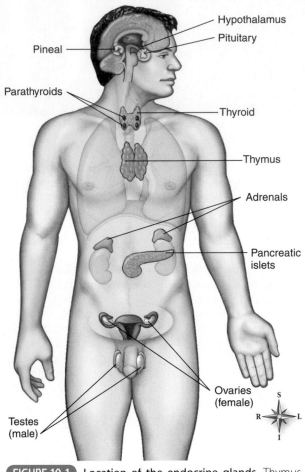

FIGURE 10-1 Location of the endocrine glands. Thymus gland is shown at maximum size at puberty.

Labels (top to bottom, left and right):
Pineal — Parathyroids — Thyroid — Thymus — Adrenals — Pancreatic islets — Ovaries (female) — Testes (male) — Hypothalamus — Pituitary

their importance is almost impossible to exaggerate. Hormones are the main regulators of metabolism, growth and development, reproduction, and many other body activities. They play important roles in maintaining homeostasis—fluid and electrolyte, acid-base, and energy balances, for example. Hormones make the difference between normalcy and many kinds of abnormalities such as dwarfism, gigantism, and sterility. They are important not only for the healthy survival of each one of us but also for the survival of the human species.

Diseases of the endocrine glands are numerous, varied, and sometimes spectacular. Tumors or other abnormalities often cause a gland to secrete too much or too little hormone. Production of too much hormone by a diseased gland is called

hypersecretion. If too little hormone is produced, the condition is called **hyposecretion.**

MECHANISMS OF HORMONE ACTION

A hormone causes its target cells to respond in particular ways; this has been the subject of intense interest and research. The two major classes of hormones—**nonsteroid hormones** and **steroid hormones**—differ in the mechanisms by which they influence target cells.

Nonsteroid Hormones

Nonsteroid hormones are whole proteins, shorter chains of amino acids, or simply versions of single amino acids. Nonsteroid hormones work according to the *second messenger mechanism.* According to this concept, a protein hormone, such as thyroid-stimulating hormone, acts as a "first messenger" (that is, it delivers its chemical message from the cells of an endocrine gland to highly specific membrane receptor sites on the target cells). This interaction between a hormone and its specific receptor site on the target cell's plasma membrane is often compared with the fitting of a unique key into a lock. (This idea is the *lock-and-key model* of chemical activity.) After the hormone is attached to its specific receptor site, a number of chemical reactions occur. These reactions activate molecules within the cell called **second messengers.** One example of this mechanism occurs when the hormone-receptor interaction changes energy-rich ATP molecules inside the cell into **cyclic adenosine monophosphate (cAMP).** cAMP serves as the second messenger, delivering information inside the cell that regulates the cell's activity. For example, cAMP causes thyroid cells to respond to thyroid-stimulating hormone by secreting a thyroid hormone such as thyroxine. cAMP is only one of several second messengers that have been discovered.

In summary, nonsteroid hormones serve as first messengers, providing communication between endocrine glands and target organs. Another molecule, such as cAMP, then acts as the second messenger, providing communication within a hormone's target cells. Figure 10-2 summarizes the mechanism of nonsteroid hormone action as explained by the second messenger hypothesis.

TABLE 10-1

Endocrine Glands, Hormones, and Their Functions

GLAND/HORMONE	FUNCTION
Anterior Pituitary	
Thyroid-stimulating hormone (TSH)	Tropic hormone Stimulates secretion of thyroid hormones
Adrenocorticotropic hormone (ACTH)	Tropic hormone Stimulates secretion of adrenal cortex hormones
Follicle-stimulating hormone (FSH)	Tropic hormone *Female:* stimulates development of ovarian follicles and secretion of estrogens *Male:* stimulates seminiferous tubules of testes to grow and produce sperm
Luteinizing hormone (LH)	Tropic hormone *Female:* stimulates maturation of ovarian follicle and ovum; stimulates secretion of estrogen; triggers ovulation; stimulates development of corpus luteum (luteinization) *Male:* stimulates interstitial cells of the testes to secrete testosterone
Growth hormone (GH)	Stimulates growth in all organs; mobilizes food molecules, causing an increase in blood glucose concentration
Prolactin (PRL) (lactogenic hormone)	Stimulates breast development during pregnancy and milk secretion (milk let-down) after pregnancy
Posterior Pituitary*	
Antidiuretic hormone (ADH)	Stimulates retention of water by the kidneys
Oxytocin (OT)	Stimulates uterine contractions at the end of pregnancy; stimulates the release of milk into the breast ducts
Hypothalamus	
Releasing hormones (RHs) (several)	Stimulate the anterior pituitary to release hormones
Inhibiting hormones (IHs) (several)	Inhibit the anterior pituitary's secretion of hormones
Thyroid	
Thyroxine (T_4) and triiodothyronine (T_3)	Stimulate the energy metabolism of all cells
Calcitonin (CT)	Inhibits the breakdown of bone; causes a decrease in blood calcium concentration
Parathyroid	
Parathyroid hormone (PTH)	Stimulates the breakdown of bone; causes an increase in blood calcium concentration
Adrenal Cortex	
Mineralocorticoids (MCs): aldosterone	Regulate electrolyte and fluid homeostasis
Glucocorticoids (GCs): cortisol (hydrocortisone)	Stimulate gluconeogenesis, causing an increase in blood glucose concentration; also have anti-inflammatory and anti-immunity, antiallergy effects
Sex hormones (androgens)	Stimulate sexual drive in the female but have negligible effects in the male
Adrenal Medulla	
Epinephrine (Epi) (adrenaline) and norepinephrine (NR)	Prolong and intensify the sympathetic nervous response during stress
Pancreatic Islets	
Glucagon	Stimulates liver glycogenolysis, causing an increase in blood glucose concentration
Insulin	Promotes glucose entry into all cells, causing a decrease in blood glucose concentration
Ovary	
Estrogens	Promotes development and maintenance of female sexual characteristics (see Chapter 20)
Progesterone	Promotes conditions required for pregnancy (see Chapter 20)
Testis	
Testosterone	Promotes development and maintenance of male sexual characteristics (see Chapter 20)

*Posterior pituitary hormones are synthesized in the hypothalamus but released from axon terminals in the posterior pituitary.

Continued

TABLE 10-1

Endocrine Glands, Hormones, and Their Functions—cont'd

GLAND/HORMONE	FUNCTION
Thymus	
Thymosins	Promote development of immune-system cells
Placenta	
Chorionic gonadotropin, estrogens, progesterone	Promote conditions required during early pregnancy
Pineal Gland	
Melatonin	Inhibits tropic hormones that affect the ovaries; may be involved in the body's internal clock
Heart (Atria)	
Atrial natriuretic hormone (ANH)	Regulates fluid and electrolyte homeostasis
Gastrointestinal (GI) Tract	
Ghrelin	Affects energy balance (metabolism)
Fat-Storing Cells	
Leptin	Controls how hungry or full we feel

Research, Issues, & Trends

Second Messenger Systems

Rapid and revolutionary discoveries about how nonsteroid hormones act on their target cells began with the pioneering work of Earl Sutherland, who received the 1971 Nobel Prize for formulating the second messenger hypothesis, and new discoveries continue to be made even today. Later, the important role of the *G protein* in getting the signal from the receptor to the enzyme that forms cAMP was discovered. Look for the G protein in Figure 10-2. More recently, the role of nitric oxide (NO) in second messenger systems has been worked out. All of these discoveries resulted in Nobel Prizes, which shows the importance the scientific community has placed on them. Why? By working out the details of how hormones work, we can more clearly understand how and why things can go wrong that affect endocrine disorders. Perhaps we may even gain new knowledge about disorders that we previously did not even know involved hormone mechanisms. Once the processes of disease mechanisms are figured out, we hope scientists will be able to design tests that can screen for such problems. Or perhaps they can develop drugs that will "fix" the broken mechanisms and cure the disease. Although this complex subject may seem like too much for you to comprehend now, you will discover that understanding how hormones act on target cells **(signal transduction)** will prepare you for the revolution in medicine that is now upon us.

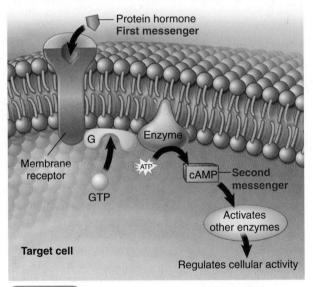

FIGURE 10-2 Mechanism of nonsteroid hormone action. The hormone acts as a "first messenger," delivering its message via the bloodstream to a membrane receptor in the target cell much like a key fits into a lock. The "second messenger" causes the cell to respond and perform its specialized function.

Steroid Hormones

The action of small, lipid-soluble steroid hormones such as estrogen does not occur by the second messenger system. Because they are lipid soluble, steroid hormones can pass intact directly through the plasma membrane of the target cell. Once inside the cell, steroid hormones pass through the cytoplasm and enter the nucleus where they bind with a receptor (according to the lock-and-key model) to form a hormone-receptor complex. This complex acts on DNA, which ultimately causes the formation of a new protein in the cytoplasm that then produces specific effects in the target cell. In the case of estrogen, for example, that effect might be breast development in the female adolescent.

Figure 10-3 summarizes this mechanism of steroid hormone action. Because it takes some time to accomplish all of the steps illustrated in the diagram, steroid hormone responses typically are slow compared to responses triggered by nonsteroid hormones.

Besides the primary effects of steroids produced by the DNA-triggering mechanism just described, steroid hormones may also trigger membrane receptors to produce a variety of secondary effects.

These secondary effects usually appear much more rapidly than do the primary steroid effects.

> ### ✓ QUICK CHECK
>
> 1. What is the chemical messenger used by the endocrine system?
> 2. How do nonsteroid hormones and steroid hormones differ? How are they alike?
> 3. What is a *second messenger* system?

REGULATION OF HORMONE SECRETION

The regulation of hormone levels in the blood depends on a highly specialized homeostatic mechanism called *negative feedback* (see Chapter 1, p. 12). The principle of **negative feedback** can be illustrated by using the hormone insulin as an exam-

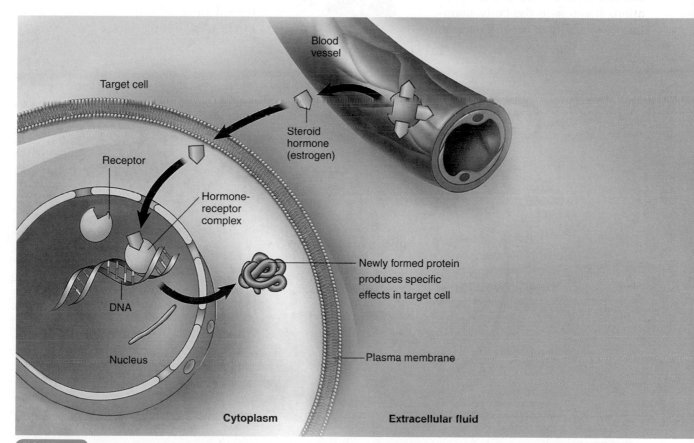

FIGURE 10-3　**Mechanism of steroid hormone action.** Steroid hormones pass through the plasma membrane and enter the nucleus to form a hormone receptor complex that acts on DNA. As a result, a new protein is formed in the cytoplasm that produces specific effects in the target cell.

ple. When released from endocrine cells in the pancreas, insulin lowers blood sugar levels. Normally, elevated blood sugar levels occur after a meal, after the absorption of sugars from the digestive tract takes place. The elevated blood sugar stimulates the release of insulin from the pancreas. Insulin then assists in the transfer of sugar from the blood into cells, causing blood sugar levels to drop. Low blood sugar levels then cause endocrine cells in the pancreas to cease the production and release of insulin. These responses are *negative*. The homeostatic mechanism is called a *negative feedback control mechanism* because it reverses the change in blood sugar level (Figure 10-4).

Positive feedback mechanisms, which are uncommon, amplify changes rather than reverse them. Usually, such amplification threatens homeostasis, but in some situations it can help the body maintain its stability. For example, during labor, the muscle contractions that push the baby through the birth canal become stronger and stronger by means of a positive feedback mechanism that regulates secretion of the hormone oxytocin (OT).

PROSTAGLANDINS

Prostaglandins (PGs), or tissue hormones, are important and extremely powerful substances found in a wide variety of tissues. They play an important role in communication and in the control of many body functions but do not meet the definition of a typical hormone. The term *tissue hormone* is appropriate because in many instances a prostaglandin is produced in a tissue and then diffuses only a short distance to act on cells within that tissue. Typical hormones influence and control activities of widely separated organs; typical prostaglandins influence activities of neighboring cells.

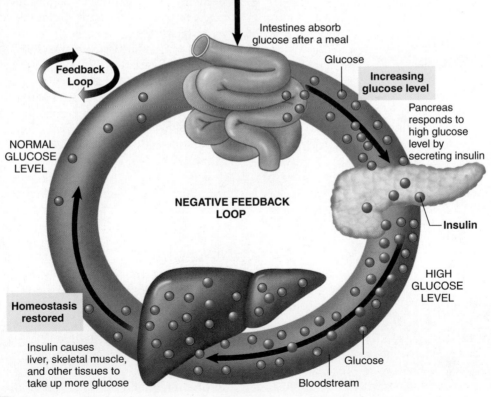

FIGURE 10-4 **Negative feedback.** The secretion of most hormones is regulated by negative feedback mechanisms that tend to reverse any deviations from normal. In this example, an increase in blood glucose triggers secretion of insulin. Because insulin promotes glucose uptake by cells, the blood glucose level is restored to its lower, normal level.

The prostaglandins in the body can be divided into several groups. Three classes of prostaglandins—prostaglandin A (PGA), prostaglandin E (PGE), and prostaglandin F (PGF)—are among the best known. PGs have profound effects on many body functions. They influence respiration, blood pressure, gastrointestinal secretions, inflammation, and the reproductive system. Researchers believe that most PGs regulate cells by influencing the production of cAMP. Although much research is yet to be done, PGs are already playing an important role in the treatment of conditions such as high blood pressure, asthma, and ulcers. In fact, many common treatments such as aspirin cause their effects by altering the functions of PGs in the body.

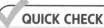

QUICK CHECK

1. How does negative feedback affect hormone levels in the blood?
2. Why are prostaglandins called *tissue hormones*?

PITUITARY GLAND

The **pituitary** (pi-TOO-i-tair-ee) **gland** is a small but mighty structure. Although no larger than a pea, it is really two glands—each a different type. One is called the *anterior pituitary gland* or **adenohypophysis** (ad-eh-no-hye-POF-i-sis), and the other is called the *posterior pituitary gland* or **neurohypophysis** (noo-roh-hye-POF-i-sis). Differences between the two glands are indicated by their names—*adeno* means "gland," and *neuro* means "nervous." The adenohypophysis has the structure of an endocrine gland, whereas the neurohypophysis has the structure of nervous tissue. Hormones secreted by the adenohypophysis serve very different functions from those released from the neurohypophysis.

The protected location of this dual gland suggests its importance. The pituitary gland lies buried deep in the cranial cavity, in the small depression of the sphenoid bone that is shaped like a saddle and called the **sella turcica** (Turkish saddle). A stemlike structure, the pituitary stalk, attaches the gland to the undersurface of the brain. More specifically, the stalk attaches the pituitary body to the hypothalamus.

Anterior Pituitary Gland Hormones

The anterior pituitary gland (adenohypophysis) secretes several major hormones. Each of the four hormones listed as a **tropic** (TROH-pik) **hormone** in Table 10-1 stimulates another endocrine gland to grow and secrete its hormones. Because the anterior pituitary gland exerts this control over the structure and function of the thyroid gland, the adrenal cortex, the ovarian follicles, and the corpus luteum, it was sometimes called the *master gland.* However, because its secretions are in turn controlled by the hypothalamus and other mechanisms, the anterior pituitary is hardly the master of body function it was once thought to be.

Thyroid-stimulating hormone (TSH) acts on the thyroid gland. As its name suggests, it stimulates the thyroid gland to increase secretion of thyroid hormone.

The **adrenocorticotropic** (ah-dree-no-kor-teh-koh-TROH-pic) **hormone (ACTH)** acts on the adrenal cortex. It stimulates the adrenal cortex to increase in size and to secrete larger amounts of its hormones, especially larger amounts of cortisol (hydrocortisone).

Follicle-stimulating hormone (FSH) stimulates the primary ovarian follicles in an ovary to start growing and to continue developing to maturity (that is, to the point of ovulation). FSH also stimulates follicle cells to secrete estrogens. In the male, FSH stimulates the seminiferous tubules to grow and form sperm.

Luteinizing (loo-tee-in-EYE-zing) **hormone (LH)** acts with FSH to perform several functions. It stimulates a follicle and ovum to complete their growth to maturity, it stimulates follicle cells to secrete estrogens, and it causes ovulation (rupturing of the mature follicle with expulsion of its ripe ovum). Because of this function, LH is sometimes called the *ovulating hormone.* Finally, LH stimulates the formation of a golden body, the corpus luteum, in the ruptured follicle; the process is called **luteinization.** This function, of course, is the one that earned LH its title of *luteinizing hormone.* As it promotes luteinization, LH stimulates the corpus luteum to produce the hormone progesterone. The male pituitary gland also secretes LH. In males, LH stimulates interstitial cells in the testes to develop and secrete testosterone, the male sex hormone.

Another important hormone secreted by the anterior pituitary gland is **growth hormone.** Growth hormone (GH) speeds up the movement of digested proteins (amino acids) out of the blood and into the cells, and this accelerates the cells' **anabolism** (build-up) (see Chapter 16) of amino acids to form tissue proteins; hence this action promotes normal growth. Growth hormone also affects fat and carbohydrate metabolism; it accelerates fat catabolism (breakdown) but slows glucose catabolism. This means that less glucose leaves the blood to enter cells, and therefore the amount of glucose in the blood increases. Thus growth hormone and insulin have opposite effects on blood glucose. Insulin decreases blood glucose, and growth hormone increases it. Too much insulin in the blood produces **hypoglycemia** (hye-poh-glye-SEE-mee-ah) (lower than normal blood glucose concentration). Too much growth hormone produces **hyperglycemia** (higher than normal blood glucose concentration).

The anterior pituitary gland also secretes **prolactin** (proh-LAK-tin) **(PRL),** or *lactogenic hormone*. During pregnancy, prolactin stimulates the breast development necessary for eventual lactation (milk secretion). Also, soon after delivery of a baby, a woman's prolactin stimulates the breasts to start secreting milk, a function suggested by prolactin's other name, lactogenic hormone.

Figure 10-5 provides a summary of anterior pituitary hormone target organs and functions.

Posterior Pituitary Gland Hormones

The posterior pituitary gland (neurohypophysis) releases two hormones—**antidiuretic** (an-tee-dye-yoo-RET-ik) **hormone (ADH)** and **oxytocin** (ahk-see-TOH-sin) **(OT).** ADH accelerates the reabsorption of water from urine in kidney tubules back into the blood. With more water moving out of the tubules into the blood, less water remains in the tubules, and therefore less urine leaves the body.

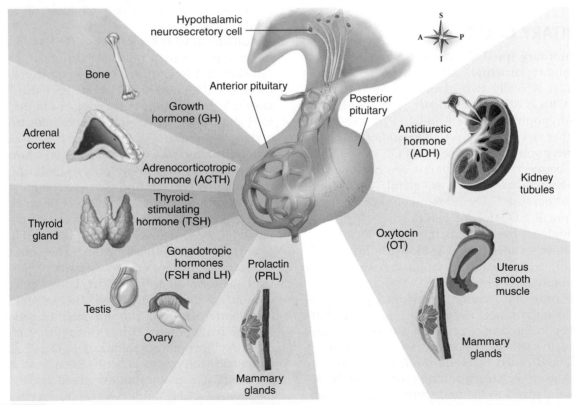

FIGURE 10-5 **Pituitary hormones.** Principal anterior pituitary hormones and their major target organs *(shaded purple)* and posterior pituitary hormones and some major target organs *(shaded blue).*

Clinical Application

Growth Hormone Abnormalities

Hypersecretion of growth hormone during the early years of life produces a condition called **gigantism** (jye-GAN-tiz-em) *(left side of photo)*. The name suggests the obvious characteristics of this condition. The child grows to giant size. Hyposecretion of the growth hormone produces pituitary **dwarfism** (DWARF-iz-em) *(right side of photo)*.

If the anterior pituitary gland secretes too much growth hormone after the normal growth years, then the disease called **acromegaly** (ak-roh-MEG-ah-lee) develops. Characteristics of this disease are enlargement of the bones of the hands, feet, jaws, and cheeks. The facial appearance typical of acromegaly results from the combination of bone and soft tissue overgrowth. A prominent forehead and large nose are characteristic. In addition, the skin is characterized by large, widened pores, and the mandible grows in length so that separation of the lower teeth commonly occurs.

The name *antidiuretic hormone* is appropriate because *anti-* means "against" and *diuretic* means "increasing the volume of urine excreted." Therefore *antidiuretic* means "acting against an increase in urine volume"; in other words, ADH acts to decrease urine volume. Hyposecretion of ADH results in **diabetes insipidus** (dye-ah-BEE-teez in-SIP-i-dus), a condition in which large volumes of urine are formed. Dehydration and electrolyte imbalances may cause serious problems unless the sufferer is treated with injections or nasal sprays containing ADH.

The posterior pituitary hormone oxytocin is secreted by a woman's body before and after she has a baby. Oxytocin stimulates contraction of the smooth muscle of the pregnant uterus and is believed to initiate and maintain labor. This is why physicians sometimes prescribe oxytocin injections to induce or increase labor. Oxytocin also performs a function important to a newborn baby. It causes the glandular cells of the breast to release milk into ducts from which a baby can obtain it by sucking. In short, oxytocin stimulates "milk letdown." Oxytocin is also thought to enhance social bonding—a function helpful in supporting the mother-infant bond.

The right side of Figure 10-5 summarizes posterior pituitary functions.

HYPOTHALAMUS

In discussing ADH and oxytocin, we noted that these hormones were *released* from the posterior lobe of the pituitary. Actual production of these two hormones occurs in the hypothalamus. Two groups of specialized neurons in the hypothalamus synthesize the posterior pituitary hormones, which then pass down along axons into the pituitary gland. Release of ADH and oxytocin into the blood is controlled by nervous stimulation.

In addition to oxytocin and ADH, the hypothalamus also produces substances called **releasing hormones (RHs)** and **inhibiting hormones (IHs).** These substances are produced in the hypothalamus and then travel directly through a specialized blood capillary system to the anterior pituitary gland, where they cause the release of anterior pituitary hormones or, in a number of instances, inhibit their production and their release into the general circulation.

The combined nervous and endocrine functions of the hypothalamus allow the nervous system to influence many endocrine functions. Therefore the hypothalamus plays a dominant role in the regulation of many body functions related to homeostasis. Examples include the regulation of body temperature, appetite, and thirst.

✓ **QUICK CHECK**

1. How are the anterior pituitary and posterior pituitary different? How are they alike?
2. What makes a hormone a *tropic* hormone?
3. Name the hormones produced by the pituitary gland.
4. How does the hypothalamus control the pituitary gland?

THYROID GLAND

Earlier in this chapter, we mentioned that some endocrine glands are not located in a body cavity. The thyroid is one of these. It lies in the neck just below the larynx (Figure 10-6).

The thyroid gland secretes two thyroid hormones, **thyroxine** (thy-ROK-sin), or **T_4**, and **triiodothyronine** (try-eye-oh-doh-THY-roh-neen), or **T_3**. It also secretes the hormone **calcitonin** (kal-si-TOH-nin) **(CT)**. Of the two thyroid hormones, T_4 is the more abundant; however, T_3 is the more potent and is considered by physiologists to be the principal thyroid hormone. One molecule of T_4 contains four atoms of iodine, and one molecule of T_3, as its name suggests, contains three iodine atoms. For T_4 to be produced in adequate amounts, the diet must contain sufficient iodine.

Most endocrine glands do not store their hormones but secrete them directly into the blood as they are produced. The thyroid gland is different in that it stores considerable amounts of the thyroid hormones in the form of a colloid compound seen in Figure 10-7. The colloid material is stored in the follicles of the gland, and when the thyroid hormones are needed, they are released from the colloid and secreted into the blood.

T_4 and T_3 influence every one of the trillions of cells in our bodies. They make them speed up their release of energy from foods. In other words, these thyroid hormones stimulate cellular metabolism. This has far-reaching effects. Because all body functions depend on a normal supply of energy, they all depend on normal thyroid secretion. Even normal mental and physical growth and development depend on normal thyroid functioning.

A   **B**

FIGURE 10-6 **Thyroid and parathyroid glands.** Note their relationship to each other and to the larynx (voice box) and trachea.

Calcitonin decreases the concentration of calcium in the blood by first acting on bone to inhibit its breakdown. With less bone being resorbed, less calcium moves out of bone into blood, and, as a result, the concentration of calcium in blood decreases. An increase in calcitonin secretion quickly follows any increase in blood calcium concentration, even if it is a slight one. This causes blood calcium concentration to decrease to its normal level. Calcitonin thus helps maintain homeostasis of blood calcium. It prevents a harmful excess of calcium in the blood, a condition called **hypercalcemia** (hye-per-kal-SEE-mee-ah), from developing.

 To learn more about thyroid secretion, go to AnimationDirect on your CD-ROM.

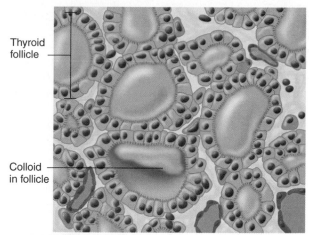

Thyroid follicle

Colloid in follicle

FIGURE 10-7 **Thyroid gland tissue.** Note that each of the follicles is filled with colloid. The colloid serves as a storage medium for the thyroid hormones.

 Clinical Application

Thyroid Hormone Abnormalities

Hyperthyroidism (hye-per-THY-royd-iz-em), or oversecretion of the thyroid hormones, dramatically increases the metabolic rate. Food material is burned by the cells at an excessive rate, and individuals who suffer from this condition lose weight, are irritable, have an increased appetite, and often show protrusion of the eyeballs due in part to edema of tissue at the back of the eye socket; see Figure A.

Hypothyroidism (hye-poh-THY-royd-iz-em), or undersecretion of thyroid hormones, can be caused by and result in a number of different conditions. Low dietary intake of iodine causes a painless enlargement of the thyroid gland called **simple goiter** (GOY-ter), shown in Figure B. This condition was once common in areas of the United States where the iodine content of the soil and water is inadequate. The use of iodized salt has dramatically reduced the incidence of simple goiter caused by low iodine intake. In simple goiter the gland enlarges to compensate for the lack of iodine in the diet necessary for the synthesis of thyroid hormones.

Hyposecretion of thyroid hormones during the formative years leads to a condition called **cretinism** (KREE-tin-iz-em). It is characterized by a low metabolic rate, retarded growth and sexual development, and, often, mental retardation. Fortunately, health screening for low thyroid function can lead to treatment before cretinism develops. Later in life, deficient thyroid hormone secretion produces the disease called **myxedema** (mik-seh-DEE-mah). The low metabolic rate that characterizes myxedema leads to lessened mental and physical vigor, weight gain, loss of hair, and swelling of tissues.

A

B

PARATHYROID GLANDS

The **parathyroid glands** are small glands. There are usually four of them, and they are found on the back of the thyroid gland (see Figure 10-6). The parathyroid glands secrete **parathyroid hormone (PTH).**

   PTH increases the concentration of calcium in the blood—the opposite effect of the thyroid gland's calcitonin. Whereas calcitonin acts to decrease the amount of calcium being resorbed from bone, PTH acts to increase it. PTH stimulates bone-resorbing cells or osteoclasts to increase their breakdown of bone's hard matrix, a process that frees the calcium stored in the matrix. The released calcium then moves out of bone into blood, and this in turn increases the blood's calcium concentration. Figure 10-8 provides a summary of the antagonistic effects of calcitonin and parathyroid hormone. This is a matter of life-and-death importance because our cells are extremely sensitive to changing amounts of blood calcium. They cannot function normally with too much or too little calcium. For example, with too much blood calcium, brain cells and heart cells soon cease to function normally; a person becomes mentally disturbed, and the heart may stop. However, with too little blood calcium, nerve cells become overactive, sometimes to such a degree that they bombard muscles with so many impulses that the muscles go into spasms.

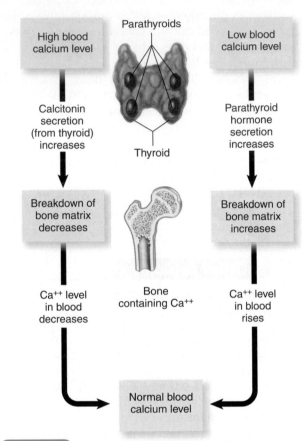

Feedback Loop

High blood calcium level

Calcitonin secretion (from thyroid) increases

Breakdown of bone matrix decreases

Ca++ level in blood decreases

Parathyroids

Thyroid

Bone containing Ca++

Low blood calcium level

Parathyroid hormone secretion increases

Breakdown of bone matrix increases

Ca++ level in blood rises

Normal blood calcium level

FIGURE 10-8 Regulation of blood calcium levels. Calcitonin and parathyroid hormones have antagonistic (opposite) effects on calcium concentration in the blood.

QUICK CHECK

1. Where are the thyroid and parathyroid glands located?
2. What gland stores its hormones for later use?
3. Calcitonin and parathyroid hormone both regulate the blood concentration of what important ion?

ADRENAL GLANDS

As you can see in Figures 10-1 and 10-9, an adrenal gland curves over the top of each kidney. From the surface an adrenal gland appears to be only one organ, but it is actually two separate endocrine glands: the *adrenal cortex* and the *adrenal medulla.* Does this two-glands-in-one structure remind you of another endocrine organ? (see p. 231). The adrenal cortex is the outer part of an adrenal gland, and the medulla is its inner part. Adrenal cortex

hormones have different names and quite different actions from adrenal medulla hormones.

Adrenal Cortex

Three different zones or layers of cells make up the **adrenal cortex** as you can see in Figure 10-9. Follow this diagram carefully as you read the following paragraph and you will easily see the special function of each layer of the adrenal cortex.

   Hormones secreted by the three cell layers or zones of the adrenal cortex are called **corticoids** (KOHR-ti-koydz). The outer zone of adrenal cortex cells secretes hormones called **mineralocorticoids** (min-er-al-oh-KOHR-ti-koydz), or **MCs** for

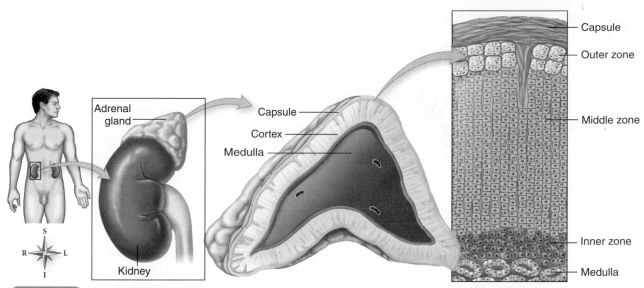

FIGURE 10-9 **The adrenal gland.** The three cell layers of the adrenal cortex are easily seen here. The outer zone cells secrete mineralocorticoids (aldosterone). The middle zone cells secrete glucocorticoids (hydrocortisone). The inner zone cells secrete sex hormones (androgens).

short. The main mineralocorticoid is the hormone **aldosterone** (AL-deh-steh-rohn *or* al-DAH-stair-ohn). The middle zone secretes **glucocorticoids** (gloo-koh-KOHR-ti-koydz), or **GCs. Cortisol,** or **hydrocortisone,** is the chief glucocorticoid. The innermost or deepest zone of the cortex secretes small amounts of *sex hormones*. Sex hormones secreted by the adrenal cortex resemble testosterone. A brief discussion of the functions of these three kinds of adrenal cortical hormones follows.

As their name suggests, mineralocorticoids help control the amount of certain mineral salts (mainly sodium chloride) in the blood. Aldosterone is the chief mineralocorticoid. Remember its main functions—to increase the amount of sodium and decrease the amount of potassium in the blood— because these changes lead to other profound changes. Aldosterone increases blood sodium and decreases blood potassium by influencing the kidney tubules. It causes them to speed up their reabsorption of sodium back into the blood so that less of it will be lost in the urine. At the same time, aldosterone causes the tubules to increase their secretion of potassium so that more of this mineral will be lost in the urine. The effects of aldosterone speed up kidney reabsorption of water.

An important role of glucocorticoids is to help maintain normal blood glucose concentration. Glucocorticoids increase **gluconeogenesis** (gloo-

koh-nee-oh-JEN-eh-sis), a process that converts amino acids or fatty acids to glucose and that is performed mainly by liver cells. Glucocorticoids act in several ways to increase gluconeogenesis. They promote the breakdown of tissue proteins to amino acids, especially in muscle cells. Amino acids thus formed move out of the tissue cells into blood and circulate to the liver. Liver cells then change them to glucose by the process of gluconeogenesis. The newly formed glucose leaves the liver cells and enters the blood. This action increases blood glucose concentration.

In addition to performing these functions— which are necessary for maintaining normal blood glucose concentration—glucocorticoids also play an essential part in maintaining normal blood pressure. They act in a complicated way to make it possible for two other hormones secreted by the adrenal medulla to partially constrict blood vessels, a condition necessary for maintaining normal blood pressure. Also, glucocorticoids act with these hormones from the adrenal medulla to produce an anti-inflammatory effect. They bring about a normal recovery from inflammations produced by many kinds of agents. The use of hydrocortisone to relieve skin rashes, for example, is based on the anti-inflammatory effect of glucocorticoids.

Another effect produced by glucocorticoids is called their *anti-immunity, antiallergy effect.*

Glucocorticoids bring about a decrease in the number of certain cells that produce antibodies, substances that make us immune to some factors and allergic to others.

When extreme stimuli act on the body, they produce an internal state or condition known as **stress.** Surgery, hemorrhage, infections, severe burns, and intense emotions are examples of extreme stimuli that bring on stress. The normal adrenal cortex responds to the condition of stress by quickly increasing its secretion of glucocorticoids. This fact is well established. What is still not known, however, is whether the increased amount of glucocorticoids helps the body cope successfully with stress. Increased glucocorticoid secretion is only one of many ways in which the body responds to stress, but it is one of the first stress responses, and it brings about many of the other stress responses. Examine Figure 10-10 to discover what stress responses are produced by a high concentration of glucocorticoids in the blood.

The sex hormones that are secreted by the inner zone are male hormones **(androgens)** similar to testosterone. These hormones are secreted in small amounts in both males and females. In females, these androgens stimulate the female sexual drive.

In males, so much testosterone is secreted by the testes that adrenal androgens are physiologically insignificant.

Adrenal Medulla

The **adrenal medulla,** or inner portion of the adrenal gland shown in Figure 10-9, secretes the hormones **epinephrine** (ep-i-NEF-rin) **(Epi)** and **norepinephrine** (nor-ep-i-NEF-rin) **(NR).** Epinephrine is also known as *adrenaline.*

Our bodies have many ways to defend themselves against enemies that threaten their well-being. A physiologist might say that the body resists stress by making many stress responses. We have just discussed increased glucocorticoid secretion. An even faster-acting stress response is increased secretion by the adrenal medulla. This occurs very rapidly because nerve impulses conducted by sympathetic nerve fibers stimulate the adrenal medulla. When stimulated, it literally squirts epinephrine and norepinephrine into the blood. As with glucocorticoids, these hormones may help the body resist or avoid stress. In other words, these hormones produce the body's "fight-or-flight" response to danger (stress). However,

FIGURE 10-10 Stress responses induced by high concentrations of glucocorticoids in blood.

Clinical Application

Adrenal Hormone Abnormalities

Injury, disease states, or malfunction of the adrenal glands can result in hypersecretion or hyposecretion of several different hormones.

Tumors of the adrenal cortex located in the middle zone of the cortex often result in the production of abnormally large amounts of glucocorticoids. The medical name for this condition is **Cushing syndrome.** Figure A shows a boy just diagnosed with Cushing syndrome. Figure B shows the same boy 4 months later, after treatment. For some reason many more women than men develop Cushing syndrome. Its most noticeable features are the so-called moon face and the buffalo hump on the upper back that develop because of redistribution of body fat. These individuals also have elevated blood sugar levels and suffer frequent infections. Surgical removal of a glucocorticoid-producing tumor may result in dramatic improvement of the moon-face symptom within 6 months.

Deficiency, or hyposecretion, of adrenal cortex hormones results in a condition called **Addison disease.** President

John F. Kennedy suffered from Addison disease, which causes reduced cortical hormone levels resulting in muscle weakness, reduced blood sugar, nausea, loss of appetite, and weight loss.

epinephrine and norepinephrine are not essential for maintaining life. On the other hand, glucocorticoids, the hormones from the adrenal cortex, are essential for life.

Suppose you suddenly faced some threatening situation. Imagine that a gunman threatened to kill you or that your doctor told you that you had to have a dangerous operation. Almost instantaneously, the medullas of your two adrenal glands would be galvanized into feverish activity. They would quickly secrete large amounts of epinephrine into your blood. Many of your body functions would seem to be supercharged. Your heart would beat faster, your blood pressure would rise, more blood would be pumped to your skeletal muscles, your blood would contain more glucose for more energy, and so on. In short, you would be geared up for strenuous activity, for "fight or flight." Epinephrine prolongs and intensifies changes in body function brought about by the stimulation of the sympathetic subdivision of the autonomic nervous system. Recall from Chapter 8 that sympathetic or adrenergic fibers release epinephrine and norepinephrine as neurotransmitter substances.

The close functional relationship between the nervous and the endocrine systems is perhaps most noticeable in the body's response to stress. In stress conditions the hypothalamus acts on the anterior pituitary gland to cause the release of ACTH, which stimulates the adrenal cortex to secrete glucocorticoids. In addition, the sympathetic subdivision of the autonomic nervous system is stimulated with the adrenal medulla, so the release of epinephrine and norepinephrine occurs to assist the body in responding to the stressful stimulus. Unfortunately, during periods of prolonged stress, glucocorticoids may have harmful side effects because they are anti-inflammatory and cause blood vessels to constrict. For example, decreased immune activity in the body may promote the spread of infections and cancer, and prolonged blood vessel constriction may lead to increased blood pressure.

 To learn more about adrenal function, go to AnimationDirect on your CD-ROM.

✓ QUICK CHECK

1. Why is the adrenal gland often thought of as two separate glands?
2. Name the hormones produced by the adrenal gland.
3. How does the pituitary gland influence adrenal function?

PANCREATIC ISLETS

All the endocrine glands discussed so far are big enough to be seen without a magnifying glass. The **pancreatic islets,** or *islets of Langerhans,* in contrast, are too tiny to be seen without a microscope. These glands are merely little clumps of cells scattered like islands in a sea among the exocrine pancreatic cells that secrete the pancreatic digestive juice (Figure 10-11).

Two of the most important kinds of cells in the pancreatic islets are the *alpha cells* (or *A cells*) and *beta cells* (or *B cells*). Alpha cells secrete a hormone called **glucagon,** whereas beta cells secrete one of the best known of all hormones, **insulin.** Glucagon accelerates a process called **glycogenolysis** (glye-koh-jeh-NOL-i-sis) in the liver. Glycogenolysis is a chemical process by which the glucose stored in the liver cells in the form of glycogen is converted to glucose. This glucose then leaves the liver cells and enters the blood. Glucagon therefore increases blood glucose concentration.

Insulin and glucagon are antagonists. In other words, insulin decreases blood glucose concentration and glucagon increases it. Insulin is the only hormone that can decrease blood glucose concentration. Other hormones, however, increase its concentration, including glucocorticoids, growth hormone, and glucagon. Insulin decreases blood glucose by accelerating its movement out of the

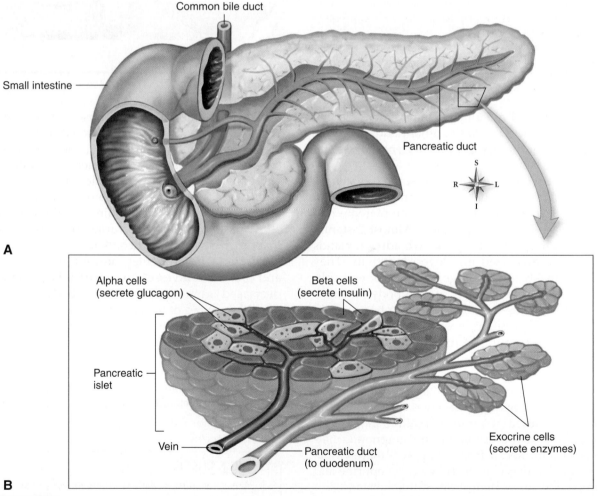

FIGURE 10-11 **Pancreas. A,** Location and structure of the pancreas (shown cut open). **B,** A pancreatic islet (of Langerhans) in cross section, showing the glucagon-producing alpha cells and insulin-producing beta cells. Notice the many exocrine cells surrounding the endocrine pancreatic islet.

blood, through cell membranes, and into cells. As glucose enters the cells at a faster rate, the cells increase their metabolism of glucose. Briefly then, insulin decreases blood glucose and increases glucose metabolism.

If the pancreatic islets secrete a normal amount of insulin, a normal amount of glucose enters the cells, and a normal amount of glucose stays behind in the blood. ("Normal" blood glucose is about 70 to 100 mg of glucose in every 100 mL of blood.) If the pancreatic islets secrete too much insulin, as they sometimes do when a person has a tumor of the pancreas, more glucose than usual leaves the blood to enter the cells, and blood glucose decreases. If the pancreatic islets secrete too little insulin, as they do in **type 1 diabetes** (dye-ah-BEE-teez) **mellitus** (MELL-i-tus), less glucose leaves the blood to enter the cells, so the blood glucose increases, sometimes to even three or more times the normal amount. Most cases of **type 2 diabetes mellitus** result from some decrease of insulin and an abnormality of the insulin receptors, preventing the normal effects of insulin on its target cells and thus also raising blood glucose levels.

Screening tests for all types of **diabetes mellitus** rely on the fact that the blood glucose level is elevated in this condition. Today, most screening is done with a simple test with a drop of blood. Subjects with a high blood glucose level are suspected of having diabetes mellitus. Testing for sugar in the urine is another common screening procedure. In diabetes mellitus, excess glucose is filtered out of the blood by the kidneys and lost in the urine, producing the condition **glycosuria** (glye-koh-SOO-ree-ah). Figure 10-12 summarizes some of the many problems that can be caused by diabetes mellitus. A quick look at these problems underscores the importance of insulin and insulin receptors in healthy bodies.

✓ QUICK CHECK

1. Name the two primary hormones of the pancreatic islets.
2. What effect does insulin have on the blood's glucose concentration?
3. How does diabetes produce glucose in the urine?

FEMALE SEX GLANDS

A woman's primary sex glands are her two ovaries. Each ovary contains two different kinds of glandular structures: the ovarian follicles and the corpus luteum. **Ovarian follicles** are little pockets in which egg cells, or **ova,** develop. Ovarian follicles also secrete **estrogen,** the "feminizing hormone." Estrogen is involved in the development and maturation of the breasts and external genitals. This hormone is also responsible for development of adult female body contours and initiation of the menstrual cycle. The **corpus luteum** chiefly secretes **progesterone** but also some estrogen. We shall save our discussion of the structure of these endocrine glands and the functions of their hormones for Chapter 20.

MALE SEX GLANDS

Some of the cells of the testes produce the male sex cells called **sperm.** Other cells in the testes, male reproductive ducts, and glands produce the liquid portion of the male reproductive fluid called **semen.** The interstitial cells in the testes secrete the male sex hormone called **testosterone** directly into the blood. These cells of the testes are therefore the male endocrine glands. Testosterone is the "masculinizing hormone." It is responsible for the maturation of the external genitals, beard growth, changes in voice at puberty, and for the muscular development and body contours typical of the male. Chapter 20 contains more information about the structure of the testes and the functions of testosterone.

 Health and Well-Being

Exercise and Diabetes Mellitus

Type 1 diabetes mellitus is characterized by high blood glucose concentration because the lack of sufficient insulin prevents glucose from entering cells. However, exercise physiologists have found that aerobic training increases the number of insulin receptors in target cells and the insulin affinity (attraction) of the receptors. This condition allows a small amount of insulin to have a greater effect than it would have otherwise had. Thus exercise reduces the severity of the diabetic condition.

All forms of diabetes benefit from properly planned exercise therapy. Not only is this form of treatment natural and cost effective, but it also helps reduce or prevent other problems such as obesity and heart disease.

FIGURE 10-12 Diabetes mellitus. The signs and symptoms of this disorder *(highlighted in yellow)* all result from decreased insulin effects.

THYMUS

The thymus is located in the mediastinum (see Figure 10-1), and in infants it may extend up into the neck as far as the lower edge of the thyroid gland. Like the adrenal gland, the thymus has a cortex and medulla. Both portions are composed largely of lymphocytes (white blood cells). As part of the body's immune system, the endocrine func-tion of the thymus is not only important but es-sential. This small structure (it weighs less than a gram at most) plays a critical part in the body's defenses against infections—its vital immunity mechanism.

The hormone **thymosin** (THY-moh-sin) is actu-ally a group of several hormones that together play an important role in the development and function of the body's immune system.

PLACENTA

The placenta functions as a temporary endocrine gland. During pregnancy, it produces **chorionic gonadotropins** (koh-ree-ON-ik goh-na-doh-TROH-pinz), so called because they are tropic hormones secreted by cells of the **chorion** (KOH-ree-on), the outermost membrane that surrounds the baby during development in the uterus. In addition to producing chorionic gonadotropins, the placenta also produces estrogen and progesterone. During the earliest weeks of pregnancy, the kidneys excrete large amounts of chorionic gonadotropins in the urine. This fact, discovered more than a half century ago, led to the development of early pregnancy tests.

PINEAL GLAND

The pineal gland is a small gland near the roof of the third ventricle of the brain (see Figure 8-9). It is named "pineal" because it resembles the pine nut (which looks like a kernel of corn). The pineal gland is easily located in a child but becomes fibrous and encrusted with calcium deposits as a person ages. The pineal gland produces a number of hormones in very small quantities, with **melatonin** being the most significant. Melatonin inhibits the tropic hormones that affect the ovaries, and it is thought to be involved in regulating the onset of puberty and the menstrual cycle in women. Because the pineal gland receives and responds to sensory information from the optic nerves, it is sometimes called the *third eye*. The pineal gland uses information regarding changing light levels to adjust its output of melatonin; melatonin levels increase during the night and decrease during the day. This cyclic variation is thought to be an important timekeeping mechanism for the body's internal clock.

OTHER ENDOCRINE STRUCTURES

Continuing research into the endocrine system has shown that nearly every organ and system has an endocrine function. Tissues in the kidneys, stomach, intestines, and other organs secrete hormones that regulate a variety of essential human functions. For example, **ghrelin** (GRAY-lin) is secreted by epithelial cells lining the stomach and boosts appetite, slows metabolism, and reduces fat burning. Ghrelin may, therefore, be involved in the development of obesity. Another example, **atrial natriuretic hormone (ANH),** is secreted by cells in the wall of the heart's atria (upper chambers). ANH is an important regulator of fluid and electrolyte homeostasis and is an antagonist to aldosterone. Aldosterone stimulates the kidney to retain sodium ions and water, whereas ANH stimulates loss of sodium ions and water.

A more recently discovered hormone is **leptin,** which is secreted by fat-storing cells throughout the body. Leptin seems to regulate how hungry or full we feel and how fat is metabolized by the body. Researchers are now looking at how leptin works with other hormones in the hopes of finding ways to treat patients with obesity, diabetes mellitus, and other disorders involving fat storage.

> ### ✓ QUICK CHECK
>
> 1. Which hormones are produced by the male and female sex glands?
> 2. Why is the placenta considered to be a gland?
> 3. Why is the pineal gland sometimes called a *time-keeper of the body?*

Science Application

Endocrinology
Frederich Banting (1891-1941) and Charles Best (1899-1978)

The undisputed heroes of endocrinology are Canadian surgeon Frederick Banting and his assistant Charles Best. Until the early twentieth century, children with type 1 diabetes mellitus died a slow, horrible death from their cells literally starving to death from lack of glucose. Acting on Banting's idea for removing insulin from the pancreatic islets of dogs, the two were the first to successfully isolate this important hormone. Chemist James Collip was able to purify the insulin sufficiently so that in 1921 their colleague, Scots physiologist John Macleod, could administer the insulin to a 14-year-old boy with diabetes. It worked! The treatment not only relieved the boy's suffering, but gave him a healthy, long life. This breakthrough, for which Banting and Macleod received the 1923 Nobel Prize, was the start of a century of rapid progress in understanding and treating endocrine disorders.

Because hormones affect so many different body functions, nearly every kind of health professional, from medical doctors to nurses to dieticians, needs to be aware of their functions. Of course, hormones and chemicals that influence hormone actions are often used in treatments, so pharmacologists and pharmacists must also have an excellent knowledge of endocrinology. Some scientists have applied principles of endocrinology in a variety of unexpected ways, including the development of early pregnancy test kits and ovulation test kits and the use of synthetic hormones in healthy people to control their fertility.

OUTLINE SUMMARY

MECHANISMS OF HORMONE ACTION

A. Endocrine glands secrete chemicals (hormones) into the blood (see Figure 10-1)
B. Hormones perform general functions of communication and control but a slower, longer-lasting type of control than that provided by nerve impulses
C. Cells acted on by hormones are called *target cells;* organs containing target cells are *target organs*
D. Nonsteroid hormones (first messengers) bind to receptors on the target cell membrane, triggering second messengers to affect the cell's activities (see Figure 10-2)
E. Steroid hormones
  1. Primary effects produced by binding to receptors within the target cell nucleus and influence cell activity by acting on DNA — a slower process than nonsteroid action (see Figure 10-3)
  2. Secondary effects may occur when steroid hormones bind to membrane receptors to rapidly trigger functional changes in the target cell

REGULATION OF HORMONE SECRETION

A. Hormone secretion is controlled by homeostatic feedback
B. Negative feedback — mechanisms that reverse the direction of a change in a physiological system (see Figure 10-4)
C. Positive feedback — (uncommon) mechanisms that amplify physiological changes

PROSTAGLANDINS

A. Prostaglandins (PGs) are powerful substances found in a wide variety of body tissues
B. PGs are often produced in a tissue and diffuse only a short distance to act on cells in that tissue
C. Several classes of PGs include prostaglandin A (PGA), prostaglandin E (PGE), and prostaglandin F (PGF)
D. PGs influence many body functions, including respiration, blood pressure, gastrointestinal secretions, and reproduction

PITUITARY GLAND (See Figure 10-5)

A. Anterior pituitary gland (adenohypophysis)
  1. Names of major hormones
    a. Thyroid stimulating hormone (TSH)
    b. Adrenocorticotropic hormone (ACTH)
    c. Follicle-stimulating hormone (FSH)
    d. Luteinizing hormone (LH)
    e. Growth hormone (GH)
    f. Prolactin (PRL) (lactogenic hormone)
  2. Functions of major hormones
    a. TSH — stimulates growth of the thyroid gland; also stimulates it to secrete thyroid hormone
    b. ACTH — stimulates growth of the adrenal cortex and stimulates it to secrete glucocorticoids (mainly cortisol)
    c. FSH — initiates growth of ovarian follicles each month in the ovary and stimulates one or more follicles to develop to the stage of maturity and ovulation; FSH also stimulates estrogen secretion by developing follicles; stimulates sperm production in the male
    d. LH — acts with FSH to stimulate estrogen secretion and follicle growth to maturity; causes ovulation; causes luteinization of the ruptured follicle and stimulates progesterone secretion by corpus luteum; causes interstitial cells in the testes to secrete testosterone in the male
    e. GH — stimulates growth by accelerating protein anabolism; also accelerates fat catabolism and slows glucose catabolism; by slowing glucose catabolism, tends to increase blood glucose to higher than normal level (hyperglycemia)
    f. PRL, or lactogenic hormone — stimulates breast development during pregnancy and secretion of milk after the delivery of the baby
B. Posterior pituitary gland (neurohypophysis)
  1. Names of hormones
    a. Antidiuretic hormone (ADH)
    b. Oxytocin
  2. Functions of hormones
    a. ADH — accelerates water reabsorption from urine in the kidney tubules into the blood, thereby decreasing urine secretion

    b. Oxytocin (OT) — stimulates the pregnant uterus to contract; may initiate labor; causes glandular cells of the breast to release milk into ducts; enhances social bonding

HYPOTHALAMUS

A. Actual production of ADH and oxytocin occurs in the hypothalamus
B. After production in the hypothalamus, hormones pass along axons into the pituitary gland
C. The secretion and release of posterior pituitary hormones is controlled by nervous stimulation
D. The hypothalamus controls many body functions related to homeostasis (temperature, appetite, and thirst)

THYROID GLAND (See Figure 10-6)

A. Names of hormones
  1. Thyroid hormones — thyroxine (T_4) and triiodothyronine (T_3)
  2. Calcitonin (CT)
B. Functions of hormones
  1. Thyroid hormones — accelerate catabolism (increase the body's metabolic rate)
  2. CT — decreases the blood calcium concentration by inhibiting breakdown of bone, which would release calcium into the blood

PARATHYROID GLANDS (See Figure 10-6)

A. Name of hormone — parathyroid hormone (PTH)
B. Function of hormone — increases blood calcium concentration by increasing the breakdown of bone with the release of calcium into the blood

ADRENAL GLANDS (See Figure 10-9)

A. Adrenal cortex
  1. Names of hormones (corticoids)
    a. Glucocorticoids (GCs) — chiefly cortisol (hydrocortisone)
    b. Mineralocorticoids (MCs) — chiefly aldosterone
    c. Sex hormones — small amounts of male hormones (androgens) secreted by adrenal cortex of both sexes

2. Three cell layers (zones)
   a. Outer layer, secretes mineralocorticoids
   b. Middle layer, secretes glucocorticoids
   c. Inner layer, secretes sex hormones
3. Mineralocorticoids — increase blood sodium and decrease body potassium concentrations by accelerating kidney tubule reabsorption of sodium and excretion of potassium
4. Functions of glucocorticoids
   a. Help maintain normal blood glucose concentration by increasing gluconeogenesis — the formation of "new" glucose from amino acids produced by the breakdown of proteins, mainly those in muscle tissue cells; also the conversion to glucose of fatty acids produced by the breakdown of fats stored in adipose tissue cells
   b. Play an essential part in maintaining normal blood pressure — make it possible for epinephrine and norepinephrine to maintain a normal degree of vasoconstriction, a condition necessary for maintaining normal blood pressure
   c. Act with epinephrine and norepinephrine to produce an anti-inflammatory effect, to bring about normal recovery from inflammations of various kinds
   d. Produce anti-immunity, antiallergy effect; bring about a decrease in the number of lymphocytes and plasma cells and therefore a decrease in the number of antibodies formed
   e. Secretion of glucocorticoid quickly increases when the body is thrown into a condition of stress; high blood concentration of glucocorticoids, in turn, brings about many other stress responses (see Figure 10-10)
B. Adrenal medulla
   1. Names of hormones — epinephrine (Epi), or adrenaline, and norepinephrine (NR)
   2. Functions of hormones — help the body resist stress by intensifying and prolonging the effects of sympathetic stimulation; increased epinephrine secretion is the first endocrine response to stress

PANCREATIC ISLETS (See Figure 10-11)
A. Names of hormones
   1. Glucagon — secreted by alpha cells
   2. Insulin — secreted by beta cells
B. Functions of hormones
   1. Glucagon increases the blood glucose level by accelerating liver glycogenolysis (conversion of glycogen to glucose)
   2. Insulin decreases the blood glucose by accelerating the movement of glucose out of the blood into cells, which increases glucose metabolism by cells

FEMALE SEX GLANDS
A. The ovaries contain two structures that secrete hormones — the ovarian follicles and the corpus luteum; see Chapter 20
B. Effects of estrogen (feminizing hormone)
   1. Development and maturation of breasts and external genitals
   2. Development of adult female body contours
   3. Initiation of menstrual cycle

MALE SEX GLANDS
A. The interstitial cells of testes secrete the male hormone testosterone; see Chapter 20
B. Effects of testosterone (masculinizing hormone)
   1. Maturation of external genitals
   2. Beard growth
   3. Voice changes at puberty
   4. Development of musculature and body contours typical of the male

THYMUS
A. Name of hormone — thymosin
B. Function of hormone — plays an important role in the development and function of the body's immune system

PLACENTA
A. Names of hormones — chorionic gonadotropins, estrogens, and progesterone
B. Function of hormones — maintain the corpus luteum during pregnancy

PINEAL GLAND

A. A small gland near the roof of the third ventricle of the brain
  1. Glandular tissue predominates in children and young adults
  2. Becomes fibrous and calcified with age
B. Called *third eye* because its influence on secretory activity is related to the amount of light entering the eyes
C. Secretes melatonin, which:
  1. Inhibits ovarian activity
  2. Regulates the body's internal clock

OTHER ENDOCRINE STRUCTURES

A. Many organs (for example, the stomach, intestines, and kidney) produce endocrine hormones
  1. Stomach lining produces ghrelin, which affects appetite and metabolism
B. The atrial wall of the heart secretes atrial natriuretic hormone (ANH), which stimulates sodium loss from the kidneys
C. Fat-storing cells secrete leptin, which controls how full or hungry we feel

NEW WORDS

acromegaly
Addison disease
adenohypophysis
adrenal cortex
adrenal medulla
adrenocorticotropic hormone (ACTH)
aldosterone
anabolism
androgen
antidiuretic hormone (ADH)
atrial natriuretic hormone (ANH)
calcitonin (CT)
chorion
chorionic gonadotropin
corpus luteum
corticoid
cortisol (hydrocortisone)
cretinism
Cushing syndrome
cyclic adenosine monophosphate (cAMP)

diabetes insipidus
diabetes mellitus
dwarfism
epinephrine (Epi) (adrenaline)
endocrine gland
exocrine gland
estrogen
follicle-stimulating hormone (FSH)
ghrelin
gigantism
glucagon
glucocorticoid (GC)
glycogenolysis
gluconeogenesis
glycosuria
growth hormone (GH)
hormone
hypercalcemia
hyperglycemia
hypersecretion
hypoglycemia
hyposecretion

inhibiting hormone (IH)
insulin
leptin
luteinization
luteinizing hormone (LH)
melatonin
mineralocorticoid (MC)
myxedema
negative feedback
neurohypophysis
nonsteroid hormone
norepinephrine (NR)
ova
ovarian follicle
oxytocin (OT)
pancreatic islets (of Langerhans)
parathyroid gland
parathyroid hormone (PTH)
pituitary gland
positive feedback
progesterone

prolactin (PRL) (lactogenic hormone)
prostaglandin
releasing hormone (RH)
second messenger
sella turcica
semen
signal transduction
simple goiter
sperm
steroid hormone
stress
target cell
testosterone
thymosin
thyroid-stimulating hormone (TSH)
thyroxine (T$_4$)
triiodothyronine (T$_3$)
tropic hormone
type 1 diabetes mellitus
type 2 diabetes mellitus

REVIEW QUESTIONS

1. Differentiate between endocrine and exocrine glands.
2. Define or explain *hormone, target cell, hypersecretion,* and *hyposecretion.*
3. Explain the mechanism of action of nonsteroid hormones.
4. Explain the mechanism of action of steroid hormones.
5. Explain and give an example of a negative feedback loop for the regulation of hormone secretion.
6. Explain and give an example of a positive feedback loop for the regulation of hormone secretion.
7. Explain the difference between prostaglandins and hormones. List some of the body functions that can be influenced by prostaglandins.
8. Describe the structure of the pituitary gland and where it is located.
9. Name the four tropic hormones released by the anterior pituitary gland and briefly explain their function.
10. Explain the function of growth hormone.
11. Explain the function of ADH.
12. Explain the function of prolactin and oxytocin.

13. Explain the function of the hypothalamus in the endocrine system.
14. Explain the difference between T_3 and T_4. What is unique about the thyroid gland?
15. Name the hormones produced by the zones or areas of the adrenal cortex.
16. Explain the function of aldosterone.
17. Explain the function of glucocorticoids.

CRITICAL THINKING

18. Explain why a second messenger system is necessary for nonsteroid hormones but not for steroid hormones.
19. Pick a body function (regulation of glucose or calcium levels in the blood) and explain how the interaction of hormones is used to help maintain homeostasis.
20. What would be the effect on the body if the thyroid gland were removed?
21. If a doctor discovered a patient had very low levels of thyroxine but high levels of TSH, would the patient's problem be in the thyroid gland or the pituitary gland? Explain your answer.

CHAPTER TEST

1. _____ glands secrete their products into ducts that empty onto a surface or into a cavity.
2. _____ glands are ductless and secrete their products, called _____, into intercellular spaces where they diffuse into the blood.
3. The two major classes of hormones are _____ hormones and _____ hormones.
4. A cell or body organ that has receptors for a hormone that triggers a reaction is called a _____.
5. One example of a second messenger system involves the conversion of ATP into _____.

6. The hormone receptors for nonsteroid hormones are located _____, whereas the receptors for steroid hormones are located _____.
7. "Tissue hormones" is another name for _____.
8. This part of the pituitary gland is made of nervous tissue: _____.
9. This part of the pituitary gland is made of glandular tissue: _____.
10. The hormone oxytocin is released by the _____ but is made in the _____.

CHAPTER TEST—cont'd

11. A tropic hormone secreted by the anterior pituitary gland is:
    a. thyroid stimulating hormone
    b. adrenocorticotropic hormone
    c. luteinizing hormone
    d. all of the above

12. Antidiuretic hormone (ADH):
    a. is made in the posterior pituitary gland
    b. accelerates water reabsorption in the kidney
    c. in high concentrations causes diabetes insipidus
    d. all of the above

13. This hormone is released by the anterior pituitary and stimulates breast development during pregnancy necessary for eventual milk production:
    a. estrogen
    b. oxytocin
    c. prolactin
    d. progesterone

14. This hormone is released by the posterior pituitary and stimulates the contraction of the pregnant uterus:
    a. estrogen
    b. oxytocin
    c. prolactin
    d. progesterone

15. Thyroxine:
    a. is symbolized by T_3
    b. is made in the thyroid gland
    c. contains less iodine than triiodothyronine
    d. all of the above

16. Calcitonin:
    a. decreases the level of calcium in the blood
    b. increases the level of calcium in the blood
    c. stimulates the release of calcium from bone tissue
    d. both b and c

Match each function or source in Column B with the corresponding hormone in Column A.

COLUMN A

17. _____ parathyroid hormone
18. _____ mineralocorticoids
19. _____ glucocorticoids
20. _____ epinephrine
21. _____ glucagon
22. _____ insulin
23. _____ chorionic gonadotropins
24. _____ melatonin
25. _____ atrial natriuretic hormone

COLUMN B

a. released by the adrenal medulla; prolongs the effect of the sympathetic nervous system
b. made in the heart; helps regulate blood sodium
c. made in the islets of Langerhans; decreases blood glucose levels
d. has the opposite effect of calcitonin
e. made by alpha cells in the pancreatic islets
f. made in the outermost layer of the adrenal cortex
g. the most significant hormone released by the pineal gland
h. the hormone made by the placenta and detected by home pregnancy tests
i. made by the middle layer of the adrenal cortex

OBJECTIVES

AFTER YOU HAVE COMPLETED THIS CHAPTER, YOU SHOULD BE ABLE TO:

1. Describe the primary functions of blood.
2. Describe the characteristics of blood plasma.
3. List the formed elements of blood and identify the most important function of each.
4. Discuss anemia in terms of red blood cell numbers and hemoglobin content.
5. Explain the steps involved in blood clotting.
6. Describe ABO and Rh blood typing.
7. Define the following medical terms associated with blood: *hematocrit, leukocytosis, leukopenia, polycythemia, sickle cell, phagocytosis, acidosis, thrombosis, erythroblastosis fetalis, serum, fibrinogen, Rh factor, anemia.*

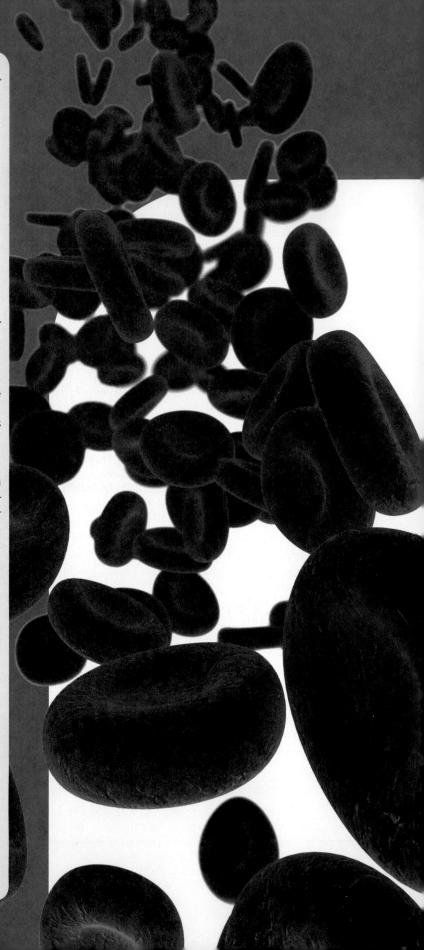

Blood 11

The next few chapters deal with *transportation* and *protection,* two of the body's most important functions. Have you ever thought of what would happen if the transportation ceased in your city or town? Or what would happen if the police, firefighters, and armed services stopped doing their jobs? Food would become scarce, garbage would pile up, and no one would protect you or your property. Stretch your imagination just a little, and you can imagine many disastrous results. Similarly, lack of transportation and protection for the cells—the "individuals" of the body—threatens the homeostasis of the body. The systems that provide these vital services for the body are the *circulatory system* and *lymphatic system.* In this chapter, we discuss the primary transportation fluid: blood. Blood not only performs vital pickup and delivery services but also provides much of the protection necessary to withstand foreign "invaders." Blood vessels and the heart are discussed in Chapter 12. The lymphatic system is discussed in Chapter 13.

BLOOD COMPOSITION

Blood is a fluid tissue that has many kinds of chemicals dissolved in it and millions upon millions of cells floating in it (Figure 11-1). The liquid (extracellular) part is called **plasma.** Suspended in the plasma are many different types of cells and cell fragments, which make up the *formed elements* of blood.

Blood Plasma

Blood plasma is the liquid part of the blood, or blood minus its formed elements. It consists of water with many substances dissolved in it. All of the chemicals needed by cells to stay alive—nutrients,

oxygen, and salts, for example—have to be brought to them by the blood. Nutrients and salts are dissolved in plasma; so, too, is a small amount of oxygen. Most of the oxygen in the blood is carried in the red blood cells as oxyhemoglobin (see p. 254). Wastes that cells must get rid of are dissolved in plasma and transported to the excretory organs. The hormones and other regulatory chemi-

FIGURE 11-1 **Components of blood.** Approximate values for the components of blood in a normal adult. Values will vary with age, sex, and nutritional status.

cals that help control cells' activities are also dissolved in plasma. As Figure 11-1 shows, the most abundant type of solute in the plasma is a group of **plasma proteins,** which constitute about 7% of the plasma by weight. These proteins include *albumins,* which help thicken and maintain the blood volume; *globulins,* which include the antibodies that help protect us from infections; and *fibrinogen* and *prothrombin,* which are necessary for blood clotting.

Blood **serum** is plasma minus its clotting factors, such as fibrinogen. Serum is obtained from whole blood by allowing it to clot in the bottom of a tube and then pouring off the liquid serum. Serum still contains antibodies, so it can be used to treat patients that have a need for specific antibodies.

Many people seem curious about how much blood they have. The amount depends on how big they are and whether they are male or female. A big person has more blood than a small person, and a man has more blood than a woman. But as a general rule, most adults probably have between 4 and 6 liters of blood. It normally accounts for about 7% to 9% of the total body weight.

Formed Elements

There are three main types and several subtypes of **formed elements:**
1. Red blood cells (RBCs), or **erythrocytes** (eh-RITH-roh-sytes)
2. White blood cells (WBCs), or **leukocytes** (LOO-koh-sytes)
   a. Granular leukocytes (have granules in their cytoplasm)
      (1) Neutrophils
      (2) Eosinophils
      (3) Basophils

TABLE 11-1

Formed Elements of the Blood

BLOOD CELL		FUNCTION	BLOOD CELL		FUNCTION
Erythrocyte		Oxygen and carbon dioxide transport	B lymphocyte		Antibody production
Neutrophil		Immune defense (phagocytosis)	T lymphocyte		Cellular immune response; destroys virally infected cells and cancer cells
Eosinophil		Defense against parasites	Monocyte		Immune defenses (phagocytosis)
Basophil		Inflammatory response	Platelet		Blood clotting

b. Nongranular leukocytes (do not have granules in their cytoplasm)
(1) Lymphocytes
(2) Monocytes
3. Platelets, or **thrombocytes** (THROM-boh-sytes)

Figure 11-1 shows the breakdown of numbers and percentages of the formed elements. Table 11-1 lists the functions of the formed elements of blood and shows what each looks like under the microscope.

It is difficult to believe how many blood cells and cell fragments there are in the body. For instance, 5,000,000 RBCs, 7,500 WBCs, and 300,000 platelets in 1 cubic millimeter (mm³) of blood (approximately 1 drop) would be considered normal RBC, WBC, and platelet counts. Because RBCs, WBCs, and platelets are continually being destroyed, the body must continually make new ones to take their place at a really staggering rate: a few million RBCs are manufactured *each second!*

Two kinds of connective tissue—**myeloid tissue** and **lymphatic tissue**—make blood cells for the body. Recall that formation of new blood cells is called *hematopoiesis.* Myeloid tissue is better known as *red bone marrow.* In the adult, it is chiefly in the sternum, ribs, and coxal (hipbones). A few other bones such as the vertebrae, clavicles, and cranial bones also contain small amounts of this important

tissue. Red bone marrow forms all types of blood cells except lymphocytes. These are formed by lymphatic tissue, which is located chiefly in the lymph nodes, thymus, and spleen.

Clinical Application

Bone Marrow Transplants

Bone marrow may be damaged by toxic chemicals or by high-dose x-ray and chemotherapy treatments. It can also be destroyed by diseases such as leukemia. Regardless of cause, if the bone marrow is severely damaged, a *bone marrow transplant* can be life saving. In this procedure, a needle is used to extract red marrow from the coxal or hipbone of a compatible donor who is under sedation, or anesthesia. The donated bone marrow is then processed and introduced into the recipient intravenously. Transplantation also may involve infusion of blood, forming *stem cells* (see Clinical Application: Stem Cells box, p. 72) harvested from the individual being treated, from a compatible donor, or from umbilical cord blood (see Research, Issues, & Trends: Freezing Umbilical Cord Blood Box, p. 476). If the recipient's immune system does not reject the new tissue or stem cells, always a danger in transplant procedures, a new colony of healthy tissue may become established in the bone marrow. As a result, destroyed or damaged myeloid tissue will be replaced and begin again to produce normal, functioning blood cells.

As blood cells mature, they move into the circulatory vessels. Erythrocytes circulate for up to 4 months before they break apart and their components are removed from the bloodstream by the spleen and liver. Granular leukocytes often have a life span of only a few days, but nongranular leukocytes may live for more than 6 months.

✓ **QUICK CHECK**

1. What are "formed elements" of blood?
2. What is the difference between blood *plasma* and blood *serum?*

Red Blood Cells

As you can see in Figure 11-2, *A*, RBCs have an unusual shape. The cell is "caved in" on both sides so that each one has a thin center and thicker edges. Notice also that mature RBCs have no nucleus. Figure 11-2 shows RBCs photographed with a scanning electron microscope. With this instrument, extremely small objects can be enlarged far more than is possible with a standard light microscope, and as you can see in the illustration, objects appear more three-dimensional. Because of the large numbers of RBCs and their unique shape, their total surface area is enormous. In fact, the total surface area of the body's RBCs provides an area larger than a football field for the exchange of oxygen and carbon dioxide between the blood and the body's cells.

RBCs perform several important functions. One essential function is to help transport carbon dioxide. Carbon dioxide (CO_2) is a harmful waste produced by the energy-producing processes of all living cells. It must be carried away from cells and to the lungs for disposal into the external environment. RBCs also transport oxygen from the lungs to other cells in the body. A red pigment called **hemoglobin** (hee-moh-GLOH-bin) in RBCs unites with oxygen to form **oxyhemoglobin** (ahk-see-hee-moh-GLOH-bin). This combined oxygen-hemoglobin complex makes possible the efficient transport of large quantities of oxygen to body cells. Hemoglobin can also carry a small proportion of the CO_2 carried by the blood, forming **carbaminohemoglobin** (kar-bam-ee-no-hee-moh-GLOH-bin).

 To learn more about RBCs, go to AnimationDirect on your CD-ROM.

Anemia

The term **anemia** (ah-NEE-mee-ah) is used to describe a number of different disease conditions caused by an inability of the blood to carry sufficient oxygen to the body cells. Anemias can result from inadequate numbers of RBCs or a deficiency of hemoglobin. Thus anemia can occur if the hemoglobin in RBCs is inadequate, even if adequate numbers of RBCs are present. **Hemorrhagic** (HEM-oh-raj-ick) **anemia** results from a decrease in the number of RBCs caused by hemorrhage resulting from, for example, accidents or bleeding

FIGURE 11-2 Comparison of normal and sickle-shaped RBCs (color-enhanced scanning electron micrographs [SEMs]). **A,** Normal RBCs. **B,** Shape of RBCs in sickle cell anemia.

ulcers. **Aplastic** (ay-PLAS-tik) **anemia** is character-ized by a reduction in RBC numbers following de-struction of the blood-forming elements in bone marrow. The cause is often related to exposure to certain toxic chemicals, high-dose irradiation (x-rays), certain drugs, and chemotherapy agents. The term **pernicious** (per-NISH-us) **anemia** is used to describe a deficiency of RBCs that results from a failure of the stomach lining to produce *"intrinsic factor"*—the substance that allows vitamin B_{12} to be absorbed from the foods we eat. Because RBC pro-duction requires adequate blood levels of this vita-min, red cell numbers will decrease in the absence of intrinsic factor even if the vitamin is present in the diet. Therefore successful long-term treatment requires repeated injections of vitamin B_{12} to main-tain normal RBC production. **Sickle cell anemia** is a severe and sometimes fatal hereditary disease caused by an abnormal type of hemoglobin. A per-son who inherits only one defective gene develops a form of the disease called **sickle cell trait.** In this condition, RBCs contain a small amount of a type of hemoglobin that is less soluble than normal (Hb S). It forms solid crystals when the blood oxygen is low, causing distortion of the RBC (see Figure 11-2, *B*). If two defective genes are inherited (one from each parent), more of the defective hemoglobin is produced and the distortion of RBCs becomes severe.

Iron is a critical component of the hemoglobin molecule. Without adequate iron in the diet, the body cannot manufacture enough hemoglobin. The result is **iron deficiency anemia,** a worldwide medical problem. If hemoglobin and RBC numbers fall below the normal levels, as they do in anemia, it starts an unhealthy chain reaction: less hemoglo-bin, less oxygen transported to cells, slower break-down and use of nutrients by cells, less energy produced by cells, decreased cellular functions. If you understand this relationship between hemo-globin and energy, you can correctly guess that an anemic person's chief complaint will probably be that he or she feels "so tired all the time."

If bone marrow produces an excess of RBCs, the result is a condition called **polycythemia** (pol-ee-sye-THEE-me-ah). The blood in individuals suffer-ing from this condition may contain so many RBCs that it may become too thick to flow properly, re-sulting in a stroke or heart attack.

Hematocrit Test

A common laboratory test called the **hematocrit** (hee-MAT-oh-krit), or **Hct,** test is a measure of the total blood volume made up by the RBCs. If whole blood is placed in a special hematocrit tube and then "spun down" in a centrifuge (Figure 11-3, *D*), the heavier formed elements will quickly settle to

FIGURE 11-3 Hematocrit tubes showing normal blood, anemia, and polycythemia. Note the buffy coat located between the packed RBCs and the plasma. **A,** A normal percentage of RBCs. **B,** Anemia (a low percentage of RBCs). **C,** Polycythemia (a high per-centage of RBCs). **D,** Photograph shows a laboratory centrifuge used to "spin down" tubes of whole blood to separate the formed elements from the plasma.

the bottom of the tube with the RBCs forced to the bottom first. The height of the RBC column is then measured after centrifugation and compared to the height of the column of the total whole blood. Normally about 45% of the blood volume consists of RBCs, and the easy-to-perform Hct test is often used to monitor RBC values. Hematocrit values tend to be higher in men than women and decrease with advancing age. As the whole blood sample is spun down, the WBCs and platelets settle out in a layer called the **buffy coat,** which can be seen between the packed RBCs on the bottom and the liquid layer of plasma above. For a patient with anemia, the percentage of RBCs drops, and for a patient with polycythemia, it increases dramatically (see Figure 11-3).

As with any test, falsely high or low Hct values sometimes occur. One cause of erroneous test results is *dehydration*—caused by excessive loss of body water. In the absence of adequate fluid replacement, it can occur in athletes who lose significant amounts of body water through heavy sweating or in individuals experiencing severe diarrhea or other illnesses that result in loss of body fluids. Would you expect the hematocrit value to increase or decrease in a person with dehydration? The answer is that the Hct would be falsely high. Why? Because in dehydration total blood volume is decreased and RBCs make up a greater proportion of the total, although their actual numbers have not increased. Overhydration has the opposite effect.

FIGURE 11-4 Leukocytes in human blood smears. A-E, Each light micrograph shows a different type of stained WBC surrounded by several smaller RBCs.

QUICK CHECK

1. What protein in blood cells carries oxygen?
2. Can you give a broad definition of *anemia?*

White Blood Cells (Leukocytes)

Recall from the listing of formed elements found in the blood (see p. 252) that the WBCs, or leukocytes, are categorized by the presence of granules (*granulocytes*) or absence of granules (*agranulocytes*) in their cytoplasm. The granulocytic WBCs include the **neutrophils** (NOO-troh-filz), **eosinophils** (ee-oh-SIN-oh-filz), and **basophils** (BAY-soh-filz) (Figure 11-4, *A-C*). The **lymphocytes** (LIM-foh-sytes) and **monocytes** (MON-oh-sytes) (Figure 11-4, *D* and *E*) are agranulocytes. The WBCs have a function that is just as vital as that of RBCs. They defend the body from cancer cells that form inside our tissues and from microorganisms that have succeeded in invading our body.

 To learn more about WBCs, go to AnimationDirect on your CD-ROM.

White Blood Cell Count

Normally, the **total WBC count**—the total number of WBCs per cubic millimeter (mm^3) of whole blood ranges between 5,000 and 9,000. A special type of WBC count called a **differential WBC count** reveals more information than simply counting the total number of all the different types of WBCs in a blood sample. In a differential WBC count, the proportions of each type of WBC are reported as percentages of the total WBC count. Because all disorders do not affect each WBC type the same way, the differential WBC count is a valuable diagnostic tool. For example, although some parasite infestations do not cause an increase in the total WBC count, they often cause an increase in the proportion of eosinophils that are present. The reason? This type of WBC specializes in defending against parasites (see Table 11-1).

The term **leukopenia** (loo-koh-PEE-nee-ah) refers to an abnormally low WBC count (less than 5,000 WBCs/mm³ of blood). A number of disease conditions may affect the immune system and decrease circulating WBC numbers. *Acquired immunodeficiency syndrome* or *AIDS,* which is discussed in Chapter 13, is one example of a disease characterized by marked leukopenia. **Leukocytosis** (loo-koh-sye-TOH-sis) refers to an abnormally high WBC count (more than 10,000 WBCs/mm³ of blood). Leukocytosis is a much more common problem than leukopenia and almost always accompanies bacterial infections.

Leukocyte Types and Functions

Granulocytes. Neutrophils are the most numerous of the active WBCs called **phagocytes** (FAG-oh-sytes), which protect the body from invading microorganisms by taking them into their own cell bodies and digesting them by the process of phagocytosis (Figure 11-5).

Eosinophils also serve as weak phagocytes. Perhaps one of their most important functions, as noted above, involves protection against infections caused by certain parasitic worms.

Basophils in peripheral blood secrete the chemical *histamine,* which is released during inflammatory reactions. Basophils also produce a potent anticoagulant called **heparin,** which helps prevent blood from clotting as it flows through the blood vessels of the body.

Agranulocytes. Monocytes are the largest leukocytes. Like neutrophils, they are aggressive phagocytes. Because of their size, they are capable of engulfing larger bacterial organisms and cancerous cells. **Macrophages** (meaning "large eater") are specialized monocytes that grow to several times their original size after migrating out of the bloodstream. They are discussed further in Chapter 13.

Lymphocytes help protect us against infections, but they do it by a process different from phagocytosis. Lymphocytes function in the immune mechanism, the complex process that makes us immune to infectious diseases. Lymphocytes called *B lymphocytes* secrete specialized proteins, called *anti-*

White blood cell

Bacteria

FIGURE 11-5 **Phagocytosis.** Diagrammatic representation of phagocytosis by a neutrophil (note the multilobed nucleus). Extension of cytoplasm envelope the bacteria, which are drawn through the cell membrane and into the cytoplasm.

bodies, which specifically act to destroy particular bacteria, viruses, or chemical toxins. *T lymphocytes* do not secrete antibodies but instead protect us by directly attacking virally infected or cancerous cells. Details of the immune system are discussed in Chapter 13.

White Blood Cell Disorders

Leukemia (loo-KEE-mee-ah) is the term used to describe a number of blood cancers affecting the WBCs. In almost every form of leukemia, marked leukocytosis, or elevated WBC levels, occurs. Leukocyte counts in excess of 100,000/mm³ in circulating blood are common. The different types of leukemia are identified as either *acute* or *chronic,* based on how quickly symptoms appear after the disease begins, and as *lymphocytic* or *myeloid* depending on the cell type involved.

Platelets and Blood Clotting

Platelets, the third main type of formed element, play an essential part in blood clotting, or *coagulation*. Your life might someday be saved just because your blood can clot. A clot plugs up torn or cut vessels and stops bleeding that otherwise might prove fatal.

The story of blood clots is the story of a chain of rapid-fire reactions. The first step in the chain is some kind of an injury to a blood vessel that makes a rough spot in its lining. (Normally the lining of blood vessels is extremely smooth.) Almost immediately, damaged tissue cells in the injured vessel wall release certain clotting factors into the plasma. These factors rapidly react with other factors already present in the plasma to form **prothrombin activator** (proh-THROM-bin AK-tiv-ayt-or). At the same time this is happening, platelets become "sticky" at the point of in-

jury and soon accumulate near the opening in the broken blood vessel, forming a soft, temporary *platelet plug.* As the platelets accumulate, they release additional clotting factors, forming even more prothrombin activator. If the normal amount of blood calcium is present, prothrombin activator triggers the next step of clotting by converting prothrombin (a protein in normal blood) to **thrombin** (THROM-bin). In the last step, thrombin reacts with **fibrinogen** (fye-BRIN-oh-jen) (a normal plasma protein) to change it to a fibrous gel called **fibrin.** Under the microscope, fibrin looks like a tangle of fine threads with RBCs caught in the tangle. This meshwork is the blood clot that forms a more long-term seal of the damaged blood vessel. Figure 11-6 illustrates the steps in the blood-clotting mechanism.

The clotting mechanism contains clues for ways to stop bleeding by speeding up blood clotting. For example, you might simply apply gauze to a bleeding surface. Its slight roughness would cause more platelets to stick together and release more clotting factors. These additional factors would then make the blood clot more quickly.

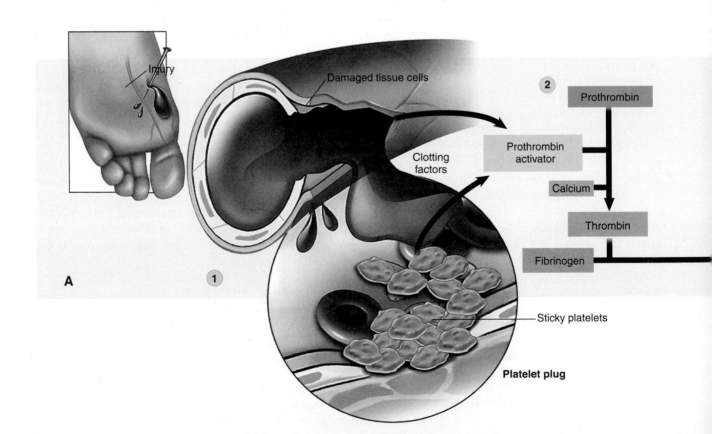

Injury

Damaged tissue cells

2

Prothrombin

Clotting factors

Prothrombin activator

Calcium

Thrombin

Fibrinogen

Sticky platelets

A

1

Platelet plug

Clinical Application

Anticoagulant Therapy

The anticoagulant Coumadin (warfarin sodium) acts by inhibiting the synthesis of prothrombin and other vitamin K–dependent clotting factors. By doing so, Coumadin decreases the ability of blood to clot and is effective in preventing repeat thromboses after a heart attack or the formation of clots after surgical replacement of heart valves. Heparin can also be used to prevent excessive blood clotting. Heparin inhibits the conversion of prothrombin to thrombin, thus preventing formation of a thrombus. The most widely used anticoagulant is low-dose (81-mg) aspirin. This readily available drug inhibits the formation of tiny platelet plugs and the subsequent formation of emboli, which may cause blockage of small blood vessels in the brain and lead to a stroke.

A laboratory test called the *prothrombin time (PT)* is often used to regulate dosage of anticoagulant drugs. In this test, thromboplastin (a blood clotting factor) and calcium are added simultaneously to a tube of the patient's plasma and a tube containing a normal control solution, and the time required for clot formation in both tubes is determined. A patient prothrombin time in excess of the standard control value (11 to 12.5 seconds) indicates the level of anticoagulant effect caused by the administered drug. Unfortunately, PT test results may vary between different clinical laboratories. Variability is often caused by differing techniques or differences in the sensitivity of reagents used. To minimize the effects of these and other variables and standardize the results of anticoagulation testing, a system called the **INR** (abbreviation for **I**nternational **N**ormalized **R**atio) has been developed. PT is reported in seconds. The INR is a mathematical calculation and is reported as a number. An INR of 0.8 to 1.2 is considered normal. In regulating anticoagulant therapy, keeping the INR between 1.5 and 3 will help ensure the prevention of unwanted blood coagulation in "at risk" individuals. By monitoring changes in the INR, a physician can adjust the dose of anticoagulant drug needed to maintain an appropriate level of anticoagulant effect.

RBCs enmeshed in fibrin

③ **Blood clot**

Fibrin mesh (blood clot)

Fibrin

B

FIGURE 11-6   Blood clotting. **A,** The extremely complex clotting mechanism can be distilled into three basic steps: *1,* release of clotting factors from both injured tissue cells and sticky platelets at the injury site (which form a temporary platelet plug); *2,* series of chemical reactions that eventually result in the formation of thrombin; and *3,* formation of fibrin and trapping of RBCs to form a clot. **B,** RBCs and WBCs entrapped in a fibrin *(yellow)* mesh during clot formation (WBCs are *blue*).

Physicians sometimes prescribe vitamin K before surgery to make sure that the patient's blood will clot fast enough to prevent hemorrhage. Vitamin K stimulates liver cells to increase the synthesis of prothrombin. More prothrombin in blood allows faster production of thrombin during clotting and thus faster clot formation.

Unfortunately, clots sometimes form in unbroken blood vessels of the heart, brain, lungs, or some other organ—a dreaded thing because they may produce sudden death by shutting off the blood supply to a vital organ. When a clot stays in the place where it formed, it is called a **thrombus** (THROM-bus), and the condition is spoken of as **thrombosis** (throm-BOH-sis). If part of the clot dislodges and circulates through the bloodstream, the dislodged part is then called an **embolus** (EM-bohlus), and the condition is called an **embolism** (EMboh-liz-em). A number of drugs are now available to help dissolve clots. *Streptokinase* and *recombinant tissue plasminogen activator (t-PA)* are drugs frequently used in a variety of conditions, including treatment of clot-induced strokes, heart attacks, and other thrombus- and embolus-induced medical emergencies. Suppose that your doctor told you that you had a clot in one of your coronary arteries. Which diagnosis would he or she make—coronary thrombosis or coronary embolism—if the physician thought that the clot had formed originally in the coronary artery as a result of the accumulation of fatty material in the vessel wall? Physicians now have effective drugs that they can use to help prevent thrombosis and embolism.

✓ QUICK CHECK

1. Name the formed elements of blood.
2. In general, what function do the WBCs perform?
3. What is the role of fibrin in blood clotting?

 To learn more about platelets and blood clotting, do to AnimationDirect on your CD-ROM.

BLOOD TYPES

ABO System

Blood types are identified by certain "self-antigens" located in the plasma membrane of the RBCs (Figure 11-7). An **antigen** (AN-ti-jen) is a substance that can activate the immune system to make certain responses, including the production of antibodies. Almost all substances that act as antigens and stimulate the immune system are foreign proteins called "non-self" antigens. That is, they are not the body's own natural self-antigens, which are found on the cell membranes of normal body cells. Instead, they are generally proteins that have entered the body from the outside by way of infection, transfusion, or some other method.

The word *antibody* can be defined in terms of what causes its formation or in terms of how it functions. Defined the first way, an **antibody** (ANti-bod-ee) is a substance made by the body in response to stimulation by an antigen. Defined according to its functions, an antibody is a substance that reacts with the antigen that stimulated its formation. Many antibodies react with their antigens to clump or **agglutinate** (ah-GLOO-tin-ayt) them. In other words, they cause their antigens to stick together in little clusters.

Every person's blood is one of the following blood types in the ABO system of typing:

1. Type A
2. Type B
3. Type AB
4. Type O

Suppose that you have type A blood (as do about 41% of Americans). The letter A stands for a certain type of "self-antigen" (a protein) in the plasma membrane of your RBCs, which has been there since birth. Because you were born with type A antigen, your body does not form antibodies to react with it. In other words, your blood plasma contains no anti-A antibodies. It does, however, contain anti-B antibodies. These antibodies are present naturally in type A blood plasma. The body did not form them in response to the presence of the B antigen. In summary, in type A blood, the RBCs contain type A antigen, and the plasma contains anti-B antibodies.

Similarly, in type B blood, the RBCs contain type B self-antigen, and the plasma contains antiA antibodies. In type AB blood, as its name indicates, the RBCs contain both type A and type B self-antigens, and the plasma contains neither anti-A nor anti-B antibodies. The opposite is true of type O blood; its RBCs contain neither type A nor type B antigens, and its plasma contains both anti-A and anti-B antibodies.

Recipient's blood		Reactions with donor's blood			
RBC antigens	Plasma antibodies	Donor type O	Donor type A	Donor type B	Donor type AB
None (Type O)	Anti-A Anti-B	No agglutination	Agglutination	Agglutination	Agglutination
A (Type A)	Anti-B	No agglutination	No agglutination	Agglutination	Agglutination
B (Type B)	Anti-A	No agglutination	Agglutination	No agglutination	Agglutination
A and B (Type AB)	(None)	No agglutination	No agglutination	No agglutination	No agglutination

FIGURE 11-7   Results of different combinations of donor and recipient blood. The left columns show the recipient's blood characteristics, and the top row shows the donor's blood type.

Normal blood   Agglutinated blood

 To learn more about blood grouping, go to AnimationDirect on your CD-ROM.

Rh System

In addition to typing blood using the ABO system, testing for the presence or absence of an additional antigen, called the *Rh antigen*, is important in blood transfusions. Testing for the presence or absence of the Rh antigen is the basis for classifying blood as being either *Rh-positive* or *Rh-negative*. In the United States, about 82% of the general population are Rh-positive; that is, the Rh antigen is present on their red cells (Table 11-2). If, for example, a person has type AB, Rh-positive blood (AB$^+$) the RBCs contain type A antigen, type B antigen, and the Rh antigen. And, a person with type O, Rh-negative blood (O$^-$) would have no type A, B, or Rh antigens located in the plasma membrane of their RBCs. The term *Rh* is used because this important blood cell antigen was first discovered in the blood of Rhesus monkeys.

Universal Donor and Universal Recipient Blood

Harmful effects or even death can result from a blood transfusion reaction if the donor's RBCs become agglutinated by antibodies in the recipient's plasma. If a donor's RBCs do not contain any A, B, or Rh antigen, they cannot be clumped by anti-A, anti-B, or anti-Rh antibodies. For this reason, the type of blood that contains no A, B, or Rh

TABLE 11-2

Blood Typing

BLOOD TYPE (ABO, Rh)	ANTIGENS PRESENT*	ANTIBODIES PRESENT*	PERCENT OF GENERAL POPULATION
O, +	Rh	A, B	35%
O, −†	None	A, B, Rh?	7%
A, +	A, Rh	B	35%
A, −	A	B, Rh?	7%
B, +	B, Rh	A	8%
B, −	B	A, Rh?	2%
AB, +‡	A, B, Rh	None	4%
AB, −	A, B	Rh?	2%

From Pagana KD, Pagana TJ: *Mosby's manual of diagnostic and laboratory tests,* ed 4, St Louis, 2010, Mosby.
*Anti-Rh antibodies *may* be present, depending on exposure to Rh antigens.
†Universal donor.
‡Universal recipient.

antigens—namely, type O, Rh-negative blood (O⁻)—can be used in an emergency as donor blood without the danger of anti-A, anti-B, or anti-Rh antibodies clumping its RBCs. Type O⁻ blood has therefore been called *universal donor blood.* Similarly, blood type AB⁺ has been called *universal recipient blood* because it contains no anti-A, anti-B, or anti-Rh antibodies in its plasma. Therefore it does not clump any donor's RBCs containing A, B, or Rh antigens. In a normal clinical setting, however, all blood intended for transfusion is not only matched carefully to the blood of the recipient for ABO and Rh compatibility but also tested further in a process called *crossmatching* for a variety of so-called "minor antigens" that may also cause certain types of transfusion reactions.

Figure 11-7 shows the results of different combinations of donor and recipient blood.

Erythroblastosis Fetalis

Plasma never naturally contains anti-Rh antibodies. But if Rh-positive blood cells are introduced into an Rh-negative person's body, anti-Rh antibodies soon appear in the blood plasma. In this fact lies the danger for a baby born to an Rh-negative mother and an Rh-positive father. If the baby inherits the Rh-positive trait from his father, the Rh factor on his RBCs may stimulate the mother's body to form anti-Rh antibodies. Then, if she later carries another Rh-positive fetus, he may develop a disease called **erythroblastosis** (eh-rith-roh-blas-TOH-sis) **fetalis** (feh-TAL-is), caused by the mother's Rh antibodies reacting with the baby's Rh-positive cells (Figure 11-8). When this occurs, large numbers of red cells in the fetus break apart or *lyse,* resulting in severe anemia and jaundice. Without treatment consisting of intra-

 Health and Well-Being

Blood Doping

A number of athletes have reportedly improved their performance by a practice called *blood boosting* or **blood doping.** A few weeks before an important event, an athlete has some blood drawn. The RBCs in this sample are separated and frozen. Just before competition, the RBCs are thawed and injected back into the athlete. The increased hematocrit that results slightly improves the oxygen-carrying capacity of the blood, which theoretically improves performance. However, in practice the effects are slight. This method is judged to be an unfair and unwise practice in athletics.

In addition to blood transfusions, injection of substances such as hormones that increase RBC levels in an attempt to improve athletic performance has also been condemned by leading authorities in the area of sports medicine and by athletic organizations around the world. "Doping" with either the naturally occurring hormone erythropoietin (EPO) or with synthetic drugs that have similar biological effects—such as Epogen and Procrit—can result in devastating medical outcomes.

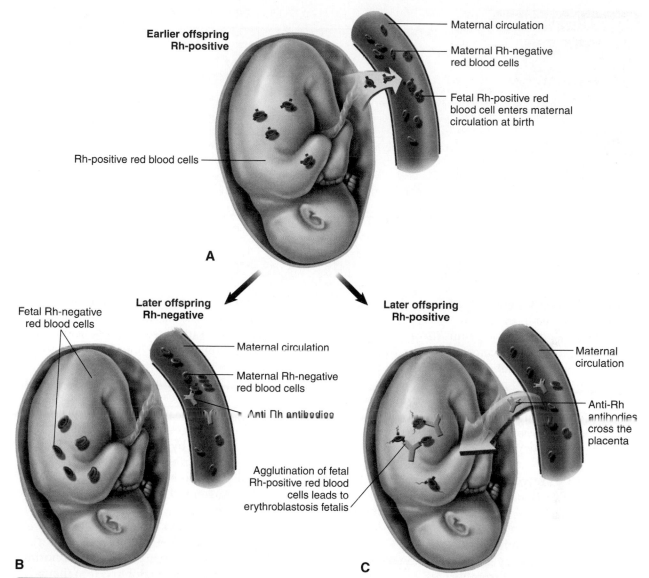

Earlier offspring Rh-positive

Maternal circulation
Maternal Rh-negative red blood cells
Fetal Rh-positive red blood cell enters maternal circulation at birth

Rh-positive red blood cells

A

Later offspring Rh-negative

Fetal Rh-negative red blood cells

Maternal circulation
Maternal Rh-negative red blood cells
Anti-Rh antibodies

Later offspring Rh-positive

Maternal circulation
Anti-Rh antibodies cross the placenta

Agglutination of fetal Rh-positive red blood cells leads to erythroblastosis fetalis

B   **C**

FIGURE 11-8 **Erythroblastosis fetalis. A,** Rh-positive blood cells enter the mother's bloodstream during delivery of an Rh-positive baby. If not treated, the mother's body will produce anti-Rh antibodies. **B,** A later pregnancy involving an Rh-negative baby is normal because there are no Rh antigens in the baby's blood. **C,** A later pregnancy involving an Rh-positive baby may result in erythroblastosis fetalis. Anti-Rh antibodies enter the baby's blood supply and cause agglutination of RBCs with the Rh antigen.

uterine transfusion or immediate exchange transfusion after birth, the condition can result in death of the baby.

All Rh-negative mothers who carry an Rh-positive baby should be treated with a protein marketed as RhoGAM. RhoGAM stops the mother's body from forming anti-Rh antibodies and thus prevents the possibility of harm to the next Rh-positive baby.

QUICK CHECK

1. What is an *antigen* in blood typing?
2. What is meant when a person's blood is described as "Rh negative"?

 To learn more about erythroblastosis fetalis, go to AnimationDirect on your CD-ROM.

Hematology
Charles Richard Drew (1904-1950)

African-American physician Charles Richard Drew was a pioneer in hematology, the study of blood. During World War II, he developed the idea of blood banks and researched the best way to store blood for transfusions to wounded soldiers. In New York, he set up the first blood bank ever, in 1941. This blood bank served as the model for a network of blood banks opened by the American Red Cross.

Many hematologists continue in Drew's footsteps, refining and perfecting the practice of blood science. Many professions benefit from this research. Phlebotomists collect blood for testing or storage, clinical laboratory technicians analyze blood samples, and many different health professionals use blood analysis and blood transfusions to help their patients. Of course, military medics still rely on blood banking technology to provide immediate aid to wounded combat and terrorism victims.

OUTLINE SUMMARY

BLOOD COMPOSITION (See Table 11-1)
A. Blood plasma
  1. Definition — blood minus its cells
  2. Composition — water containing many dissolved substances (for example, nutrients, salts, and hormones)
  3. Amount of blood — varies with size and sex; 4 to 6 liters about average; about 7% to 9% of body weight
B. Formed elements
  1. Types
    a. RBCs (erythrocytes)
    b. WBCs (leukocytes)
      (1) Granular leukocytes — neutrophils, eosinophils, and basophils
      (2) Nongranular leukocytes — lymphocytes and monocytes
    c. Platelets, or thrombocytes
  2. Count
    a. RBCs — 4.5 to 5 million per mm³ of blood
    b. WBCs — 5,000 to 10,000 per mm³ of blood
    c. Platelets — 300,000 per mm³ of blood
  3. Formation — red bone marrow (myeloid tissue) forms all blood cells except some lymphocytes and monocytes, which are formed by lymphatic tissue in the lymph nodes, thymus, and spleen
C. RBCs
  1. Structure — disk-shaped, without nuclei
  2. Functions — transport oxygen and carbon dioxide

3. Anemia — inability of blood to carry adequate oxygen to tissues due to (1) inadequate RBC numbers or (2) a deficiency of hemoglobin
  a. Types
    (1) Hemorrhagic — decreased RBC numbers caused by blood loss (hemorrhage)
    (2) Aplastic — decreased RBC numbers caused by destruction of blood-forming elements
    (3) Pernicious — lack of intrinsic factor in stomach reduces availability of vitamin B₁₂ needed for RBC production
    (4) Sickle cell — inherited defective gene or genes produce an abnormal type of hemoglobin (HbS) that is less able to carry oxygen
4. Polycythemia — abnormally high RBC count
5. Hematocrit test — medical test in which a centrifuge is used to separate whole blood into formed elements and liquid fraction (see Figure 11-3)
  a. Buffy coat is WBC and platelet fraction
  b. Normal RBC level is about 45%
  c. Erroneous test result can be caused by dehydration
D. WBCs (leukocytes)
  1. General function — defense
  2. WBC count
    a. Differential WBC count reveals proportions of each type of WBC

   b. Leukopenia — abnormally low WBC count
   c. Leukocytosis — abnormally high WBC count
 3. Neutrophils and monocytes carry out phagocytosis
 4. Lymphocytes produce antibodies (B lymphocytes) or directly attack foreign cells (T lymphocytes)
 5. Eosinophils protect against parasitic worms
 6. Basophils produce heparin, which inhibits clotting
E. WBC disorders
 1. Leukemia — cancer
   a. Elevated WBC count
   b. Cells do not function properly
F. Platelets and blood clotting (see Figure 11-6)
 1. Platelets play an essential role in blood clotting
 2. Blot clot formation
   a. Clotting factors released at the injury site produce prothrombin activator
   b. Prothrombin activator and calcium convert prothrombin to thrombin
   c. Thrombin reacts with fibrinogen and triggers formation of fibrin, which traps RBCs to form a clot

BLOOD TYPES
A. ABO system (see Figure 11-7)
 1. Antigen — substance that can activate immune system
 2. Antibody — substance made by body in response to stimulation by an antigen
 3. Blood types
   a. Type A blood — type A self-antigens in RBCs; anti–B type antibodies in plasma
   b. Type B blood — type B self-antigens in RBCs; anti–A type antibodies in plasma
   c. Type AB blood — type A and type B self-antigens in RBCs; no anti-A or anti-B antibodies in plasma
   d. Type O blood — no type A or type B self-antigens in RBCs; both anti-A and anti-B antibodies in plasma
B. Rh system
 1. Rh-positive blood — Rh factor antigen present in RBCs
 2. Rh-negative blood — no Rh factor present in RBCs; no anti-Rh antibodies present naturally in plasma; anti-Rh antibodies, however, appear in the plasma of Rh-negative persons if Rh-positive RBCs have been introduced into their bodies
C. Universal donor and universal recipient blood
 1. Type O Rh-negative — universal donor blood
 2. Type AB Rh-positive — universal recipient blood
D. Hemolytic disease of the newborn or erythroblastosis fetalis — may occur when Rh-negative mother carries a second Rh-positive fetus; caused by mother's Rh antibodies reacting with the fetus's Rh-positive cells

NEW WORDS

agglutinate	erythroblastosis fetalis	leukemia	plasma protein
albumin	erythrocyte	leukocyte	platelet
anemia	fibrin	leukocytosis	polycythemia
antibody	fibrinogen	leukopenia	prothrombin
antigen	formed elements	lymphocyte	prothrombin activator
aplastic anemia	globulins	macrophage	serum
basophil	hematocrit (Hct)	monocyte	sickle cell anemia
buffy coat	hemoglobin	myeloid	sickle cell trait
carbaminohemoglobin	hemorrhagic anemia	neutrophil	thrombin
differential WBC count	heparin	oxyhemoglobin	thrombocyte
embolism	International Normal-ized Ratio (INR)	pernicious anemia	thrombosis
embolus	iron deficiency anemia	phagocyte	thrombus
eosinophil		plasma	total WBC count

REVIEW QUESTIONS

1. Name several substances found in blood plasma.
2. Explain the function of albumins, globulins, and fibrinogen.
3. What is the difference between serum and plasma?
4. What two types of connective tissue form blood cells? Where are they found and what do each of them form?
5. Describe the structure of an RBC. What advantage does the unique shape of the RBC have?
6. What is anemia? Give two possible causes of anemia and identify two specific types.
7. What is the buffy coat?
8. Explain the function of neutrophils and monocytes.
9. Explain the function of lymphocytes.
10. What is leukemia? How is it classified?
11. Explain the function of eosinophils and basophils.
12. Explain fully the process of blood clot formation.
13. Differentiate between a thrombus and an embolus.
14. Explain how type A blood differs from type B blood.
15. Explain the cause of erythroblastosis fetalis.

CRITICAL THINKING

16. Explain how heparin inhibits blood clot formation.
17. Differentiate between the process of blood clot formation and the process of blood agglutination.
18. Why is the first Rh-positive baby born to an Rh-negative mother usually unaffected?

CHAPTER TEST

1. The liquid part of the blood is called
   _____.

2. Three important plasma proteins are
   _____, _____, and _____.

3. Blood plasma without the clotting factors is
   called _____.

4. The three types of formed elements in the
   blood are _____, _____, and
   _____.

5. The two types of connective tissue that
   make blood cells are _____ and
   _____.

6. The red pigment in RBCs that carries
   oxygen is called _____.

7. The term _____ is used to describe a
   number of disease conditions caused by the
   inability of RBCs to carry a sufficient
   amount of oxygen.

8. If the body produces an excess of RBCs, the
   condition is called _____.

9. These WBCs are the most numerous of the
   phagocytes: _____.

10. These WBCs produce antibodies to fight
    microbes: _____.

11. Prothrombin activator and the mineral
    _____ in the blood convert prothrom-
    bin to thrombin in blood clot formation.

12. Thrombin converts the inactive plasma
    protein _____ into a fibrous gel called
    _____.

13. Vitamin _____ stimulates the liver to
    increase the synthesis of prothrombin.

14. A _____ is an unneeded blood clot that
    stays in the place where it was formed.

15. If part of a blood clot is dislodged and circu-
    lates through the bloodstream, it is called
    an _____.

16. _____ is a foreign substance that can
    cause the body to produce an antibody.

17. A person with type AB blood has _____
    antigens on the blood cells and _____
    antibodies in the plasma.

18. A person with type B blood has _____
    antigens on the blood cells and _____
    antibodies in the plasma.

19. Type _____ blood is considered the uni-
    versal donor.

20. Type _____ blood is considered the uni-
    versal recipient.

21. A condition called _____ can develop if
    an Rh-negative mother produces antibodies
    against an Rh-positive fetus.

OBJECTIVES

AFTER YOU HAVE COMPLETED THIS CHAPTER, YOU SHOULD BE ABLE TO:

1. Discuss the location, size, and position of the heart in the thoracic cavity and identify the heart chambers, valves, and sounds.
2. Trace blood through the heart and compare the functions of the heart chambers on the right and left sides.
3. List the anatomical components of the heart conduction system and discuss the features of a normal electrocardiogram.
4. Explain the relationship between blood vessel structure and function.
5. Trace the path of blood through the systemic, pulmonary, hepatic portal, and fetal circulations.
6. Identify and discuss the primary factors involved in the generation and regulation of blood pressure and explain the relationships between these factors.

The Cardiovascular System 12

The system that supplies our body's transportation needs is the **cardiovascular system.** We need such a system to make sure that each cell is surrounded by fluid that is constantly replenished with oxygen, water, and nutrients as they are used up by a cell. And we need to continually remove waste products from extracellular fluid as they are released from cells. A circulating stream of blood can pick substances from various parts of the body and deliver them to others, thus allowing your body to move substances around in a way that helps you maintain a relative constancy of our internal environment. Clearly, circulation of the blood is critical to maintaining a homeostatic balance in your body.

We begin the study of the cardiovascular system with the heart—the pump that keeps blood moving through a closed circuit of blood vessels. Details related to heart structure will be followed by a discussion of how the heart functions. This chapter concludes with a study of the vessels through which blood flows as a result of the pumping action of the heart. As a group, these vessels are multipurpose structures. Some allow for rapid movement of blood from one body area to another. Others, such as the microscopic capillaries, permit the movement or exchange of many substances between the blood and fluid surrounding body cells. Chapter 13 covers the lymphatic system and immunity topics that relate in many ways to the structure and functions of the cardiovascular system. Together the network of cardiovascular and lymphatic vessels make up what is often called the *circulatory system*.

STUDY TIPS

To make the study of the cardiovascular system more efficient, we suggest these tips:

1. Before studying Chapter 12, review the synopsis of the cardiovascular system in Chapter 4. Chapter 12 deals with the heart, which is the pump that moves the blood, and the vessels, which are the tubing that carries the blood.
2. The prefix *cardio-* refers to the heart; in Chapter 7 you learned that *myo-* means muscle. *Myocardium* is the heart muscle.
3. The arteries and veins are composed of three layers of tissue. There is a difference in thickness in these vessels because the arteries carry blood under higher pressure. Arteries and veins carry blood in opposite directions— arteries away from the heart, veins toward the heart. Capillaries need to be thin-walled because this is where the exchange of material between the blood and the tissues takes place.
4. A liquid moves from high to low pressure, so it is logical that the blood pressure in the cardiovascular system is highest just after leaving the heart and is lowest just before returning to the heart.
5. The structures of the heart can be learned with flash cards. The location of the semilunar valves should be easy to remember because their names tell you where they are. It is harder to remember where the tricuspid and mitral valves are because the names do not help. An easier way to remember them is to use their other names: the right and left atrioventricular valves, respectively. This name tells you exactly where they are: between the atria and ventricles on the right or left side. Blood moves through the cardiovascular system in one direction, from the right heart, to the lungs, to the left heart, to the rest of the body, and back to the right heart.
6. If you are asked to learn the sequence of blood flow through the heart, don't forget the valves. Heart conduction may make more sense if you remember that atria contract from the top down, but ventricles must contract from the bottom up.

Continued on page 270.

HEART

Location, Size, and Position

No one needs to be told where the heart is or what it does. Everyone knows that the heart is in the chest, that it beats night and day to keep the blood flowing, and that if it stops, life stops.

Most of us probably think of the heart as being located on the left side of the body. As you can see in Figure 12-1, the heart is located between the lungs in the lower portion of the mediastinum. Draw an imaginary line through the middle of the trachea in Figure 12-1 and continue the line down through the thoracic cavity to divide it into right and left halves. Note that about two thirds of the mass of the heart is to the left of this line and one third is to the right.

The heart is often described as a triangular organ, shaped and sized roughly like a closed fist. In Figure 12-1 you can see that the **apex,** or blunt point, of the lower edge of the heart lies on the diaphragm, pointing toward the left. Physicians and nurses often listen to the heart sounds by placing a stethoscope on the chest wall directly over the apex of the heart. Sounds of the so-called *apical beat* are easily heard in this area (that is, in the space between the fifth and sixth ribs on a line even with the midpoint of the left clavicle).

The heart is positioned in the thoracic cavity between the sternum in front and the bodies of the thoracic vertebrae behind. Because of this placement, it can be compressed or squeezed by application of pressure to the lower portion of the body of the sternum using the heel of the hand. Rhythmic compression of the heart in this way can maintain blood flow in cases of cardiac arrest and, if combined with effective artificial respiration, the resulting procedure, called **cardiopulmonary resuscitation (CPR),** can be lifesaving.

 To learn more about the location of the heart, go to AnimationDirect on your CD-ROM.

Anatomy

Heart Chambers

If you cut open a heart, you can see many of its main structural features (Figure 12-2). This organ is hollow, not solid. A partition divides it into right and left sides. The heart contains four cavities, or hollow chambers. The two upper chambers are called **atria** (AY-tree-ah) (*singular,* **atrium**), and the two lower chambers are called **ventricles** (VEN-tri-kulz).

The atria are smaller than the ventricles, and their walls are thinner and less muscular. Atria are often called *receiving chambers* because blood enters the heart through veins that open into these upper cavities. Eventually, blood is pumped from the heart into arteries that exit from the ventricles; therefore, the ventricles are sometimes referred to as the *discharging chambers* of the heart.

Each heart chamber is named according to its location. There are right and left atrial chambers above and right and left ventricular chambers below.

The wall of each heart chamber is composed of cardiac muscle tissue, usually referred to as the **myocardium** (my-oh-KAR-dee-um). The septum between the atrial chambers is called the *interatrial septum;* the *interventricular septum* separates the ventricles.

Each chamber of the heart is lined by a thin layer of very smooth tissue called the **endocardium** (en-doh-KAR-dee-um) (see Figure 12-2). Inflammation of this lining is referred to as **endocarditis** (en-doh-kar-DYE-tis). If inflamed, the endocardial lining can become rough and abrasive to red blood cells passing over its surface. Blood flowing over a

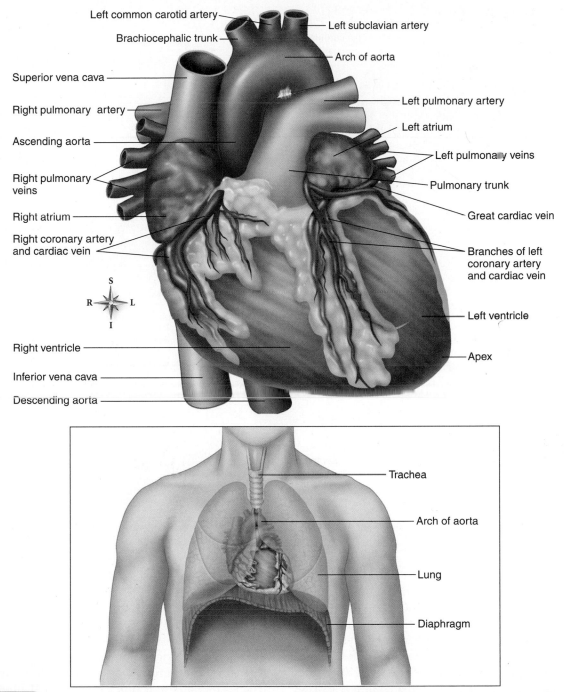

Left common carotid artery
Brachiocephalic trunk
Left subclavian artery
Arch of aorta
Superior vena cava
Right pulmonary artery
Left pulmonary artery
Left atrium
Ascending aorta
Left pulmonary veins
Right pulmonary veins
Pulmonary trunk
Right atrium
Great cardiac vein
Right coronary artery and cardiac vein
Branches of left coronary artery and cardiac vein
Left ventricle
Right ventricle
Apex
Inferior vena cava
Descending aorta

S
R · L
I

Trachea
Arch of aorta
Lung
Diaphragm

FIGURE 12-1 **The heart.** The heart and major blood vessels viewed from the front (anterior). *Inset* shows the relationship of the heart to other structures in the thoracic cavity.

rough surface is subject to clotting, and a **thrombus** (THROM-bus), or clot, may form (see Chapter 11). Unfortunately, rough spots caused by endocarditis or injuries to blood vessel walls often cause the release of platelet factors. The result is often the formation of a fatal blood clot.

 To learn more about the chambers of the heart, go to AnimationDirect on your CD-ROM.

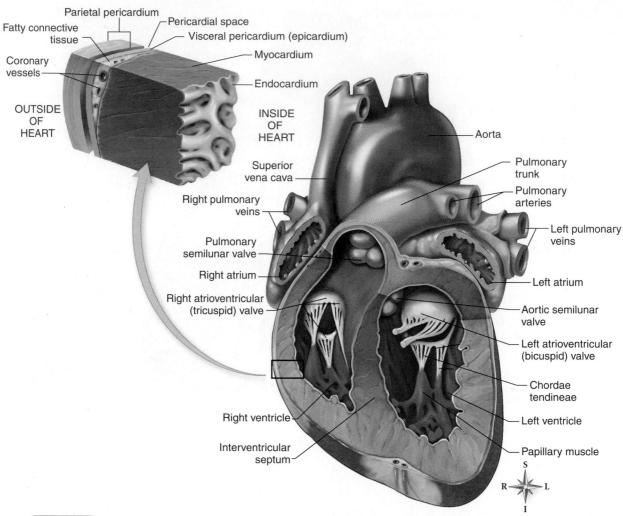

FIGURE 12-2 An internal view of the heart. *Inset* shows a cross-section of the heart wall, including the pericardium.

Covering Sac, or Pericardium

The heart has a covering and a lining. Its covering, called the **pericardium** (pair-i-KAR-dee-um), consists of two layers of fibrous tissue with a small space in between them. The inner layer of the pericardium is called the **visceral pericardium** or **epicardium** (ep-i-KAR-dee-um). It covers the heart the way an apple skin covers an apple. The outer layer of pericardium is called the **parietal pericardium.** It fits around the heart like a loose-fitting sack, allowing enough room for the heart to beat.

It is easy to remember the difference between the *endocardium*, which lines the heart chambers, and the *epicardium*, which covers the surface of the heart (see Figure 12-2), if you understand the meaning of the prefixes *endo-* and *epi-*. *Endo-* comes from the Greek word meaning "inside" or "within," and *epi-* comes from the Greek word meaning "upon" or "on."

The two pericardial layers slide against each other without friction when the heart beats because these are serous membranes with moist, not dry, surfaces. A thin film of pericardial fluid furnishes the lubricating moistness between the heart and its enveloping pericardial sac.

If the pericardium becomes inflamed, a condition called **pericarditis** (pair-i-kar-DYE-tis) results.

Heart Action

The heart serves as a muscular pumping device for distributing blood to all parts of the body.

Contraction of the heart is called **systole** (SIS-toh-lee), and relaxation is called **diastole** (dye-ASS-toh-lee). When the heart beats (that is, when it contracts), the atria contract first (atrial systole), forcing blood into the ventricles. Once filled, the two ventricles contract (ventricular systole) and force blood out of the heart (Figure 12-3). For the heart to be efficient in its pumping action, more than just the rhythmic contraction of its muscular fibers is required. The direction of blood flow must

FIGURE 12-3 **Heart action. A,** During atrial systole (contraction), cardiac muscle in the atrial wall contracts, forcing blood through the atrioventricular (AV) valves and into the ventricles. Bottom illustration shows superior view of all four valves, with semilunar (SL) valves closed and AV valves open. **B,** During ventricular systole that follows, the AV valves close, and blood is forced out of the ventricles through the semilunar valves and into the arteries. Bottom illustration shows superior view of SL valves open and AV valves closed.

be directed and controlled. This is accomplished by four sets of valves located at the entrance and near the exit of the ventricles.

Heart Valves

The two valves that separate the atrial chambers above from the ventricles below are called **atrioventricular** (ay-tree-oh-ven-TRIK-yoo-lar) **(AV) valves.** The left AV valve is the **bicuspid valve,** or **mitral** (MY-tral), **valve,** located between the left atrium and ventricle. The left AV valve is the **tricuspid valve** located between the right atrium and ventricle. The AV valves prevent backflow of blood into the atria when the ventricles contract. Locate the AV valves in Figures 12-2 and 12-3. Note that a number of stringlike structures called **chordae tendineae** (KOHR-dee ten-DIN-ee) attach the AV valves to the wall of the ventricles.

The **semilunar** (sem-i-LOO-nar) **(SL) valves** are located between the two ventricular chambers and the large arteries that carry blood away from the heart when contraction occurs (see Figure 12-3). The ventricles, like the atria, contract together; therefore, the two SL valves open and close at the same time. The pulmonary SL valve is located at the beginning of the pulmonary artery and allows blood going to the lungs to flow out of the right ventricle but prevents it from flowing back into the ventricle. The aortic SL valve is located at the beginning of the aorta and allows blood to flow out of the left ventricle up into the aorta but prevents backflow into this ventricle.

Heart Sounds

If a stethoscope is placed on the anterior chest wall, two distinct sounds can be heard. They are rhythmical and repetitive sounds that are often described as *lub dup.*

The first, or *lub,* sound is caused by the vibration and abrupt closure of the AV valves as the ventricles contract. Closure of the AV valves prevents blood from rushing back up into the atria during contraction of the ventricles. This first sound is of longer duration and lower pitch than the second. The pause between this first sound and the *dup,* or second, sound is shorter than that after the second sound and the *lub dup* of the next systole. The second heart sound is caused by the closing of both the SL valves when the ventricles undergo diastole (relax).

Blood Flow Through the Heart

The heart acts as two separate pumps. The right atrium and the right ventricle perform a task quite different from the left atrium and the left ventricle. When the heart "beats," first the atria contract simultaneously. This is atrial systole. After the ventricles fill with blood, they, too, contract together during ventricular systole. Although the atria contract as a unit, followed by the ventricles below, the right and left sides of the heart act as separate pumps. As we study the blood flow through the heart, the separate functions of the two pumps will become clearer.

Note in Figure 12-3 that blood enters the right atrium through two large veins called the **superior vena** (VEE-nah) **cava** (KAY-vah) and **inferior vena cava.** The right heart pump receives oxygen-poor blood from the veins. After entering the right atrium, it is pumped through the right AV, or tricuspid valve, and enters the right ventricle. When the ventricles contract, blood in the right ventricle is pumped through the pulmonary SL valve into the **pulmonary artery** and eventually to the lungs, where oxygen is added and carbon dioxide is lost.

As you can see in Figure 12-3, blood rich in oxygen returns to the left atrium of the heart through four **pulmonary veins.** It then passes through the left AV, or bicuspid valve, into the left ventricle. When the left ventricle contracts, blood is forced through the aortic SL valve into the **aorta** (ay-OR-tah) and is distributed to the body as a whole.

As you can tell from Figure 12-4, the two sides of the heart actually pump blood through two separate "circulations" and function as two separate pumps. The *pulmonary circulation* involves movement of blood from the right ventricle to the lungs, and the *systemic circulation* involves movement of blood from the left ventricle throughout the body as a whole. The pulmonary and systemic circulations are discussed later in this chapter.

Blood Supply to the Heart Muscle

To sustain life, the heart must pump blood throughout the body on a regular and ongoing basis. As a result, the heart muscle, or myocardium, requires a constant supply of blood containing nutrients and oxygen to function effectively. The delivery of oxygen and nutrient-rich arterial blood to cardiac muscle tissue and the return of

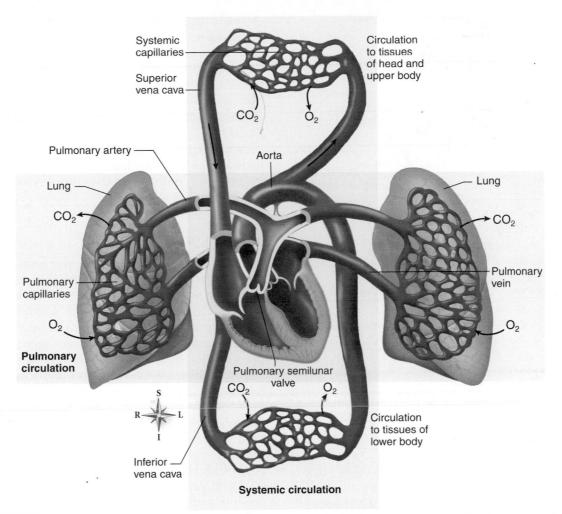

FIGURE 12-4 Blood flow through the cardiovascular system. In the pulmonary circulatory route, blood is pumped from the right side of the heart to the gas-exchange tissues of the lungs. In the systemic circulation, blood is pumped from the left side of the heart to all other tissues of the body.

oxygen-poor blood from this active tissue to the venous system are called **coronary circulation.**

Blood flows into the heart muscle by way of two small vessels—the right and left **coronary arteries.** The coronary arteries are the aorta's first branches (Figure 12-5). The openings into these small vessels lie behind the flaps of the aortic SL valve. During ventricular systole, the myocardium is contracting and putting pressure on the coronary arteries, so little blood can enter them. However, during ventricular diastole, blood that backs up behind the aortic SL valve can flow easily into the coronary arteries.

In both coronary thrombosis and coronary **embolism** (EM-boh-liz-em), a blood clot occludes

or plugs up some part of a coronary artery. Blood cannot pass through the occluded vessel and so cannot reach the heart muscle cells it normally supplies. Deprived of oxygen, these cells soon become damaged or die. In medical terms, **myocardial** (my-oh-KAR-dee-al) **infarction** (in-FARK-shun) **(MI),** or tissue death, occurs.

Myocardial infarction, also referred to as a "heart attack," is a common cause of death during middle and late adulthood. Recovery from a myocardial infarction is possible if the amount of heart tissue damaged was small enough so that the remaining undamaged heart muscle can pump blood effectively enough to supply the needs of the rest of the heart and the body.

A

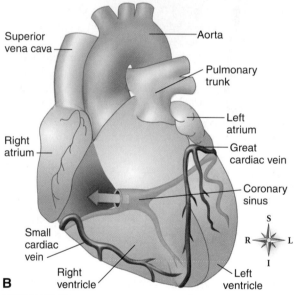

B

FIGURE 12-5 Coronary circulation. **A,** Arteries. **B,** Veins. Both are anterior views of the heart. Vessels near the anterior surface are more darkly colored than those of the posterior surface seen through the heart.

The term **angina** (an-JYE-nah) **pectoris** (PECK-tor-is) is used to describe the severe chest pain that occurs when the myocardium is deprived of adequate oxygen. It is often a warning that the coronary arteries are no longer able to supply enough blood and oxygen to the heart muscle.

Coronary bypass surgery is a common treatment for those who suffer from severely restricted coronary artery blood flow. In this procedure, veins or arteries are "harvested" or removed from other areas of the body and used to bypass partial blockages in coronary arteries (Figure 12-6). Another treatment used to improve coronary blood flow is *angioplasty*, a procedure in which a device is inserted into a blood vessel to open a channel for blood flow.

After blood has passed through the capillary beds in the myocardium, it flows into **cardiac veins,** which empty into the **coronary sinus** and finally into the right atrium.

Cardiac Cycle

The beating of the heart is a regular and rhythmic process. Each complete heartbeat is called a **cardiac cycle** and includes the contraction (systole) and relaxation (diastole) of atria and ventricles. Each cycle takes about 0.8 seconds to complete if the heart is beating at an average rate of about 72 beats per minute. The term **stroke volume** refers to the volume of blood ejected from the ventricles during each beat. **Cardiac output,** or the volume of blood pumped by one ventricle per minute, averages about 5 liters in a normal, resting adult.

> ✓ **QUICK CHECK**
>
> 1. What are the functions of the atria and ventricles of the heart?
> 2. What coverings does the heart have? What is the heart's lining called?
> 3. What are systole and diastole of the heart?
> 4. What are the two major "circulations" of the body?

Conduction System of the Heart

Cardiac muscle fibers can contract rhythmically on their own. However, they must be coordinated by electrical signals (impulses) if the heart is to pump effectively.

Although the rate of the cardiac muscle's rhythm is controlled by autonomic nerve signals, the heart has its own built-in conduction system for coordinating contractions during the cardiac cycle. The most important thing to realize about this conduction system is that all of the cardiac muscle fibers in each region of the heart are electrically linked together. The *intercalated disks* that were first

Single bypass

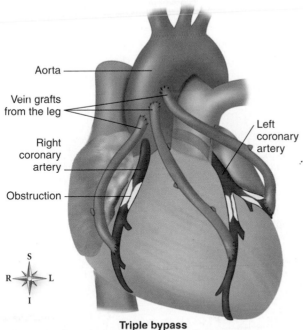

Triple bypass

FIGURE 12-6   Coronary bypass. In coronary bypass surgery, blood vessels are "harvested" from other parts of the body and used to construct detours around blocked coronary arteries. Artificial vessels can also be used.

introduced in Chapter 3 (see Figure 3-22, p. 63) are actually connections that electrically join muscle fibers into a single unit that can conduct an impulse through the entire wall of a heart chamber without stopping. Thus both atrial walls will contract at about the same time because all of their fibers are electrically linked. Likewise, both ventricular walls will contract at about the same time.

Four structures embedded in the wall of the heart specialize in generating strong impulses and conduct them rapidly to certain regions of the heart wall. Thus they make sure that the atria contract and then the ventricles contract in an efficient manner. The structures that make up this conduction system of the heart are as follows:

1. **Sinoatrial** (sye-no-AY-tree-al) **node,** which is sometimes called the SA node or the **pacemaker**
2. **Atrioventricular** (ay-tree-oh-ven-TRIK-yoo-lar) **node,** or **AV node**
3. **AV bundle,** or **bundle of His**
4. **Purkinje** (pur-KIN-jee) **fibers**

Impulse conduction normally starts in the heart's pacemaker, namely, the SA node. From there, it spreads, as you can see in Figure 12-7, in all directions through the atria. This causes the atrial fibers to contract. When impulses reach the AV node, it is triggered to relay its own impulse by way of the bundle of His and Purkinje fibers to the ventricles, causing them to contract. Normally, therefore, a ventricular beat follows each atrial beat.

Various conditions such as endocarditis or myocardial infarction, however, can damage the heart's conduction system and thereby disturb its rhythmic beating. One such disturbance is the condition commonly called *heart block*. Impulses are blocked from getting through to the ventricles, resulting in the ventricles beating at a much slower rate than normal. A physician may treat heart block by implanting in the heart an artificial pacemaker, an electrical device that causes ventricular contractions at a rate fast enough to maintain an adequate circulation of blood.

Electrocardiogram

The specialized structures of the heart's conduction system generate tiny electrical currents that spread through surrounding tissues to the surface of the body. This fact is of great clinical significance

FIGURE 12-7 **Conduction system of the heart.** Specialized cardiac muscle cells in the wall of the heart rapidly conduct an electrical impulse throughout the myocardium. The signal is initiated by the SA node (pacemaker) and spreads to the rest of the atrial myocardium and to the atrioventricular (AV) node. The AV node then initiates a signal that is conducted through the ventricular myocardium by way of the AV bundle (of His) and Purkinje fibers.

FIGURE 12-8 **Events represented by the electrocardiogram (ECG).** It is nearly impossible to illustrate the invisible, dynamic events of heart conduction in a few cartoon panels or "snapshots," but the sketches here give you an idea of what is happening in the heart as the ECG is recorded.

because these electrical signals can be picked up from the body surface and transformed into visible tracings by an instrument called an **electrocardiograph** (ee-lek-troh-KAR-dee-oh-graf).

The **electrocardiogram** (ee-lek-troh-KAR-dee-oh-gram) is the graphic record of the heart's electrical activity. This chart is also called an **ECG**—or **EKG** when spoken aloud. Skilled interpretation of these ECG records may sometimes make the difference between life and death. A normal ECG tracing is shown in Figure 12-8.

A normal ECG tracing has three very characteristic deflections, or waves, called the **P wave,** the **QRS complex,** and the **T wave.** These deflections represent the electrical activity that regulates the contraction or relaxation of the atria or ventricles. The term **depolarization** describes the electrical activity that triggers contraction of the heart muscle. **Repolarization** begins just before the relaxation phase of cardiac muscle activity. In the normal ECG shown in Figure 12-8, the small P wave occurs with depolarization of the atria. The QRS complex occurs as a result of depolarization of the ventricles, and the T wave results from electrical activity generated by repolarization of the ventricles. You may wonder why no visible record of atrial repolarization is noted in a normal ECG. The reason is simply that the deflection is very small

and is hidden by the large QRS complex that occurs at the same time.

Damage to cardiac muscle tissue that is caused by a myocardial infarction or disease affecting the heart's conduction system results in distinctive changes in the ECG. Therefore, ECG tracings are extremely valuable in the diagnosis and treatment of heart disease.

> ✓ **QUICK CHECK**
> 1. What structure is the natural "pacemaker" of the heart?
> 2. What information is in an electrocardiogram?

BLOOD VESSELS

Types

Arterial blood is pumped from the heart through a series of large distribution vessels—the **arteries.** The largest artery in the body is the aorta. Arteries subdivide into vessels that become progressively smaller and finally become tiny **arterioles** (ar-TEER-ee-ohlz) that control the flow into microscopic exchange vessels called **capillaries** (KAP-i-lair-eez). In the so-called *capillary beds,* the exchange of nutrients and respiratory gases occurs between

FIGURE 12-8, cont'd

Health and Well-Being

Changes in Blood Flow During Exercise

Not only does the overall rate of blood flow increase during exercise, but also the relative blood flow through the different organs of the body changes. During exercise, blood is routed away from the kidneys and digestive organs and toward the skeletal muscles, cardiac muscle, and skin. Rerouting of blood is accomplished by contracting precapillary sphincters in some tissues (thus reducing blood flow) while relaxing precapillary sphincters in other tissues (thus increasing blood flow). How can homeostasis be better maintained by these changes? One reason is that glucose and oxygen

levels drop rapidly in muscles as they use up these substances to produce energy for exercising. Increased blood flow restores normal levels of glucose and oxygen more rapidly. Blood that has been warmed up in active muscles flows to the skin for cooling. This helps keep the body temperature from getting too high. Can you think of other ways this change in blood flow helps maintain homeostasis? Typical changes in organ blood flow with exercise are shown in the illustration. The *red bar* in each pair shows the resting blood flow; the *blue bar* shows the flow during exercise.

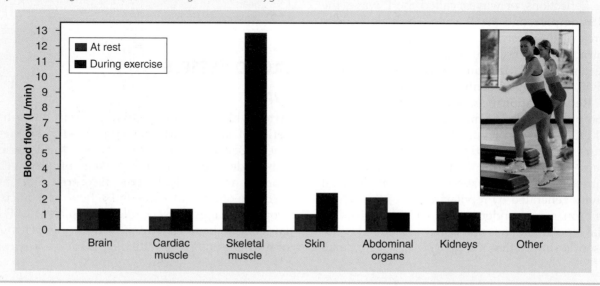

the blood and tissue fluid around the cells. Blood exits or is drained from the capillary beds and then enters the small **venules** (VEN-yoolz), which join with other venules and increase in size, becoming **veins.** The largest veins are the superior vena cava and the inferior vena cava.

As noted previously (see Figure 12-4), arteries carry blood away from the heart and toward capillaries. Veins carry blood toward the heart and away from capillaries, and capillaries carry blood from the tiny arterioles into tiny venules. The aorta carries blood out of the left ventricle of the heart, and the venae cavae return blood to the right atrium after the blood has circulated through the body.

Structure

Arteries, veins, and capillaries differ in structure. Three coats, or layers, are found in both arteries and veins (Figure 12-9). The outermost layer is

called the **tunica externa** (or *tunica adventitia*). This outer layer is made of connective tissue fibers, which reinforce the wall of the vessel so that it will not burst under pressure.

Figure 12-9 shows that smooth muscle tissue is found in the middle layer, or **tunica media,** of arteries and veins. However, this muscle layer is much thicker in arteries than it is in veins. Why is this important? Because the thicker muscle layer in the artery wall is able to resist great pressures generated by ventricular systole. In arteries, the tunica media plays a critical role in maintaining blood pressure and controlling blood distribution. This is a smooth muscle, so it is controlled by the autonomic nervous system. The tunica media also includes a thin layer of elastic fibrous tissue.

An inner layer of endothelial cells called the **tunica intima** lines arteries and veins. The tunica intima is actually a single layer of squamous epithelial cells called **endothelium** (en-doh-THEE-lee-um)

ARTERY

Elastic tissue

Tunica intima
(endothelium)

Tunica media
(smooth muscle layer
and elastic tissue)

- Thicker in arteries
- Thinner in veins

Tunica externa
(connective tissue)

- Thinner than tunica media in arteries
- Thickest layer in veins

VEIN

Venous valve

Basement membrane

Smooth muscle

A   B

FIGURE 12-9   **Artery and vein.** Schematic drawings of an artery, **A,** and a vein, **B,** show comparative thicknesses of the three layers: the outer layer or *tunica externa*, the muscle layer or *tunica media*, and the *tunica intima* made of endothelium. Note that the muscle and outer layer are much thinner in veins than in arteries and that veins have valves.

that lines the inner surface of the entire cardiovascular system.

As you can see in Figure 12-9, veins have a unique structural feature not present in arteries. They are equipped with one-way valves that prevent the backflow of blood.

When a surgeon cuts into the body, only arteries, arterioles, veins, and venules can be seen. Capillaries cannot be seen because they are microscopic. The most important structural feature of capillaries is their extreme thinness—only one layer of flat, endothelial cells composes the capillary membrane. Instead of three layers or coats, the capillary wall is composed of only one—the tunica intima. Substances such as glucose, oxygen, and wastes can quickly pass through it on their way to or from cells.

Smooth muscle cells called **precapillary sphincters** guard the entrances to the capillaries and determine how much blood will flow into each capillary, as you can see in Figure 12-10.

From heart

Arteriole
Endothelium
Smooth muscle fiber

Precapillary sphincters (relaxed) — **Capillary bed**

Capillary

Smooth muscle fiber

Thoroughfare channel

Endothelium
Venule

To heart

FIGURE 12-10   **Capillaries.** Capillaries are microscopic, thin-walled vessels that form networks joining arterioles to venules. Smooth muscles wrapping around the entrances to capillaries (precapillary sphincters) act as valves that control local blood flow.

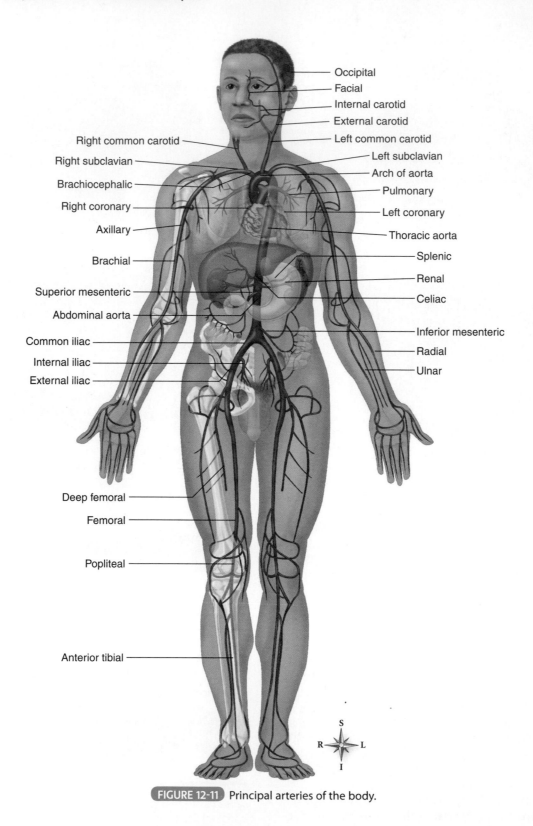

FIGURE 12-11 Principal arteries of the body.

Functions

Arteries, veins, and capillaries have different functions.

Arteries and arterioles distribute blood from the heart to capillaries in all parts of the body. In addition, by constricting or dilating, arterioles help maintain arterial blood pressure at a normal level.

Venules and veins collect blood from capillaries and return it to the heart. They also serve as blood reservoirs because they carry blood under lower pressure (than arteries) and can expand to hold a larger volume of blood or constrict to hold a much smaller amount.

Capillaries function as exchange vessels. For example, glucose and oxygen move out of the blood in capillaries into interstitial fluid and then on into cells. Carbon dioxide and other substances move in the opposite direction (that is, into the capillary blood from the cells). Fluid is also exchanged between capillary blood and interstitial fluid (see Chapter 18).

Study Figure 12-11 and Table 12-1 to learn the names of the main arteries of the body and Figure 12-12 and Table 12-2 for the names of the main veins.

QUICK CHECK

1. What are the two main types of blood vessels in the body? How are they different?
2. Can you describe the three major layers of a large blood vessel?
3. What are capillaries?

CIRCULATION OF BLOOD

Systemic and Pulmonary Circulation

The term *blood circulation* is self-explanatory, meaning that blood flows through vessels that are arranged in a complete circuit or circular pattern.

Blood flow from the left ventricle of the heart through blood vessels to all parts of the body and back to the right atrium of the heart has already been referred to as the **systemic circulation.** The left ventricle pumps blood into the aorta. From there, it flows into arteries that carry it into the tissues and organs of the body. As indicated in Figure 12-13, within each structure, blood moves from arteries to arterioles to capillaries. There, the vital two-way exchange of substances occurs between blood and cells. Next, blood flows out of each organ's capillary beds by way of its venules and then

---

TABLE 12-1

The Major Systemic Arteries

ARTERY	TISSUES SUPPLIED	ARTERY	TISSUES SUPPLIED
Head and Neck		**Abdomen—cont'd**	
Occipital	Posterior head and neck	Superior mesenteric	Small intestine; upper half of the large intestine
Facial	Mouth, pharynx, and face	Inferior mesenteric	Lower half of the large intestine
Internal carotid	Anterior brain and meninges		
External carotid	Superficial neck, face, eyes, and larynx	**Upper Extremity**	
		Axillary	Axilla (armpit)
Common carotid	Head and neck	Brachial	Arm
Vertebral	Brain and meninges	Radial	Lateral side of the hand
		Ulnar	Medial side of the hand
Thorax			
Left subclavian	Left upper extremity	**Lower Extremity**	
Brachiocephalic	Head, neck, and upper extremity	Internal iliac	Pelvic viscera, genitalia, and rectum
Arch of aorta	Branches to head, neck, and upper extremities	External iliac	Lower trunk and lower extremity
Coronary	Heart muscle	Deep femoral	Deep thigh muscles
		Femoral	Thigh
Abdomen		Popliteal	Knee and leg
Celiac	Stomach, spleen, and liver	Anterior tibial and posterior tibial	Leg
Splenic	Spleen		
Renal	Kidneys		

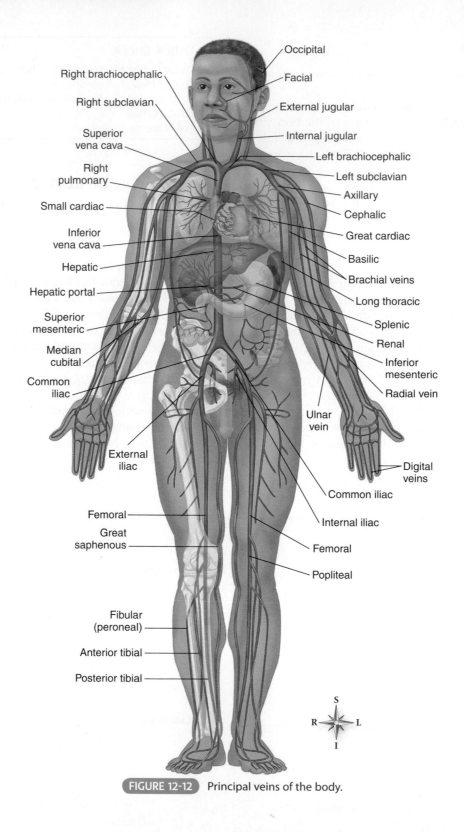

Occipital

Right brachiocephalic

Facial

Right subclavian

External jugular

Superior vena cava

Internal jugular

Right pulmonary

Left brachiocephalic

Left subclavian

Small cardiac

Axillary

Inferior vena cava

Cephalic

Hepatic

Great cardiac

Hepatic portal

Basilic

Superior mesenteric

Brachial veins

Median cubital

Long thoracic

Common iliac

Splenic

Renal

Inferior mesenteric

Radial vein

Ulnar vein

External iliac

Digital veins

Femoral

Common iliac

Great saphenous

Internal iliac

Femoral

Popliteal

Fibular (peroneal)

Anterior tibial

Posterior tibial

FIGURE 12-12 Principal veins of the body.

TABLE 12-2

The Major Systemic Veins

VEIN	TISSUES DRAINED	VEIN	TISSUES DRAINED
Head and Neck		**Upper Extremity**	
Facial and anterior facial	Anterior and superficial face	Cephalic	Lateral arm
External jugular	Superficial tissues of the head and neck	Axillary	Axilla and arm
		Basilic	Medial arm
Internal jugular	Sinuses of the brain	Median cubital	Cephalic vein (to basilic vein)
		Radial	Lateral forearm
Thorax		Ulnar	Medial forearm
Brachiocephalic	Head, neck, upper extremity		
Subclavian	Upper extremity	**Lower Extremity**	
Superior vena cava	Head, neck, and upper extremities	External iliac	Lower limb
Pulmonary	Lungs	Internal iliac	Pelvic viscera
Cardiac	Heart	Femoral	Thigh
Inferior vena cava	Lower body	Great saphenous	Leg
		Small saphenous	Foot
Abdomen		Popliteal	Leg
Hepatic	Liver	Peroneal (fibular)	Foot
Long thoracic	Abdominal and thoracic muscles	Anterior tibial	Deep anterior leg and dorsal foot
Hepatic portal	Intestines and nearby internal organs	Posterior tibial	Deep posterior leg and plantar aspect of foot
Splenic	Spleen		
Superior mesenteric	Small intestine and most of the colon		
Inferior mesenteric	Descending colon and rectum		

its veins to drain eventually into the inferior or superior venae cavae. These two great veins return venous blood to the right atrium of the heart.

At that point, the blood is short of coming full circle back to its starting point in the left ventricle. To reach the left ventricle and start on its way again, it must first flow through another circuit, referred to earlier as the **pulmonary circulation.** Observe in Figure 12-13 that venous blood moves from the right atrium to the right ventricle and then to the pulmonary artery to lung arterioles and capillaries. There, the exchange of gases between the blood and air takes place, converting the deep crimson color typical of venous blood to the scarlet color of arterial blood. This oxygenated blood then flows through lung venules into four pulmonary veins and returns to the left atrium of the heart. From the left atrium, it enters the left ventricle, from which it will once again be pumped throughout the body in the systemic circulation.

 To learn more about pulmonary circulation and systemic circulation, go to AnimationDirect on your CD-ROM.

Hepatic Portal Circulation

The term **hepatic portal circulation** refers to the route of blood flow through the liver. Veins from the spleen, stomach, pancreas, gallbladder, and intestines do not pour their blood directly into the inferior vena cava as do the veins from other abdominal organs. Instead, blood flow from these organs is funneled to the liver by means of the hepatic portal vein (Figure 12-14). The blood then passes through the liver before it reenters the regular venous return pathway to the heart. Blood leaves the liver by way of the hepatic veins, which drain into the inferior vena cava.

As noted in Figure 12-13, most of the blood flows from arteries to arterioles to capillaries to venules to veins and back to the heart. Blood flow that is diverted to the hepatic portal circulation, however, does not follow this direct route. The diverted venous blood, instead of returning directly to the heart, is sent instead through a second capillary bed in the liver. The hepatic portal vein shown in Figure 12-14 is located between two capillary beds—one located in the digestive organs and the other in the liver. Once blood exits from

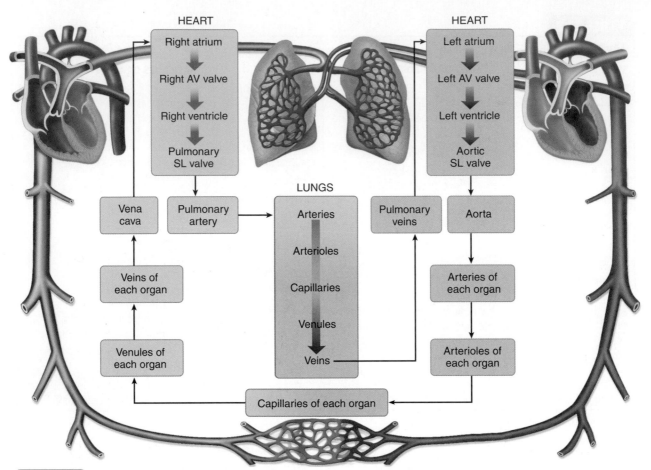

HEART

Right atrium

Right AV valve

Right ventricle

Pulmonary SL valve

FIGURE 12-13 Diagram of blood flow in the cardiovascular system. Blood leaves the heart through arteries and then travels through arterioles, capillaries, venules, and veins before returning to the opposite side of the heart. Compare this figure with Figure 12-4.

the liver capillary beds, it returns to the systemic blood pathway returning to the right atrium of the heart.

The detour of venous blood through a second capillary bed in the liver before its return to the heart serves some valuable purposes. For example, when nutrients from a meal are being absorbed, the blood in the portal vein contains a higher-than-normal concentration of glucose. Recall from Chapter 10 (Figure 10-4, p. 230) that such high glucose levels trigger the secretion of insulin from pancreatic islets. Influenced by insulin, liver cells remove the excess glucose and store it as glycogen. Therefore blood leaving the liver usually has a somewhat normal blood glucose concentration. Liver cells also remove and detoxify various poisonous substances that may be present in the blood. The hepatic portal system is an excellent

example of how "structure follows function" in helping the body maintain homeostasis.

Fetal Circulation

Circulation in the body before birth differs from circulation after birth because the fetus must secure oxygen and nutrients from maternal blood instead of from its own lungs and digestive organs.

For the exchange of nutrients and oxygen to occur between fetal and maternal blood, specialized blood vessels must carry the fetal blood to the **placenta** (plah-SEN-tah), where the exchange occurs, and then return it to the fetal body. Three vessels (shown in Figure 12-15 as part of the **umbilical cord**) accomplish this purpose. They are the two small **umbilical arteries** and a single, much larger **umbilical vein.** The movement of

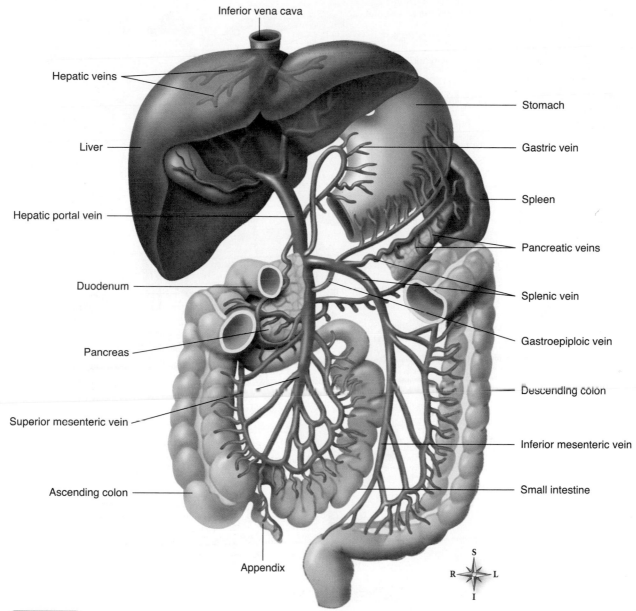

FIGURE 12-14 **Hepatic portal circulation.** In this very unusual circulation, a vein is located between two capillary beds. The hepatic portal vein collects blood from capillaries in visceral structures located in the abdomen and empties it into the liver. Hepatic veins return blood to the inferior vena cava. (Organs are not drawn to scale here.)

blood in the umbilical vessels may seem unusual at first in that the umbilical vein carries oxygenated blood, and the umbilical artery carries oxygen-poor blood. Remember that arteries are vessels that carry blood away from the heart, whereas veins carry blood toward the heart, regardless of the oxygen content these vessels may have.

Another structure unique to fetal circulation is called the **ductus venosus** (DUK-tus veh-NOH-sus). As you can see in Figure 12-15, it is actually a continuation of the umbilical vein. It serves as a shunt, allowing most of the blood returning from the placenta to bypass the immature liver of the developing fetus and empty directly into the inferior vena cava.

Two other structures in the developing fetus allow most of the blood to bypass the developing lungs, which remain collapsed until birth. The

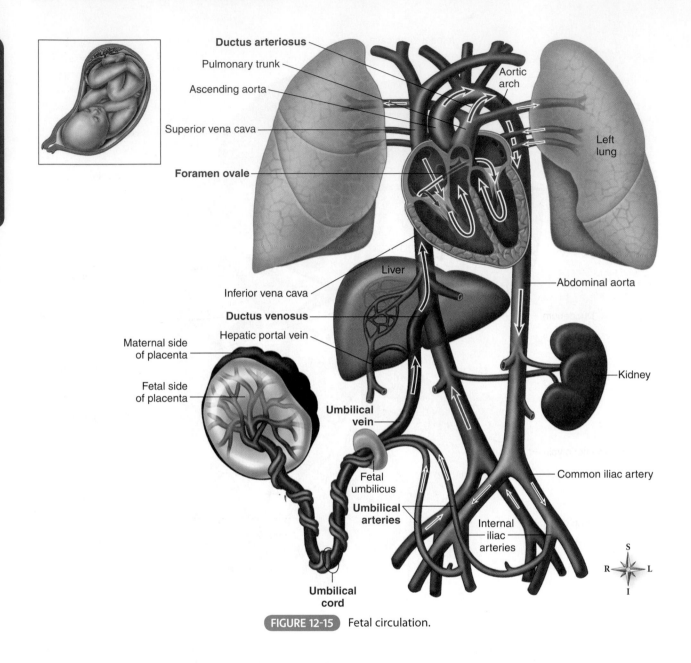

FIGURE 12-15 Fetal circulation.

foramen ovale (foh-RAY-men oh-VAL-ee) shunts blood from the right atrium directly into the left atrium, and the **ductus arteriosus** (DUK-tus ar-teer-ee-OH-sus) connects the aorta and the pulmonary artery.

At birth, the baby's specialized fetal blood vessels and shunts must be rendered nonfunctional. When the newborn infant takes its first deep breaths, the cardiovascular system is subjected to increased pressure. The result is closure of the fo-ramen ovale and rapid collapse of the umbilical blood vessels, the ductus venosus, and ductus arteriosus.

✓ **QUICK CHECK**

1. How do systemic and pulmonary circulations differ?
2. What is the hepatic portal circulation?
3. How is fetal circulation different from adult circulation?

BLOOD PRESSURE

Defining Blood Pressure

A good way to explain blood pressure might be to first answer a few questions about it. What is blood pressure? Just what the words indicate— blood pressure is the pressure or "push" of blood as it flows through the cardiovascular system.

Where does blood pressure exist? It exists in all blood vessels, but it is highest in the arteries and lowest in the veins. In fact, if we list blood vessels in order according to the amount of blood pressure in them and draw a graph, as in Figure 12-16, the graph looks like a hill, with aortic blood pressure at the top and vena caval pressure at the bottom. This blood pressure "hill" is spoken of as the **blood pressure gradient.**

More precisely, the blood pressure gradient is the difference between two blood pressures. The blood pressure gradient for the entire systemic circulation is the difference between the average or mean blood pressure in the aorta and the blood pressure at the termination of the venae cavae where they join the right atrium of the heart. The mean blood pressure in the aorta, given in Figure 12-16, is 100 millimeters of mercury (mm Hg), and the pressure at the termination of the venae cavae is 0. Therefore, with these typical normal figures, the systemic blood pressure gradient is 100 mm Hg (100 minus 0).

Why is it important to understand how blood pressure functions? The blood pressure gradient is vitally involved in keeping the blood flowing. When a blood pressure gradient is present, blood circulates; conversely, when a blood pressure

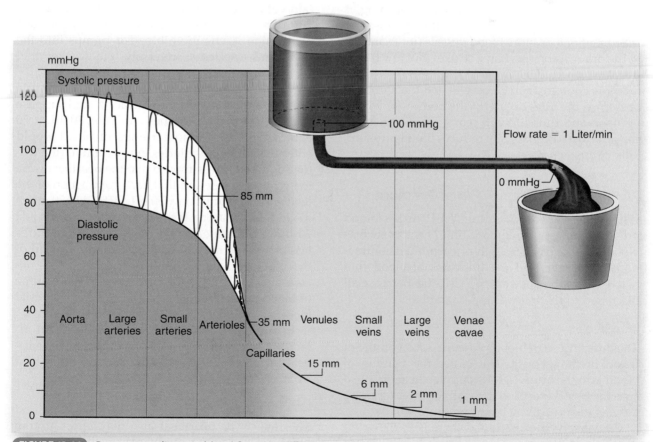

FIGURE 12-16   **Pressure gradients in blood flow.** Blood flows down a "blood pressure hill" from arteries, where blood pressure is highest, into arterioles, where it is somewhat lower, into capillaries, where it is still lower, and so on. All numbers on the graph indicate blood pressure measured in millimeters of mercury (mm Hg). The broken line, starting at 100 mm Hg, represents the average pressure in each part of the cardiovascular system

gradient is not present, blood does not circulate. For example, suppose that the blood pressure in the arteries were to decrease to a point at which it became equal to the average pressure in arterioles. The result would be that there would be no blood pressure gradient between arteries and arterioles, and therefore no force would be available to move blood out of arteries into arterioles. Circulation would stop, in other words, and very soon life itself would cease. That is why when arterial blood pressure is observed to be falling rapidly, whether during surgery or in some other circumstance, emergency measures must be started quickly to try to reverse this fatal trend.

What we have just said may start you wondering about why high blood pressure (meaning, of course, high arterial blood pressure) and low blood pressure are bad for circulation. High blood pressure, or **hypertension** (hye-per-TEN-shun) **(HTN),** is bad for several reasons. For one thing, if blood pressure becomes too high, it may cause the rupture of one or more blood vessels (for example, in the brain, as happens in a stroke). But low blood pressure can be dangerous too. If arterial pressure falls low enough, then blood will not flow through, or *perfuse*, the vital organs of the body. Circulation of blood and thus life will cease. Massive hemorrhage, which dramatically reduces blood pressure, kills in this way.

Factors That Influence Blood Pressure

What causes blood pressure? What makes blood pressure change from time to time? Factors such as blood volume, the strength of each heart contraction, heart rate, and the thickness of blood that help explain the answers to these questions are all discussed in the following paragraphs.

Blood Volume

The direct cause of blood pressure is the volume of blood in the vessels. The larger the volume of blood is in the arteries, for example, the more pressure the blood exerts on the walls of the arteries, or the higher the arterial blood pressure will be.

Conversely, the less blood there is in the arteries, the lower the blood pressure tends to be. Hemorrhage demonstrates this relationship between blood volume and blood pressure. Hemorrhage is a pronounced loss of blood, and this decrease in the volume of blood causes blood pressure to drop. In fact, the major sign of hemorrhage is a rapidly falling blood pressure. Another example is the fact that *diuretics*—drugs that promote water loss by increasing urine output—are often used to treat hypertension (high blood pressure). As water is lost from the body, blood volume decreases, and thus blood pressure decreases to a lower level.

The volume of blood in the arteries is determined by how much blood the heart pumps into the arteries and how much blood the arterioles drain out of them. The diameter of the arterioles plays an important role in determining how much blood drains out of arteries into arterioles.

Strength of Heart Contractions

The strength and the rate of the heartbeat affect cardiac output and therefore blood pressure. Each time the left ventricle contracts, it squeezes a certain volume of blood (the stroke volume) into the aorta and into other arteries. The stronger each contraction is, the more blood it pumps into the aorta and arteries. Conversely, the weaker that each contraction is, the less blood it pumps.

Suppose that one contraction of the left ventricle pumps 70 mL of blood into the aorta, and suppose that the heart beats 70 times a minute; 70 mL $\times$ 70 equals 4900 mL. Almost 5 liters of blood would enter the aorta and arteries every minute (the cardiac output). Now suppose that the heartbeat were to become weaker and that each contraction of the left ventricle pumps only 50 mL instead of 70 mL of blood into the aorta. If the heart still contracts just 70 times a minute, it will obviously pump much less blood into the aorta—only 3500 mL instead of the more normal 4900 mL per minute. This decrease in the heart's output decreases the volume of blood in the arteries, and the decreased arterial blood volume decreases arterial blood pressure.

In summary, the strength of the heartbeat affects blood pressure in this way: a stronger heartbeat increases blood pressure, and a weaker beat decreases it.

Heart Rate

The rate of the heartbeat also may affect arterial blood pressure. You might reason that when the heart beats faster, more blood enters the aorta, and therefore the arterial blood volume and blood pressure would increase.

This is true only if the stroke volume does not decrease sharply when the heart rate increases. Often, however, when the heart beats faster, each contraction of the left ventricle takes place so rapidly that it has little time to fill with blood and therefore squeezes out much less blood than usual into the aorta.

For example, suppose that the heart rate speeded up from 70 to 100 times per minute and that, at the same time, its stroke volume decreased from 70 mL to 40 mL. Instead of a cardiac output of 70 × 70 or 4900 mL per minute, the cardiac output would have changed to 100 × 40 or 4000 mL per minute. Arterial blood volume decreases under these conditions, and therefore blood pressure also decreases, even though the heart rate has increased.

What generalization, then, can we make? We can say only that an increase in the rate of the heartbeat increases blood pressure, and a decrease in the rate decreases blood pressure. But whether a change in the heart rate actually produces a similar change in blood pressure depends on whether the stroke volume also changes and in which direction.

Blood Viscosity

Another factor that needs to be mentioned in connection with blood pressure is the viscosity of blood, or in plainer language, its thickness. If blood becomes less viscous than normal, blood pressure decreases. For example, if a person suffers a hemorrhage, fluid moves into the blood from the interstitial fluid. This dilutes the blood and decreases its viscosity, and blood pressure then falls because of the decreased viscosity. After hemorrhage, transfusion of whole blood or plasma is preferred to infusion of saline solution. The reason is that saline solution is not a viscous liquid and so cannot keep blood pressure at a normal level.

In a condition called *polycythemia*, the number of red blood cells increases beyond normal and thus increases blood viscosity. This in turn increases blood pressure. Polycythemia can occur when oxygen levels in the air decrease and the body attempts to increase its ability to attract oxygen to the blood, as happens in working at high altitudes.

Resistance to Blood Flow

A factor that has a huge impact on local blood pressure gradients, and thus on blood flow, is any factor that changes the resistance to blood flow. The term **peripheral** (peh-RIF-er-al) **resistance** describes any force that acts against the flow of blood in a blood vessel. Viscosity of blood, for example, affects peripheral resistance by influencing the ease with which blood flows through blood vessels.

Another factor that affects peripheral resistance is the tension in muscles of the blood vessel wall (Figure 12-17). When these muscles are relaxed,

Decreased resistance

(diameter = 2)

Smooth muscle relaxation

Smooth muscle cell

(diameter = 1)

Normal resting tone

Increased resistance

(diameter = 1/2)

Smooth muscle contraction

FIGURE 12-17   Vasomotor mechanism. Changes in smooth muscle tension in the wall of an arteriole influence the resistance of the vessel to blood flow. Relaxation of muscle results in decreased resistance; contraction of muscle results in increased resistance.

resistance is low and therefore blood pressure is low—thus blood may flow easily down its pressure gradient and into the vessel. When vessel wall muscles are contracted, however, resistance increases and therefore so does the blood pressure—thus the pressure gradient is reduced and blood will not flow so easily into the vessel. Such adjustment of muscle tension in vessel walls to control blood pressure, and therefore blood flow, is often called the **vasomotor mechanism** (vay-soh-MOH-tor MEK-ah-niz-em).

Fluctuations in Blood Pressure

No one's blood pressure stays the same all the time. It fluctuates, even in a perfectly healthy individual. For example, it goes up when a person exercises strenuously. Not only is this normal, but the increased blood pressure serves a good purpose. It increases circulation to bring more blood to muscles each minute and thus supplies them with more oxygen and food for more energy.

A normal arterial blood pressure is below 120/80, or 120 mm Hg systolic pressure (as the ventricles contract) and 80 mm Hg diastolic pressure (as the ventricles relax). Remember, however, that what is "normal" varies somewhat among individuals and also varies with age.

The venous blood pressure, as you can see in Figure 12-16, is very low in the large veins and falls almost to 0 by the time blood leaves the venae cavae and enters the right atrium. The venous blood pressure within the right atrium is called the **central venous pressure.** This pressure level is important because it influences the pressure that exists in the large peripheral veins. If the heart beats strongly, the central venous pressure is low as blood enters and leaves the heart chambers efficiently. However, if the heart is weakened, central venous pressure increases, and the flow of

---

Clinical Application

Blood Pressure Readings

A device called a **sphygmomanometer** (sfig-moh-mah-NAH-meh-ter) is often used to measure blood pressures in both clinical and home health care situations. The traditional sphygmomanometer is an inverted tube of mercury (Hg) with a balloonlike air cuff attached via an air hose. The air cuff is placed around a limb, usually the subject's upper arm as shown in the figure. A stethoscope sensor is placed over a major artery (the *brachial artery* in the figure) to listen for the arterial pulse. A hand-operated pump fills the air cuff, increasing the air pressure and pushing the column of mercury higher. While listening through the stethoscope, the operator opens the air cuff's outlet valve and slowly reduces the air pressure around the limb. Loud, tapping *Korotkoff sounds* suddenly begin when the cuff pressure measured by the mercury column equals the **systolic pressure**—often below 120 mm Hg. As the air pressure surrounding the arm continues to decrease, the Korotkoff sounds disappear. The pressure measurement at which the sounds disappear is equal to the **diastolic pressure**—often 70 to 80 mm Hg. The subject's blood pressure is then expressed as systolic pressure (the maximum arterial pressure during each cardiac cycle) over the diastolic pressure (the minimum arterial pressure), such as 120/80 (read "one-twenty over eighty"). The final reading can then be compared with the expected value, which is based on the patient's age and various other indi-vidual factors. Mercury sphygmomanometers have been replaced in many clinical settings by nonmercury devices that similarly measure the maximum and minimum arterial blood pressures. In home health care settings, patients are often taught how to monitor their own blood pressure.

blood into the right atrium is slowed. As a result, a person suffering heart failure, who is sitting at rest in a chair, often has distended external jugular veins as blood "backs up" in the venous network.

Five mechanisms help keep venous blood moving back through the cardiovascular circuit and into the right atrium. They are the following:

1. Continued beating of the heart, which pumps blood through the entire cardiovascular system
2. Adequate blood pressure in the arteries, to push blood to and through the veins
3. Semilunar valves in the veins that ensure continued blood flow in one direction (toward the heart)
4. Contraction of skeletal muscles, which squeeze veins, producing a kind of pumping action
5. Changing pressures in the chest cavity during breathing that produce a kind of pumping action in the veins in the thorax

PULSE

What you feel when you take a **pulse** is an artery expanding and then recoiling alternately. To feel a pulse, you must place your fingertips over an artery that lies near the surface of the body and over a bone or other firm base. The pulse is a valuable clinical sign. It can provide information, for example, about the rate, strength, and rhythmicity of the heartbeat. It is also easily determined with little or no danger or discomfort. The nine major "pulse points" are named after the arteries over which they are felt. Locate each pulse point on Figure 12-18 and on your own body.

Three pulse points are located on each side of the head and neck: (1) over the superficial temporal artery in front of the ear, (2) the common carotid artery in the neck along the front edge of the sternocleidomastoid muscle, and (3) over the facial artery at the lower margin of the mandible at a point below the corner of the mouth.

A pulse is also detected at three points in the upper limb: (1) in the axilla over the axillary artery, (2) over the brachial artery at the bend of the elbow along the inner or medial margin of the biceps brachii muscle, and (3) at the radial artery at the wrist. The so-called radial pulse is the most

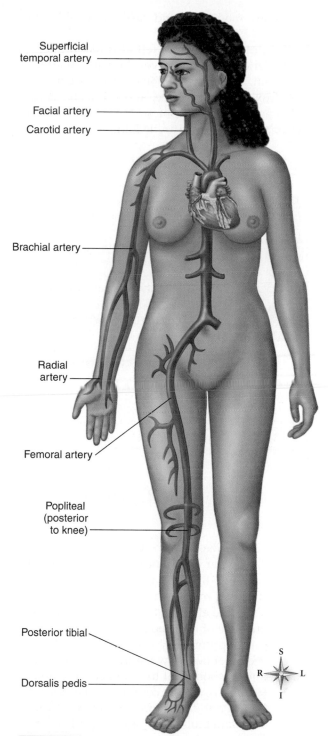

FIGURE 12-18   Pulse points. Each pulse point is named after the artery with which it is associated.

frequently monitored and easily accessible in the body.

The pulse also can be felt at three locations in the lower extremity: (1) over the femoral artery in the groin, (2) at the popliteal artery behind and just proximal to the knee, and (3) at the dorsalis pedis artery on the front surface of the foot, just below the bend of the ankle joint.

> ✓ **QUICK CHECK**
>
> 1. How does the blood pressure gradient explain blood flow?
> 2. Name four factors that influence blood pressure.
> 3. Does a person's blood pressure stay the same all the time?
> 4. Where are the places on your body that you can likely feel your pulse?

Science Application

Cardiology
Willem Einthoven (1860–1927)

Cardiology, the study and treatment of the heart, owes much to Dutch physiologist Willem Einthoven and his invention of the modern electrocardiograph in 1903. Einthoven's first major contribution was the invention of a machine that could record electrocardiograms (ECGs) with far greater sensitivity than the crude machines of the nineteenth century. Then, with the help of British physician Lewis Thomas, Einthoven demonstrated and named the P, Q, R, S, and T waves and proved that these waves precisely record the electrical activity of the heart (see Figure 12-7). In 1905, he even invented a way that ECG data could be sent from a patient over the telephone to his laboratory where they could be recorded and analyzed—a technique now called *telemetry*. His detailed studies of ECG recordings changed the practice of heart medicine forever. In fact, his invention was later applied to the study of nerve impulses and led to breakthrough discoveries in the neurosciences.

Cardiologists today still use modern versions of Einthoven's machine to diagnose heart disorders. Of course, biomedical engineers continue to develop refinements to electrocardiograph equipment and to invent new machines to monitor heart function. In fact, engineers and designers have worked with cardiologists to develop artificial heart valves, artificial pacemakers, and even artificial hearts. Along with all of this medical equipment being used in cardiology, and medicine in general, are many technicians working to keep it all in good repair.

OUTLINE SUMMARY

HEART
A. Location, size, and position
1. Triangular organ located in mediastinum with two thirds of the mass to the left of the body midline and one third to the right; the apex on the diaphragm; shape and size of a closed fist (see Figure 12-1)
2. Cardiopulmonary resuscitation (CPR) — the heart lies between the sternum in front and the bodies of the thoracic vertebrae behind; rhythmic compression of the heart between the sternum and vertebrae can maintain blood flow during cardiac arrest; if combined with artificial respiration procedure, it can be lifesaving

B. Anatomy
1. Heart chambers (see Figure 12-2)
   a. Two upper chambers called *atria* (receiving chambers) — right and left atria
   b. Two lower chambers called *ventricles* (discharging chambers) — right and left ventricles
   c. Wall of each heart chamber is composed of cardiac muscle tissue called *myocardium*
   d. Endocardium — smooth lining of heart chambers — inflammation of endocardium called *endocarditis*
2. Covering sac, or pericardium
   a. Pericardium is a two-layered fibrous sac with a lubricated space between the two layers
   b. Inner layer called *visceral pericardium* or *epicardium*
   c. Outer layer called *parietal pericardium*
3. Heart action
   a. Contraction of the heart is called *systole*
   b. Relaxation is called *diastole*

4. Heart valves (see Figure 12-3)
   a. Valves keep blood flowing through the heart and prevent backflow
   b. Consist of two atrioventricular (AV) and two semilunar (SL) valves
      (1) Tricuspid — at the opening of the right atrium into the ventricle
      (2) Bicuspid (mitral) — at the opening of the left atrium into the ventricle
      (3) Pulmonary semilunar — at the beginning of the pulmonary artery
      (4) Aortic semilunar — at the beginning of the aorta

C. Heart sounds
   1. Two distinct heart sounds in every heartbeat or cycle — "lub dup"
   2. First sound (lub) is caused by the vibration and closure of AV valves during contraction of the ventricles
   3. Second sound (dub) is caused by the closure of the semilunar valves during relaxation of the ventricles

D. Blood flow through the heart (see Figure 12-4)
   1. The heart acts as two separate pumps — the right atrium and right ventricle performing different functions from the left atrium and left ventricle
   2. Sequence of blood flow: venous blood enters the right atrium through the superior and inferior venae cavae — passes from the right atrium through the tricuspid valve to the right ventricle; from the right ventricle it passes through the pulmonary semilunar valve to the pulmonary artery to the lungs — blood moves from the lungs to the left atrium, passing through the bicuspid (mitral) valve to the left ventricle; blood in the left ventricle is pumped through the aortic semilunar valve into the aorta and is distributed to the body as a whole

E. Blood supply to the heart muscle
   1. Blood, which supplies oxygen and nutrients to the myocardium of the heart, flows through the right and left coronary arteries (see Figure 12-5); called *coronary circulation*
   2. Blockage of blood flow through the coronary arteries is called *myocardial infarction (heart attack)*
   3. Angina pectoris — chest pain caused by inadequate oxygen to the heart

4. Coronary bypass surgery — veins from other parts of the body are used to bypass blockages in coronary arteries (see Figure 12-6)

F. Cardiac cycle
   1. Heartbeat is regular and rhythmic — each complete beat is called a *cardiac cycle* — average is about 72 beats per minute
   2. Each cycle, about 0.8 seconds long, is subdivided into systole (contraction phase) and diastole (relaxation phase)
   3. Stroke volume — volume of blood ejected from one ventricle with each beat
   4. Cardiac output — amount of blood that one ventricle can pump each minute; average is about 5 liters per minute at rest

G. Conduction system of the heart (see Figure 12-7)
   1. Intercalated disks are electrical connectors that join all the cardiac muscle fibers in a region together so that they receive their impulse, and thus contract, at about the same time
   2. Specialized conduction system structures generate and transmit the electrical impulses that result in contraction of the heart
      a. SA (sinoatrial) node, the pacemaker — located in the wall of the right atrium near the opening of the superior vena cava
      b. AV (atrioventricular) node — located in the right atrium along the lower part of the interatrial septum
      c. AV bundle (bundle of His) — located in the septum of the ventricle
      d. Purkinje fibers — located in the walls of the ventricles

H. Electrocardiogram (see Figure 12-8)
   1. The tiny electrical impulses traveling through the heart's conduction system can be picked up on the surface of the body and transformed into visible tracings by a machine called an *electrocardiograph*
   2. The visible tracing of these electrical signals is called an *electrocardiogram*, or *ECG*
   3. The normal ECG has three deflections or waves
      a. P wave — associated with depolarization of the atria

b. QRS complex — associated with depolarization of the ventricles

c. T wave — associated with repolarization of the ventricles

BLOOD VESSELS

A. Types
 1. Arteries — carry blood away from the heart and toward capillaries
 2. Veins — carry blood toward the heart and away from veins
 3. Capillaries — carry blood from the arterioles to the venules

B. Structure (see Figure 12-9)
 1. Arteries
    a. Tunica intima — inner layer of endothelial cells
    b. Tunica media — smooth muscle with some elastic tissue, thick in arteries; important in blood pressure regulation
    c. Tunica externa — thin layer of fibrous elastic connective tissue
 2. Capillaries — microscopic vessels with only one layer — tunica intima
 3. Veins
    a. Tunica intima — inner layer; valves prevent retrograde movement of blood
    b. Tunica media — smooth muscle; thin in veins
    c. Tunica externa — heavy layer of fibrous connective tissue in many veins

C. Functions
 1. Arteries — distribution of nutrients, gases, etc., with movement of blood under high pressure; assist in maintaining the arterial blood pressure
 2. Capillaries — serve as exchange vessels for nutrients, wastes, and fluids
 3. Veins — collect blood for return to the heart; low pressure vessels

D. Names of main arteries — see Figure 12-11 and Table 12-1

E. Names of main veins — see Figure 12-12 and Table 12-2

CIRCULATION OF BLOOD

A. Systemic and pulmonary circulation
 1. Blood circulation — refers to the flow of blood through all the vessels, which are arranged forming a complete circuit or circular pattern (see Figure 12-13)
 2. Systemic circulation
    a. Carries blood throughout the body
    b. Path goes from left ventricle through aorta, smaller arteries, arterioles, capillaries, venules, venae cavae, to right atrium
 3. Pulmonary circulation
    a. Carries blood to and from the lungs
    b. Arteries deliver deoxygenated blood to the lungs for gas exchange
    c. Path goes from right ventricle through pulmonary arteries, lungs, pulmonary veins, to left atrium

B. Special circulatory plans
 1. Hepatic portal circulation (see Figure 12-14)
    a. Unique blood route through the liver
    b. Vein (hepatic portal vein) exists between two capillary beds
    c. Assists with homeostasis of blood glucose levels
 2. Fetal circulation (see Figure 12-15)
    a. Refers to circulation before birth
    b. Modifications required for fetus to efficiently secure oxygen and nutrients from the maternal blood
    c. Unique structures include the placenta, umbilical arteries and vein, ductus venosus, ductus arteriosus, and foramen ovale

BLOOD PRESSURE

A. Defining blood pressure — push, or force, of blood in the blood vessels
 1. Highest in arteries, lowest in veins (see Figure 12-16)
 2. Blood pressure gradient causes blood to circulate — liquids can flow only from the area where pressure is higher to where it is lower

B. Factors that influence blood pressure
 1. Blood volume — the larger the volume, the more pressure is exerted on vessel walls
 2. Strength of heart contractions — affect cardiac output; stronger heartbeat increases pressure; weaker beat decreases it
 3. Heart rate — increased rate increases pressure; decreased rate decreases pressure

4. Blood viscosity (thickness) — less-than-normal viscosity decreases pressure, more-than-normal viscosity increases pressure
5. Resistance to blood flow (peripheral resistance) — affected by many factors, including the vasomotor mechanism (vessel muscle contraction/relaxation) (see Figure 12-17)

C. Fluctuations in blood pressure
   1. Blood pressure varies within normal range
   2. Normal average arterial blood pressure is 120/80
   3. Venous blood pressure within right atrium called *central venous pressure*

4. Venous return of blood to the heart depends on five mechanisms:
   a. A strongly beating heart
   b. An adequate arterial blood pressure
   c. Valves in the veins
   d. Pumping action of skeletal muscles as they contract
   e. Changing pressures in the chest cavity caused by breathing

PULSE

A. Definition — alternate expansion and recoil of the blood vessel wall
B. Nine major "pulse points" named after arteries over which they are felt (see Figure 12-18)

NEW WORDS

angina pectoris
aorta
apex
arteriole
artery
atrioventricular (AV) bundle (of His)
atrioventricular (AV) node
atrioventricular (AV) valve
atrium (pl. atria)
bicuspid valve (mitral valve)
blood pressure gradient
capillary
cardiac cycle
cardiac output
cardiac vein
cardiopulmonary resuscitation (CPR)
cardiovascular system

central venous pressure
chordae tendineae
coronary artery
coronary bypass surgery
coronary circulation
coronary sinus
depolarization
diastole
diastolic pressure
ductus arteriosus
ductus venosus
electrocardiogram (ECG or EKG)
electrocardiograph
embolism
endocarditis
endocardium
endothelium
epicardium (visceral pericardium)
foramen ovale

hepatic portal circulation
hypertension (HTN)
mitral valve
myocardial infarction (MI)
myocardium
P wave
pericarditis
pericardium (parietal and visceral)
peripheral resistance
placenta
precapillary sphincter
pulmonary artery
pulmonary circulation
pulmonary vein
pulse
Purkinje fiber
QRS complex
repolarization
semilunar (SL) valve

sinoatrial node (pacemaker)
sphygmomanometer
stroke volume
systemic circulation
systole
systolic pressure
T wave
thrombus
tricuspid valve
tunica externa
tunica intima
tunica media
umbilical artery
umbilical cord
umbilical vein
vasomotor mechanism
vein
vena cava (superior and inferior)
ventricle
venule

REVIEW QUESTIONS

1. Describe the heart and its position in the body.
2. Name the four chambers of the heart.
3. What is the myocardium? What is the endocardium?
4. Describe the two layers of the pericardium. What is the function of pericardial fluid?
5. Define *systole* and *diastole*.
6. Name and give the location of the four heart valves.
7. Trace the flow of blood from the superior vena cava to the aorta.
8. What is angina pectoris?
9. Differentiate between stroke volume and cardiac output.
10. Trace the path and name the structures involved in the conduction system of the heart.
11. Name and describe the main types of blood vessels in the body.
12. Name the three tissue layers that make up arteries and veins.
13. Describe systemic circulation and pulmonary circulation.
14. Name and briefly explain the four factors that influence blood pressure.
15. List the five mechanisms that keep the venous blood moving toward the right atrium.
16. Name four locations in the body where the pulse can be felt.

CRITICAL THINKING

17. Explain how the traces on an ECG relate to what is occurring in the heart.
18. Explain hepatic portal circulation. How is it different from typical systemic circulation, and what advantages are gained from this type of circulation?
19. Explain the differences between normal postnatal circulation and fetal circulation. Based on the environment of the fetus, explain how these differences make fetal circulation more efficient.
20. Explain why a pressure difference must exist between the aorta and the right atrium.

CHAPTER TEST

1. _____ are the thicker chambers of the heart, which are sometimes called the *discharging chambers.*
2. The _____ are the thinner chambers of the heart, which are sometimes called the *receiving chambers* of the heart.
3. Cardiac muscle tissue is called _____.
4. The ventricles of the heart are separated into right and left sides by the _____.
5. The thin layer of tissue lining the interior of the heart chambers is called the _____.
6. Another term for the visceral pericardium is the _____.
7. Contraction of the heart is called _____.
8. Relaxation of the heart is called _____.
9. The heart valve located between the right atrium and right ventricle is called the _____ valve.
10. The term _____ refers to the volume of blood ejected from the ventricle during each beat.
11. The _____ is the pacemaker of the heart and causes the contraction of the atria.
12. The _____ are extensions of the atrioventricular fibers and cause the contraction of the ventricles.
13. The ECG tracing that occurs when the ventricles depolarize is called the _____.
14. The ECG tracing that occurs when the atria depolarize is called the _____.
15. The _____ are the blood vessels that carry blood back to the heart.
16. The _____ are the blood vessels that carry blood away from the heart.
17. The _____ are the microscopic blood vessels in which substances are exchanged between the blood and tissues.

18. The innermost layer of tissue in an artery is called the _____.
19. The outermost layer of tissue in an artery is called the _____.
20. Systemic circulation involves the moving of blood throughout the body; _____ involves moving blood from the heart to the lungs and back.
21. The two structures in the developing fetus that allow most of the blood to bypass the lungs are the _____ and the _____.
22. The strength of the heart contraction and blood volume are two factors that influence blood pressure. Two other factors that influence blood pressure are _____ and _____.
23. Place the following structures in their proper order in blood flow through the heart by putting a 1 in front of the first structure the blood would pass through and ending with a 10 in front of the last structure the blood would pass through.
    a. _____ left atrium
    b. _____ tricuspid valve (right atrioventricular valve)
    c. _____ right ventricle
    d. _____ pulmonary vein
    e. _____ aortic semilunar valve
    f. _____ mitral valve (left atrioventricular valve)
    g. _____ left ventricle
    h. _____ pulmonary artery
    i. _____ right atrium
    j. _____ pulmonary semilunar valve

OBJECTIVES

AFTER YOU HAVE COMPLETED THIS CHAPTER, YOU SHOULD BE ABLE TO:

1. Describe the generalized functions of the lymphatic system and list the primary lymphatic structures.
2. Discuss and compare nonspecific and specific immunity, natural and artificial immunity, and active and passive immunity.
3. Discuss the major types of immune system molecules and indicate how antibodies and complement proteins function.
4. Discuss and contrast the development and functions of B and T cells.
5. Compare and contrast humoral and cell-mediated immunity.

The Lymphatic System and Immunity 13

All of us live in a hostile and dangerous environment. Each day we are faced with potentially harmful toxins, disease-causing bacteria, viruses, and even cells from our own bodies that have been transformed into cancerous invaders. Fortunately, we are protected from this staggering variety of differing biological enemies by a remarkable set of defense mechanisms. We refer to this protective "safety net" as the **immune system.**

This system is characterized by structural components, the lymphatic organs, and by a functional group of defensive cells and molecules that protect us from infection and disease. This chapter begins with an overview of the lymphatic system, discussing vessels that help maintain fluid balance and lymphoid tissues that help defend the internal environment.

We then discuss the basic principles of immunity and the ways that highly specialized cells and molecules provide us with effective and very specific resistance to disease.

THE LYMPHATIC SYSTEM

Lymph and Lymphatic Vessels

Maintaining the constancy of the fluid around each body cell is possible only if numerous homeostatic mechanisms function effectively together in a controlled and integrated response to changing conditions. We know from Chapter 12 that the cardiovascular system plays a key role in bringing many needed substances to cells and then removing the waste products that accumulate as a result of metabolism. This exchange of substances between blood and tissue fluid occurs in capillary beds. Many additional substances that cannot enter or return through the capillary walls, including ex-

STUDY TIPS

To make the study of the lymphatic system and immunity more efficient, we suggest these tips:

1. Before starting Chapter 13, review the synopsis of the lymphatic system in Chapter 4.
2. The lymphatic system is the "drainage" system of the body. Plasma is pushed out of the capillaries and washes over the tissue cells. The fluid carries bacteria and cellular debris into the open-ended capillaries in the lymphatic system. The fluid is then called *lymph*. It is carried to the lymph node, where it is filtered, cleaned, and carried in the ducts back to the blood. Keep this process in mind when you study the structures of the lymphatic system.
3. Several specific organs make up the lymphatic system. Flash cards with their names, locations, and functions will help you learn them.
4. The immune system is divided into nonspecific immunity and specific immunity, according to differences in function. If you keep this division of immune function "styles" in mind, immunity becomes easier to understand.
5. The immune system is divided into nonspecific and specific immunity. Most of the nonspecific immunity is fairly simple; the most complex part is the inflammatory response, so study that well.
6. Specific immunity can be classified as natural or artificial depending on how the body was exposed to the antigen, and active or passive depending on how much work the body had to do to develop the response. The natural, active immune response is divided into two parts also: humoral immunity and cell-mediated immunity. Humoral immunity is mediated by B lymphocytes, or B cells. They stay in the lymph node and secrete antibodies into the blood, a body humor. They also form memory cells for lifelong immunity. T lymphocytes, or T cells, provide the cell-mediated immunity. They leave the lymph node and actively engage the antigen.
7. In your study groups, use flash cards to quiz each other on the terms and structures of the lymphatic and immune systems.

Continued on page 302.

STUDY TIPS—cont'd

8. Discuss the process of how lymph is formed, filtered, and returned to the blood.
9. Discuss nonspecific immunity, especially the inflammatory response.
10. Discuss what type of immunity getting a vaccination or coming down with the disease would be.
11. Discuss the steps in humoral and cell-mediated immunity.
12. Go over the questions in the back of the chapter and discuss possible test questions.

cess fluid and protein molecules, are returned to the blood as **lymph.**

Lymph is a fluid formed in the tissue spaces that is transported by way of **lymphatic vessels** to eventually reenter the bloodstream carried by the cardiovascular system. Thus the lymphatic system is an important partner of the *cardiovascular system*—both vital components of the *circulatory system*.

In addition to lymph and the lymphatic vessels, the lymphatic system includes lymph nodes and specialized lymphatic organs such as the thymus and spleen (Figure 13-1). Such lymphatic organs help to filter the body's fluids, removing harmful particles before they can cause significant damage to other parts of the body.

Lymph forms in this way: blood plasma filters out of the capillaries into the microscopic spaces between tissue cells because of the pressure generated by the pumping action of the heart. There, the liquid is called **interstitial fluid,** or tissue fluid. Much of the interstitial fluid goes back into the blood by the same route it came out (that is, through the capillary membrane). The remainder of the interstitial fluid enters the lymphatic system before it returns to the blood. The fluid, called *lymph* at this point, enters a network of tiny blind-ended tubes distributed in the tissue spaces. These tiny vessels, called **lymphatic capillaries**, permit excess tissue fluid and some other substances such as dissolved protein molecules to leave the tissue spaces. Figure 13-2 shows the role of the lymphatic system in fluid homeostasis.

Lymphatic and blood capillaries are similar in many ways. Both types of vessels are microscopic and both are formed from sheets that consist of a cell layer of simple squamous epithelium called *endothelium* (en-doh-THEE-lee-um). The flattened endothelial cells that form blood capillaries, however, fit tightly together so that large molecules cannot enter or exit from the vessel. The "fit" between endothelial cells forming the lymphatic capillaries is not as tight. As a result, they are more porous and allow larger molecules, including proteins and other substances, as well as the fluid itself, to enter the vessel and eventually return to the general circulation.

The movement of lymph in the lymphatic vessels goes one way only. Unlike blood, lymph does not flow over and over again through vessels that form a circular route. The lymphatic vessels often have a "beaded" appearance, resulting from the presence of valves that assist in maintaining a one-way flow of lymph. These valves, similar to those in veins, sometimes cause lymph to back up behind them and cause swellings that look like beads.

Lymph flowing through the lymphatic capillaries next moves into successively larger and larger vessels sometimes called *lymphatic venules* and *veins*. These lymphatic vessels eventually empty into one of two terminal vessels called the **right lymphatic duct** and the **thoracic duct,** which empty their lymph into the blood in large veins in the neck region.

Lymph from about three fourths of the body eventually drains into the thoracic duct, which is the largest lymphatic vessel in the body. Lymph from the right upper extremity and from the right side of the head, neck, and upper torso flows into the right lymphatic duct (Figure 13-3). Note in Figure 13-1 that the thoracic duct in the abdomen has an enlarged pouchlike structure called **cisterna chyli** (sis-TER-nah KYE-lye), which serves as a temporary holding area for lymph moving toward its point of entry into the veins.

Lymphatic capillaries in the wall of the small intestine are given the special name of **lacteals** (LAK-tee-alz). They transport fats obtained from food to the bloodstream and are discussed further in Chapter 15.

 To learn more about lymph and lymphatic vessels, go to AnimationDirect on your CD-ROM.

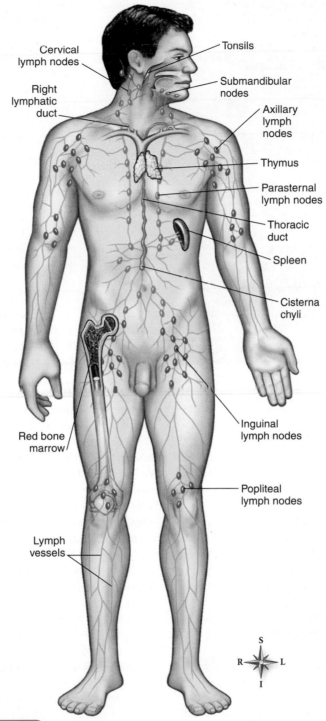

Cervical lymph nodes

Tonsils

Right lymphatic duct

Submandibular nodes

Axillary lymph nodes

Thymus

Parasternal lymph nodes

Thoracic duct

Spleen

Cisterna chyli

Red bone marrow

Inguinal lymph nodes

Popliteal lymph nodes

Lymph vessels

FIGURE 13-1 **The lymphatic system.** Principal organs of the lymphatic system.

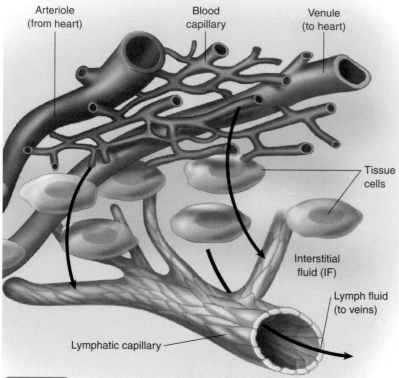

FIGURE 13-2 Role of lymphatic system in fluid homeostasis. Fluid from blood plasma that is not reabsorbed by blood vessels drains into lymphatic vessels. Lymphatic drainage prevents accumulation of too much tissue fluid.

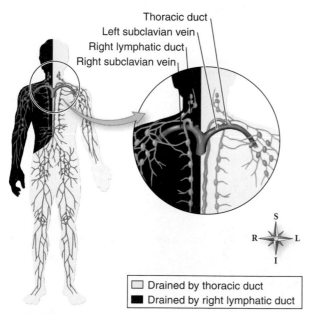

FIGURE 13-3 Lymph drainage. The right lymphatic duct drains lymph from the upper right quarter of the body into the right subclavian vein at its junction with the internal jugular vein. The thoracic duct drains lymph from the rest of the body into the left subclavian vein at its junction with the internal jugular vein.

Lymph Nodes

As lymph moves from its origin in the tissue spaces toward the thoracic or right lymphatic ducts and then into the venous blood, it is filtered by moving through **lymph nodes,** which are located in clusters along the pathway of lymphatic vessels. Some of these nodes may be as small as a pinhead, and others may be as large as a lima bean. With the exception of comparatively few single nodes, most lymph nodes occur in groups or clusters in certain areas (Figures 13-1 and 13-5). Figure 13-1 shows the locations of the clusters of greatest clinical importance. The structure of the lymph nodes makes it possible for them to perform two important immune functions: defense and white blood cell formation.

Lymph nodes are *lymphoid organs* because they contain *lymphoid tissue,* which is a mass of developing lymphocytes and related cells. Lymphoid organs such as lymph nodes, tonsils, thymus, and spleen are important structural components of the immune system because they provide immune defense and development of immune cells.

Defense Function: Biological Filtration

Figure 13-4 shows the structure of a typical lymph node. In this example, a small node located next to an infected hair follicle is shown filtering bacteria from lymph. Lymph nodes perform biological filtration, a process in which cells (phagocytic cells in this case) alter the contents of the filtered fluid. Biological filtration of bacteria and other abnormal cells by phagocytosis prevents local infections from spreading.

Figure 13-4 shows that lymph enters the node through four **afferent** (Latin "to carry toward") **lymphatic vessels.** These vessels deliver lymph to the node. Once lymph enters the node, it "percolates" slowly through spaces called *sinuses* that surround *nodules* found in the outer (cortex) and inner

A

FIGURE 13-4 Lymph node structure and function. A, Structure of a lymph node. B, Inset shows diagrammatic representation of a skin section in which an infection surrounds a hair follicle. The yellow areas represent dead and dying cells (pus). The black dots around the yellow areas represent bacteria. Bacteria entering the node via the afferent lymphatics are filtered out.

B

the node through a single **efferent** (Latin "to carry away from") **lymphatic vessel.**

Clusters of lymph nodes allow a very effective biological filtration of lymph flowing from specific body areas. Figure 13-5 shows an x-ray image called a *lymphangiogram* (lim-FAN-jee-oh-gram). A special dye was injected into the soft tissues that drain the part of the lymphatic network that appears in the image. You can see that the dyed lymph appears in the vessels and nodes of the inguinal and pelvic regions.

Knowledge of lymph node location and function is important in clinical medicine. A surgeon uses knowledge of lymph node function when removing lymph nodes under the arms (axillary nodes) and in other nearby areas during an operation for breast cancer. These nodes may contain cancer cells filtered out of the lymph drained from the breast. Cancer of the breast is one of the most

(medullary) areas of the node (see Figure 13-4). In passing through the node, lymph is filtered so that bacteria, cancer cells, and damaged tissue cells are removed and prevented from entering the blood and circulating all over the body. Lymph exits from

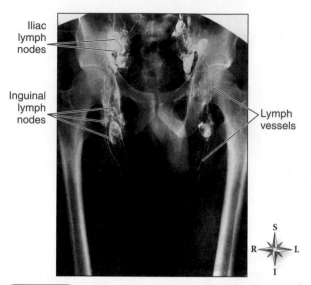

Iliac lymph nodes

Inguinal lymph nodes

Lymph vessels

FIGURE 13-5 **Lymphangiogram.** Dye material was injected into the soft tissues below the area visualized in the x ray.

common forms of this disease in women. Unfortunately, cancer cells from a single tumorous growth in the breast often spread to other areas of the body through the lymphatic system. Figure 13-6 shows how lymph from the breast drains into many different and widely placed nodes.

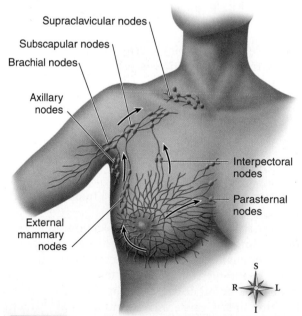

Supraclavicular nodes

Subscapular nodes

Brachial nodes

Axillary nodes

Interpectoral nodes

Parasternal nodes

External mammary nodes

FIGURE 13-6 **Lymphatic drainage of the breast.** Note the extensive network of nodes that receive lymph from the breast.

Health and Well-Being

Effects of Exercise on Immunity

Exercise physiologists have found that moderate exercise increases the number of white blood cells (WBCs), specifically granular leukocytes and lymphocytes. Not only is the number of circulating immune cells higher after exercise, but the activity of sensitized T cells is also increased. But at the same time, research also shows that strenuous exercise may actually inhibit immune function. Nevertheless, moderate exercise such as walking, when engaged in immediately after a trauma such as surgery, is often encouraged because of its immunity-strengthening effects.

To learn more about lymph nodes, go to AnimationDirect on your CD-ROM.

Thymus

As you can see in Figure 13-1, the **thymus** (THY-muss) is a small lymphoid tissue organ located in the mediastinum, extending upward in the midline of the neck. It is composed of lymphocytes in a meshlike framework. The thymus, also called the *thymus gland,* is largest at puberty and even then weighs only about 35 or 40 grams—a little more than an ounce.

Although small in size, the thymus plays a central and critical role in the body's vital immunity mechanism. First, it is a source of lymphocytes before birth and is then especially important in the "maturation," or development, of a type of lymphocyte that then leaves the thymus and circulates to the spleen, tonsils, lymph nodes, and other lymphoid tissues. These **T lymphocytes,** or **T cells,** are critical to the functioning of the immune system and are discussed later. A group of hormones secreted by the thymus called **thymosins** (THY-moh-sinz) influences the development of T cells.

The thymus appears to complete much of its work early in childhood, reaching its maximum size at puberty. The thymus tissue is then gradually replaced by fat and connective tissue, a process called *involution.* By age 60, the thymus is about half its maximum size and is virtually gone by age 80 or so.

Tonsils

Masses of lymphoid tissue called *tonsils* are located in a protective ring under the mucous membranes in the mouth and back of the throat (Figure 13-7). They help protect against bacteria that may invade tissues in the area around the openings between the nasal and oral cavities. The **palatine**

tonsils are located on each side of the throat. The **pharyngeal tonsils,** known as **adenoids** (AD-ch noydz) when they become swollen, are near the posterior opening of the nasal cavity. A third type of tonsil, the **lingual tonsils,** is near the base of the tongue. The tonsils serve as the first line of defense from the exterior and as such are subject to chronic infection. In rare cases, they may be removed surgically if antibiotic therapy is not successful at treating the chronic infection or if swelling impairs breathing.

Spleen

The **spleen** is the largest lymphoid organ in the body. It is located high in the upper left quadrant of the abdomen lateral to the stomach (see Figures 13-1 and 1-6). Although the spleen is protected by the lower ribs, it can be injured by abdominal trauma. The spleen has a very rich blood supply and may contain more than 500 mL (about 1 pint) of blood. If the spleen is damaged and bleeding, surgical removal, called a **splenectomy** (spleh-NEK-toh-mee), may be required to stop the loss of blood.

After entering the spleen, blood flows through dense, pulplike accumulations of lymphocytes. As blood flows through the pulp, the spleen removes by filtration and phagocytosis many bacteria and other foreign substances, destroys worn out red blood cells and salvages the iron found in hemoglobin for future use, and serves as a reservoir for

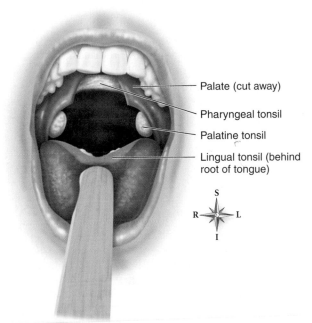

Palate (cut away)

Pharyngeal tonsil

Palatine tonsil

Lingual tonsil (behind root of tongue)

S
R —⊛— L
I

FIGURE 13-7   **Location of the tonsils.** Small segments of the roof and floor of the mouth have been removed to show the protective ring of tonsils (lymphoid tissue) around the internal opening of the nose and throat.

Clinical Application

Allergy

The term **allergy** is used to describe hypersensitivity of the immune system to relatively harmless environmental antigens. One in six Americans has a genetic predisposition to an allergy. Immediate allergic responses involve antigen-antibody reactions that trigger the release of histamine, kinins, and other inflammatory substances. These responses usually cause symptoms such as a runny nose, conjunctivitis, and hives. In some cases, these substances may cause constriction of airways, relaxation of blood vessels, and irregular heart rhythms that can lead to a life-threatening condition called **anaphylactic** (an-ah-fih-LAK-tik) **shock.** Delayed allergic responses, on the other hand, involve cell-mediated immunity. In contact dermatitis, for example, T-lymphocytes trigger events that lead to local skin inflammation a few hours or even days after initial exposure.

blood that can be returned to the cardiovascular system when needed.

 To learn more about the spleen, go to AnimationDirect on your CD-ROM.

✓ **QUICK CHECK**

1. How does the lymphatic system return fluid to the blood?
2. What is the role of lymph nodes in the body?
3. Why is the thymus important for immunity?

THE IMMUNE SYSTEM

Function of the Immune System

The body's defense mechanisms protect us from disease-causing microorganisms that invade our bodies, from foreign tissue cells that may have been transplanted into our bodies, and from our own cells when they have turned malignant or cancerous. The body's overall defense system is called the *immune system*. The immune system makes us immune—that is, able to resist these threats to our health and survival.

In the lymphatic system, we have seen many organs that provide defense: lymph nodes, tonsils, thymus, and spleen. The immune system is not simply a small group of organs working together. Instead, it is an interactive network of many organs and billions of freely moving cells and trillions of free-floating molecules in many different areas of the body.

Nonspecific Immunity

Nonspecific immunity is maintained by mechanisms that attack any irritant or abnormal substance that threatens the internal environment. In other words, nonspecific immunity confers general protection rather than protection from certain kinds of threatening cells or chemicals. Because we are born with nonspecific defenses that do not require prior exposure to a harmful substance or threatening cell, nonspecific immunity is often called **innate immunity.**

There are many types of nonspecific immune defenses in the body. The skin and mucous membranes, for example, are nonspecific mechanical barriers that prevent entry into the body by bacteria and many other substances such as toxins and harmful chemicals. Tears and mucus also contribute to nonspecific immunity. Tears wash harmful substances from the eyes, and mucus traps foreign material that may enter through the respiratory tract. Phagocytosis of bacteria by white blood cells (WBCs) is a nonspecific form of immunity.

The **inflammatory response** is a set of nonspecific responses that often occurs in the body. In the example shown in Figure 13-8, bacteria cause tissue damage that, in turn, triggers the release of mediators from any of a variety of immune cells. Some of the mediators attract WBCs to the area. Many of these factors produce the characteristic signs of inflammation: heat, redness, pain, and swelling. These signs are caused by increased blood flow (resulting in heat and redness) and vascular permeability (resulting in tissue swelling and the pain that it causes) in the affected region.

TABLE 13-1		
Nonspecific and Specific Immunity		
	NONSPECIFIC IMMUNITY	**SPECIFIC IMMUNITY**
Synonyms	Innate immunity, native immunity, genetic immunity	Adaptive immunity, acquired immunity
Specificity	Not specific—recognizes variety of nonself or abnormal cells and particles	Specific—recognizes certain antigens on certain cells or particles
Speed of reaction	Rapid—immediate up to several hours	Slower—several hours to several days
Memory	None—same response to repeated exposures to same antigen	Yes—enhanced response to repeated exposures to same antigen
Chemicals	Complement proteins, interferons, others	Antibodies, various signaling chemicals
Cells	Phagocytes (neutrophils, macrophages, dendritic cells)	Lymphocytes (B cells and T cells)

Such changes help phagocytic WBCs reach the general area and enter the affected tissue.

As you can see in Table 13-1, nonspecific immune responses are more rapid than specific immune responses.

Specific Immunity

Specific immunity includes protective mechanisms that confer very specific protection against certain types of threatening microorganisms or other toxic materials. Specific immunity involves memory and the ability to recognize and respond to certain harmful substances or bacteria. Because it is able to adapt to newly encountered "enemies," specific immunity is often called **adaptive immunity.**

In specific immunity, when the body is first attacked by particular bacteria or viruses, disease symptoms may occur as the body fights to destroy the threatening organism. However, if the body is exposed a second time to the same threatening organism, no serious symptoms occur because the organism is destroyed quickly—the person is said to be *immune* to that particular organism. Immunity to one type of disease-causing bacteria or virus does not protect the body against others. Immunity can be very selective.

As Table 13-1 shows, specific immune responses are slow compared to nonspecific immune responses. However, specific immune responses have memory—the ability to produce a stronger, faster response to repeated exposure to the same antigen. Table 13-1 summarizes other important features of both types of immunity, some of which will be discussed later in this chapter.

Specific immunity may be classified as either "natural" or "artificial" depending on how the body is exposed to the harmful agent (Table 13-2). Natural exposure is not deliberate and occurs in the course of everyday living. We are naturally exposed to many disease-causing agents on a regular basis. Artificial exposure is called **immunization** and is the deliberate exposure of the body to a potentially harmful agent.

Natural and artificial immunity may be "active" or "passive." Active immunity occurs when an individual's own immune system responds to a harmful agent, regardless of whether that agent was naturally or artificially encountered. Passive immunity results when immunity to a disease that

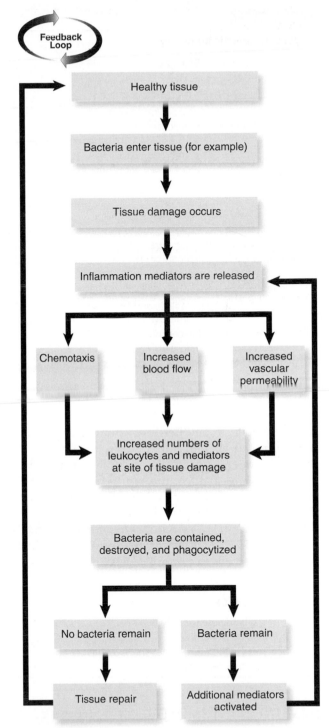

FIGURE 13-8 **Inflammatory response.** In this example, bacterial infection triggers a set of responses that tend to inhibit or destroy the bacteria.

TABLE 13-2

Types of Specific Immunity

TYPE	EXAMPLE
Natural immunity	Exposure to the causative agent is not deliberate, happens naturally in course of living.
Active immunity	A child develops measles and acquires an immunity to a subsequent infection.
Passive immunity	A fetus receives protection from the mother through the placenta, or an infant receives protection via the mother's milk.
Artificial immunity	Exposure to the causative agent is deliberate.
Active immunity	Injection of the causative agent, such as a vaccination against polio, activates the immune system and thus confers immunity.
Passive immunity	Injection of protective material (antibodies) that was developed by another individual's immune system is given.

has developed in another individual or animal is transferred to an individual who was not previously immune. For example, antibodies in a mother's milk confer passive immunity to her nursing infant. Active immunity generally lasts longer than passive immunity. Passive immunity, although temporary, provides immediate protection. Table 13-2 lists the various forms of specific immunity and gives examples of each.

> ### ✓ QUICK CHECK
> 1. What is the difference between *specific immunity* and *nonspecific immunity*?
> 2. Can you outline the changes that occur in the body's inflammatory response?

IMMUNE SYSTEM MOLECULES

The immune system functions because of adequate amounts of defensive protein molecules and protective cells. The protein molecules critical to immune system functioning are called **antibodies** (AN-ti-bod-eez) and **complement** (KOM-pleh-ment) proteins.

Antibodies

Definition

Antibodies are protein compounds that are normally present in the body. A defining characteristic of an antibody molecule is the uniquely shaped concave regions, called **combining sites,** on its surface. Another defining characteristic is the ability of an antibody molecule to combine with a specific compound called an **antigen** (AN-ti-jen).

All antigens are compounds whose molecules have small regions on their surfaces that are uniquely shaped to fit into the combining sites of a specific antibody molecule as precisely as a key fits into a specific lock. Antigens are often protein molecules embedded in the surface membranes of threatening or diseased cells, such as microorganisms or cancer cells.

Functions

In general, antibodies produce **humoral,** or **antibody-mediated, immunity** by changing the antigens in a way that prevents them from harming the body (Figure 13-9). To do this, an antibody must first bind to its specific antigen. This forms an antigen-antibody complex. The antigen-antibody complex then acts in one or more ways to make the antigen, or the cell on which it is present, harmless.

For example, if the antigen is a toxin (that is, a substance poisonous to body cells), the toxin is neutralized or made nonpoisonous by becoming part of an antigen-antibody complex. Or if antigens are molecules in the surface membranes of threatening cells, when antibodies combine with them, the resulting antigen-antibody complexes may **agglutinate** the enemy cells (that is, make them stick together in clumps). Then macrophages or the other phagocytes can rapidly destroy them by ingesting and digesting large numbers of them at one time.

Another important function of antibodies is promotion and enhancement of phagocytosis. Certain antibody fractions help promote the attachment of phagocytic cells to the object they will engulf. As a result, the contact between the phagocytic cell and its victim is enhanced, and the object is more easily ingested. This process contributes to the efficiency of immune system phagocytic cells, which is described on p. 312. Probably the most important way in which antibodies act is a process

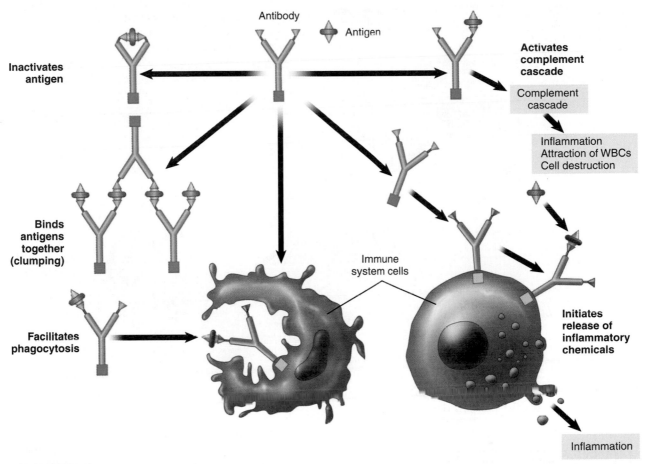

FIGURE 13-9   **Antibody function.** Antibodies produce humoral immunity by binding to specific antigens to form antigen-antibody complexes. These complexes produce a variety of changes that inactivate or kill threatening cells.

called the **complement cascade.** Often when antigens that are molecules on an antigenic or foreign cell's surface combine with antibody molecules, they change the shape of the antibody molecule slightly but just enough to expose two previously hidden regions. These are called **complement-binding sites.** The exposure of the complement-binding sites of an antibody that is attached to an antigen on the surface of a threatening cell then permits complement proteins to initiate a series of events that kill the cell. The next section describes these events.

Complement Proteins

Complement is the name used to describe a group of protein enzymes normally present in an inactive state in blood. These proteins may be activated by exposure of complement-binding sites on antibod-ies when they attach to antigens. The result is formation of highly specialized protein molecules that target foreign cells for destruction. The process is a rapid-fire cascade or sequence of events collectively called the **complement cascade.** The end result of this process is that doughnut-shaped protein rings (complete with a hole in the middle) are formed and literally bore holes in the foreign cell!

The tiny holes allow sodium to rapidly diffuse into the cell. Water follows, through the process of osmosis. The cell literally bursts as the internal osmotic pressure increases (Figure 13-10).

Complement proteins also serve other roles in the immune system, such as attracting immune cells to a site of infection, activating immune cells, marking foreign cells for destruction, and increasing permeability of blood vessels. Complement proteins also play a vital role in producing the inflammatory response.

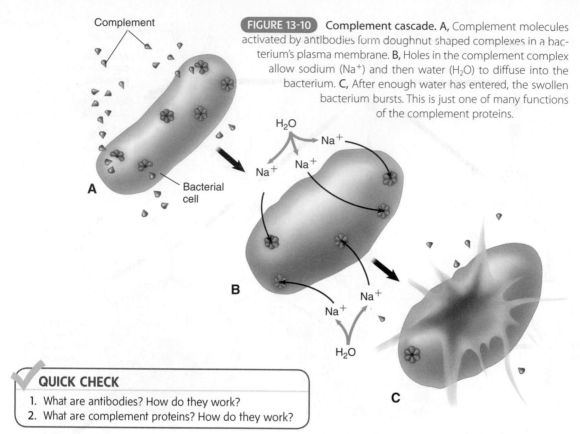

Complement

FIGURE 13-10 Complement cascade. **A,** Complement molecules activated by antibodies form doughnut shaped complexes in a bacterium's plasma membrane. **B,** Holes in the complement complex allow sodium (Na^+) and then water (H_2O) to diffuse into the bacterium. **C,** After enough water has entered, the swollen bacterium bursts. This is just one of many functions of the complement proteins.

H_2O

Na^+

Na^+ Na^+

A   Bacterial cell

B

Na^+

Na^+

H_2O

C

✓ QUICK CHECK

1. What are antibodies? How do they work?
2. What are complement proteins? How do they work?

IMMUNE SYSTEM CELLS

The primary cells of the immune system include the following:

1. Phagocytes
   a. Neutrophils
   b. Monocytes
   c. Macrophages
2. Lymphocytes
   a. T lymphocytes
   b. B lymphocytes

Phagocytes

Phagocytic WBCs are an important part of the immune system. In Chapter 11, phagocytes were described as cells derived from the bone marrow that carry on phagocytosis, or ingestion and digestion of foreign cells or particles.

Antibody molecules that bind to and coat certain foreign particles help macrophages function effectively. They serve as "flags" that alert the macrophage to the presence of foreign material, infectious bacteria, or cellular debris. They also help bind the phagocyte to the foreign material so that it can be engulfed more effectively (Figure 13-11).

Two important phagocytes are neutrophils and monocytes (see Figure 11-4, p. 256). These blood phagocytes migrate out of the blood and into the tissues in response to an infection.

The neutrophils are functional but short lived in the tissues. The pus found at some infection sites is mostly dead neutrophils.

Once in the tissues, monocytes develop into phagocytic cells called **macrophages** (MAK-roh-fay-jez). Most macrophages then "wander" through the tissues to engulf bacteria wherever they find them.

Another type of phagocytic cell is called the **dendritic cell (DC).** These highly branched (*dendrite* "branch") cells are produced in bone marrow and are released into the bloodstream. Some remain in the blood, but many migrate to tissues in contact with the external environment—the skin, respiratory lining, digestive lining, and so on. Resident DCs in these barrier regions help protect us from threatening particles and cells.

Research, Issues, & Trends

Monoclonal Antibodies

Techniques that have permitted biologists to produce large quantities of pure and very specific antibodies have resulted in dramatic advances in medicine. As a new medical technology, the development of **monoclonal antibodies** has been compared in importance with advances in recombinant DNA or genetic engineering.

Monoclonal antibodies are specific antibodies produced or derived from a population or culture of identical, or *monoclonal,* cells. In the past, antibodies produced by the immune system against a specific antigen had to be "harvested" from serum containing literally hundreds of other antibodies. The total amount of a specific antibody that could be recovered was very limited, so the cost of recovery was high. Monoclonal antibody techniques are based on the ability of immune system cells to produce individual antibodies that bind to and react with very specific antigens. We know, for example, that if the body is exposed to the varicella virus of chickenpox, white blood cells (WBCs) will produce an antibody that will react very specifically with that virus and no other.

With monoclonal antibody techniques, lymphocytes that are produced by the body after the injection of a specific antigen are "harvested" and then "fused" with other cells that have been transformed to grow and divide indefinitely in a tissue culture medium. These fused, or hybrid, cells, called **hybridomas** (hye-brid-OH-mahz), continue to produce the same antibody produced by the original lymphocyte. The result is a rapidly growing population of identical, or monoclonal, cells that produce large quantities of a very specific antibody. Monoclonal antibodies have now been produced against a wide array of different antigens, including disease-producing organisms and various types of cancer cells.

The availability of very pure antibodies against specific disease-producing agents is the first step in the commercial preparation of diagnostic tests that can be used to identify viruses, bacteria, and even specific cancer cells in the blood or other body fluids. The use of monoclonal antibodies may serve as the basis for specific treatment of many human diseases.

Monoclonal antibodies are also used in over-the-counter early pregnancy test kits. The antibodies in such kits bind to the hormone *human chorionic gonadotropin* (hCG), found in the urine of women in the early stages of pregnancy. When the antibodies in the kit bind to hCG molecules, they trigger a chemical reaction that produces a color change.

FIGURE 13-11 **Phagocytosis.** This series of scanning electron micrographs shows the progressive steps in phagocytosis of damaged red blood cells (RBCs) by a macrophage. **A,** RBCs *(R)* attach to the macrophage *(M)*. **B,** Plasma membrane of the macrophage begins to enclose the RBCs. **C,** The RBCs are almost totally ingested by the macrophage.

Macrophages and DCs perform another important immune function besides destruction of threatening cells and particles. They also act as **antigen-presenting cells (APCs).** Macrophages and DCs ingest a cell or particle, remove its antigens, and display some of them on their cell surfaces. The displayed antigens can then be presented to other immune cells to trigger additional, specific immune responses.

Lymphocytes

The most numerous cells of the immune system are the lymphocytes; they are ultimately responsible for antibody production. Several million strong, lymphocytes continually patrol the body, searching out any enemy cells that may have entered. Lymphocytes circulate in the body's fluids. Huge numbers of them wander vigilantly throughout most of its tissues. Lymphocytes densely populate the body's widely scattered lymph nodes and its other lymphatic tissues, especially the thymus gland in the chest and the spleen and liver in the abdomen.

There are two major types of lymphocytes, sometimes designated as *B* and *T lymphocytes* but usually called **B cells** and T cells. Each type of lymphocyte has a different set of roles to play in immunity.

Development of B Cells

All lymphocytes that circulate in the tissues arise from primitive cells in the bone marrow called *stem cells* and go through two stages of development. The first stage of B-cell development—transformation of stem cells into immature B cells—occurs in the liver and bone marrow before birth but only in the bone marrow in adults. Because this process was first discovered in a bird organ called the *bursa*, these cells were named *B cells.*

Immature B cells are small lymphocytes that have synthesized and inserted into their cytoplasmic membranes numerous molecules of one specific kind of antibody (Figure 13-12).

After they mature, B cells eventually leave the tissue where they were formed. Each mature, but inactive, B cell carries a different type of antibody. The various B cells then enter the blood and are transported to their new place of residence, chiefly the lymph nodes.

The second stage of B-cell development changes a mature, inactive B cell into an activated B cell. Not all B cells undergo this change. They do so only if an inactive B cell comes in contact with certain nonself or abnormal molecules—antigens—whose shape fits into the shape of the B cell's surface antibody molecules. If this happens, the antigens lock onto the antibodies and, by so doing, change the inactive B cell into an activated B cell. B-cell activation also requires a chemical signal from another immune cell—a type of T cell. Then the activated B cell, by dividing rapidly and repeatedly, develops into clones of many identical cells—all having the same type of antibody. A **clone** is a family of many identical cells, all descended from one cell.

Each clone of B cells is made up of two kinds of cells, **plasma cells** (also called **effector cells**) and

Stem cells

Develop shortly before and after birth into

Immature B cells
Small lymphocytes with antibody molecules in cytoplasmic membranes

Mature B cells migrate to lymph nodes, liver, and spleen; binding of antigen to antibody on surfaces of inactive B cells and chemical signal from T cells changes them into

FIGURE 13-12 **B-cell development.** B-cell development takes place in two stages. *First stage:* Shortly before and after birth, stem cells develop into immature B cells, which then mature into inactive B cells that migrate to lymphoid organs. *Second stage* (occurs only if the inactive B cell contacts its specific antigen): Inactive B cell develops into activated B cell, which divides rapidly and repeatedly to form a clone of plasma cells and a clone of memory cells. Plasma cells secrete antibodies capable of combining with the specific antigen that caused an inactive B cell to develop into an active B cell. Stem cells maintain a constant population of newly differentiating inactive B cells.

memory cells, as you can see in Figure 13-12. Plasma cells secrete huge amounts of antibody into the blood—reportedly, 2,000 antibody molecules per second by each plasma cell for every second of the four days that it lives. Antibodies circulating in the blood constitute an enormous, mobile, ever-on-duty army.

Memory cells can secrete antibodies but do not immediately do so. They remain in reserve in the lymph nodes until they are contacted by the same antigen that led to their formation. Then, very quickly, the memory cells develop into plasma cells and secrete large numbers of antibodies. Memory cells, in effect, seem to "remember" their ancestor-activated B cell's encounter with its appropriate antigen. They stand ready, at a moment's notice, to produce antibodies that will combine with this antigen.

Function of B Cells

B cells function indirectly to produce humoral immunity. Recall that humoral immunity is resistance to disease organisms produced by the actions of antibodies binding to specific antigens while circulating in body fluids. Activated B cells develop into plasma cells. **Plasma cells** secrete antibodies into the blood; they are the "antibody factories" of the body. These antibodies, like other proteins manufactured for extracellular use, are formed on the endoplasmic reticulum of the cell.

Development of T Cells

T cells are lymphocytes that have undergone their first stage of development in the thymus gland. Stem cells from the bone marrow seed the thymus, and shortly before and after birth, they develop into T cells. The newly formed T cells stream out of the thymus into the blood and migrate chiefly to

FIGURE 13-13 T-cell development. The first stage takes place in the thymus gland shortly before and after birth. Stem cells maintain a constant population of newly differentiating cells as they are needed. The second stage occurs only if a T cell contacts an antigen, which combines with certain proteins on the T cell's surface.

FIGURE 13-14 T cells. The purple cells seen in this scanning electron microscope view are T cells attacking a much larger cancer cell. The cells are a significant part of our defense against cancer and other types of foreign cells.

the lymph nodes, where they take up residence. Embedded in each T cell's cytoplasmic membrane are protein molecules shaped to fit only one specific kind of antigen molecule.

The second stage of T-cell development takes place when and if a T cell comes into contact with its specific antigen. If this happens, the antigen binds to the protein on the T cell's surface, thereby changing the T cell to an activated T cell (Figure 13-13). As with B cells, T cells must also receive a chemical signal from another T cell to become activated. Likewise, T cells also produce a clone of identical cells, all able to react with the same antigen. And as with B cells, T cells form a group of *effector cells* along with *memory cells*. The effector T cells actively engage in immune responses, whereas the memory T cells do not. Later, if more effector T cells are needed, the memory T cells can produce additional clones that include more effector T cells.

Functions of T Cells

Activated T cells produce cell-mediated immunity. As the name suggests, **cell-mediated immunity** is resistance to disease organisms that results from the actions of cells—chiefly, sensitized T cells. Some activated T cells kill infected cells and tumor cells directly (Figure 13-14). When bound to antigens, these *cytotoxic (sye-toh-TOK-sik) T cells* release a substance that acts as a specific and lethal poison against the abnormal cell.

Activated T cells called *helper T cells* produce their deadly effects indirectly by means of compounds that they release into the area around enemy cells. Among these is a substance that attracts macrophages into the vicinity of the enemy cells.

Memory cells

Subsequent exposure to antigen
changes memory cells to

Effector cells

Kill infected cells
and tumor cells;
trigger B and
T-cell activation;
regulate various
immune functions

The assembled macrophages then destroy the cells
by phagocytosing (ingesting and digesting) them
(Figure 13-15). Helper T cells also release the
chemicals needed to help trigger the activation of
B cells. Activated *regulatory T cells* help shut down
an immune reaction after the antigens have been
destroyed and also help prevent inappropriate immune reactions.

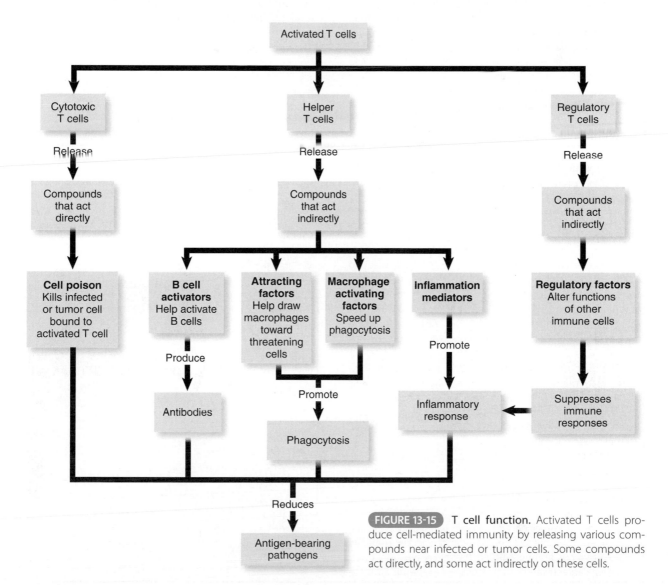

FIGURE 13-15   **T cell function.** Activated T cells produce cell-mediated immunity by releasing various compounds near infected or tumor cells. Some compounds
act directly, and some act indirectly on these cells.

Clinical Application

Human Immunodeficiency Virus Infection

Infection by **HIV** (**human immunodeficiency virus**) is a worldwide health concern. HIV infection has reached epidemic proportions in many countries, thus qualifying as a *pandemic.*

HIV, a retrovirus, contains RNA that undergoes reverse transcription inside infected cells to form its own DNA. The viral DNA often becomes part of the cell's DNA. When the viral DNA is activated, it directs the synthesis of its own RNA and protein coat, thus "stealing" raw materials from the cell. When this occurs in certain T cells, the cell is destroyed, and immunity is impaired. As the T cell dies, it releases new retroviruses that can spread the HIV infection.

Although HIV can invade several types of cells, it has its most obvious effects in a certain type of T cell called a *CD4+* T cell. When T-cell function is impaired, infectious organisms and cancer cells can grow and spread much more easily than normal. Unusual conditions, such as *pneumocystosis* (a protozoan infection) and *Kaposi sarcoma* (a type of skin cancer), may also appear. Because their immune systems are deficient, AIDS patients may eventually die from one of these infections or cancers.

HIV infection sometimes progresses to a collection of symptoms called **AIDS,** or **acquired immunodeficiency syndrome.** After infection with HIV, an untreated person may not show signs of AIDS for months or years. This is because the immune system can hold the infection at bay for a long time before finally succumbing to it.

There are several strategies for preventing the development of AIDS. Many agencies are trying to reduce the incidence of AIDS by educating people about how to avoid contact with the HIV retrovirus. HIV is spread by means of direct contact of body fluids, so preventing such contact reduces HIV transmission. Sexual relations, contaminated blood transfusions, and intravenous use of contaminated needles are the usual modes of HIV transmission. HIV can also be a *perinatal infection,* that is, an infection passing from mother to infant during birth. Many researchers are working on HIV vaccines. Like many viruses, such as those that cause the common cold, HIV changes rapidly enough to make development of a vaccine difficult at best.

Another way to inhibit the progress of an HIV infection is by means of chemicals such as azidothymidine (AZT) and ritonavir (Norvir) that block HIV's ability to reproduce within infected cells. A "cocktail" of several antiviral drugs working together greatly reduces the number of virus particles in a patient's blood, thus reducing the effects of HIV infection. More than 100 such compounds in various combinations are being evaluated for use in halting the progress of HIV infections.

Research, Issues, & Trends

Mucosal Immunity

The *mucosal immune system* is a complex system of defense distinct from the systemic (internal) immune system, which has been discussed in most of this chapter. It is an innate (nonspecific) and adaptive (specific) system that is found within the mucous barriers of the body: digestive tract, urinary/reproductive tracts, respiratory tract, exocrine ducts, conjunctiva (eye covering), middle ear, and so on. The immune cells that make up the mucosal immune system are located mainly in or near *mucosal-associated lymphoid tissue (MALT).*

The main functions of the mucosal immune system involve preventing pathogens from colonizing the mucous surfaces of the body, preventing the accidental absorption of antigens from outside the body, and preventing inappropriate or intense responses of the systemic immune system to these external antigens.

Understanding the mucosal immune system and its cooperation with the systemic (internal) immune system promises to reveal new strategies of immunization. For example, researchers have found that immunizing through the bloodstream activates only the internal (systemic) B cells and T cells. Thus a pathogen would have to actually enter the internal environment before this type of specific immunity could protect us. Immunization of the mucosal lymphocytes, however, can activate both mucosal and systemic lympho-cytes, providing a more thorough type of protection. Another advantage of mucosal immunization is that it is easier to administer to patients than immunizations injected under the skin or into the bloodstream. For example, immunization can be delivered by nasal sprays or drops instead of "shots."

Science Application

Vaccines
Edward Jenner (1749–1823)

English surgeon Edward Jenner changed the world forever in 1789 when he inoculated his young son and two others against the terrible viral disease smallpox. Using material from the blisters of a patient with the milder disease swinepox, he was able to trigger immunity to smallpox—the world's first vaccination. Later, in 1796, he found that vaccination with material from cowpox blisters worked even better in protecting people from smallpox. A disease that had formerly killed millions of people worldwide eventually disappeared from the human population in the twentieth century because of Jenner's pioneering efforts.

In this century, interest in smallpox vaccinations has resurfaced because of the threat of smallpox as a weapon. Immunologists are at work improving on this important vaccine to protect people against such weapons. They also continue to work on vaccines for other infectious diseases such as AIDS and even disorders such as heart disease and cancer. Many health care professionals use vaccines in their practice to boost the immune systems of their clients. Many physicians also treat disorders of the immune system itself. For example, immune deficiencies such as AIDS, allergies such as "hay fever," and autoimmune disorders such as lupus and rheumatoid arthritis are treated every day by physicians and other health professionals.

OUTLINE SUMMARY

THE LYMPHATIC SYSTEM (See Figure 13-1)

A. Lymph — fluid in the tissue spaces that carries protein molecules and other substances back to the blood

B. Lymphatic vessels — permit only one-way movement of lymph
1. Lymphatic capillaries — tiny blind-ended tubes distributed in tissue spaces (see Figure 13-2)
   a. Microscopic in size
   b. Sheets consisting of one cell layer of simple squamous epithelium
   c. Poor "fit" between adjacent cells results in porous walls
   d. Called *lacteals* in the intestinal wall (fat transportation from food to bloodstream)
2. Right lymphatic duct (see Figure 13-3)
   a. Drains lymph from the right upper extremity and right side of head, neck, and upper torso
3. Thoracic duct
   a. Largest lymphatic vessel
   b. Has an enlarged pouch along its course, called *cisterna chyli*
   c. Drains lymph from about three fourths of the body (see Figure 13-3)

C. Lymph nodes
1. Filter lymph (see Figure 13-4)
2. Located in clusters along the pathway of lymphatic vessels (see Figures 13-1, 13-5, and 13-6)
3. Lymphoid tissue — mass of lymphocytes and related cells inside a lymphoid organ; provides immune function and development of immune cells
4. Lymph nodes and other lymphoid organs have functions that include defense and WBC formation
5. Flow of lymph: to node via several afferent lymphatic vessels and drained from node by a single efferent lymphatic vessel

D. Thymus
1. Lymphoid tissue organ located in mediastinum
2. Total weight of 35 to 40 grams — a little more than an ounce
3. Plays a vital and central role in immunity
4. Produces T lymphocytes, or T cells
5. Secretes hormones called *thymosins*, which influence T-cell development
6. Lymphoid tissue is replaced by fat (during childhood) in the process called *involution*

E. Tonsils (see Figure 13-7)
1. Composed of three masses of lymphoid tissue around the openings of the mouth and throat
   a. Palatine tonsils ("the tonsils")
   b. Pharyngeal tonsils (also known as *adenoids*)
   c. Lingual tonsils
2. Subject to chronic infection
3. Enlargement of pharyngeal tonsils may impair breathing

F. Spleen
1. Largest lymphoid organ in body
2. Located in upper left quadrant of abdomen
3. Often injured by trauma to abdomen
4. Surgical removal called *splenectomy*
5. Functions include phagocytosis of bacteria and old RBCs; acts as a blood reservoir

THE IMMUNE SYSTEM
A. Protects body from pathological bacteria, foreign tissue cells, and cancerous cells
B. Made up of defensive cells and molecules
C. Nonspecific immunity (Table 13-1)
1. Also called *innate immunity* because it does not require prior exposure to an antigen
2. Skin — mechanical barrier to bacteria and other harmful agents
3. Tears and mucus — wash eyes and trap and kill bacteria
4. Inflammation — attracts immune cells to site of injury, increases local blood flow, increases vascular permeability; promotes movement of WBCs to site of injury or infection (see Figure 13-8)
D. Specific immunity (see Tables 13-1 and 13-2)
1. Also called *adaptive immunity* because of its ability to recognize, respond to, and remember harmful substances or bacteria
2. Types of specific immunity
a. Natural immunity — exposure to causative agent is not deliberate
(1) Active — active disease produces immunity
(2) Passive — immunity passes from mother to fetus through placenta or from mother to child through mother's milk
b. Artificial immunity — exposure to causative agent is deliberate
(1) Active — vaccination results in activation of immune system
(2) Passive — protective material developed in another individual's immune system and given to previously nonimmune individual

IMMUNE SYSTEM MOLECULES
A. Antibodies
1. Protein compounds with specific combining sites
2. Combining sites attach antibodies to specific antigens (foreign proteins), forming an antigen-antibody complex — called *humoral*, or *antibody-mediated, immunity* (see Figure 13-9)
3. Antigen-antibody complexes may do the following:
a. Neutralize toxins
b. Clump or agglutinate enemy cells
c. Promote phagocytosis
B. Complement proteins
1. Group of proteins normally present in blood in inactive state
2. Complement cascade
a. Important mechanism of action for antibodies
b. Causes cell lysis by permitting entry of water through a defect created in the plasma membrane (see Figure 13-10)
3. Also perform other functions (*examples:* attracting immune cells to a site of infection, activating immune cells, marking foreign cells for destruction, increasing permeability of blood vessels), the inflammatory response

IMMUNE SYSTEM CELLS
A. Phagocytes
1. Ingest and destroy foreign cells or other harmful substances via phagocytosis (see Figure 13-11)
2. Types
a. Neutrophils — short-lived phagocytic cells
b. Monocytes — develop into phagocytic macrophages and migrate to tissues (see Figure 13-15)
c. Dendritic cells (DCs) — often found at or near external surfaces
3. Macrophages and DCs act as antigen-presenting cells (APCs) by displaying ingested antigens on their outer surface to trigger specific immune cells
B. Lymphocytes
1. Most numerous of immune system cells
2. Development of B cells — primitive stem cells migrate from bone marrow and go through two stages of development (see Figure 13-12)
a. First stage — stem cells develop into immature B cells
(1) Takes place in the liver and bone marrow before birth and in the bone marrow only in adults

(2) B cells are small lymphocytes with antibody molecules (which they have synthesized) in their plasma membranes

(3) After they mature, inactive B cells migrate chiefly to lymph nodes

b. Second stage — inactive B cell develops into activated B cell

(1) Initiated by inactive B cell's contact with antigens, which bind to its surface antibodies, plus signal chemicals from T cells

(2) Activated B cell, by dividing repeatedly, forms two clones of cells — plasma (effector) cells and memory cells

(3) Plasma cells secrete antibodies into blood; memory cells are stored in lymph nodes

(4) If subsequent exposure to antigen that activated B cell occurs, memory cells become plasma cells and secrete antibodies

3. Function of B cells — indirectly, B cells produce humoral immunity

a. Activated B cells develop into plasma cells

b. Plasma cells secrete antibodies into the blood

c. Circulating antibodies produce humoral immunity (see Figure 13-12)

4. Development of T cells — stem cells from bone marrow migrate to thymus gland (see Figure 13-13)

a. First stage — stem cells develop into T cells

(1) Occurs in thymus during few months before and after birth

(2) T cells migrate chiefly to lymph nodes

b. Second stage — T cells develop into activated T cells

(1) Occurs when, and if, antigen binds to T cell's surface proteins and a chemical signal is received from another T cell

(2) As with B cells, clones made up of effector cells and memory cells are formed

5. Functions of T cells — produce cell-mediated immunity (see Figures 13-14 and 13-15)

a. Cytotoxic T cells — kill infected or tumor cells by releasing a substance that poisons infected or tumor cells

b. Helper T cells — release chemicals that attract and activate macrophages to kill cells by phagocytosis; produce chemicals that help activate B cells

c. Regulatory T cells — release chemicals to suppress immune responses

NEW WORDS

acquired immunodeficiency syndrome (AIDS)	clone	immune system	palatine tonsils
adenoid	combining site	immunization	pharyngeal tonsils
afferent lymphatic vessel	complement	inflammatory response	plasma cell (effector B cell)
agglutinate	complement-binding site	interferon (IF)	right lymphatic duct
anaphylactic shock	complement cascade	interstitial fluid	specific immunity (adaptive immunity)
antibodies	dendritic cell (DC)	lacteal	spleen
antigen	effector cells	lingual tonsils	splenectomy
antigen-presenting cell (APC)	efferent lymphatic vessel	lymph	T cell (T lymphocyte)
B cell (B lymphocyte)	human immunodeficiency virus (HIV)	lymph node	thoracic duct
cell-mediated immunity	humoral immunity (antibody-mediated immunity)	lymphatic capillary	thymosin
cisterna chyli	hybridoma	lymphatic vessel	thymus
		macrophage	
		memory cell	
		monoclonal antibody	
		nonspecific immunity (innate immunity)	

REVIEW QUESTIONS

1. Define *lymph* and explain its function.
2. Name the two lymphatic ducts and the areas of the body each of them drain.
3. Describe the structure of the lymph node.
4. Explain the defense function of the lymph node.
5. Where is the thymus gland? What are its functions?
6. Name the three pairs of tonsils and give the location of each.
7. Give the location and function of the spleen.
8. Explain the types of nonspecific immunity.
9. Name and differentiate between the four types of specific immunity.
10. What are antibodies? What are antigens?
11. Explain the role of complement in the immune system.
12. Explain the role of macrophages in the immune system.
13. Explain the development and functioning of B cells.
14. Explain the development and functioning of T cells.

CRITICAL THINKING

15. Differentiate between lymphatic capillaries and blood capillaries. Explain how the differences in structure relate to their function.
16. Explain the role of lymph nodes in the possible spread of cancer.

CHAPTER TEST

1. _____ is the fluid that leaves the blood capillaries and is not returned to the blood.
2. Lymph from about three fourths of the body drains into the _____.
3. Lymph from the right upper extremity and the right side of the head drains into the _____.
4. The enlarged, pouchlike structure in the abdomen that serves as a storage area for lymph is called the _____.
5. The function of the _____ is to filter and clean the lymph.
6. The many lymphatic vessels that enter the lymph node are called the _____ vessels. The single vessel leaving the lymph node is called the _____ vessel.
7. The thymus gland is the site of maturation for these WBCs: _____. It also produces the hormone _____.
8. The three pairs of tonsils are the _____ tonsils, the _____ tonsils, and the _____ tonsils.
9. The largest lymphoid organ is the _____.

CHAPTER TEST—cont'd

10. The signs of _____ are heat, redness, pain, and swelling.
11. _____ kills threatening cells by drilling holes in their plasma membrane, which disrupts the sodium and water balance.
12. Macrophages were originally _____ that migrated into the tissues.
13. The immunity that develops against polio after receiving a polio vaccination is an example of:
    a. active natural immunity
    b. passive natural immunity
    c. active artificial immunity
    d. passive artificial immunity
14. The immunity that is given to the fetus or newborn by the immune system of the mother is an example of:
    a. active natural immunity
    b. passive natural immunity
    c. active artificial immunity
    d. passive artificial immunity
15. The immunity that comes from the injection of antibodies made by another individual's immune system is an example of:
    a. active natural immunity
    b. passive natural immunity
    c. active artificial immunity
    d. passive artificial immunity

16. The immunity that develops after a person has had a disease is an example of:
    a. active natural immunity
    b. passive natural immunity
    c. active artificial immunity
    d. passive artificial immunity

If the following statement describes the development or functioning of a B cell, write a B in front of it. If it describes the development or functioning of a T cell, write a T in front of it.

17. _____ produces antibodies
18. _____ some develop into plasma cells
19. _____ the main cell involved in cell-mediated immunity
20. _____ the main cell involved in humoral immunity
21. _____ develops in the thymus gland
22. _____ moves to the site of the antigen and releases cell poison
23. _____ divides rapidly into clones once it is activated
24. _____ releases a substance that attracts macrophages
25. _____ some of these cells develop into memory cells

OBJECTIVES

AFTER YOU HAVE COMPLETED THIS CHAPTER, YOU SHOULD BE ABLE TO:

1. Discuss the generalized functions of the respiratory system.
2. List the major organs of the respiratory system and describe the functions of each.
3. Compare, contrast, and explain the mechanism responsible for the exchange of gases that occurs during internal and external respiration.
4. List and discuss the volumes of air exchanged during pulmonary ventilation.
5. Identify and discuss the mechanisms that regulate respiration.

The Respiratory System 14

No one needs to be told how important the **respiratory system** is. The respiratory system serves the body much as a lifeline to an oxygen tank serves a deep-sea diver. Think how panicked you would feel if suddenly your lifeline became blocked—if you could not breathe for a few seconds! Of all the substances that cells and therefore the body as a whole must have to survive, oxygen is by far the most crucial. A person can live a few weeks without food, a few days without water, but only a few minutes without oxygen. Constant removal of carbon dioxide from the body is just as important for survival as a constant supply of oxygen.

The organs of the respiratory system are designed to perform two basic functions: they serve as an *air distributor* and as a *gas exchanger* for the body. The respiratory system ensures that oxygen is supplied to, and carbon dioxide is removed from, the body's cells. The process of respiration therefore is an important **homeostatic mechanism.** By constantly supplying adequate oxygen and by removing carbon dioxide as it forms, the respiratory system helps maintain a constant environment that enables your body cells to function effectively.

In addition to air distribution and gas exchange, the respiratory system effectively *filters, warms,* and *humidifies* the air we breathe. Respiratory organs or organs closely associated with the respiratory system, such as the **sinuses,** also influence speech or sound production and make possible the sense of smell, or **olfaction** (ohl-FAK-shun). In this chapter, the structural plan of the respiratory system is considered first, then the respiratory organs are discussed individually, and finally some facts about gas exchange and

STUDY TIPS

To make the study of the respiratory system more efficient, we suggest these tips:

1. Before you begin or during your more in-depth study of the respiratory system, take time to briefly review helpful information presented in Chapter 2 (chemical reactions and pH), Chapter 3 (diffusion), Chapter 4 (synopsis of respiratory system), Chapter 5 (serous membranes), Chapter 11 (red blood cell [RBC] and hemoglobin functions), and Chapter 12 (systemic vs. pulmonary circulation).

2. Think of the respiratory system as a series of tubes serving as an air distribution system. The distribution tubes resemble an "upside-down tree" with the trachea as the trunk and the bronchial tubes being the branches. Ultimately, the very smallest tubes end in millions of tiny, thin-walled sacs (alveoli) that serve as air exchangers for movement of oxygen and carbon dioxide. Discuss the difference between the respiratory mucosa and the respiratory membrane.

3. Learn how to correlate the movement of air into and out of the lungs (breathing or pulmonary ventilation) with measurement of pressure changes in the chest cavity. To move air in or out of the lungs, the pressure of the chest cavity must be lowered or raised. Changes in pressure are caused by changes in the size (volume) of the thorax, which, in turn, are caused by alternate contraction and relaxation of the inspiratory (diaphragm/external intercostal) and expiratory (internal intercostal and abdominal) respiratory muscles. Expiration can also occur because the elastic nature of lung tissue causes them to "recoil" as air leaves the alveoli, thus assisting in expiration. Flash cards can help you learn the names and definitions of the various pulmonary volumes and types of breathing.

4. In your study group, define the term *partial pressure* of a gas and discuss how the partial pressure of oxygen and of carbon dioxide influence the exchange of these gases in the lungs and tissues. Remember, gases diffuse "down their partial pressure gradients." Flash cards can help you review the various ways that oxygen and carbon dioxide are transported in the blood and can also help you learn the names and locations of the control centers and specialized receptors that influence respiration.

Continued on page 326.

the nervous system's control of respiration are discussed.

STRUCTURAL PLAN

Respiratory organs include the **nose, pharynx** (FAIR-inks), **larynx** (LAIR-inks), **trachea** (TRAY-kee-ah), **bronchi** (BRONG-kye), and **lungs.** The basic structural design of this organ system is that of a tube with many branches ending in millions of extremely tiny, very thin-walled sacs called **alveoli** (al-VEE-oh-lye). Figure 14-1 shows the extensive branching of the "respiratory tree" in both lungs. Think of this air distribution system as an "upside-down tree." The trachea, or windpipe, then becomes the trunk and the bronchial tubes the branches. This idea is developed further when the types of bronchi and the alveoli are studied in more detail later in the chapter. A network of capillaries fits like a hairnet around each microscopic alveolus. Incidentally, this is a good place for us to think again about a principle already mentioned several times—namely, that structure and function are intimately related. The function of alveoli—in fact, the function of the entire respiratory system—is to distribute air close enough to blood for a gas exchange to take place between air and blood. The passive transport process of *diffusion,*

Clinical Application

Oxygen Therapy

Oxygen therapy is the administration of oxygen to individuals suffering from **hypoxia** (hye-POCK-see-ah)—an insufficient oxygen supply to the tissues. Individuals with certain respiratory problems, such as emphysema, may require supplemental oxygen in order to maintain a normal lifestyle.

Oxygen (O_2) in the form of compressed gas is commonly stored in and dispensed from small, green, metal cylinders or tanks. Because the oxygen dispensed from such tanks is often cold and dry, it may need to be warmed and moistened, generally by bubbling the released gas through water, to prevent damage to the respiratory tract. Supplemental oxygen is delivered through a mask or tubes that lead into the nasal passage (nasal prongs).

Supplemental (and generally very expensive) oxygen is now being dispensed for recreational purposes at trendy "oxygen bars." Delivery is at low flow levels and, although considered safe for healthy individuals, has more psychological than measurable physiological effects. Breathing supplemental oxygen for short periods after strenuous exercise is another nonmedical application of oxygen therapy. Although it may shorten recovery times for some athletes, it seldom provides more than transitory benefits.

Some endurance athletes, such as cyclists and long-distance runners who perform at high altitudes, have used "low oxygen level" or "hypoxic tents" to reduce available O_2 levels over longer periods of sleep or rest to mimic available oxygen levels at high altitudes. The intent is to obtain the physiological advantage of long-term high-altitude training (increased RBC production) without the inconvenience of actually training at high altitudes prior to competition. Many sport-sanctioning groups have now questioned the ethics of this type of extended-use oxygen level manipulation as a training technique or have banned the practice outright as a form of "doping" (see Health and Well-Being: Blood Doping box, p. 262).

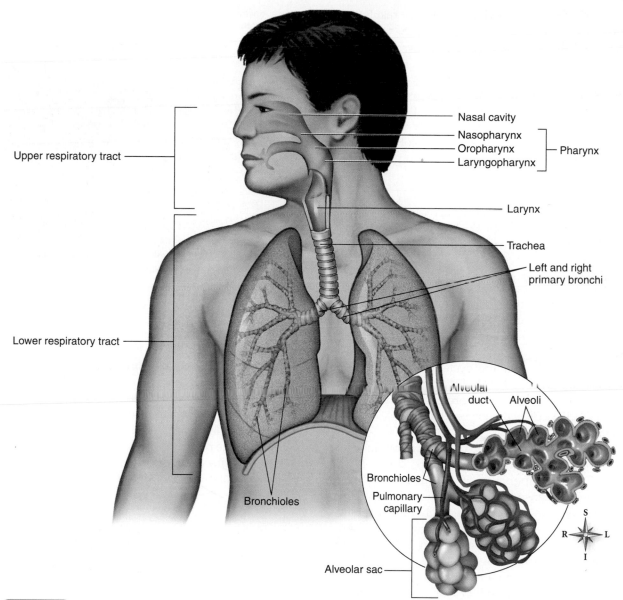

Upper respiratory tract

Nasal cavity

Nasopharynx
Oropharynx
Laryngopharynx

Pharynx

Larynx

Trachea

Left and right
primary bronchi

Lower respiratory tract

Alveolar
duct

Alveoli

Bronchioles

Pulmonary
capillary

Bronchioles

Alveolar sac

S
R   L
I

FIGURE 14-1   Structural plan of the respiratory organs showing the pharynx, trachea, bronchi, and lungs. *Inset* shows the alveolar sacs where the exchange of oxygen and carbon dioxide takes place through the walls of the grapelike alveoli. Capillaries surround the alveoli.

which was described in Chapter 3, is responsible for the exchange of gases that occurs in the respiratory system. You may want to review the discussion of diffusion on pp. 45-46 before you study the mechanism of gas exchange that occurs in the lungs and body tissues.

 To learn more about alveoli, go to AnimationDirect on your CD-ROM.

RESPIRATORY TRACTS

The respiratory system is often divided into upper and lower tracts or divisions to assist in the description of symptoms associated with common respiratory problems such as a cold. The organs of the upper respiratory tract are located outside of the thorax, or chest cavity, whereas those in the lower tract or division are located almost entirely within it. The **upper respiratory tract** is composed of the nose, pharynx, and larynx. The **lower respiratory tract,** or division, consists of the trachea, all segments of the bronchial tree, and the lungs. The designation *upper respiratory infection*, or URI, is often used to describe what many patients call a "head cold." Typically the symptoms of an upper respiratory infection involve the sinuses, nasal cavity, pharynx, and larynx, whereas the symptoms of what is often referred to as a "chest cold" are similar to pneumonia and involve the organs of the lower respiratory tract.

 To learn more about the bronchial tree, go to AnimationDirect on your CD-ROM.

RESPIRATORY MUCOSA

Before beginning the study of individual organs in the respiratory system, it is important to review the histology or microscopic anatomy of the **respiratory mucosa**—the membrane that lines most of the air distribution tubes in the system. The respiratory mucosa is covered by pseudostratified columnar epithelium rich in mucus-producing goblet cells. Hairlike cilia cover the exposed surface of the epithelial cells.

Recall that in addition to serving as air distribution passageways or gas exchange surfaces, the anatomical components of the respiratory tract and lungs cleanse, warm, and humidify inspired air. Air entering the nose is generally contaminated with one or more common irritants; examples include insects, dust, pollen, and bacterial organisms. A remarkably effective air purification mechanism removes almost every form of contaminant before inspired air reaches the alveoli, or terminal air sacs, in the lungs.

The layer of protective mucus that covers a large portion of the membrane that lines the respiratory tree serves as the most important air purification mechanism. More than 125 mL of respiratory mucus is produced daily. It forms a continuous sheet called a *mucous blanket*, which covers the lining of the air distribution tubes in the respiratory tree. This layer of cleansing mucus moves upward to the pharynx from the lower portions of the bronchial tree on millions of hairlike cilia that cover the epithelial cells in the respiratory mucosa (Figure 14-2). The microscopic cilia that cover epithelial

Pseudostratified ciliated epithelium   Mucus   Cilia   Goblet cell

Mucous gland   Submucosa

FIGURE 14-2 Respiratory mucosa lining the trachea. A layer of mucus covers the hairlike cilia.

cells in the respiratory mucosa beat or move only in one direction. The result is upward movement of mucus toward the pharynx in a process sometimes called the *mucociliary escalator*. Cigarette smoke paralyzes these cilia and results in accumulations of **mucus** and the typical smoker's cough, which is an effort to clear the secretions. Respiratory mucosa lining the passageways of the nasal cavity also sweep covering mucus with its trapped airborne contaminants toward the pharynx.

 To learn more about respiratory mucosa, go to AnimationDirect on your CD-ROM.

✔ QUICK CHECK

1. What are the primary functions of the respiratory system?
2. Can you distinguish the upper respiratory tract from the lower respiratory tract?
3. What is the role of the respiratory membrane?

NOSE

Air enters the respiratory tract through the **external nares** (NAY-reez), or nostrils. It then flows into the right and left **nasal cavities,** which are lined by respiratory mucosa. A partition called the **nasal septum** separates these two cavities.

The surface of the nasal cavities is moist from mucus and warm from blood flowing just under it. Nerve endings responsible for the sense of smell (olfactory receptors) are located in the nasal mucosa. The word part *para* means "by the side of" or "near"; *nasal* refers to the nose, and *sinus* (SYE-nus) refers to a space or cavity located in some solid structure such as a bone. The **paranasal sinuses** are appropriately named. They are spaces or cavities located inside the frontal, maxillary, sphenoidal, and ethmoid bones, which are located close to the nose. The paranasal sinuses all drain into the nasal cavities (Figure 14-3). Because the mucosa that lines the sinuses is continuous with the mucosa that lines the nose, sinus infections, called **sinusitis** (sye-nyoo-SYE-tis), often develop from colds in which the nasal mucosa is inflamed. The paranasal sinuses are lined with a mucous membrane that assists in the production of mucus for the respiratory tract. In addition, these hollow spaces help lessen the weight of the skull bones and serve as resonant chambers for the production of sound.

Two ducts from the **lacrimal sacs** (LAK-ri-mal saks) also drain into the nasal cavity, as Figure 14-3 shows. The lacrimal sacs collect tears from the corner of each eyelid and drain them into the nasal cavity.

Note in Figure 14-4 that three shelf-like structures called **conchae** (KONG-kee) protrude into the nasal cavity on each side. The mucosa-covered conchae greatly increase the surface over which air must flow as it passes through the nasal cavity. As air moves over the conchae and through the nasal cavities, it is warmed and humidified. This helps explain why breathing through the nose is more effective in humidifying inspired air than is breathing through the mouth. If an individual who is ill requires supplemental oxygen, it is first bubbled through water to reduce the amount of moisture that would otherwise have to be removed from the lining of the respiratory tree to humidify it. Administration of "dry" oxygen pulls water from the mucosa and results in respiratory discomfort and irritation.

PHARYNX

The **pharynx** is the structure that many of us call the throat. It is about 12.5 cm (5 inches) long and can be divided into three portions (see Figure 14-4). The uppermost part of the tube just behind the nasal cavities is called the **nasopharynx** (nay-zoh-FAIR-inks). The portion behind the mouth is called the **oropharynx** (oh-roh-FAIR-inks). The last or lowest segment is called the **laryngopharynx** (lah-ring-go-FAIR-inks). The pharynx as a whole serves the same purpose for the respiratory and digestive tracts as a hallway serves for a house. Air and food pass through the pharynx on their way to the lungs and the stomach, respectively. Air enters the pharynx from the two nasal cavities and leaves it by

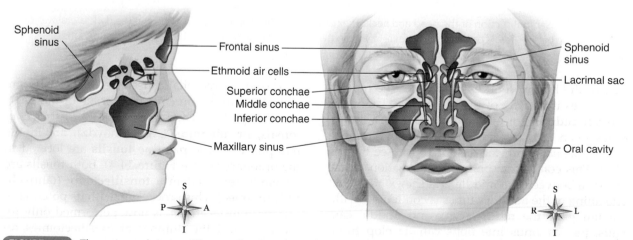

FIGURE 14-3   The paranasal sinuses. The anterior view shows the anatomical relationship of the paranasal sinuses to each other and to the nasal cavity. *Inset* is a lateral view of the position of the sinuses.

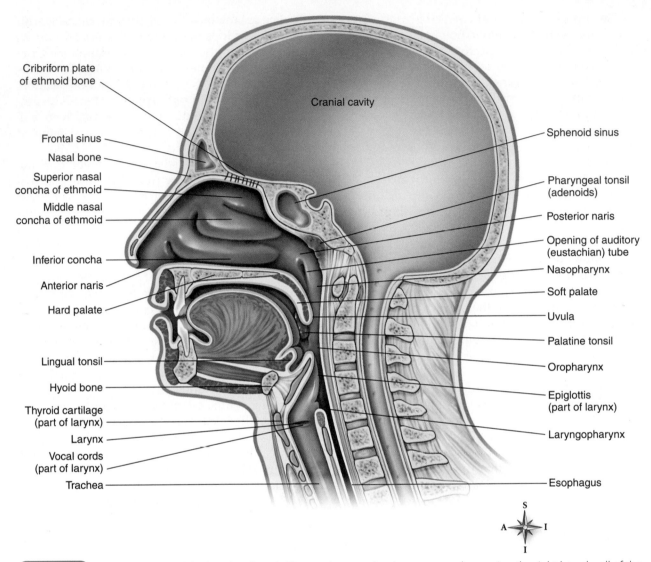

Cribriform plate
of ethmoid bone

Cranial cavity

Frontal sinus

Nasal bone

Superior nasal
concha of ethmoid

Middle nasal
concha of ethmoid

Inferior concha

Anterior naris

Hard palate

Lingual tonsil

Hyoid bone

Thyroid cartilage
(part of larynx)

Larynx

Vocal cords
(part of larynx)

Trachea

Sphenoid sinus

Pharyngeal tonsil
(adenoids)

Posterior naris

Opening of auditory
(eustachian) tube

Nasopharynx

Soft palate

Uvula

Palatine tonsil

Oropharynx

Epiglottis
(part of larynx)

Laryngopharynx

Esophagus

FIGURE 14-4 **Sagittal section of the head and neck.** The nasal septum has been removed, exposing the right lateral wall of the nasal cavity so that the nasal conchae can be seen. Note also the divisions of the pharynx and the position of the tonsils.

way of the larynx; food enters it from the mouth and leaves it by way of the esophagus. The right and left **auditory,** or **eustachian** (yoo-STAY-shun), **tubes** open into the nasopharynx; they connect the middle ears with the nasopharynx (see Figure 14-4). This connection permits equalization of air pressure between the middle and the exterior ear. The lining of the auditory tubes is continuous with the lining of the nasopharynx and middle ear. Thus, just as sinus infections can develop from colds in which the nasal mucosa is inflamed, middle ear infections can develop from inflammation of the nasopharynx.

Masses of lymphatic tissue called **tonsils** are embedded in the mucous membrane of the pharynx (see p. 307). The **pharyngeal** (fah-RIN-jee-al) **tonsils,** or **adenoids** (AD-eh-noydz), are in the nasopharynx. The **palatine tonsils** are located in the oropharynx (see Figure 14-4). Both tonsils are generally removed in a **tonsillectomy** (tahn-sih-LEK-toh-mee). This procedure, with its potentially serious complications, is now performed only reluctantly, and the number of tonsillectomies reported each year continues to decrease. Physicians now recognize the value of lymphatic tissue in the body defense mechanism and delay removal of the tonsils—even in cases of inflammation, or **tonsillitis**—unless antibiotic treatment is ineffective. When the pharyngeal tonsils become swollen, they are referred to as *adenoids*. Such swelling caused by infections may make it difficult or impossible for air to travel from the nose into the throat. In these cases the individual is forced to breathe through his or her mouth.

LARYNX

The **larynx,** or voice box, is located just below the pharynx. It is composed of several pieces of cartilage. You know the largest of these (the *thyroid cartilage*) as the "Adam's apple" (Figure 14-5).

Two short fibrous bands, the **vocal cords,** stretch across the interior of the larynx. Muscles that attach to the larynx cartilages can pull on these cords in such a way that they become tense or relaxed. When they are tense, the voice is high pitched; when they are relaxed, it is low pitched.

The space between the vocal cords is the **glottis.** Another cartilage, the **epiglottis** (ep-i-GLOT-is) partially covers the opening of the larynx (see Figure 14-5). The epiglottis acts like a trapdoor, closing off the larynx during swallowing and preventing food from entering the trachea.

TRACHEA

The **trachea,** or windpipe, is a tube about 11 cm (4.5 inches) long that extends from the larynx in the neck to the bronchi in the chest cavity (Figures 14-1 and 14-6). The trachea performs a number of vital functions. Certainly one of its most important roles is to furnish part of the open passageway through which air can reach the lungs from the outside. Additional functional significance is related to the fact that the trachea is lined by the typical respiratory mucosa, which contains numerous mucus-producing glands and is covered by cilia. The glands help produce part of

FIGURE 14-5 **The larynx. A,** Sagittal section of the larynx. **B,** Superior view of the larynx. **C,** Photograph of the larynx taken with an endoscope (optical device) inserted through the mouth and pharynx to the epiglottis.

Posterior view

- Trachea
- Primary bronchii
- Secondary bronchi
- Diaphragm
- Hyaline cartilage (tracheal ring)
- Smooth muscle
- Fibrous connective tissue
- Connective tissue covering
- Mucous coat

(Inset labels)
- Mucous coat
- Smooth muscle
- Cartilage
- Connective tissue

FIGURE 14-6 **Cross section of the trachea.** *Inset* at top shows from where the section was cut. The scanning electron micrograph shows the tip of one of the C-shaped cartilage rings.

the blanket of mucus that is continually moved by the beating cilia in one direction—upward and toward the pharynx—as part of the "mucociliary escalator" mechanism. Therefore, in addition to its role in air distribution, the trachea serves a protective function by production and movement of mucus important in trapping and eliminating airborne contaminants.

By pushing with your fingers against your throat about an inch above the sternum, you can feel the shape of the trachea or windpipe. Only if you use considerable force can you squeeze it closed. Nature has taken precautions to keep this lifeline open. Its framework is made of an almost noncollapsible material—15 or 20 C-shaped rings of cartilage placed one above the other with only a little soft tissue between them (see Figure 14-6).

Despite the structural safeguard of cartilage rings, closing of the trachea sometimes occurs. A tumor or an infection may enlarge the lymph nodes of the neck so much that they squeeze the trachea shut, or a person may aspirate (breathe in) a piece of food or something else that blocks the windpipe. Because air has no other way to get to the lungs, complete tracheal obstruction causes death in a matter of minutes. Suffocation from all causes, including choking on food and other substances caught in the trachea, kills more than 4,000

people each year and is the fifth major cause of accidental death in the United States.

> **QUICK CHECK**
> 1. What are the paranasal sinuses? What is their role?
> 2. What are the three divisions of the pharynx?
> 3. What is the scientific term for the voice box?
> 4. What keeps the trachea from collapsing?

BRONCHI, BRONCHIOLES, AND ALVEOLI

Recall that one way to picture the thousands of air tubes that make up the lungs is to think of an upside-down tree. The trachea is the main trunk of this tree; the right bronchus (the tube leading into the right lung) and the left bronchus (the tube leading into the left lung) are the trachea's first branches, or **primary bronchi.** In each lung, they branch into smaller, or **secondary, bronchi** (*singular,* bronchus) whose walls, as with those of the trachea and bronchi, are kept open by rings of cartilage for air passage. These bronchi divide into smaller and smaller tubes, ultimately branching into tiny tubes whose walls contain only smooth muscle. These very small passageways are called **bronchioles.** The bronchioles subdivide into microscopic tubes called **alveolar ducts,** which resemble the main stem of a bunch of grapes (Figure 14-7). Each alveolar duct ends in several **alveolar sacs,** each of which resembles a cluster of grapes, and the wall of each alveolar sac is made up of numerous **alveoli,** each of which resembles a single grape.

Alveoli are very effective in promoting the rapid and effective exchange of oxygen and carbon dioxide between blood circulating through the lung capillaries and alveolar air. Once again, structure and function are closely related. Two characteristics about the structure of alveoli assist in diffusion and make them able to perform this function admirably. First, the wall of each alveolus is made up of a single layer of simple squamous epithelial cells—and so are the walls of the capillaries that surround and lie in contact with them. This means that, between the blood in the capillaries and the air in each alveolus, there is a barrier less than 1 micron thick. This extremely thin barrier is called the **respiratory membrane** (Figure 14-8). Second, there

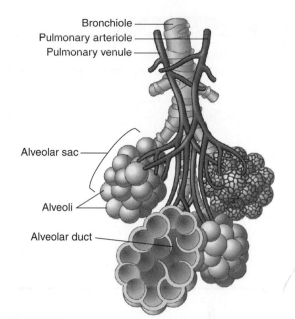

FIGURE 14-7   **Alveoli.** Bronchioles subdivide to form tiny tubes called *alveolar ducts*, which end in clusters of alveoli called *alveolar sacs.*

FIGURE 14-8   **The gas-exchange structure of the lung.** Each alveolus is continually ventilated with fresh air. *Inset* shows a magnified view of the respiratory membrane composed of the alveolar wall (surfactant, epithelial cells, and basement membrane), interstitial fluid, and the wall of a pulmonary capillary (basement membrane and endothelial cells). The gases, CO_2 (carbon dioxide) and O_2 (oxygen), diffuse across the respiratory membrane.

Infant Respiratory Distress Syndrome

Infant respiratory distress syndrome, or **IRDS,** is a serious, life-threatening condition that often affects prematurely born infants or those who weigh less than 2.2 kg (5 lb) at birth. IRDS is the leading cause of death among premature infants in the United States, claiming more than 5,000 premature babies each year. The disease, characterized by a lack of **surfactant** in the alveolar air sacs, affects 50,000 babies annually.

Surfactant is manufactured by specialized cells in the walls of the alveoli. Surfactant reduces the surface tension of the fluid on the free surface of the alveolar walls and permits easy movement of air into and out of the lungs. The ability of the body to manufacture this important substance is not fully developed until shortly before birth—normally about 38 weeks after conception.

In newborn infants who are unable to manufacture surfactant, many air sacs collapse during expiration because of the increased surface tension. The effort required to reinflate these collapsed alveoli is much greater than that needed to reinflate normal alveoli with adequate surfactant. The baby soon develops labored breathing, and symptoms of respiratory distress appear shortly after birth.

In the past, treatment of IRDS was limited to keeping the alveoli open so that delivery and exchange of oxygen and carbon dioxide could occur. To accomplish this, a tube was inserted into the respiratory tract, and oxygen-rich air was delivered under sufficient pressure to keep the alveoli from collapsing at the end of expiration. A newer treatment involves delivering air under pressure and applying prepared surfactant directly into the baby's airways by means of a tube.

are millions of alveoli. This means that together they make an enormous surface (approximately 100 square meters, an area many times larger than the surface area of the entire body) where large amounts of oxygen and carbon dioxide can rapidly be exchanged. The surface of the respiratory membrane inside each alveolus is covered by a substance called **surfactant** (sur-FAK-tant). This important substance helps reduce surface tension in the alveoli and keeps them from collapsing as air moves in and out during respiration. Note the difference in appearance between the surfactant-producing cells and the flattened alveolar epithelial cells shown in Figure 14-8. Do not confuse the *respiratory membrane* separating air in the alveoli from blood in the surrounding pulmonary capillaries with the *respiratory mucosa* (see Figure 14-2) that lines the tubes of the respiratory tree.

 To learn more about the respiratory membrane, go to AnimationDirect on your CD-ROM.

LUNGS AND PLEURA

The **lungs** are fairly large organs. Note in Figure 14-9 that the right lung has three lobes and the left lung has two. Figure 14-9 shows the relationship of the lungs to the rib cage at the end of a normal expiration. The narrow, superior position of each lung, up under the collarbone, is the apex; the

broad, inferior portion resting on the diaphragm is the base.

The **pleura** covers the outer surface of the lungs and lines the inner surface of the rib cage. The pleura resembles other serous membranes in structure and function. As with the peritoneum or pericardium, the pleura is an extensive, thin, moist, slippery membrane. It lines a large, closed cavity of the body and covers the organs located within it. The parietal pleura lines the walls of the thoracic cavity; the visceral pleura covers the lungs, and the intrapleural space lies between the two pleural membranes (Figure 14-10). **Pleurisy** is an inflammation of the pleura that causes pain when the pleural membranes rub together.

Normally the intrapleural space contains just enough fluid to make both portions of the pleura moist and slippery and able to glide easily against each other as the lungs expand and deflate with each breath. **Pneumothorax** (noo-moh-THOH-raks) is the presence of air in the intrapleural space on one side of the chest. The additional air increases the pressure on the lung on that side and causes it to collapse. While collapsed, the lung does not function in breathing.

QUICK CHECK

1. What are bronchi? What is their role?
2. What is the function of the alveoli?
3. Can you describe the structure and function of the pleura?

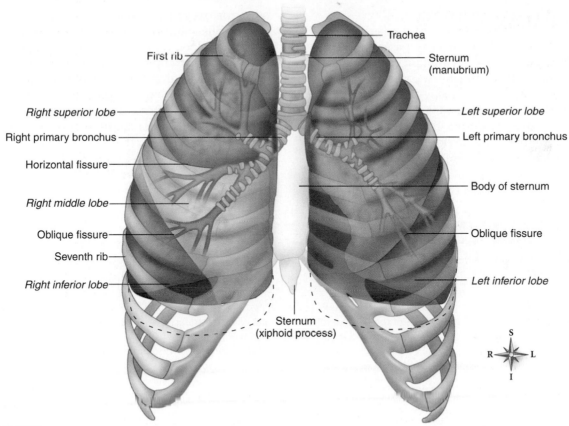

FIGURE 14-9   **Lungs.** The trachea is an airway that branches to form an inverted tree of bronchi and bronchioles. Note that the right lung has three lobes and the left lung has two lobes.

FIGURE 14-10   **Lungs and pleura.** *Inset* shows from where in the body this transverse section of the thorax was cut. A serous membrane lines the thoracic wall (parietal pleura) and then folds inward near the bronchi to cover the lung (visceral pleura). The intrapleural space contains a small amount of serous pleural fluid.

RESPIRATION

Respiration means exchange of gases (oxygen and carbon dioxide) between a living organism and its environment. If the organism consists of only one cell, gases can move directly between it and the environment. If, however, the organism consists of billions of cells, as do our bodies, most of its cells are too far from the air for a direct exchange of gases. To overcome this difficulty, a pair of organs— the lungs—provides a place where air and a circulating fluid (blood) can come close enough to each other for oxygen to move out of the air into the blood while at the same time carbon dioxide moves out of the blood into air. Breathing, or **pulmonary ventilation,** is the process that moves air into and out of the lungs. It makes possible the exchange of gases between air in the lungs and in the blood. This exchange is often called *external respiration.* In addition, exchange of gases occurs between the blood and the cells of the body—a process called *internal respiration.* **Cellular respiration** refers to the actual use of oxygen by cells in the process of metabolism, which is discussed in Chapter 16.

Research, Issues, & Trends

Lung Volume Reduction Surgery

Lung volume reduction surgery (LVRS) is a "treatment of last resort" for severe cases of emphysema. It involves the removal of 20% to 30% of each lung. Diseased tissue is generally removed from the upper, or apical, areas of the superior lobes. Evidence from a number of large clinical trials has now shown that the LVRS procedure may benefit or at least help stabilize selected emphysema patients whose lung function continues to decline despite aggressive pulmonary rehabilitation efforts and other, more conservative forms of treatment.

More than 2 million Americans, who are older than age 50 and current or former smokers, have emphysema—a major cause of disability and death in the United States. Emphysema is one of a number of conditions classified as a **chronic obstructive pulmonary disease,** or COPD. Although lung damage caused by emphysema is irreversible, in some cases the disease may be halted or its progression slowed by LVRS. In the end stages of this chronic disease, breathing becomes labored as the lungs fill with large, ir-

regular spaces resulting from the enlargement and rupture of many alveoli (see illustration). The LVRS procedure removes part of the diseased lung tissue and increases available space in the pleural cavities. As a result, the diaphragm and other respiratory muscles can more effectively move air into and out of the remaining lung tissue, thereby improving pulmonary function and making breathing easier.

LVRS may reduce the need for lung transplantation procedures and augment the effectiveness of such supporting medical treatments as nutritional supplementation and exercise training in the treatment of selected late-stage emphysema patients. Newer and less invasive techniques involving smaller incisions and specialized video equipment inserted into the thoracic cavity (video-assisted thoracic surgery) are now being used for many LVRS procedures. As a result, the relatively long hospital stays and home recovery periods previously required after more traditional openchest surgery have been shortened.

A **B**

Emphysema. The effects of emphysema can be seen in these scanning electron micrographs of lung tissue. **A,** Normal lung with many small alveoli. **B,** Lung tissue affected by emphysema. Notice that the alveoli have merged into larger air spaces, thereby reducing the surface area available for gas exchange.

Mechanics of Breathing

Pulmonary ventilation, or breathing, has two phases. **Inspiration,** or inhalation, moves air into the lungs, and **expiration,** or exhalation, moves air out of the lungs. The lungs are enclosed within the thoracic cavity. Thus changes in the shape and size of the thoracic cavity result in changes in the air pressure within that cavity and in the lungs. This difference in air pressure causes the movement of air into and out of the lungs. Air moves from an area where pressure is high to an area where pressure is lower. Respiratory muscles are responsible for the changes in the shape of the thoracic cavity that cause the air movements involved in breathing.

Inspiration

Inspiration occurs when the chest cavity enlarges. As the thorax enlarges, the lungs expand along with it, and air rushes into them and down into the alveoli. Muscles of respiration that are classified as **inspiratory muscles** include the **diaphragm** (DYE-ah-fram) and the external intercostals. The diaphragm is the dome-shaped muscle separating the abdominal cavity from the thoracic cavity. The diaphragm flattens out when it contracts during inspiration. Instead of protruding up into the chest cavity, it moves down toward the abdominal cavity. Thus the contraction or flattening of the diaphragm makes the chest cavity longer from top to bottom. The diaphragm is the most important muscle of inspiration. Nerve impulses passing through the **phrenic nerve** stimulate the diaphragm to contract. The external intercostal muscles are located between the ribs. When they contract, they enlarge the thorax by increasing the size of the cavity from front to back and from side to side. Contraction of the inspiratory muscles increases the volume of the thoracic cavity and reduces the air pressure within it, drawing air into the lungs (Figure 14-11).

Expiration

Quiet expiration is ordinarily a passive process that begins when the inspiratory muscles relax. The thoracic cavity then returns to its smaller size. The elastic nature of lung tissue also causes these organs to "recoil" and decrease in size as air leaves the alveoli and flows outward through the respiratory passageways. When we speak, sing, or do heavy work, we may need more forceful expiration to increase the rate and depth of ventilation. During more forceful expiration, the **expiratory muscles** (internal intercostals and abdominal muscles) contract. When contracted, the internal intercostal muscles depress the rib cage and decrease the front-to-back size of the thorax. Contraction of the abdominal muscles pushes the abdominal organs against the underside of the diaphragm, thus elevating it and making it more "dome shaped." The result is to further shorten or decrease the top-to-bottom size of the thoracic cavity. As the thoracic cavity decreases in size, the air pressure within it increases and air flows out of the lungs (see Figure 14-11).

FIGURE 14-11 **Mechanics of breathing.** During *inspiration*, the diaphragm contracts, increasing the volume of the thoracic cavity. This increase in volume results in a decrease in pressure, which causes air to rush into the lungs. During *expiration*, the diaphragm returns to an upward position, reducing the volume in the thoracic cavity. Air pressure increases then, forcing air out of the lungs. *Insets* show the classic model in which a jar represents the rib cage, a rubber sheet represents the diaphragm, and a balloon represents the lungs.

Exchange of Gases in Lungs (External Respiration)

Blood pumped from the right ventricle of the heart enters the pulmonary artery and eventually enters the lungs. It then flows through the thousands of tiny pulmonary capillaries that are in close proximity to the air-filled alveoli (see Figure 14-1). **External respiration,** or the exchange of gases between the blood and alveolar air, occurs by diffusion.

The amounts or concentrations of some blood substances are measured in terms of weight. Reporting how many milligrams of a particular substance are present in 100 mL of blood (mg/dL) is one example. However, the concentration of a particular gas in air or within the blood is expressed as the *pressure* exerted by that gas and is reported in millimeters of mercury (mm Hg). Recall from Chapter 12 that blood pressure levels are also reported in mm Hg. Several different gases are present in both air and blood. The total pressure of all gases present in an air or blood sample is, of course, the sum of the pressures exerted by each of the gases present. Because the pressure of the so-called *respiratory gases*—oxygen (O_2) and carbon dioxide (CO_2)—in air or blood constitutes only a part of the total pressure present, their concentration is reported as a **partial pressure (P).** The symbol used to designate partial pressure is the capital letter P preceding the chemical symbol for the gas. For respiratory gases the symbols Po_2 and Pco_2 are used. Measurement of the partial pressure of a number of blood gases is important in the diagnosis and treatment of many disease conditions.

Diffusion is a passive process resulting in movement down a concentration, or partial pressure, gradient (i.e., substances move from an area of high concentration or partial pressure to an area of lower concentration or partial pressure of the diffusing substance). O_2 is continually removed from the blood and used by the body cells. By the time blood flows into the pulmonary capillaries, it has a Po_2 of about 40 mm Hg. Because alveolar air is rich in oxygen (Pco_2 100 mm Hg), diffusion causes movement of oxygen from the area of high partial pressure (alveolar air) to the area of lower partial pressure (capillary blood). Put another way, oxygen diffuses "down" its partial pressure gradient.

Diffusion of carbon dioxide also occurs between blood in pulmonary capillaries and alveolar air. Blood flowing through the pulmonary capil-laries is high in CO_2, having a Pco_2 of 46 mm Hg. The Pco_2 of alveolar air is about 40 mm Hg. Therefore diffusion of CO_2 results in its movement from an area of high partial pressure in the pulmonary capillaries to an area of lower partial pressure in alveolar air. Then from the alveoli, carbon dioxide leaves the body in expired air (Figure 14-12).

Exchange of Gases in Tissues (Internal Respiration)

The exchange of gases that occurs between blood in systemic capillaries and the body cells is called internal respiration. As you would expect, the direction of movement of oxygen and carbon dioxide during internal respiration is just the opposite of that noted in the exchange that occurs during external respiration, when gases are exchanged between the blood in the pulmonary capillaries and the air in alveoli. During the process of internal respiration, oxygen molecules move rapidly out of the blood through the systemic capillary membrane into the interstitial fluid and on into the cells that make up the tissues. At the same time, carbon dioxide molecules leave the cells, diffuse through the interstitial fluid and then enter the systemic capillaries, eventually being transported to the lungs for elimination from the body. The oxygen is used by the cells in their metabolic activities. Diffusion results in the movement of oxygen from an area of high partial pressure in the systemic capillaries (Po_2 100 mm Hg) to an area of lower partial pressure (Po_2 40 mm Hg) in the cells where it is needed. Diffusion is also responsible for the movement of CO_2 from an area of high partial pressure in the cells (Pco_2 46 mm Hg) to an area of lower partial pressure (Pco_2 43 mm Hg) in the systemic capillaries. Simply stated, during internal respiration, oxygenated blood enters systemic capillaries and is changed into deoxygenated blood as it flows through them. In the process of losing oxygen, the waste product carbon dioxide is picked up and transported to the lungs for removal from the body.

Blood Transportation of Gases

Blood transports the respiratory gases, oxygen and carbon dioxide, either in a dissolved state or combined with other chemicals. Immediately on entering the blood, both oxygen and carbon

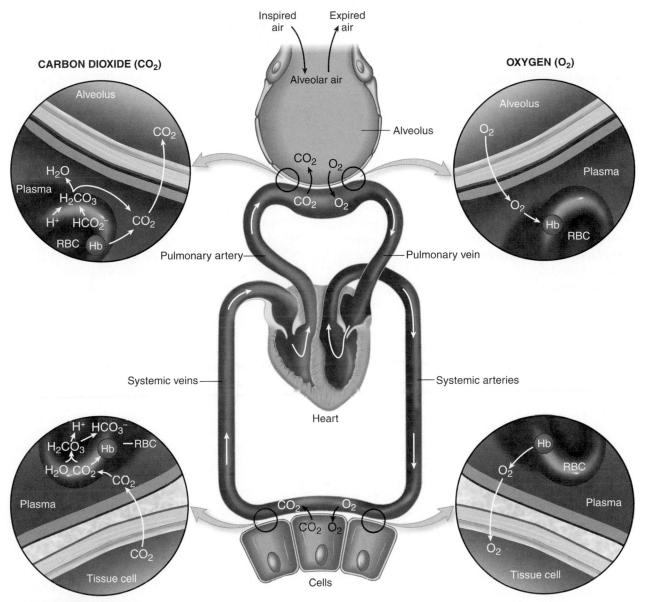

FIGURE 14-12 **Exchange of gases in pulmonary and systemic capillaries.** The *right insets* show O_2 diffusing out of alveolar air into blood and associating with hemoglobin (Hb) in pulmonary capillaries to form oxyhemoglobin. In systemic capillaries, oxyhemoglobin dissociates, releasing O_2, which diffuses from the red blood cells (RBCs) and then crosses the capillary wall to reach the tissue cells. As the *left insets* show, CO_2 diffuses in the opposite direction (into RBCs), and some of it associates with Hb to form carbaminohemoglobin. However, most CO_2 combines with water to form carbonic acid (H_2CO_3), which dissociates to form H^+ and HCO_3^- (bicarbonate) ions. Back in the pulmonary capillaries, CO_2 dissociates from the bicarbonate and carbaminohemoglobin molecules and diffuses out of blood into alveolar air.

dioxide dissolve in the plasma, but because fluids can hold only small amounts of gas in solution, most of the oxygen and carbon dioxide rapidly form a chemical union with hemoglobin, another plasma protein found in the blood, or water. Once gas molecules are bound to another molecule, their plasma concentration (partial pressure) decreases and more gas can diffuse into the plasma. In this way, comparatively large volumes of the gases can be transported.

Transport of Oxygen

Only very limited amounts of oxygen can be dissolved in the blood. Of the total amount of oxygen that blood can transport, about 20.4 mL in 100 mL of blood, only about 1.5% or 0.3 mL is actually dissolved. Many times that amount, about 21.1 mL, combines with the hemoglobin (Hb) in 100 mL of blood to form **oxyhemoglobin** (ahk-see-hee-moh-GLOH-bin) (HbO$_2$) so that it can be carried to the tissues and used by the body cells.

To combine with hemoglobin, oxygen must first diffuse into the RBCs to form oxyhemoglobin. Hemoglobin molecules are large proteins that contain four iron-containing **heme** components, each of which is capable of combining with an oxygen molecule. In many ways each hemoglobin molecule acts as a kind of "oxygen sponge." Oxygen associates with hemoglobin rapidly—so rapidly, in fact, that about 97% of the blood's hemoglobin has united with oxygen and become "oxygenated blood" by the time it leaves the pulmonary capillaries to return to the heart. Oxygenated blood is found in the systemic arteries and pulmonary veins. Normally, oxygenated blood is 97% "saturated." So-called deoxygenated blood, found in the systemic veins and pulmonary arteries, is about 75% saturated with oxygen. The difference in oxygen saturation results from the release of oxygen from oxyhemoglobin to supply the body cells. Therefore the chemical combination of oxygen and hemoglobin is said to be "reversible" with oxyhemoglobin formation or oxygen release dependent on the partial pressure of oxygen driving the reaction.

Summing up, we can say that oxygen travels in two forms: (1) as dissolved O$_2$ in the plasma and (2) as a combination of O$_2$ and hemoglobin (oxyhemoglobin). Of these two forms of transport, oxyhemoglobin carries the most of the total oxygen transported by the blood.

Transport of Carbon Dioxide

Carbon dioxide is a by-product of cellular metabolism and plays an important and necessary role in regulating the pH of body fluids. However, if it accumulates in the body beyond normal limits (40 to 50 mm Hg in venous blood), it can quickly become toxic. Elimination of excess CO$_2$ from the body occurs when it enters the alveoli and is expelled during expiration. For this to occur, CO$_2$ must be transported in the blood to the lungs in one of three forms:

1. As **dissolved carbon dioxide (CO$_2$).** About 10% of the total amount of carbon dioxide is carried in the dissolved form. It is this dissolved CO$_2$ that produces the Pco$_2$ of blood plasma.

2. As **carbaminohemoglobin** (karb-am-ee-no-hee-moh-GLOH-bin). About 20% of the total CO$_2$ transported in the blood is in the form of carbaminohemoglobin. It is formed by the union of carbon dioxide, hemoglobin, and certain other plasma proteins. The formation of this compound is accelerated by an increase in Pco$_2$ and slowed by a decrease in Pco$_2$.

3. As **bicarbonate ions** (HCO$_3^-$). About 70% of the total CO$_2$ transported in the blood is carried in the form of bicarbonate ions. When CO$_2$ dissolves in water (as in blood plasma), some of the CO$_2$ molecules associate with water (H$_2$O) to form carbonic acid (H$_2$CO$_3$). Once formed, some of the H$_2$CO$_3$ molecules dissociate to form hydrogen (H$^+$) and bicarbonate (HCO$_3^-$) ions. The speed of this process is quite slow when it occurs in the plasma, but the rate of reaction increases dramatically within RBCs because of the presence of an enzyme called *carbonic anhydrase* (kar-BON-ik an-HYE-drays). The reaction is summarized by the following chemical equation:

$$\underset{\substack{\text{Carbon} \\ \text{dioxide}}}{CO_2} + \underset{\text{Water}}{H_2O} \xrightleftharpoons[]{\text{Carbonic anhydrase}} \underset{\substack{\text{Carbonic} \\ \text{acid}}}{H_2CO_3}$$

$$\Updownarrow$$

$$\underset{\substack{\text{Hydrogen} \\ \text{ion}}}{H^+} + \underset{\substack{\text{Bicarbonate} \\ \text{ion}}}{HCO_3^-}$$

Note that the arrows go in both directions. This indicates that the reaction is *reversible*—it can go in either direction. If bicarbonate is being formed, CO$_2$ molecules entering into plasma can continually be removed from the blood and transported to the lungs. And, when the process is reversed in the lungs, CO$_2$ can be released to enter the alveolar air and then be exhaled.

 To learn more about gas exchange, go to AnimationDirect on your CD-ROM.

Volumes of Air Exchanged in Pulmonary Ventilation

A special device called a **spirometer** is used to measure the amount of air exchanged in breathing. Figure 14-13 illustrates the various pulmonary volumes, which can be measured as a subject breathes into a spirometer. We take 500 mL (about a pint) of air into our lungs with each normal inspiration and expel it with each normal expiration. Because this amount comes and goes regularly like the tides of the sea, it is referred to as the **tidal volume (TV).** The largest amount of air that we can breathe out in one expiration is known as the **vital capacity (VC).** In young men, this is normally about 4,800 mL. Tidal volume and vital capacity are frequently measured in patients with lung disease such as emphysema or heart problems, conditions

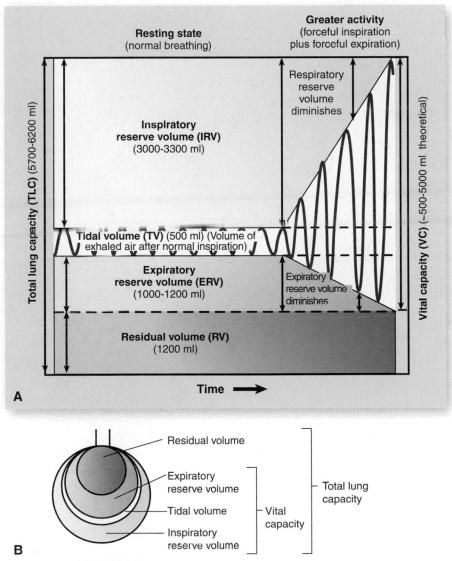

FIGURE 14-13 **Pulmonary ventilation volumes.** The chart in **A** shows a tracing like that produced with a spirometer. The diagram in **B** shows the pulmonary volumes as relative proportions of an inflated balloon (see Figure 14-11). During normal, quiet breathing, about 500 mL of air is moved into and out of the respiratory tract, an amount called the *tidal volume.* During forceful breathing (like that during and after heavy exercise), an extra 3,300 mL can be inspired (the inspiratory reserve volume), and an extra 1,000 mL or so can be expired (the expiratory reserve volume). The largest volume of air that can be moved in and out during ventilation is called the *vital capacity.* Air that remains in the respiratory tract after a forceful expiration is called the *residual volume.*

Health and Well-Being

Maximum Oxygen Consumption

Exercise physiologists use **maximum oxygen consumption** ($VO_{2\,max}$) as a predictor of a person's capacity to do aerobic exercise. An individual's $VO_{2\,max}$ represents the amount of oxygen taken up by the lungs, transported to the tissues, and used to do work. $VO_{2\,max}$ is determined largely by hereditary factors, but aerobic (endurance) training can increase it by as much as 35%. Many endurance athletes are now using $VO_{2\,max}$ measurements to help them determine and then maintain their peak condition.

To help supply cells with more oxygen when they are doing more work, automatic adjustments occur not only in respirations but also in circulation. Most notably, the heart beats faster and harder and therefore pumps more blood throughout the body each minute. This means that the millions of RBCs make more round trips between the lungs and tissues each minute and so deliver more oxygen per minute to tissue cells.

Working cells not only require more oxygen, they also produce more waste products such as carbon dioxide and certain metabolic acids. The increase in respirations during exercise shows us how the body automatically regulates its vital functions. By increasing the rate and depth of respiration, we can adjust to the varying demands for increased oxygen while increasing the elimination of metabolic waste products in expired air to maintain homeostasis.

Normal respiration depends on proper functioning of the muscles of respiration. These muscles are stimulated by nervous impulses that originate in **respiratory control centers** located in the medulla and pons of the brain. These centers are in turn regulated by a number of inputs from receptors located in varying areas of the body. These receptors can sense the need for changing the rate or depth of respirations to maintain homeostasis. Certain receptors sense carbon dioxide or oxygen levels, whereas others sense blood acid levels or the amount of stretch in lung tissues. The two most important control centers are in the medulla and are called the **inspiratory center** and the **expiratory center.** Centers in the pons have a modifying function. Under rest conditions, neurons in the inspiratory and expiratory centers "fire" at a rate that will produce a normal breathing rate of about 12 to 18 breaths a minute.

The depth and rate of respiration can be influenced by many "inputs" to the respiratory control centers from other areas of the brain or from specialized receptors located outside of the central nervous system (see Figure 14-14).

Clinical Application

Sudden Infant Death Syndrome

Sudden infant death syndrome (SIDS) is the third-ranking cause of infant death and accounts for about 1 in 9 of the nearly 30,000 infant deaths reported each year in the United States. Sometimes called "crib-death," SIDS occurs most frequently in babies with no obvious medical problems who are younger than 3 months of age. The exact cause of death can seldom be determined, even after extensive testing and autopsy.

SIDS occurs at a higher rate in African American and Native American babies than in white, Hispanic, or Asian infants, although the reasons remain a mystery. Regardless of infant ethnicity, recent data suggest that certain precautions, such as having babies sleep only on their backs and keeping cribs free of pillows or plush toys that might partially cover the nose or mouth, may reduce the incidence of SIDS. Also important is the elimination of smoking during pregnancy and protecting infants from exposure to "secondhand" cigarette smoke after birth. Although the exact cause of SIDS remains unknown, genetic defects involving the structure and function of the respiratory system or unusual physiological responses to common flu or cold viruses may also play a role in this tragic problem.

that often lead to abnormal volumes of air being moved in and out of the lungs.

Observe the area in Figure 14-13 that represents the **expiratory reserve volume (ERV).** This is the amount of air that can be forcibly exhaled after expiring the tidal volume. Compare this with the area in Figure 14-13 that represents the **inspiratory reserve volume (IRV).** The IRV is the amount of air that can be forcibly inspired over and above a normal inspiration. As the tidal volume increases, the ERV and IRV decrease. Note in Figure 14-13 that VC is the total of tidal volume, inspiratory reserve volume, and expiratory reserve volume—or expressed in another way: VC = TV + IRV + ERV. **Residual volume (RV)** is simply the air that remains in the lungs after the most forceful expiration.

> ### ✓ QUICK CHECK
>
> 1. How does the diaphragm operate during inspiration? During expiration?
> 2. In what form does oxygen travel in the blood? What form of carbon dioxide?
> 3. What is the vital capacity? How is it measured?

REGULATION OF RESPIRATION

We know that the body uses oxygen to obtain energy for the work it has to do. The more work the body does, the more oxygen it needs to be delivered to its millions of cells. One way this is accomplished is by increasing the rate and depth of respirations. Although we may take only 12 to 18 breaths a minute when we are not moving about, we take considerably more than that when we are exercising. Not only do we take more breaths, but our tidal volume also increases.

Cerebral Cortex

The cerebral cortex in the brain can influence respiration by modifying the rate at which neurons "fire" in the inspiratory and expiratory centers of the medulla. In other words, an individual may voluntarily speed up or slow down the breathing rate or greatly change the pattern of respiration during activities. This ability permits us to change respiratory patterns and even to hold our breath for short periods to accommodate activities such as speaking, eating,

or underwater swimming. This voluntary control of respiration, however, has limits. As discussed in a later section, other factors such as blood carbon dioxide levels are much more powerful in controlling respiration than is conscious control. Regardless of cerebral intent to the contrary, we resume breathing when our bodies sense the need for more oxygen or if carbon dioxide levels increase to certain levels.

Reflexes That Influence Respiration

Chemoreflexes

Chemoreceptors (kee-moh-ree-SEP-torz) located in the **carotid** and **aortic bodies** are specialized receptors that are sensitive to increases in blood carbon dioxide level and decreases in blood oxygen level. They also can sense and respond to increasing blood acid levels. The carotid body receptors are found at the point where the common carotid arteries divide, and the aortic bodies are small clusters of chemosensitive cells that lie adjacent to the aortic arch near the heart (Figure 14-14). When stimulated by increasing levels of blood carbon dioxide, decreasing oxygen levels, or increasing

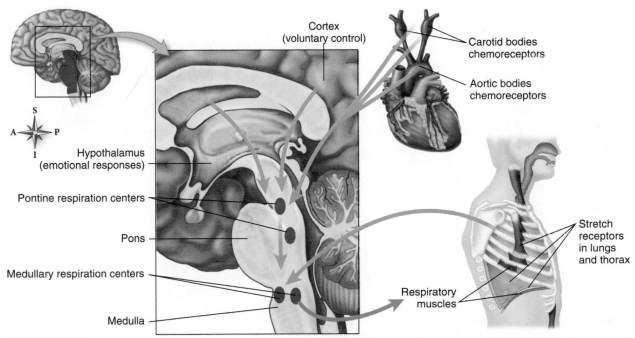

FIGURE 14-14   **Regulation of respiration.** Respiratory control centers in the brainstem control the basic rate and depth of breathing. The brainstem also receives input from other parts of the body: information from chemoreceptors and stretch receptors can alter the basic breathing pattern, as can emotional and sensory input. Despite these controls, the cerebral cortex can override the "automatic" control of breathing to some extent to accomplish activities such as singing or blowing up a balloon. *Green arrows* show how regulatory information flows into the respiratory control centers. The *purple arrow* shows the flow of regulatory information from the control centers to the respiratory muscles that drive breathing.

blood acidity, these receptors send nerve impulses to the respiratory regulatory centers that in turn modify respiratory rates. The blood P_{CO_2} level is the most powerful stimulus driving respiration.

Pulmonary Stretch Reflexes

Specialized stretch receptors in the lungs are located throughout the pulmonary airways and in the alveoli (see Figure 14-14). Nervous impulses generated by these receptors influence the normal pattern of breathing and protect the respiratory system from excess stretching caused by harmful overinflation. When the tidal volume of air has been inspired, the lungs are expanded enough to stimulate stretch receptors that then send inhibitory impulses to the inspiratory center. Relaxation of inspiratory muscles occurs, and expiration follows. After expiration, the lungs are sufficiently deflated to inhibit the stretch receptors, and inspiration is then allowed to start again.

TYPES OF BREATHING

Several terms are used to describe breathing patterns. **Eupnea** (YOOP-nee-ah), for example, refers to a normal respiratory rate. During eupnea, the need for oxygen and carbon dioxide exchange is being met, and the individual is usually not aware of the breathing pattern. The terms **hyperventilation** and **hypoventilation** describe very rapid and deep or slow and shallow respirations, respectively. Hyperventilation sometimes results from a conscious voluntary effort preceding exertion or from psychological factors—"hysterical hyperventilation." **Dyspnea** (DISP-nee-ah) refers to labored or difficult breathing and is often associated with hypoventilation. If breathing stops completely for a brief period, regardless of cause, it is called **apnea** (AP-nee-ah). *Sleep apnea* is a condition that results in brief but often frequent stops in breathing during sleep. It is often caused by enlarged tonsil tissue and may necessitate tonsillectomy. Failure to resume breathing after a prolonged period of apnea is called **respiratory arrest.**

> **QUICK CHECK**
> 1. Where are the respiratory control centers located?
> 2. What is a chemoreceptor? How does it influence breathing?
> 3. What is hyperventilation? Hypoventilation?

Science Application

Respiratory Medicine
Henry Heimlich (b. 1920)

The name of American physician Henry Heimlich is known to many people around the world because of the Heimlich maneuver, which he developed in 1974 to save the lives of people who are choking. What many do not know is that Heimlich has made important breakthroughs throughout his life. For example, after witnessing a soldier die after being shot in the chest in 1945, he went on to develop the Heimlich chest drain valve that drains blood and air out of the chest. In 1980, he developed a tiny tube called the Heimlich MicroTrach™, which can be inserted into the trachea under local anesthesia and used in oxygen therapy (see Clinical Application: Oxygen Therapy box, p. 326). Later, he developed a method for teaching stroke victims who were fed through a tube to swallow again.

Although modified to reflect current knowledge and medical practice, many of Heimlich's techniques and medical instrument discoveries are still being used nearly 40 years after he first introduced the lifesaving procedure that bears his name. Today, countless physicians, nurses, respiratory therapists, emergency medical technicians, paramedics, police, firefighters, and even ordinary citizens trained in first aid continue to benefit from the work of this pioneering physician.

OUTLINE SUMMARY

STRUCTURAL PLAN

A. Basic plan of respiratory system would be similar to an inverted tree if it were hollow; leaves of the tree would be comparable to alveoli, with the microscopic sacs enclosed by networks of capillaries (see Figure 14-1)

B. Passive transport process of diffusion is responsible for the exchange of gases that occurs during respiration.

RESPIRATORY TRACTS

A. Upper respiratory tract — nose, pharynx, and larynx
B. Lower respiratory tract — trachea, bronchial tree, and lungs

RESPIRATORY MUCOSA

A. Specialized membrane that lines the air distribution tubes in the respiratory tree (see Figure 14-2)
B. More than 125 mL of mucus produced each day forms a "mucous blanket" over much of the respiratory mucosa
C. Mucus serves as an air purification mechanism by trapping inspired irritants such as dust and pollen
D. Cilia on mucosal cells beat in only one direction, moving mucus upward to pharynx for removal

NOSE

A. Structure
   1. Nasal septum separates interior of nose into two cavities
   2. Mucous membrane lines nose
   3. Frontal, maxillary, sphenoidal, and ethmoidal sinuses drain into nose (see Figure 14-3)
B. Functions
   1. Warms and moistens inhaled air
   2. Contains sense organs of smell

PHARYNX

A. Structure (see Figure 14-4)
   1. Pharynx (throat) about 12.5 cm (5 inches) long
   2. Divided into nasopharynx, oropharynx, and laryngopharynx
   3. Two nasal cavities, mouth, esophagus, larynx, and auditory tubes all have openings into pharynx
   4. Pharyngeal tonsils and openings of auditory tubes open into nasopharynx; tonsils found in oropharynx
   5. Mucous membrane lines pharynx
B. Functions
   1. Passageway for food and liquids
   2. Air distribution; passageway for air

LARYNX

A. Structure (see Figure 14-5)
   1. Several pieces of cartilage form framework
      a. Thyroid cartilage (Adam's apple) is largest
      b. Epiglottis partially covers opening into larynx
   2. Mucous lining
   3. Vocal cords stretch across interior of larynx
B. Functions
   1. Air distribution; passageway for air to move to and from lungs
   2. Voice production

TRACHEA

A. Structure (see Figure 14-6)
   1. Tube about 11 cm (4.5 inches) long that extends from larynx into the thoracic cavity
   2. Mucous lining
   3. C-shaped rings of cartilage hold trachea open
B. Function — passageway for air to move to and from lungs
C. Obstruction
   1. Blockage of trachea occludes the airway and, if complete, causes death in minutes
   2. Tracheal obstruction causes more than 4,000 deaths annually in the United States

BRONCHI, BRONCHIOLES, AND ALVEOLI

A. Structure
   1. Trachea branches into right and left bronchi
   2. Each bronchus branches into smaller and smaller tubes eventually leading to bronchioles
   3. Bronchioles end in clusters of microscopic alveolar sacs, the walls of which are made up of alveoli (see Figure 14-7)
B. Function
   1. Bronchi and bronchioles — air distribution; passageway for air to move to and from alveoli
   2. Alveoli — exchange of gases between air and blood (see Figure 14-8)

LUNGS AND PLEURA

A. Structure (see Figure 14-9)
   1. Size — large enough to fill the chest cavity, except for middle space occupied by heart and large blood vessels

2. Apex — narrow upper part of each lung, under collarbone
3. Base — broad lower part of each lung; rests on diaphragm
4. Pleura — moist, smooth, slippery membrane that lines chest cavity and covers outer surface of lungs; reduces friction between the lungs and chest wall during breathing (see Figure 14-10)

B. Function — breathing (pulmonary ventilation)

RESPIRATION

A. Mechanics of breathing (see Figure 14-11)
   1. Pulmonary ventilation includes two phases called *inspiration* (movement of air into lungs) and *expiration* (movement of air out of lungs)
   2. Changes in size and shape of thorax cause changes in air pressure within that cavity and in the lungs
   3. Air pressure differences actually cause air to move into and out of the lungs

B. Inspiration
   1. Active process — air moves into lungs
   2. Inspiratory muscles include diaphragm and external intercostals
      a. Diaphragm flattens during inspiration — increases top-to-bottom length of thorax
      b. External intercostals contraction elevates the ribs — increases the size of the thorax from the front to the back and from side to side
   3. Increase in the size of the chest cavity reduces pressure within it; air then enters the lungs

C. Expiration
   1. Quiet expiration is ordinarily a passive process
   2. During expiration, thorax returns to its resting size and shape
   3. Elastic recoil of lung tissues aids in expiration
   4. Expiratory muscles used in forceful expiration are internal intercostals and abdominal muscles
      a. Internal intercostals — contraction depresses the rib cage and decreases the size of the thorax from the front to back
      b. Contraction of abdominal muscles elevates the diaphragm, thus decreasing size of the thoracic cavity from the top to bottom
   5. Reduction in the size of the thoracic cavity increases its pressure and air leaves the lungs

D. Exchange of gases in lungs (see Figure 14-12)
   1. Carbaminohemoglobin breaks down into carbon dioxide and hemoglobin
   2. Carbon dioxide moves out of lung capillary blood into alveolar air and out of body in expired air
   3. Oxygen moves from alveoli into lung capillaries
   4. Hemoglobin combines with oxygen, producing oxyhemoglobin

E. Exchange of gases in tissues
   1. Oxyhemoglobin breaks down into oxygen and hemoglobin
   2. Oxygen moves out of tissue capillary blood into tissue cells
   3. Carbon dioxide moves from tissue cells into tissue capillary blood
   4. Hemoglobin combines with carbon dioxide, forming carbaminohemoglobin

F. Blood transportation of gases
   1. Transport of oxygen
   2. Transport of carbon dioxide
   3. Volumes of air exchanged in pulmonary ventilation (see Figure 14-13)
      a. Volumes of air exchanged in breathing can be measured with a spirometer
      b. Tidal volume (TV) — amount normally breathed in or out with each breath
      c. Vital capacity (VC) — greatest amount of air that one can breathe out in one expiration
      d. Expiratory reserve volume (ERV) — amount of air that can be forcibly exhaled after expiring the tidal volume
      e. Inspiratory reserve volume (IRV) — amount of air that can be forcibly inhaled after a normal inspiration
      f. Residual volume (RV) — air that remains in the lungs after the most forceful expiration
      g. Rate — usually about 12 to 18 breaths a minute; much faster during exercise

REGULATION OF RESPIRATION (See Figure 14-14)

A. Regulation of respiration permits the body to adjust to varying demands for oxygen supply and carbon dioxide removal
   1. Most important central regulatory centers in medulla are called *respiratory control centers* (inspiratory and expiratory centers)
   2. Under resting conditions, nervous activity in the respiratory control centers produces a normal rate and depth of respirations (12 to 18 per minute)
B. Respiratory control centers in the medulla are influenced by "inputs" from receptors located in other body areas.
C. Cerebral cortex — voluntary (but limited) control of respiratory activity
D. Receptors that influence respiration
   1. Chemoreceptors respond to changes in carbon dioxide, oxygen, and blood acid levels — located in carotid and aortic bodies
   2. Pulmonary stretch receptors — respond to the stretch in lungs, thus protecting respiratory organs from overinflation

TYPES OF BREATHING

A. Eupnea — normal breathing
B. Hyperventilation — rapid and deep respirations
C. Hypoventilation — slow and shallow respirations
D. Dyspnea — labored or difficult respirations
E. Apnea — stopped respiration
F. Respiratory arrest — failure to resume breathing after a period of apnea

NEW WORDS

alveolar duct	expiratory reserve	lower respiratory tract	respiratory membrane
alveolar sac	volume (ERV)	maximum oxygen	respiratory mucosa
alveoli	glottis	consumption	sinusitis
aortic body	heme	paranasal sinuses	spirometer
apnea	hyperventilation	partial pressure (P)	surfactant
bronchi (sg, bronchus)	hypoventilation	pharynx	tidal volume (TV)
bronchioles	hypoxia	phrenic nerve	tonsillectomy
carbaminohemoglobin	infant respiratory	pleurisy	trachea
carotid body	distress syndrome	pneumothorax	upper respiratory tract
conchae	(IRDS)	pulmonary ventilation	vital capacity (VC)
dyspnea	inspiratory reserve	residual volume (RV)	
epiglottis	volume (IRV)	respiration	
eupnea	larynx	respiratory arrest	

REVIEW QUESTIONS

1. Differentiate between the respiratory membrane and the respiratory mucosa.
2. List the functions of the paranasal sinuses.
3. What is the function of the auditory tube?
4. What is the function of the epiglottis?
5. Describe, in decreasing order of size, the structures that make up the air tubes of the lung.
6. Describe the pleura. What is the function of pleural fluid?
7. Differentiate between external respiration, internal respiration, and cellular respiration.
8. Explain the mechanical process of inspiration.
9. Explain the mechanical process of expiration.
10. Define the term *partial pressure (P)* of a gas and explain how the partial pressure of oxygen (Po_2) and carbon dioxide (Pco_2) influence their diffusion.

REVIEW QUESTIONS

11. Explain how gas is exchanged between the lung and the blood, and between the blood and the tissues.
12. How is oxygen carried in the blood? How is carbon dioxide carried in the blood?
13. Name and explain the volumes that make up vital capacity.
14. Explain the function of chemoreceptors in regulating respiration.
15. Explain the function of stretch receptors in the lung.

CRITICAL THINKING

16. Explain the effect smoking has on the body's ability to remove trapped material in the respiratory mucosa.
17. The developing fetus does not produce lung surfactant until late in its development. Explain what problem a premature infant would have if born before surfactant had been produced.
18. Explain the role of other systems in the regulation of respiration.

CHAPTER TEST

1. The organs of the respiratory system are designed to perform two basic functions: _____ and _____.
2. The upper respiratory tract consists of the _____, the _____, and the _____.
3. The lower respiratory tract consists of the _____, the _____, and the _____.
4. The membrane that separates the air in the alveoli from the blood in the surrounding capillaries is called the _____.
5. The membrane that lines most of the air distribution tubes in the respiratory system is called the _____.
6. The frontal, maxillary, sphenoidal, and ethmoidal cavities make up the _____.

CHAPTER TEST—cont'd

7. The _____ sacs drain tears into the nasal cavity.
8. The _____ protrude into the nasal cavities and function to warm and humidify the air.
9. The _____ is the structure that can also be called the *throat*.
10. The _____ is also called the *voice box*.
11. The _____ is the large air tube in the neck.
12. The four progressively smaller air tubes that connect the trachea and the alveolar sacs are the _____, _____, _____, and the _____.
13. A _____ is a substance made by the lungs to help reduce the surface tension of water in the alveoli.
14. The right lung is made up of _____ lobes, whereas the left lung is made up of _____ lobes.
15. The exchange of gases between the blood and the tissues is called _____.
16. The exchange of gases between the blood and the air in the lungs is called _____.

17. The _____ is the most important muscle in respiration.
18. Oxygen is carried in the blood as _____.
19. Carbon dioxide can be carried in the blood as the _____ ion or combined with hemoglobin as _____.
20. The inspiratory and expiratory centers are located in this part of the brain: _____.
21. _____ are the receptors that inhibit the inspiratory center that keeps the lungs from overexpanding.
22. _____ are the receptors that modify respiratory rates by responding to the amount of carbon dioxide, oxygen, or acid levels in the blood.
23. The amount of air that is moved in and out of the lung during normal breathing is called _____ volume.
24. The three volumes that make up vital capacity are _____, _____, and _____.
25. The volume included in total lung capacity but not vital capacity is _____ volume.

OBJECTIVES

AFTER YOU HAVE COMPLETED THIS CHAPTER, YOU SHOULD BE ABLE TO:

1. List in sequence each of the component parts or segments of the alimentary canal from the mouth to the anus and identify the accessory organs of digestion.
2. List and describe the four layers of the wall of the alimentary canal. Compare the lining layer in the esophagus, stomach, small intestine, and large intestine.
3. Discuss the basics of protein, fat, and carbohydrate digestion and give the end products of each process.
4. Define and contrast mechanical and chemical digestion.
5. Define *peristalsis*, *bolus*, *chyme*, *jaundice*, *ulcer*, and *diarrhea*.

The Digestive System 15

All of us enjoy a good meal! Food preferences differ widely between cultures and individuals, but there is no doubt that the sight, smell, taste, texture, and especially the nutrient content of the foods we eat contribute in many ways to our quality of life. Although we do not "live to eat," we certainly must "eat to live." The ingestion of food is the first step in an important and complex biological process that begins when we consume a meal. How we process the food we eat so that nutrients can be extracted and then absorbed for use by the millions of body cells for energy is a requirement for life and is called **digestion.** That critical process is dependent on the normal structure and function of the digestive system organs (Table 15-1 and Figure 15-1).

After we have explored the various mechanisms of the digestive process and learned about the anatomy, placement, and functions of the digestive organs in this chapter, we will be ready for Chapter 16, which discusses the fate of nutrients after they have been absorbed.

OVERVIEW OF THE DIGESTIVE PROCESS

The principal structure of the **digestive system** is an irregular tube, open at both ends, called the **alimentary** (al-i-MEN-tar-ee) **canal** or the **gastrointestinal** (GAS-troh-in-TESS-tih-nul) **(GI) tract**. In the adult, this hollow tube is about 9 meters (29 feet) long. Think of the tube as a passageway that extends through the body like a hallway through a building. Thus the food we eat and even the nutrient materials released by the digestive process are not truly "part of the body" until they

TABLE 15-1

Organs of the Digestive System

MAIN ORGAN	ACCESSORY ORGAN
Mouth	Teeth and tongue
	Salivary glands
	Parotid
	Submandibular
	Sublingual
Pharynx (throat)	
Esophagus	
Stomach	
Small intestine	Liver
Duodenum	Gallbladder
Jejunum	Pancreas
Ileum	
Large intestine	Vermiform appendix
Cecum	
Colon	
Ascending colon	
Transverse colon	
Descending colon	
Sigmoid colon	
Rectum	
Anal canal	

have passed through the wall of the GI tract and entered the internal environment.

To accomplish the functions of making nutrients available to each cell of the body, the digestive system uses various mechanisms (Table 15-2). First, complex foods must be taken into the GI tract in a process called **ingestion.** Then, the ingested food material must be broken down into simpler nutrients in the process that gives this system its name: **digestion.** The breakdown, or digestion, of food material is both *mechanical* and *chemical* in nature. The teeth are used to physically break down large chunks of food before it is swallowed. The churning of food in the stomach then continues the mechanical digestive process. To physically break down large chunks of food into smaller bits and to move it along the tract, movement or **motility** of the GI wall is required. In chemical digestion, large food molecules are reduced to smaller molecules. This process requires **secretion** of digestive enzymes and other products into the lumen of the GI tract. After the digestive processes have altered the physical and chemical composition of ingested food, the resulting

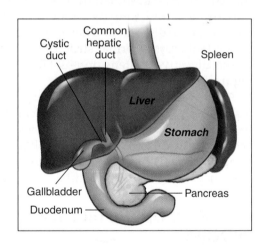

FIGURE 15-1 Location of digestive organs.

TABLE 15-2

Primary Mechanisms of the Digestive System

MECHANISM	DESCRIPTION
Ingestion	Process of taking food into the mouth, starting it on its journey through the digestive tract
Digestion	A group of processes that break complex nutrients into simpler ones, thus facilitating their absorption; *mechanical* digestion physically breaks large chunks into small bits; *chemical digestion* breaks molecules apart
Motility	Movement by the muscular components of the digestive tube, including processes of mechanical digestion; examples include *peristalsis* and *segmentation*
Secretion	Release of digestive juices (containing enzymes, acids, bases, mucus, bile, or other products that facilitate digestion); some digestive organs also secrete endocrine hormones that regulate digestion or metabolism of nutrients
Absorption	Movement of digested nutrients through the gastrointestinal (GI) mucosa and into the internal environment
Elimination	Excretion of the residues of the digestive process (feces) from the rectum, through the anus; defecation
Regulation	Coordination of digestive activity (motility, secretion, etc.)

nutrients are ready for the process of **absorption,** or movement through the GI mucosa into the internal environment. Part of the digestive system, the rectum, serves also as an organ of **elimination,** ridding the body of waste material, or **feces** (FEE seez), resulting from the digestive process. **Regulation** of activities such as motility and secretion is required to coordinate the various mechanisms of digestion.

WALL OF THE DIGESTIVE TRACT

The digestive tract has been described as a tube that extends from the mouth to the anus. The wall of this digestive tube is fashioned of four layers of tissue (Figure 15-2). The inside, or hollow space within the tube, is called the **lumen.** The four layers, named from the inside coat to the outside of the tube, are as follows:

1. Mucosa or mucous membrane
2. Submucosa
3. Muscularis
4. Serosa

Although the same four tissue coats form every organ of the alimentary tract, their structure varies from organ to organ. The **mucosa** of the esophagus, for example, is composed of tough and stratified abrasion-resistant epithelium. The mucosa of the remainder of the tract is a delicate layer of simple columnar epithelium designed for absorption and secretion. The mucus produced by either type of epithelium coats the lining of the alimentary canal.

The **submucosa,** as the name implies, is a connective tissue layer that lies just below the mucosa. It contains many blood vessels and nerves. The two layers of muscle tissue called the **muscularis** (see Figure 15-2) have an important role to play in producing motility or movement of the GI tract during the digestive process. **Peristalsis** (pair-i-STAL-sis) is a rhythmic, wavelike contraction of the gut wall caused by alternating contraction and relaxation of the circular and longitudinal muscle layers in the muscularis. This type of sequenced contraction squeezes and pushes ingested food material forward through the digestive tube's internal pathway (Figure 15-3). In addition to peristalsis type contractions, alternating contraction of the circular layer of the muscularis within a single region, or segment, of the GI tract also produces a "back-and-forth" type of intestinal motility called **segmentation** (Figure 15-4). As peristaltic movement pushes food down the GI tract, segmentation contractions further assist in mixing food with digestive juices and helps continue the mechanical breakdown of larger food particles.

Peristalsis and segmentation can occur in an alternating sequence. When this happens, food is churned and mixed as it slowly progresses along the GI tract in close contact with the intestinal mucosa, which facilitates absorption of nutrients.

The **serosa** is the outermost covering or coat of the digestive tube. In the abdominal cavity, this serosa covering is call the *visceral peritoneum.* The loops of the digestive tract are anchored to the posterior wall of the abdominal cavity by a

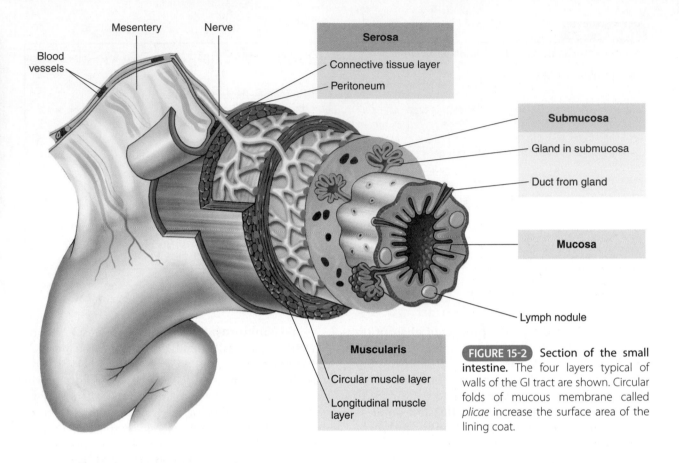

Serosa
- Connective tissue layer
- Peritoneum

Submucosa
- Gland in submucosa
- Duct from gland

Mucosa

Mesentery

Nerve

Blood vessels

Lymph nodule

Muscularis
- Circular muscle layer
- Longitudinal muscle layer

FIGURE 15-2 Section of the small intestine. The four layers typical of walls of the GI tract are shown. Circular folds of mucous membrane called *plicae* increase the surface area of the lining coat.

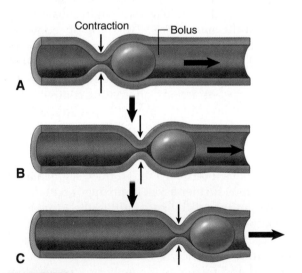

Contraction — Bolus

A

B

C

FIGURE 15-3 **Peristalsis.** Peristalsis is a progressive type of movement in which material is propelled from point to point along the GI tract. **A,** A ring of contraction occurs where the GI wall is stretched, and the bolus is pushed forward. **B,** The moving bolus triggers a ring of contraction in the next region that pushes the bolus even farther along. **C,** The ring of contraction moves like a wave along the GI tract to push the bolus forward.

Contraction Bolus

A

B

C

FIGURE 15-4 **Segmentation.** Segmentation is a back-and-forth action that breaks apart chunks of food and mixes in digestive juices. **A,** Ringlike regions of contraction occur at intervals along the GI tract. **B,** Previously contracted regions relax and adjacent regions now contract, effectively "chopping" the contents of each segment into smaller chunks. **C,** The location of the contracted regions continues to alternate back and forth, chopping and mixing the contents of the GI lumen.

large double fold of peritoneal tissue called the **mesentery** (MEZ-en-tair-ee).

MOUTH

The **mouth,** or **oral cavity,** is a hollow chamber with a roof, a floor, and walls. Food enters, or rather is ingested into, the digestive tract through the mouth, and the process of digestion begins immediately. As with the remainder of the digestive tract, the mouth is lined with mucous membrane. It may be helpful for you to review the structure and function of mucous membranes in Chapter 5. Typically, mucous membrances line hollow organs, such as the digestive tube, that open to the exterior of the body. Mucus produced by the lining of the GI tract protects the epithelium from digestive juices and lubricates food passing through the lumen.

The roof of the mouth is formed by the **hard** and **soft palates** (see Figure 15-4). The hard palate is a bony structure in the anterior or front portion of the mouth formed by parts of the palatine and maxillary bones. The soft palate is located above the posterior or rear portion of the mouth. It is soft because it consists chiefly of muscle. Hanging down from the center of the soft palate is a cone-shaped structure, the **uvula** (YOO-vyoo-lah). If you look in the mirror, open your mouth wide, and say "Ah," you can see your uvula. The uvula and the soft palate prevent any food and liquid from entering the nasal cavities above the mouth.

The floor of the mouth consists of the tongue and its muscles. The tongue is made of skeletal muscle covered with mucous membrane. It is anchored to bones in the skull and to the hyoid bone in the neck. A thin membrane called the **frenulum** (FREN-yoo-lum) attaches the tongue to the floor of the mouth. Occasionally a person is born with a frenulum that is too short to allow free movements of the tongue (Figure 15-5, *C*). Individuals with this condition cannot enunciate words normally. Note in Figure 15-5, *A*, that the tongue can be divided into a blunt rear portion called the *root*, a pointed *tip*, and a central *body*.

✓ **QUICK CHECK**

1. What is the alimentary canal?
2. What kinds of processing does food undergo in the body?
3. Describe the layers of the digestive tract's wall.
4. What is the uvula? What does it do?

Typical Tooth

A typical tooth can be divided into three main parts: crown, neck, and root. The **crown** is the portion that is exposed and visible in the mouth. It is covered by enamel—the hardest tissue in the body. Enamel is ideally suited to withstand the grinding that occurs during the chewing of hard and brittle foods. In addition to being covered by enamel, the outer shell of each tooth is covered by two other dental tissues—dentin and cementum (Figure 15-6). Dentin makes up the greatest proportion of the tooth shell. It is covered by enamel in the crown and by cementum in the neck and root areas. The center of the tooth contains a pulp cavity that consists of connective tissue, blood and lymphatic vessels, and sensory nerves.

The **neck** of a tooth is the narrow portion, shown in Figure 15-6, that joins the crown of the tooth to the root. It is surrounded by the pink *gingival* or *gum* tissue. A general term for mild, localized, and often transitory inflammation of the gums or gingiva is called **gingivitis** (jin-ji-VYE-tis).

The **root** of the tooth fits into the bony socket that surrounds it in either the upper or lower jaw bone. A fibrous **periodontal** (pair-ee-oh-DON-tull) **membrane** lines each tooth socket and anchors the tooth to the bone. **Periodontitis** (pair-ee-oh-don-TYE-tis) is a generalized and serious type of inflammation and infection. It is often a complication of untreated gingivitis. As the infection worsens, it will cause loss of both periodontal membrane and bone, resulting in loosening and eventually complete loss of teeth. Periodontitis is the leading cause of tooth loss among adults. Tooth decay, or **dental caries,** is a disease of the enamel, dentin, and cementum of teeth that results in the formation of a permanent defect called a **cavity.** The incidence of gingivitis, dental caries, and periodontitis can be reduced by good dental health practices, which include regular and thorough brushing and flossing of the teeth.

Types of Teeth

The shape and placement of the teeth (see Figure 15-5, *B*) assist in their functions. The four major types of teeth are as follows:

1. Incisors (in-SYE-zorz)
2. Canines (KAY-nynez) or cuspids
3. Premolars (PREE-moh-larz) or bicuspids
4. Molars (MOH-larz) or tricuspids

FIGURE 15-5 **Mouth cavity and tongue. A,** Mouth cavity showing hard and soft palates, tongue surface, and uvula. **B,** Types of adult teeth, undersurface of tongue showing frenulum, sublingual gland, and opening of sublingual duct. **C,** Photograph shows an abnormally short lingual frenulum, which may result in faulty speech.

In humans, a set of 20 teeth called **deciduous** (de-SID-u-us) or **baby teeth** erupt between about 6 to 30 months of age. Although the time frame may vary somewhat, these teeth are generally lost between ages 6 and 13 years old. The first permanent teeth to appear, called the first or "6-year" molars erupt before all of the baby teeth are lost. When a young adult is somewhere between 17 and 24 years old, the deciduous teeth have all been shed and completely replaced with a full set of 32 **permanent teeth.** The third molars or "wisdom

teeth" are the last of the permanent teeth to appear.

Locate the four types of teeth in Figure 15-5, *B,* which shows the full set of 32 permanent teeth. In the deciduous set of 20 teeth, there are no premolars and only two pairs of molars in each jaw. Note that the incisors have very sharp cutting edges while the canine or cuspid teeth have more pointed ends well suited for piercing and tearing. The flat premolars and molars with their two or three grinding "cusps" provide a large surface

Clinical Application

Malocclusion

Malocclusion of the teeth occurs when missing teeth create wide spaces in the dentition, when teeth overlap, or when malposition of one or more teeth prevents correct alignment of the maxillary and mandibular dental arches (Figures A and B). Malocclusion that results in protrusion of the upper front teeth, causing them to hang over the lower front teeth, is called *overbite* (Figure *A*), whereas the positioning of the lower front teeth outside the upper front teeth is called *underbite* (Figure *B*).

Dental malocclusion may cause significant problems and chronic pain in the functioning of the temporomandibular joint, contribute to the generation of headaches, or complicate routine mastication of food. Fortunately, even severe malocclusion problems can be corrected by the use of braces and other dental appliances. Orthodontics (or-thoh-DON-tiks) is that branch of dentistry that deals with the prevention and correction of positioning irregularities of the teeth and malocclusion.

FIGURE 15-6 Longitudinal section of a tooth. A molar is sectioned to show its bony socket and details of its three main parts: crown, neck, and root. Enamel (over the crown) and cementum (over the neck and root) surround the dentin layer. The pulp contains nerves and blood vessels.

area to effectively crush ingested food material. Together, the teeth provide for effective chewing or **mastication** (mas-ti-KAY-shun) of a wide variety and size of ingested food.

SALIVARY GLANDS

Three pairs of salivary glands—the parotids, submandibulars, and sublinguals—secrete most (about 1 liter) of the saliva produced each day in the adult. The salivary glands (Figure 15-7) are typical of the accessory glands associated with the digestive system. They are located outside of the digestive tube itself and must convey their exocrine secretions by way of ducts into the tract.

Some salivary secretions are said to be **serous** in nature if they are thin, watery, and free of mucus. Serous-type saliva, produced by serous-type secretory cells (see Figure 15-7, *B*), contains the digestive enzyme **salivary amylase** (AM-eh-lays). This enzyme begins the chemical digestion of carbohydrates. Another type of saliva is thick and rich in mucus but contains no enzymes. Mucous-type saliva, which is thick and slippery, is produced by mucous-type secretory cells (see Figure 15-7, *B*). This type of saliva serves the important function of lubricating food during mastication, thus allowing it to pass with less friction through the esophagus and into the stomach. Some saliva is a mixture of both serous- and mucous-type secretions.

The **parotid** (pah-ROT-id) **glands,** the largest of the salivary glands, lie just below and in front of each ear at the angle of the jaw—an interesting anatomical position because it explains why people

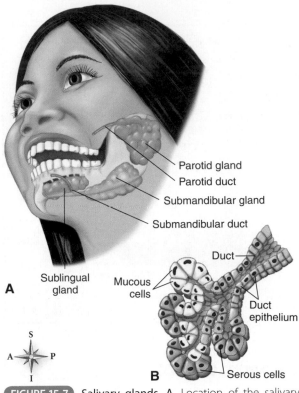

A

Parotid gland
Parotid duct
Submandibular gland
Submandibular duct
Sublingual gland

Duct
Mucous cells
Duct epithelium

B
Serous cells

S
A ✦ P
I

who have mumps (an infection of the parotid gland) often complain that it hurts when they open their mouths or chew; these movements squeeze the tender, inflamed gland. To see the openings of the parotid ducts, look in a mirror at the insides of your cheeks opposite the second molar tooth on either side of the upper jaw. The parotids contain only serous type secretory cells, which produce a watery, or serous, type of saliva containing enzymes but not mucus.

Submandibular (sub-man-DIB-yoo-lar) **glands** (see Figure 15-7, *A*) are called *mixed* or *compound* salivary glands because they contain both serous (enzyme) and mucus-producing secretory cells (see Figure 15-7, *B*). These glands are located just below the mandibular angle, are irregular in form, and are about the size of a walnut. The submandibular ducts open into the mouth on either side of the lingual frenulum.

Sublingual (sub-LING-gwal) **glands** are the smallest of the main salivary glands. They lie in front of the submandibular glands, under the mucous membrane covering the floor of the mouth. Each sublingual gland opens via 10 to 15 ducts into the floor of the mouth. Unlike the other salivary glands, the sublingual glands produce only a mucous type of saliva.

 To learn more about the mouth and associated structures in mechanical digestion, go to AnimationDirect on your CD-ROM.

PHARYNX

The **pharynx** (FAIR-inks) is a tubelike structure made of muscle and lined with mucous membrane. Note its location in Figure 15-1. Because of its location behind the nasal cavities and mouth, it functions as part of the respiratory and digestive systems. Air must pass through the pharynx on its way to the lungs, and food must pass through it on its way to the stomach. Recall that the pharynx as a whole is subdivided into three anatomical components: *nasopharynx, oropharynx,* and *laryngopharynx.* You may want to review the anatomy of the pharynx in Chapter 4, pp. 77 to 80 and illustrated in detail in Figure 14-4 on p. 330. Of the three anatomical divisions, the oropharynx is actively and most directly involved in the digestive process because of its important role in a specialized and coordinated type of GI tract motility involved in swallowing. The swallowing of food is called **deglutition** (deg-loo-TISH-un). First, mastication involves voluntary movements that result in formation of a ball or bolus of food in the mouth that is then moved involuntarily through the oropharynx and then into the esophagus and, finally, into the stomach. Swallowing is a complex process requiring the coordination of pharyngeal muscles and other muscles and structures in the head and neck. *Regulation* of voluntary swallowing movements is dependent on nervous impulses originating in the motor cortex of the cerebrum. Involuntary movements are regulated by impulses originating in the swallowing or "deglutition center" located in the medulla and pons of the brainstem (see Figure 8-9, *B*).

 To learn more about the pharynx, go to AnimationDirect on your CD-ROM.

Clinical Application

Gastroesophageal Reflux Disease

The terms *heartburn* and *acid indigestion* are often used to describe a number of unpleasant symptoms experienced by more than 60 million Americans each month. Backward flow of stomach acid up into the esophagus causes these symptoms, which typically include burning and pressure behind the breastbone. The term **gastroesophageal reflux disease (GERD)** is now used to better describe this very common and sometimes serious medical condition.

In its simplest form, GERD produces mild symptoms that occur only infrequently (twice a week or less). In these cases, avoiding problem foods or beverages, stopping smoking, or losing weight if needed may solve the problem. Additional treatment with over-the-counter antacids or nonprescription-strength acid-blocking medications may also be used. More severe and frequent episodes of GERD can trigger asthma attacks, cause severe chest pain (which can mimic the pain of a heart attack), result in bleeding, or promote a narrowing (stricture) or chronic irritation of the esophagus. In these cases, more powerful inhibitors of stomach acid production may be added to the treatment prescribed. As a last resort, a surgical procedure called *fundoplication* is performed to strengthen the sphincter. The procedure involves wrapping a layer of the upper stomach wall around the sphincter and terminal esophagus to lessen the possibility of acid reflux. If GERD is left untreated, serious pathological (precancerous) changes in the esophageal lining may develop—a condition called *Barrett esophagus.*

ESOPHAGUS

The **esophagus** (eh-SOF-ah-gus) is the muscular, mucus-lined tube that connects the pharynx with the stomach. It is about 25 centimeters (10 inches) long. The esophagus serves as a dynamic passageway for food, pushing the food toward the stomach. The production of mucus by glands in the mucosal lining lubricates the tube to permit easier passage of food moving toward the stomach.

To learn more about the esophagus, go to AnimationDirect on your CD-ROM.

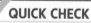

QUICK CHECK

1. What are the four major types of teeth?
2. What digestive enzyme is found in saliva?
3. What roles do the pharynx and esophagus play in the digestive tract?

STOMACH

The **stomach** (Figure 15-8; see Figure 15-13, *A*) lies in the upper part of the abdominal cavity just under the diaphragm. It serves as a pouch that food enters after it has been chewed, swallowed, and passed through the esophagus. The stomach looks small after it is emptied, not much bigger than a large sausage, but it expands considerably after a large meal. Have you ever felt so uncomfortably full after eating that you could not take a deep breath? If so, it probably meant that your stomach was so full of food that it occupied more space than usual and thus pushed up against the diaphragm. This made it hard for the diaphragm to contract and move downward as much as necessary for a deep breath to be taken.

After food has entered the stomach by passing through the muscular **lower esophageal sphincter** (eh-soff-eh-jee-al SFINK-ter) **(LES),** also called the *cardiac sphincter,* at the lower end of the esophagus, the digestive process continues. Sphincters are rings of muscle tissue. The cardiac sphincter keeps food from reentering the esophagus when the stomach contracts. Occasionally, the opening in the diaphragm that permits the passage of the esophagus into the abdomen is enlarged. This may permit a bulging of the end of the esophagus and part or even all of the stomach upward through the diaphragm and into the chest. The condition, called a **hiatal hernia** (hye-AY-tal HER-nee-ah), may result in backward movement or reflux of stomach contents into the lower portion of the esophagus. The resulting symptoms are referred to as **gastroesophageal reflux disease,** or **GERD.**

Contraction of the stomach's muscular walls mixes the food thoroughly with the gastric juice and breaks it down into a semisolid mixture called **chyme** (kyme). Gastric juice contains hydrochloric acid and enzymes that function in the digestive process. Chyme formation is a continuation of the mechanical digestive process that begins in the mouth.

Note in Figure 15-8 that there are three layers of smooth muscle in the stomach wall. The

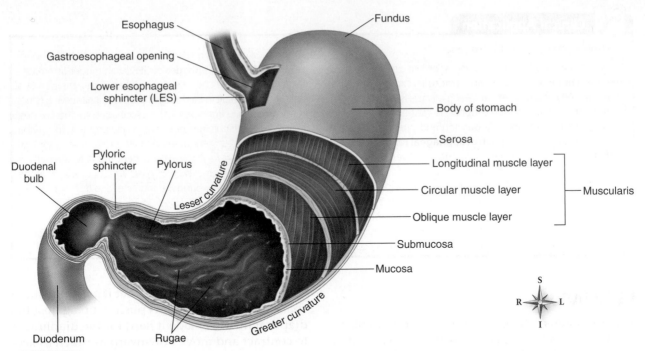

FIGURE 15-8 **Stomach.** A portion of the anterior wall has been cut away to reveal the three muscle layers of the stomach wall. Notice that the mucosa lining the stomach forms folds called *rugae*.

muscle fibers that run lengthwise, around, and obliquely make the stomach one of the strongest internal organs—well able to break up food into tiny particles and to mix them thoroughly with gastric juice to form chyme. Stomach muscle contractions result in peristalsis, which propels food down the digestive tract. Mucous membrane lines the stomach; it contains thousands of microscopic **gastric glands** that secrete gastric juice and hydrochloric acid into the stomach. When the stomach is empty, its lining lies in folds called **rugae** (ROO-gee).

The three divisions of the stomach shown in Figure 15-8 are the *fundus, body,* and *pylorus* (pye-LOR-us). The **fundus** is the enlarged portion to the left of and above the opening of the esophagus into the stomach. The **body** is the central part of the stomach, and the **pylorus** is its lower narrow section, which joins the first part of the small intestine. Partial digestion occurs after food is held in the stomach by the **pyloric** (pye-LOR-ik) **sphincter** muscle. The smooth muscle fibers of the sphincter stay contracted most of the time and thereby close off the opening of the pylorus into the small intestine. Note also in Figure 15-8 that the upper right border of the stomach is known as the *lesser curvature,* and the

lower left border is called the *greater curvature.* After food has been mixed in the stomach, chyme begins its passage through the pyloric sphincter into the first part of the small intestine.

 To learn more about the stomach, go to AnimationDirect on your CD-ROM.

QUICK CHECK

1. What is chyme?
2. How does a sphincter muscle help the stomach perform its function?
3. What are the main divisions of the stomach?

SMALL INTESTINE

The **small intestine** seems to be misnamed if you look at its length—it is roughly 7 meters (20 feet) long. However, it is noticeably smaller in diameter than the large intestine, so in this respect its name is appropriate. Different names identify different sections of the small intestine. In the order in which food passes through them, they are the **duodenum** (doo-oh-DEE-num), **jejunum** (jeh-JOO-num), and **ileum** (IL-ee-um).

The mucous lining of the small intestine, as with that of the stomach, contains thousands of microscopic glands. These **intestinal glands** secrete the intestinal digestive juice. Another structural feature of the lining of the small intestine makes it especially well suited to absorption of food and water: It is not perfectly smooth, as it appears to the naked eye. Instead, the intestinal lining is arranged into multiple circular folds called **plicae** (PLYE-kee) (Figures 15-2 and 15-9). These folds are themselves covered with thousands of tiny "fingers" called **villi** (VIL-eye). Under the microscope, the villi can be seen projecting into the hollow interior of the intestine. Inside each villus lies a rich network of blood capillaries that absorb the products of carbohydrate and protein digestion (sugars and amino acids). Millions and millions of villi jut inward from the mucous lining. Imagine the lining as perfectly smooth without any villi; think how much less surface area there would be for contact between capillaries and intestinal lining. Consider what an advantage a large contact area offers for faster absorption of nutrients from the intestine into the blood and lymph—one more illustration that structure and function are intimately related.

FIGURE 15-9 **Small intestine.** Note that the folds of mucosa are covered with villi and that each villus is covered with epithelium, which increases the surface area for absorption of food.

Clinical Application

Treatment of Ulcers

Current statistics show that about 1 in 10 individuals in the United States will suffer from either a gastric (stomach) or duodenal ulcer in the lifetime. These craterlike lesions, which destroy areas of stomach or intestinal lining, cause gnawing or burning pain and may ultimately result in hemorrhage, perforation, scarring, and other serious medical complications. Long-term use of certain pain medications such as aspirin and ibuprofen, called *nonsteroidal antiinflammatory agents* (NSAIDs), can cause ulcers. However, we now know that most gastric and duodenal ulcers result from infection with the *Helicobacter pylori (H. pylori)* bacterium. This is especially so if the infected individual has a genetic predisposition to ulcer development. *H. pylori* infection is diagnosed by biopsy, breath, or blood antibody tests.

Knowing that most ulcers are caused by a bacterial organism led to his or her development of a number of treatment programs that were designed to eradicate the bacteria by use of antibiotics while simultaneously blocking or reducing stomach acid secretion. Currently, the standard antibiotic-based treatment used most frequently to both heal ulcers and prevent recurrences is called *triple therapy*. It is successful in 80% to 95% of cases and requires that three medications be taken concurrently for 2 weeks. Triple therapy combines bismuth subsalicylate (Pepto-Bismol™) with two antibiotics. The same types of antisecretory drugs used to reduce stomach acid in GERD are also used in ulcer therapy.

Note also in Figure 15-9 that each villus in the intestine contains a lymphatic vessel, or **lacteal** (LAK-tee-al), that absorbs lipid or fat materials from the chyme passing through the small intestine. In addition to the thousands of villi that increase surface area in the small intestine, each villus is itself covered by epithelial cells, which have a brushlike border composed of **microvilli.** The microvilli further increase the surface area of each villus for absorption of nutrients.

Most of the chemical digestion occurs in the first subdivision of the small intestine or duodenum. The duodenum is C-shaped (Figure 15-10) and curves around the head of the pancreas. The acid chyme enters the bulb of the duodenum from the stomach. This area is the site of frequent

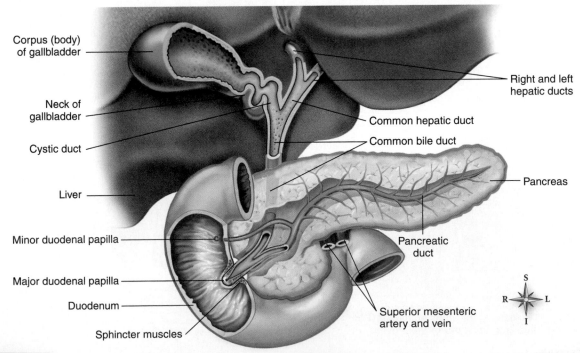

FIGURE 15-10 **Gallbladder and bile ducts.** Obstruction of the hepatic, or common, bile duct by stone or spasm blocks the exit of bile from the liver, where it is formed, and prevents bile from being ejected into the duodenum.

ulceration (duodenal ulcers). The middle third of the duodenum contains the openings of ducts that empty pancreatic digestive juice and bile from the liver into the small intestine. As you can see in Figure 15-10, the two openings are called the **minor** and **major duodenal papillae** (pah-PIL-ee). Occasionally a gallstone blocks the major duodenal papilla, causing symptoms such as severe pain, jaundice, and digestive problems. Smooth

muscle in the wall of the small intestine contracts to produce peristalsis, the wavelike contraction that moves food through the tract.

LIVER AND GALLBLADDER

The liver is so large that it fills the entire upper right section of the abdominal cavity and even extends partway into the left side. Because its cells

 Clinical Application

Gallstones and Weight Loss

Gallstones are solid clumps of material (mostly cholesterol) that form in the gallbladder of 1 in 10 Americans (Figure A). Some gallstones never cause problems and are called *silent gallstones*, whereas others produce painful symptoms or other medical complications and are called *symptomatic gallstones*. Gallstones often form when the cholesterol concentration in bile becomes excessive, causing crystallization or precipitation to occur. Stone formation is much more likely to occur if the gallbladder does not empty regularly and chemically imbalanced or cholesterol-laden bile remains in the gallbladder for long periods.

The relationship of dieting and weight loss to gallstone formation is currently under intense scrutiny. Physicians have known for years that, in severely obese individuals (BMI, or body mass index, greater than 40), the liver produces higher levels of cholesterol and the risk of developing gallstones is increased. However, only recently have scientists established with certainty that significant and rapid weight loss greatly increases the risk of symptomatic gallstone formation that may require surgery—a procedure called **cholecystectomy** (kohl-eh-sis-TEK-toh-mee).

Surgical procedures used for producing weight loss, such as restrictive gastric banding (vertical-banded gastroplasty), the LAP-BAND® Adjustable Gastric Banding (LAGB®) System, or more extensive bypass operations (for example, Roux-en-Y gastric bypass [RGB]), almost always result in rapid

postsurgical weight loss, but more than one third of these patients develop gallstones. Unfortunately, individuals who choose nonsurgical approaches to achieve significant and rapid weight loss, such as very–low-calorie or ultra–low-fat or carbohydrate diets, also experience higher rates of gallstone formation. In these cases, stone formation is related to imbalances in bile chemistry and delayed emptying or incomplete gallbladder contractions.

If surgery is required for removal of symptomatic gallstones, *laparoscopic* (LAP-ah-roh-skop-ic) *techniques* have now made the need for open abdominal surgical procedures less common. Laparoscopic surgery means using instruments to gain access to internal body content through "punched holes" rather than through the traditional incision. To punch the holes, a trocar (a sharp, pointed rod inside a tube) is inserted through the skin. Once inside the body cavity, the rod is removed but the tube remains in place. Then, instruments, lights, and gases may be inserted into the cavity as needed to conduct the surgery. In the case of laparoscopic cholecystectomy surgery, four or five holes are created. Figure B shows the most common locations for abdominal cavity access. Gallstones can sometimes be treated (dissolved) over time or prevented from developing in individuals experiencing rapid weight loss by oral administration of a naturally occurring bile constituent called *ursodeoxycholic acid* (Actigall™, ursodial, others).

secrete a substance called **bile** into ducts, the liver is classified as an exocrine gland; in fact, it is the largest gland in the body.

Look again at Figure 15-10. First, identify the hepatic ducts. They drain bile out of the liver, a fact suggested by the name "hepatic," which comes from the Greek word for liver *(hepar)*. Next, notice the duct that drains bile into the small intestine (duodenum), the common bile duct. It is formed by the union of the common hepatic duct with the cystic duct.

Chemically, bile contains significant quantities of cholesterol and substances *(bile salts)* that act as detergents to mechanically break up, or **emulsify** (eh-MUL-seh-fye), fats. Because fats form large globules, they must be broken down, or emulsified, into smaller particles to increase the surface area to aid digestion. In addition to emulsification of fats, bile that is eliminated from the body in the feces serves as a mechanism for excreting cholesterol from the body. Both emulsification of fats and elimination of cholesterol from the body are primary functions of bile.

When chyme containing lipid or fat enters the duodenum, it initiates a mechanism that contracts the gallbladder and forces bile into the small intestine. Fats in chyme stimulate or "trigger" the secretion of the hormone **cholecystokinin** (koh-lee-sis-toh-KYE-nin), or **CCK,** from the intestinal mucosa of the duodenum. This hormone then stimulates the contraction of the gallbladder, and consequently bile flows into the duodenum. Secretion of CCK is a good example of a hormone acting to regulate GI motility. Between meals, a lot of bile moves up the cystic duct into the gallbladder on the undersurface of the liver. The gallbladder thus concentrates and stores bile produced in the liver.

Visualize a gallstone blocking the common bile duct shown in Figure 15-10. Bile could not then drain into the duodenum. Feces would then appear gray-white because the pigments from bile give feces its characteristic color. Furthermore, excessive amounts of bile would be absorbed into the blood. A yellowish skin discoloration called **jaundice** (JAWN-dis) would result. Obstruction of the common hepatic duct also leads to jaundice. Because bile cannot then drain out of the liver, excessive amounts of it are absorbed. Because bile is not resorbed from the gallbladder, no jaundice occurs if the cystic duct is blocked.

PANCREAS

The pancreas lies behind the stomach in the concavity produced by the C shape of the duodenum (see Figure 15-10). A less scientific but definitely more poetic and colorful description of the location of the pancreas was written by an anatomist hundreds of years ago. He wrote about the "romance of the abdomen" and stated that the pancreas was located "lying in the arms of the duodenum." A good example, perhaps, of how textbook descriptions can change over time!

The pancreas is both an exocrine gland that secretes pancreatic juice into ducts and an endocrine gland that secretes hormones into the blood. Pancreatic juice is the most important digestive juice. It contains enzymes that digest all three major kinds of foods. It also contains sodium bicarbonate, an alkaline substance that neutralizes the hydrochloric acid in the gastric juice that enters the intestines. Pancreatic juice enters the duodenum of the small intestine at the same place that bile enters. As you can see in Figure 15-10, the common bile and pancreatic ducts open into the duodenum at the major duodenal papilla.

Between the cells that secrete pancreatic juice into ducts lie clusters of cells that have no contact with any ducts. These are the **pancreatic islets (of Langerhans),** which contain the cells that secrete the hormones of the pancreas described in Chapter 10 (see Figure 10-11 on p. 240). Locate the pancreas and nearby structures in Figure 15-11, which shows a transverse section of the abdomen of a human cadaver.

> ✓ **QUICK CHECK**
> 1. What are the main divisions of the small intestine?
> 2. What is bile and where does it come from?
> 3. What is the role of the gallbladder?
> 4. Is the pancreas an exocrine gland or an endocrine gland?

LARGE INTESTINE

The **large intestine** is only about 1.5 meters (5 feet) in length. As the name implies, however, it has a much larger diameter than the small intestine. It forms the lower or terminal portion of the digestive tract. Undigested and unabsorbed food material enters the large intestine after passing through

Anterior

Inferior vena cava   Abdominal aorta   Stomach   Pancreas

Right

Liver

Vertebral bone

Right kidney

Left

Intestine

Peritoneal space

Left kidney

Posterior

FIGURE 15-11   **Horizontal (transverse) section of the abdomen.** The photograph of a cadaver section shows the relative position of some of the major digestive organs of the abdomen. Such a view is typical in images obtained by methods such as computed tomography (CT) scanning and magnetic resonance imaging (MRI).

a sphincter-like structure (Figure 15-12) called the **ileocecal** (il-ee-oh-SEE-kal) **valve.** The word *chyme* is no longer appropriate in describing the contents of the large intestine. Chyme, which has the consistency of soup and is found in the small intestine, changes to the consistency of fecal matter as water and salts are reabsorbed during its passage through the small intestine. During its movement through the large intestine, material that escaped digestion in the small intestine is acted on by bacteria. As a result of this bacterial action, additional nutrients may be released from cellulose and other fibers and absorbed. In addition to their digestive role, bacteria in the large intestine have other important functions. They are responsible for the synthesis of vitamin K needed for normal blood clotting and for the production of some of the B-complex vitamins. After they are formed, these vitamins are absorbed from the large intestine and enter the blood.

Although some absorption of water, salts, and vitamins occurs in the large intestine, this segment of the digestive tube is not as well suited for absorption as is the small intestine. Salts, especially sodium, are absorbed by active transport, and water is moved into the blood by osmosis. No villi are present in the mucosa of the large intestine. As a result, much less surface area is available for absorption, and the efficiency and speed of movement of substances through the wall of the large intestine are lower than in the small intestine. Normal passage of material through the large intestine takes about 3 to 5 days. If the rate of passage of material quickens, the consistency of the stools or fecal material becomes more and more fluid, and **diarrhea** (dye-ah-REE-ah) results. If the time of passage through the large intestine is prolonged beyond 5 days, the feces loses volume and becomes more solid because of excessive water absorption. This reduces stimulation of the bowel emptying reflex, resulting in retention of feces, a condition called **constipation** (kon-sti-PAY-shun).

The subdivisions of the large intestine are listed below in the order in which food material or feces passes through them.

1. Cecum
2. Ascending colon
3. Transverse colon

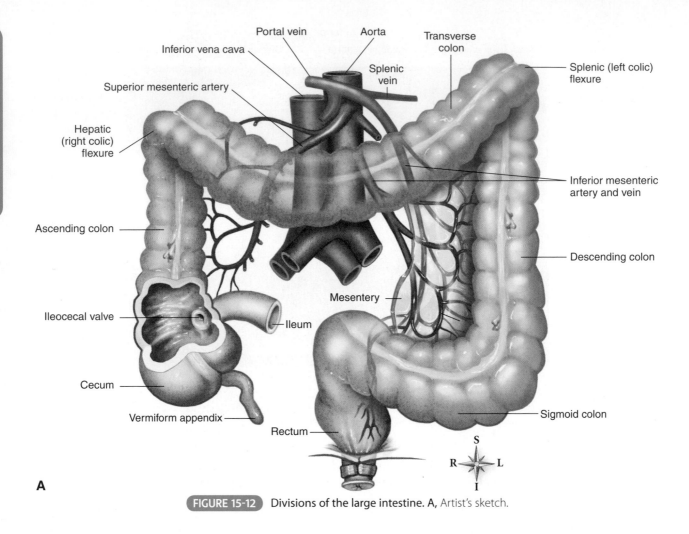

Portal vein

Aorta

Transverse colon

Inferior vena cava

Splenic vein

Splenic (left colic) flexure

Superior mesenteric artery

Hepatic (right colic) flexure

Inferior mesenteric artery and vein

Ascending colon

Descending colon

Mesentery

Ileocecal valve

Ileum

Cecum

Vermiform appendix

Sigmoid colon

Rectum

S

R — L

I

A

FIGURE 15-12 Divisions of the large intestine. A, Artist's sketch.

4. Descending colon
5. Sigmoid colon
6. Rectum
7. Anal canal

These areas can be studied (see Figure 15-12) and identified by tracing the passage of material from its point of entry into the large intestine at the ileocecal valve to its elimination from the body through the external opening called the **anus.**

Note in Figure 15-12 that the ileocecal valve opens into a pouchlike area called the **cecum** (SEE-kum). The opening itself is about 5 or 6 cm (2 inches) above the beginning of the large intestine. Food residue in the cecum flows upward on the right side of the body in the **ascending colon.** The **hepatic** (heh-PAT-ik) or **right colic flexure** is the bend between the ascending colon and the **transverse colon,** which extends across the front of the abdomen from right

to left. The **splenic** or **left colic flexure** marks the point where the **descending colon** turns downward on the left side of the abdomen. The **sigmoid** (SIG-moyd) **colon** is the S-shaped segment that terminates in the **rectum.** The terminal portion of the rectum is called the **anal canal,** which ends at the external opening, or anus.

Two sphincter muscles stay contracted to keep the anus closed except during defecation. Smooth or involuntary muscle composes the *inner anal sphincter,* but striated, or voluntary, muscle composes the *outer anal sphincter.* This anatomical fact sometimes becomes highly important from a practical standpoint. For example, often after a person has had a stroke, the voluntary anal sphincter at first becomes paralyzed. This means, of course, that the individual has no control at that time over bowel movements.

Hepatic (right colic) flexure

Ascending colon

Ileocecal valve

Cecum

Ileum

Splenic (left colic) flexure

Transverse colon

Descending colon

Sigmoid colon

Rectum

B

FIGURE 15-12, cont'd B, Lower GI study x-ray film showing segments of the colon, rectum, and anal canal.

 To learn more about the large intestine, go to AnimationDirect on your CD-ROM.

APPENDIX

The **vermiform** (VERM-i-form) **appendix** (ah-PEN-diks) (Latin *vermiformis* from *vermis* "worm" and *forma* "shape") is, as the name implies, a wormlike, tubular structure. Although it serves no important digestive function in humans, it contains lymphatic tissue and may play a minor role in the immunological defense mechanisms of the body described in Chapter 13. Note in Figure 15-12 that the appendix is directly attached to the cecum. The appendix contains a blind, tubelike interior lumen that communicates with the lumen of the large intestine 3 cm (1 inch) below the opening of

the ileocecal valve into the cecum. If the mucous lining of the appendix becomes inflamed, the resulting condition is the well-known affliction, **appendicitis** (ah-pen-di-SYE-tis). As you can see in Figure 15-12, the appendix is very close to the rectal wall. For patients with suspected appendicitis, a physician often evaluates the appendix by performing a digital rectal examination.

PERITONEUM

The **peritoneum** (pair-i-toh-NEE-um) is a large, moist, slippery sheet of serous membrane that lines the abdominal cavity and covers the organs located in it, including most of the digestive organs. The parietal layer of the peritoneum lines the abdominal cavity. The visceral layer of the peritoneum forms the outer, or covering, layer of each abdominal organ. The small space between the parietal and visceral layers is called the **peritoneal space**. It contains just enough peritoneal fluid to keep both layers of the peritoneum moist and able to slide freely against each other during breathing and digestive movements (Figure 15-13). Organs outside of the peritoneum are said to be retroperitoneal.

Extensions

The two most prominent extensions of the peritoneum are the mesentery and the greater omentum. The **mesentery** (MEZ-en-tair-ee), an extension between the parietal and visceral layers of the peritoneum, is shaped like a giant, pleated fan. Its smaller edge attaches to the lumbar region of the posterior abdominal wall, and its long, loose outer edge encloses most of the small intestine, anchoring it to the posterior abdominal wall. The **greater omentum** is a pouchlike extension of the visceral peritoneum from the lower edge of the stomach, part of the duodenum, and the transverse colon.

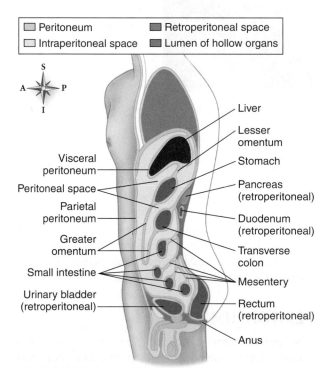

FIGURE 15-13 **Peritoneum.** The parietal layer of the peritoneum lines the abdominopelvic cavity and then extends in a continuous sheet as a series of mesenteries to form the visceral layer that covers abdominal organs.

Legend:
- Peritoneum
- Intraperitoneal space
- Retroperitoneal space
- Lumen of hollow organs

Labels:
- Visceral peritoneum
- Peritoneal space
- Parietal peritoneum
- Greater omentum
- Small intestine
- Urinary bladder (retroperitoneal)
- Liver
- Lesser omentum
- Stomach
- Pancreas (retroperitoneal)
- Duodenum (retroperitoneal)
- Transverse colon
- Mesentery
- Rectum (retroperitoneal)
- Anus

Shaped like a large apron, it hangs down over the intestines, and because spotty deposits of fat give it a lacy appearance, it has been nicknamed the *lace apron*. It usually envelops a badly inflamed appendix, walling it off from the rest of the abdominal organs.

X-Ray Studies of the Gastrointestinal (GI) Tract

Barium sulfate solution is referred to as a *contrast medium* that is **radiopaque** (ray-dee-oh-PAYK). This simply means that it does not permit passage of x rays. Barium shows up in x-ray images as a high-contrast, white outline of the structure that it fills and is often used in x-ray examinations to help visualize the various hollow segments of the GI tract. The normal x-ray images in Figure 15-14 show three areas of the GI tract that have been outlined or filled with barium. The barium solution has either been swallowed (*barium swallow*) or introduced into the lower segments of the tract by enema. The barium swallow is used in *upper GI x-ray studies* to visualize the esophagus, stomach, and small intestines, and the barium enema is used in *lower GI x-ray studies* to visualize the segments of the colon, rectum, and anal canal.

> ### ✔ QUICK CHECK
> 1. What is the role of the large intestine?
> 2. Name the divisions of the large intestine.
> 3. Where is the appendix?
> 4. What are mesenteries? What is their function?

DIGESTION

Digestion, a complex process that occurs in the alimentary canal, consists of physical and chemical changes that prepare food for absorption. *Mechanical digestion* breaks food into tiny particles, mixes them with digestive juices, moves them along the alimentary canal, and finally eliminates the digestive wastes from the body. Note that one or more types of GI motility such as chewing (mastication), swallowing (deglutition), peristalsis (see Figure 15-3), segmentation-type movements (see Figure 15-4), or defecation are closely associated in some way with mechanical digestion. *Chemical digestion* breaks down large, nonabsorbable food molecules

FIGURE 15-14 Barium-enhanced x-ray examination of the gastrointestinal (GI) tract. **A,** Upper GI study x-ray film of the lower esophagus, stomach, and duodenum. **B,** X-ray film of small intestine following barium swallow.

into smaller, absorbable nutrient molecules that are able to pass through the intestinal mucosa into blood and lymph (Figure 15-15). Chemical digestion consists of numerous chemical reactions catalyzed by enzymes in saliva, gastric juice, pancreatic juice, and intestinal juice.

Enzymes and Chemical Digestion

Enzymes (EN-zymez) are specialized protein molecules that act as *catalysts* (KAT-ah-lists). That is, they speed up specific chemical reactions without themselves being changed or consumed during the reaction process. During chemical digestion, certain enzymes very selectively speed up the breakdown of specific nutrient molecules and no others. Enzymes responsible for speeding up the breakdown of fats, for example, have no effect on carbohydrates or proteins. The names of many enzymes end with the suffix *-ase* combined with the word that describes the type of substance involved in the chemical reaction. Lip*ase* (LYE-payse), for example, is a fat-digesting enzyme that acts on lipids (fats) and prote*ase* (PROH-tee-ayse) enzymes serve to break down protein nutrients into smaller molecules. The breakdown process is called **hydrolysis** (hye-DROHL-i-sis)—an important type of chemi-

cal reaction first discussed in Chapter 2. Recall that during hydrolysis, enzymes speed up reactions that add water (hydro) to chemically break up or split (lysis) larger molecules into smaller molecules (see Figure 2-4 on p. 23).

Carbohydrate Digestion

Very little digestion of carbohydrates (starches and sugars) occurs before food reaches the small intestine. Salivary amylase usually has little time to do its work because so many of us swallow our food so fast. Gastric juice contains no carbohydrate-digesting enzymes. But after the food reaches the small intestine, pancreatic and intestinal juice enzymes digest the starches and sugars. A pancreatic enzyme (amylase) starts the process by breaking down polysaccharides such as starches into disaccharides (double sugars). Three intestinal enzymes—maltase, sucrase, and lactase—digest disaccharides by changing them into monosaccharides (simple sugars). Maltase digests maltose (malt sugar), sucrase digests sucrose (ordinary cane sugar), and lactase digests lactose (milk sugar). The end products of carbohydrate digestion are the monosaccharides, the most abundant of which is glucose.

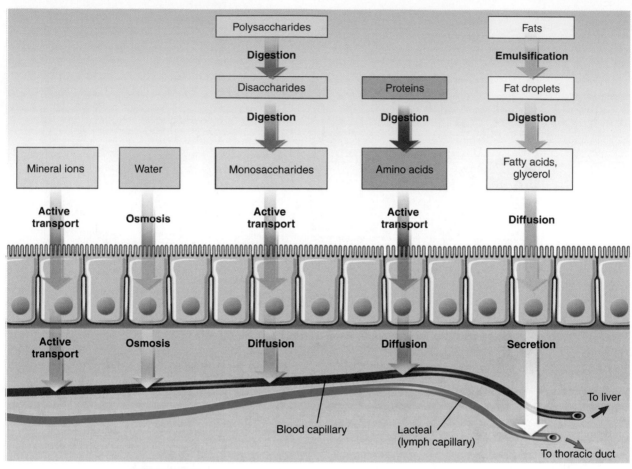

Active
transport

Osmosis

Active
transport

Active
transport

Diffusion

FIGURE 15-15 Digestion and absorption of nutrients, minerals, and water.

Protein Digestion

Protein digestion starts in the stomach. Pepsin, an enzyme in the gastric juice, causes the giant protein molecules to break up into somewhat simpler compounds. Pepsinogen (pep-SIN-oh-jen), a component of gastric juice, is converted into active pepsin enzyme by hydrochloric acid (also in gastric juice). In the intestine, other enzymes (trypsin in the pancreatic juice and peptidases in the intestinal juice) finish the job of protein digestion. Every protein molecule is made up of many amino acids joined together. When enzymes have split up the large protein molecule into its separate amino acids, protein digestion is completed. Hence the end product of protein digestion is amino acids. For obvious reasons, the amino acids are also referred to as *protein building blocks.*

Fat Digestion

Very little carbohydrate and fat digestion occurs before food reaches the small intestine. Most fats are undigested until after emulsification by bile in the duodenum (that is, fat droplets are broken into very small droplets). After this takes place, pancreatic lipase splits up the fat molecules into fatty acids and glycerol (glycerin). The end products of fat digestion, then, are fatty acids and glycerol.

Table 15-3 summarizes the main facts about chemical digestion. When carbohydrate digestion has been completed, starches (polysaccharides) and double sugars (disaccharides) have been changed mainly to glucose, a simple sugar (monosaccharide). The end products of protein digestion, on the other hand, are amino acids. Fatty acid and glycerol are the end products of fat digestion.

TABLE 15-3

Chemical Digestion

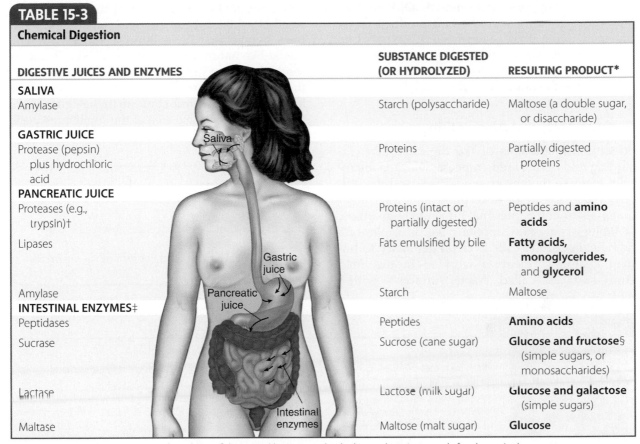

DIGESTIVE JUICES AND ENZYMES	SUBSTANCE DIGESTED (OR HYDROLYZED)	RESULTING PRODUCT*
SALIVA		
Amylase	Starch (polysaccharide)	Maltose (a double sugar, or disaccharide)
GASTRIC JUICE		
Protease (pepsin) plus hydrochloric acid	Proteins	Partially digested proteins
PANCREATIC JUICE		
Proteases (e.g., trypsin)†	Proteins (intact or partially digested)	Peptides and **amino acids**
Lipases	Fats emulsified by bile	**Fatty acids, monoglycerides,** and **glycerol**
Amylase	Starch	Maltose
INTESTINAL ENZYMES‡		
Peptidases	Peptides	**Amino acids**
Sucrase	Sucrose (cane sugar)	**Glucose and fructose**§ (simple sugars, or monosaccharides)
Lactase	Lactose (milk sugar)	**Glucose and galactose** (simple sugars)
Maltase	Maltose (malt sugar)	**Glucose**

*Substances in boldface type are end products of digestion (that is, completely digested nutrients ready for absorption).
†Secreted in inactive form (trypsinogen); activated by enterokinase, an enzyme in the intestinal brush border.
‡Brush-border enzymes.
§Glucose is also called *dextrose*; fructose is also called *levulose*.

 To learn more about the initiation of mechanical digestion, go to AnimationDirect on your CD-ROM.

ABSORPTION

After food is digested, the resulting nutrients are absorbed and move through the mucous membrane lining of the small intestine into the blood and lymph (see Figure 15-15). In other words, nutrient **absorption** is the process by which molecules of amino acids, glucose, fatty acids, and glycerol go from the inside of the intestines into the circulating fluids of the body. Absorption of nutrients is just as essential as digestion of foods. The reason is fairly obvious. As long as food stays in the intestines, it

cannot nourish the millions of cells that compose all other parts of the body. Their lives depend on the absorption of digested food and its transportation to them by the circulating blood.

Many important minerals, such as sodium, are actively transported through the intestinal mucosa. Water follows by osmosis. Other nutrients, such as monosaccharides and amino acids, are also actively transported through the intestinal mucosa and diffuse into the blood of capillaries in the intestinal villi. Fatty acids and glycerol diffuse into the absorptive cells of the GI tract and then are secreted into the lymphatic vessels or lacteals found in intestinal villi.

The "water-soluble vitamins" (vitamin C and the B vitamins) are dissolved in water and absorbed primarily from the small intestine. The "fat-soluble vitamins" (vitamins A, D, E, and K) are absorbed along with the end products of fat digestion in the small intestine and then pass into the lacteals. Bacterial action in the colon also produces some vitamin K that is absorbed through the lining of the large intestine.

Surface Area and Absorption

Structural adaptations of the digestive tube, including folds in the lining mucosa, villi, and microvilli, increase the absorptive surface and the efficiency and speed of absorption and transfer of materials from the intestinal lumen to body fluids.

Biologists are now applying the principles of a new field of study called **fractal geometry** to human anatomy. Scientists working in this field study surfaces—called "fractal surfaces"—with a seemingly infinite area, such as the lining of the small intestine. Fractal surfaces have bumps that have bumps that have bumps, and so on. The fractal-like nature of the intestinal lining is represented in Figure 15-9. The plicae (folds) have villi, the villi have microvilli, and even the microvilli have bumps that cannot be seen in the figure. Thus the absorptive surface area of the small intestine is almost limitless.

> ### ✓ QUICK CHECK
>
> 1. What is the difference between mechanical and chemical digestion?
> 2. In what form are carbohydrates absorbed into the bloodstream?
> 3. What must happen to fat before it can be chemically digested?

Science Application

Gastroenterology
William Beaumont (1785–1853)

Analyzing the word *gastroenterology* tells you it is the study (*-ology*) and treatment of the stomach (*gastro-*) and the intestines (*-entero-*). One of the pioneering gastroenterologists was the American physician William Beaumont. In 1822, the young Québécois trapper Alexis St. Martin was shot with a musket near the Army hospital in Michigan where Beaumont was working. Beaumont treated his wound but expected St. Martin to die. St. Martin recovered and lived a long life even though the wound did not heal properly. For his entire life, there remained an open hole in his abdomen leading directly into the stomach. St. Martin allowed Beaumont to study gastric secretion through the opening. Over many years, Beaumont made careful observations about how the stomach works. Many of his conclusions are still valid and serve as the foundation for modern gastroenterology.

Of course, many physicians and nurses specialize in gastroenterology today. However, many health care providers such as health care technicians and nursing assistants still need a basic knowledge of digestive structure and function in order to care for patients effectively. In addition, even those in dietetics, nutrition, and food service benefit by knowledge of the principles of digestion.

OUTLINE SUMMARY

OVERVIEW OF THE DIGESTIVE SYSTEM
(See Figure 15-1 and Table 15-1)
A. Irregular tube called *alimentary canal* or *gastrointestinal (GI) tract* and accessory organs of digestion
B. Food must first be digested and absorbed

PRIMARY MECHANISMS OF THE DIGESTIVE SYSTEM (See Table 15-2)
A. Ingestion — complex foods taken into the GI tract

B. Digestion — group of processes that break complex nutrients into simpler ones
   1. Mechanical digestion — breakup of large chunks of food into smaller bits
   2. Chemical digestion — breaks large molecules into smaller ones
C. Motility — a number of GI movements resulting from muscular contraction
D. Secretion — release of digestive juices and hormones that facilitate digestion

E. Absorption — movement of digested nutrients into the internal environment of the body

F. Regulation — neural, hormonal, and other mechanisms that regulate digestive activity

WALL OF THE DIGESTIVE TRACT (See Figure 15-2)

A. Digestive tract described as tube that extends from mouth to anus

B. Wall of the digestive tube is formed by four layers of tissue:
   1. Mucosa — type varies depending on GI location (tough and stratified or delicate and simple epithelium); mucus production
   2. Submucosa — connective tissue layer
   3. Muscularis — circular, longitudinal, and oblique (in stomach) layers of muscle important in GI motility
      a. Peristalsis — "wavelike" movement pushes food down the tract (see Figure 15-3)
      b. Segmentation — "back-and-forth" movement (see Figure 15-4)
   4. Serosa — serous membrane that covers the outside of abdominal organs; it attaches the digestive tract to the wall of the abdominopelvic cavity by forming folds called *mesenteries*

MOUTH

A. Roof — formed by hard palate (parts of maxillary and palatine bones) and soft palate, an arch-shaped muscle separating mouth from pharynx; uvula, a downward projection of soft palate (see Figure 15-5)

B. Floor — formed by tongue and its muscles; papillae, small elevations on mucosa of tongue; taste buds, found in many papillae; lingual frenulum, fold of mucous membrane that helps anchor tongue to floor of mouth (see Figure 15-5)

C. Typical tooth (see Figure 15-6)
   1. Three main parts — crown, neck, and root
   2. Enamel, which covers the crown, is hardest tissue in body

D. Types of teeth — incisors, canines (cuspids), premolars (bicuspids), and molars (tricuspids)

E. Twenty teeth in deciduous or baby set; average age for cutting first tooth about 6 months; set complete at about 30 months of age

F. Thirty-two teeth in permanent set; 6 years about average age for starting to cut first permanent tooth; set complete usually between ages of 17 and 24 years (see Figure 15-5)

SALIVARY GLANDS (Figure 15-7)

A. Saliva — exocrine gland secretion flows into ducts
   1. Serous type — watery and contains enzymes (salivary amylase) but no mucus
      a. Produced by serous type secretory cells (see Figure 15-7, B)
   2. Mucous type — thick, slippery, and contains mucus but no enzymes
      a. Lubricates food during mastication
      b. Produced by mucous type secretory cells (see Figure 15-7, B)

B. Parotid glands (see Figure 15-7)
   1. Largest salivary glands
   2. Produces serous type saliva
   3. Mumps — infection of parotids

C. Submandibular glands (see Figure 15-7)
   1. Mixed-gland — produces both serous- and mucous-type saliva (see Figure 15-7, B)
   2. Located below mandibular angle
   3. Ducts open on either side of lingual frenulum

D. Sublingual glands (see Figure 15-7)
   1. Produce only mucous-type saliva
   2. Multiple ducts open into floor of mouth

PHARYNX

A. Anatomical components: nasopharynx, oropharynx, laryngopharynx (see anatomical description in Chapter 4 and Figure 14-4)

B. Oropharynx — most involved segment in digestive process of swallowing or deglutition
   1. Regulation of deglutition movements via motor cortex of cerebrum (voluntary) and "deglutition center" of brainstem (involuntary)

ESOPHAGUS

A. Connects pharynx to stomach

B. Dynamic passageway for food

C. Food enters stomach by passing through lower esophageal sphincter (LES), or cardiac sphincter

STOMACH (See Figure 15-8)

A. Size — expands after large meal; about size of large sausage when empty

B. Food enters stomach through cardiac sphincter

C. Pyloric sphincter muscle closes opening between pylorus (lower part of stomach) and duodenum

D. Wall — many smooth muscle fibers; contractions produce churning movements (peristalsis)

E. Lining — mucous membrane; many microscopic glands secrete gastric juice and hydrochloric acid into stomach; mucous membrane lies in folds (rugae) when stomach is empty

SMALL INTESTINE (See Figure 15-9)

A. Size — about 7 meters (20 feet) long but only 2 cm or so in diameter

B. Divisions
   1. Duodenum
   2. Jejunum
   3. Ileum

C. Wall — contains smooth muscle fibers that contract to produce peristalsis and segmentation movements

D. Lining — mucous membrane; many microscopic glands (intestinal glands) secrete intestinal juice; villi (microscopic finger-shaped projections from surface of mucosa into intestinal cavity) contain blood and lymph capillaries

LIVER AND GALLBLADDER

A. Size and location — liver is largest gland; fills upper right section of abdominal cavity and extends over into left side

B. Liver secretes bile

C. Ducts (see Figure 15-10)
   1. Hepatic — drains bile from liver
   2. Cystic — duct by which bile enters and leaves gallbladder
   3. Common bile — formed by union of hepatic and cystic ducts; drains bile from hepatic or cystic ducts into duodenum

D. Gallbladder
   1. Location — undersurface of the liver
   2. Function — concentrates and stores bile produced in the liver
   3. Bile serves to emulsify fats

PANCREAS

A. Exocrine gland that lies behind stomach

B. Functions
   1. Pancreatic cells secrete pancreatic juice (most important digestive juice) into pancreatic ducts; main duct empties into duodenum
   2. Pancreatic islets (of Langerhans) — cells not connected with pancreatic ducts; secrete hormones glucagon and insulin into the blood

LARGE INTESTINE (See Figure 15-12)

A. Divisions
   1. Cecum
   2. Colon — ascending, transverse, descending, and sigmoid
   3. Rectum

B. Food enters through ileocecal valve; external opening called anus

C. Wall — contains smooth muscle fibers that contract to produce churning, peristalsis, and defecation

D. Lining — mucous membrane

APPENDIX

A. Blind tube off cecum

B. No important digestive functions in humans

PERITONEUM (See Figure 15-14)

A. Definitions — peritoneum, continuous serous membrane lining abdominal cavity and covering abdominal organs; parietal layer of peritoneum lines abdominal cavity; visceral layer of peritoneum covers abdominal organs; peritoneal space lies between parietal and visceral layers

B. Extensions — largest are the mesentery and greater omentum
   1. Mesentery is extension of parietal peritoneum, which attaches most of small intestine to posterior abdominal wall
   2. Greater omentum, or "lace apron," hangs down from lower edge of stomach and transverse colon over intestines

C. X-ray studies of the GI tract—radiopaque contrast medium used to help visualize structures in study images

DIGESTION (See Table 15-3)

A. Definition — transforms foods into substances that can be absorbed and used by cells
   1. Mechanical digestion — chewing (mastication), swallowing (deglutition), and peristalsis break food into tiny particles, mix them well with digestive juices, and move them along the digestive tract
   2. Chemical digestion — breaks up large food molecules into compounds that have smaller molecules; brought about by digestive enzymes (see Figure 15-15)
B. Enzymes and chemical digestion
   1. Enzymes are specialized protein molecules that act as catalysts
   2. Breakdown process called hydrolysis
C. Carbohydrate digestion — mainly in small intestine
   1. Pancreatic amylase — breaks polysaccharides down to disaccharides
   2. Intestinal juice enzymes
      a. Maltase — changes maltose to glucose
      b. Sucrase — changes sucrose to glucose
      c. Lactase — changes lactose to glucose
D. Protein digestion—starts in stomach; completed in small intestine
   1. Gastric juice enzyme *pepsin* partially digests proteins
   2. Pancreatic enzyme, *trypsin*, continues digestion of proteins
   3. Intestinal enzymes, *peptidases*, complete digestion of partially digested proteins and convert them to amino acids
E. Fat digestion
   1. Bile contains no enzymes but emulsifies fats (breaks fat droplets into very small droplets)
   2. Pancreatic lipase changes emulsified fats to fatty acids and glycerol in small intestine

ABSORPTION

A. Definition — process by which digested food moves from intestine into blood or lymph
B. Foods and most water, minerals, and vitamins are absorbed from small intestine; some water and vitamin K also absorbed from large intestine
C. Surface area absorption
   1. Structural adaptations increase absorptive surface area
   2. Fractal geometry — study of fragmented geometric irregular shapes such as those in lining of intestine

NEW WORDS

alimentary canal	feces	lower esophageal	peritoneum
anus	fractal geometry	sphincter (LES)	plica (pl. plicae)
appendicitis	frenulum	lumen	pyloric sphincter
bile	gallstones	malocclusion	radiopaque
cardiac sphincter	gastroesophageal	mastication	rugae
cholecystectomy	reflux disease	mesentery	salivary amylase
cholecystokinin (CCK)	(GERD)	microvilli	segmentation
chyme	gingivitis	mucosa	serosa
deciduous (baby) teeth	greater omentum	muscularis	serous saliva
defecation	hepatic (right colic)	oral (mouth) cavity	splenic (left colic)
deglutition	flexure	pancreatic islets (of	flexure
dental caries (cavity)	hiatal hernia	Langerhans)	submucosa
digestion	hydrolysis	periodontal membrane	ulcer
duodenal papilla	ileocecal valve	periodontitis	uvula
emulsify	jaundice	peristalsis	veriform appendix
enzymes	lacteal	peritoneal space	villus (pl. villi)

REVIEW QUESTIONS

1. Name and describe the four layers of the wall of the GI tract.
2. What is the function of the uvula and soft palate?
3. Explain the function of the different types of teeth.
4. Describe the three main parts of a tooth.
5. Name the three pairs of salivary glands and describe where the duct from each enters the mouth.
6. What are the functions of the cardiac and pyloric sphincter muscles?
7. Define *peristalsis*.
8. Explain how bile from the liver and gallbladder reaches the small intestine. What is the function of cholecystokinin?
9. What is contained in pancreatic juice?
10. What do the bacteria in the large intestine contribute to the body?
11. List the seven subdivisions of the large intestine.
12. Describe the mesentery and the greater omentum.
13. Differentiate between mechanical digestion and chemical digestion.
14. Briefly describe the process of carbohydrate digestion.
15. Briefly describe the process of fat digestion.
16. Briefly describe the process of protein digestion.
17. Explain the process of absorption. What function do the lacteals have in absorption?

CRITICAL THINKING

18. What structures in the small intestine increase the internal surface area? What advantage is gained by this increase in surface area?
19. Bile does not cause a chemical change; what is the effect of bile on fat and why does this make fat digestion more efficient?
20. Some people are lactose intolerant. This means they are unable to digest lactose sugar. What enzyme is probably not functioning properly and what types of food should these people try to avoid?

CHAPTER TEST

1. Food undergoes three kinds of processing in the body. All cells perform metabolism, but _____ and _____ are performed by the digestive system.
2. The _____ layer of the wall of the GI tract produces peristalsis.
3. The _____ layer of the wall of the GI tract contains blood vessels and nerves.
4. _____ is the innermost layer of the wall of the GI tract.
5. _____ is the outermost layer of the wall of the GI tract.
6. The _____ and _____ prevent food and liquid from entering the nasal cavity above the mouth when food is swallowed.
7. The three main parts of a tooth are _____, _____, and _____.
8. The names of the three pairs of salivary glands are the _____, the _____, and the _____.

CHAPTER TEST—cont'd

9. The tube connecting the pharynx and the stomach is the _____.

10. The three divisions of the stomach are the _____, the _____, and the _____.

11. The three divisions of the small intestine are the _____, the _____, and the _____.

12. The tiny, fingerlike projections covering the plicae of the small intestine are called _____.

13. The lymphatic vessel in the villi is called the _____.

14. The common bile duct is formed by the union of the _____ from the liver and the _____ from the gallbladder.

15. The part of the large intestine between the ascending and descending colon is the _____.

16. The part of the large intestine between the descending colon and the rectum is called the _____.

17. The two most prominent extensions of the peritoneum are the _____ and the _____.

18. The process by which digested food is moved from the digestive system to the circulating fluids is called _____.

Match each statement in Column B with its corresponding term in Column A.

COLUMN A

19. _____ emulsification
20. _____ amylase
21. _____ pepsin
22. _____ cholecystokinin
23. _____ peptidase
24. _____ cystic
25. _____ trypsin
26. _____ simple sugars
27. _____ amino acids
28. _____ liver
29. _____ lipase
30. _____ glycerol

COLUMN B

a. This enzyme is made in the pancreas and digests fat.
b. This enzyme is made in the small intestine and digests protein.
c. This gland produces bile.
d. This is the final end product of protein digestion.
e. Bile has this effect on fat droplets.
f. This enzyme is made in an inactive form in the pancreas and digests protein.
g. This is the final end product of carbohydrate digestion.
h. This is one of the final end products of fat digestion.
i. This enzyme is made in both the salivary gland and the pancreas and digests starch.
j. This enzyme is made in the stomach in an inactive form and digests protein.
k. This hormone stimulates the contraction of the gallbladder.
l. This duct connects the gallbladder to the common bile duct.

OBJECTIVES

AFTER YOU HAVE COMPLETED THIS CHAPTER, YOU SHOULD BE ABLE TO:

1. Define and contrast catabolism and anabolism.
2. Describe the metabolic roles of carbohydrates, fats, proteins, vitamins, and minerals.
3. Define basal metabolic rate and list some factors that affect it.
4. Discuss the physiological mechanisms that regulate body temperature.

Nutrition and Metabolism 16

Nutrition and metabolism are words that are often used together—but what do they mean? **Nutrition** is a term that refers to the food (nutrients) that we eat and the nutrients they contain. Proper nutrition requires a balance of the three basic food types: *carbohydrates*, *fats*, and *proteins*, plus essential *vitamins* and *minerals*. Malnutrition is a deficiency or imbalance in the consumption of food, vitamins, and minerals. To promote good health, Canada and the United States provide individualized online food guides that help a person determine the proper amounts and balance of nutrients (Figure 16-1).

A good phrase to remember in connection with the word **metabolism** is "use of foods" because basically this is what metabolism is—the use the body makes of foods after they have been digested, absorbed, and circulated to cells. It uses them in two ways: as an energy source and as building blocks for making complex chemical compounds. Before they can be used in these two ways, foods have to be *assimilated*. **Assimilation** occurs when food molecules enter cells and undergo many chemical changes there. All the chemical reactions that release energy from food molecules make up the process of **catabolism,** a vital process because it is the only way that the body has of supplying itself with energy for doing any work. Catabolism breaks food molecules down into smaller molecules and releases energy in the process. The many chemical reactions that build food molecules into more complex chemical compounds constitute the process of **anabolism.** Catabolism and anabolism make up the process of metabolism.

STUDY TIPS

To make the study of nutrition and metabolism more efficient, we suggest these tips:

1. This chapter begins with an explanation of the functions of the liver and the importance of the portal system, both of which were discussed previously in Chapters 12 and 15, so review that material before beginning this chapter.
2. The process of metabolism refers to the body's use of food. Fats and carbohydrates are used primarily for energy.
3. Carbohydrate metabolism begins with glycolysis. *Glyco-* refers to carbohydrates, and *-lysis* means "to destroy or break down," and the process does exactly that.
4. The end products of glycolysis enter the citric acid (or Krebs) cycle, which produces many high-energy molecules. The electron transfer system converts these high-energy molecules into adenosine triphosphate (ATP).
5. ATP is the only energy source your body can use directly. The energy is stored in the bonds between the phosphates in the molecule, and these phosphates can be broken off to release energy and replaced to store energy.
6. Fat and protein molecules can be modified so they can also enter the citric acid cycle.
7. The term *nonessential amino acids* does not mean your body doesn't need these amino acids; nonessential amino acids are necessary for you to live, but your body has the ability to make the nonessential amino from other amino acids.
8. Vitamins and minerals assist in enzyme function.
9. You can learn the names and functions of the vitamins and minerals from flash cards. In your study group, go over the flash cards for vitamins and minerals.
10. Metabolic rates describe how quickly the food is used. Basal metabolic rate is the amount of food you use just to stay alive and awake. The total metabolic rate depends on how active you are.
11. Discuss the ways heat can be lost from the body.

Continued on page 380.

FIGURE 16-1 **Food guide.** Canada, the United States, and many other countries provide online, individualized food guides that help people determine proper amounts and a healthy balance of nutrients. The website www.ChooseMyPlate.gov is hosted by the United States Department of Agriculture (USDA).

This chapter explores many of the basic ideas about why certain nutrients are necessary for survival and how they are used by the body.

ROLES OF THE LIVER

As we discussed in Chapter 15, the liver plays an important role in the mechanical digestion of lipids because it secretes *bile.* As you recall, bile breaks large fat globules into smaller droplets of fat that are more easily broken down.

In addition, the liver performs other functions necessary for healthy survival. The liver plays a major role in the metabolism of all three kinds of foods. For example, the liver helps maintain a normal blood glucose concentration by storing glucose when it is overly abundant and then releasing the glucose into the blood as needed. Many complex

chemical reactions regulated by many different hormones assist in these storage and release processes.

Liver cells carry on the first steps of protein and fat metabolism. Liver cells also synthesize several kinds of protein compounds. These proteins, when released into the blood, are called the *blood proteins* or **plasma proteins**. Prothrombin and fibrinogen, two of the plasma proteins formed by liver cells, play essential parts in blood clotting (see p. 258). Another protein made by liver cells, albumin, helps maintain normal blood volume.

The liver can detoxify various poisonous substances such as bacterial products and certain drugs. The liver can also store several useful substances, notably iron and vitamins A and D.

The liver is assisted by an interesting structural feature of the blood vessels that supply it. As you may recall from Chapter 12, the hepatic portal vein delivers blood directly from the gastrointestinal tract to the liver (see Figure 12-14). This arrangement allows blood that has just absorbed nutrients and other substances to be processed by the liver before being distributed throughout the body. Thus excess nutrients and vitamins can be stored and toxins can be efficiently removed from the bloodstream before the blood reaches other areas of the body.

QUICK CHECK

1. What are the three basic food types?
2. What is metabolism?
3. Describe the functions of the liver.

NUTRIENT METABOLISM

Carbohydrate Metabolism

Carbohydrates are the preferred energy food of the body. The larger carbohydrate molecules are composed of smaller "building blocks," primarily *glucose* (see Chapter 2). Human cells catabolize (break down) glucose rather than other substances as long as enough glucose enters them to supply their energy needs.

Three series of chemical reactions, occurring in a precise sequence, make up the process of glucose catabolism. **Glycolysis** (glye-KOHL-i-sis) is the first series of reactions, **citric acid cycle** (or *Krebs cycle*) is the second series, and **electron transfer system (ETS)** is the third.

Glycolysis, the first step of glucose catabolism, occurs in the cytoplasm of each cell of the body. As Figure 16-2 shows, glycolysis breaks down glucose (a six-carbon molecule) into two *pyruvic acids* (three-carbon molecules). Glycolysis releases a small amount of energy—enough to generate two ATP molecules—but requires no oxygen to do so. We thus say that it is an **anaerobic** (an-air-OH-bik) process.

Each pyruvic acid molecule may then move into a mitochondrion—one of the cell's tiny "battery chargers" that transfers much more of the nutrient energy to ATP. After pyruvic acid is broken down into the two-carbon acetyl molecule, *coenzyme A (CoA)* escorts it into the citric acid cycle. The citric acid cycle releases high-energy electrons as it breaks down the acetyl CoA (two carbons) to carbon dioxide (only one carbon), using enzymes located inside the mitochondrion.

The chemical reactions of glycolysis and the citric acid cycle release energy stored in the glucose molecule. More than half of the released energy is in the form of high-energy electrons. The electron transport system, embedded in the inner folds of the mitochondrion, transfers the energy from these electrons to molecules of ATP. Up to 36 molecules of ATP can be generated in the mitochondrion for every original glucose molecule that enters this metabolic pathway. The rest of the energy originally stored in the glucose molecule is released as heat, which contributes to a person's body temperature.

The metabolic pathway inside the mitochondrion, in contrast to glycolysis, is an oxygen-using or **aerobic** (air-OH-bik) process. A cell cannot operate the citric acid cycle or electron transport system—where most of energy of glucose is released—without oxygen.

ATP serves as the direct source of energy for doing cellular work in all kinds of living organisms from one-cell plants to billion-cell animals, including man. Among biological compounds, therefore, ATP ranks as one of the most important.

The energy transferred to ATP molecules differs in two ways from the energy stored in food molecules: the energy in ATP molecules is not stored but is released almost instantaneously, and it can be used directly to do cellular work. Release of energy from food molecules occurs much more slowly because it accompanies the long series of chemical reactions that make up the process of catabolism. Energy released from food molecules

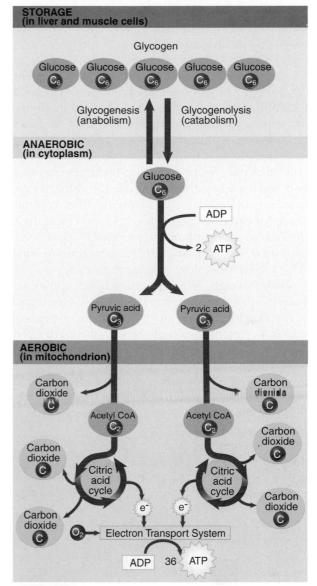

FIGURE 16-2 **Metabolism of glucose.** Glucose can be stored as subunits of glycogen in liver and muscle cells until needed to make ATP. After glycogen is split apart, each glucose molecule undergoes glycolysis in the cytoplasm. Glycolysis splits one molecule of glucose (six carbon atoms) into two molecules of pyruvic acid (three carbon atoms each) and produces enough energy to generate two ATPs. Each pyruvic acid is converted to the two-carbon acetyl molecule, which is escorted by coenzyme A (CoA) into the citric acid cycle in the mitochondrion. The citric acid cycle breaks apart each pyruvic acid molecule into three carbon dioxide molecules (one carbon atom each) and many high-energy electrons. The electron transport system (also in the mitochondrion) uses energy from these electrons to generate up to 36 ATPs in the presence of oxygen (O_2).

cannot be used directly for doing cellular work. It must first be transferred to ATP molecules and then be explosively released from them.

As Figure 16-3 shows, ATP is made up of an adenosine group and three phosphate groups. The capacity of ATP to store large amounts of energy is found in the high-energy bonds that hold the phosphate groups together, illustrated as curvy lines. When a phosphate group breaks off of the molecule, an adenosine diphosphate (ADP) molecule and free phosphate group result. Energy that had been holding the phosphate bond together is freed to do cellular work (muscle fiber contractions, for example). As you can see in Figure 16-3, the ADP and phosphate are reunited by the energy produced by carbohydrate catabolism, making ATP a reusable energy-storage molecule.

Only enough ATP for immediate cellular requirements is made at any one time. Glucose that is not needed is built up (by anabolic processes) into larger molecules that are stored for later use. Glucose anabolism is called **glycogenesis** (glye-koh-JEN-eh-sis). Carried on chiefly by liver and muscle cells, glycogenesis consists of a series of reactions that join glucose molecules together, like many beads in a necklace, to form *glycogen*, a compound sometimes called *animal starch*.

Later, when the glucose stored as glycogen is needed to make ATP, a process called **glycogenolysis** (glye-koh-jen-AH-lis-is) breaks down glycogen chains in the liver or muscle cells to release individual glucose molecules. Glycogenolysis is an example of catabolism.

Something worth noting is that the amount of nutrients in the blood normally does not change very much, not even when we go without food for many hours, when we exercise and use a lot of food for energy, or when we sleep and use little food for energy. The amount of glucose in our blood, for example, usually stays at about 80 to 110 milligrams (mg) in 100 milliliters (mL) of blood when we are "fasting" between meals.

Several hormones help regulate carbohydrate metabolism to keep blood glucose at a normal level. Insulin is one of the most important of these. It acts in some way not yet definitely known to make glucose leave the blood and enter the cells at a more rapid rate. As insulin secretion increases, more glucose leaves the blood and enters the cells. The amount of glucose in the blood therefore decreases as the rate of glucose metabolism in cells increases (see p. 240). Too little insulin secretion, such as occurs in people with diabetes mellitus, produces the opposite effects. Less glucose leaves the blood and enters the cells. More glucose therefore remains in the blood, and less glucose is metabolized by cells. In other words, high blood glucose (hyperglycemia) and a low rate of glucose metabolism characterize insulin deficiency. Insulin is the only hormone that lowers the blood glucose level. Several other hormones, on the other hand, increase it. Growth hormone secreted by the anterior pituitary gland, hydrocortisone secreted by the adrenal cortex, epinephrine secreted by the adrenal medulla, and glucagon secreted by the pancreatic islets are four of the most important hormones that increase blood glucose. More information about these hormones appears in Chapter 10.

FIGURE 16-3 Adenosine triphosphate (ATP). **A,** The structure of adenosine triphosphate (ATP). A single adenosine group (A) has three attached phosphate groups (P). The high-energy bonds between the phosphate groups can release chemical energy to do cellular work. **B,** ATP energy cycle. ATP stores energy in its last high-energy phosphate bond. When that bond is later broken, energy is released to do cellular work. The adenosine diphosphate (ADP) and phosphate groups that result can be resynthesized into ATP, capturing additional energy from nutrient catabolism.

Health and Well-Being

Carbohydrate Loading

A number of athletes and others who must occasionally sustain endurance exercise for a significant period practice **carbohydrate loading,** or **glycogen loading.** As with liver cells, some skeletal muscle fibers can take up and store glucose in the form of glycogen. By ceasing intense exercise and switching to a diet high in carbohydrates 2 or 3 days before an endurance event, an athlete can cause the skeletal muscles to store almost twice as much glycogen as usual. This allows the muscles to sustain aerobic exercise for up to 50% longer than usual. The concept of carbohydrate loading has been used to promote the use of "energy bar" sport snacks.

 To learn more about glycolysis, go to AnimationDirect on your CD-ROM.

 To learn more about the citric acid cycle, go to AnimationDirect on your CD-ROM.

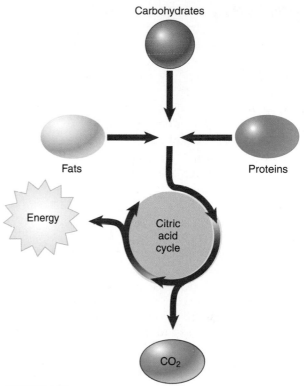

FIGURE 16-4 Catabolism of nutrients. Fats, carbohydrates, and proteins can be converted to products that enter the citric acid cycle to yield energy.

Fat Metabolism

Fats, like carbohydrates, are primarily energy foods. If cells do not have adequate amounts of glucose to catabolize, they immediately shift to the catabolism of fats for energy.

Fats are broken down into fatty acids and glycerol, and then each of these is converted into a chemical form that can enter the citric acid cycle. This happens normally when a person goes without carbohydrates for many hours. It happens abnormally in untreated diabetic individuals. Because of an insulin deficiency, too little glucose enters the cells of a diabetic person to supply all energy needs. The result is that the cells catabolize fats to make up the difference (Figure 16-4).

In all persons, fats not needed for catabolism are instead anabolized (built up) to form triglycerides and stored in adipose tissue.

Protein Metabolism

In a healthy person, proteins are catabolized to release energy to a very small extent. When fat reserves are low, as they are in the starvation that accompanies certain eating disorders such as anorexia nervosa, the body can start to use its protein

molecules as an energy source. Specifically, the amino acids that make up proteins are each broken apart to yield an amine group that is converted to a form of glucose that can enter the citric acid cycle. After a shift to reliance on protein catabolism as a major energy source occurs, death may quickly follow because vital proteins in the muscles and nerves are catabolized (see Figure 16-4).

A more common situation in normal bodies is protein anabolism, the process by which the body builds **amino acids** into complex protein compounds (for example, enzymes and proteins that form the structure of the cell). Proteins are assembled from a pool of 20 different kinds of amino acids. If any one type of amino acid is deficient, vital proteins cannot be synthesized—a serious health threat.

One way your body maintains a constant supply of amino acids is by making them from other compounds already present in the body. Only about half of the required 20 types of amino acids can be made by the body, however. The remaining types of amino acids must be supplied in the diet.

TABLE 16-1

Amino Acids

ESSENTIAL (INDISPENSABLE)	NONESSENTIAL (DISPENSABLE)
Histidine*	Alanine
Isoleucine	Arginine
Leucine	Asparagine
Lysine	Aspartic acid
Methionine	Cysteine
Phenylalanine	Glutamic acid
Threonine	Glutamine
Tryptophan	Glycine
Valine	Proline
	Serine
	Tyrosine†

*Essential in infants and, perhaps, adult males.
†Can be synthesized from phenylalanine and therefore is nonessential as long as phenylalanine is in the diet.

Essential amino acids are those that must be in the diet. *Nonessential amino acids* can be missing from the diet because they can be made by the body (Table 16-1).

QUICK CHECK

1. How are aerobic and anaerobic processes different? How are they alike?
2. How is energy transferred from glucose to ATP?
3. How are proteins used once they are absorbed into the body?
4. What are essential amino acids?

VITAMINS AND MINERALS

One glance at the label of any packaged food product reveals the importance we place on vitamins and minerals. We know that carbohydrates, fats, and proteins are used by our bodies to build important molecules and to provide energy. So why do we need vitamins and minerals?

First, let us discuss the importance of vitamins. **Vitamins** are organic molecules needed in small quantities for normal metabolism throughout the body. Most vitamin molecules attach to enzymes or *coenzymes* (molecules that assist enzymes) and help them work properly. Many enzymes are totally useless without the appropriate vitamins to activate them. Some vitamins play other important roles in the body. For example, a form of vitamin A plays an important role in detecting light in the sensory cells of the retina. Vitamin D can be converted to a hormone that helps regulate calcium homeostasis in the body. And vitamin E acts as an *antioxidant* that prevents highly reactive molecules called *free radicals* from damaging DNA and molecules in cell membranes.

Most vitamins cannot be made by the body, so we must eat them in our food. The body can store fat-soluble vitamins—A, D, E, and K—in the liver for later use. Because the body cannot store water-soluble vitamins such as B vitamins and vitamin C, they must be continually supplied in the diet. Vitamin deficiencies can lead to severe metabolic problems. Table 16-2 lists some of the better known vitamins, their sources, functions, and symptoms of deficiency.

Minerals are just as important as vitamins. Minerals are inorganic elements or salts found naturally in the earth. As with vitamins, mineral ions can attach to enzymes and help them work. Minerals also function in a variety of other vital chemical reactions. For example, sodium, calcium, and other minerals are required for nerve conduction and for contraction in muscle fibers. Without these minerals, the brain, heart, and respiratory tract would cease to function. Information about some of the more important minerals is summarized in Table 16-3.

METABOLIC RATES

The **basal metabolic rate (BMR)** is the rate at which food is catabolized under basal conditions (that is, when the individual is resting but awake, is not digesting food, and is not adjusting to a cold external temperature). Or, stated differently, the BMR is the number of calories of heat that must be produced per hour by catabolism just to keep the body alive, awake, and comfortably warm. To provide energy for muscular work and digestion and absorption of food, an additional amount of food must be catabolized. The amount of additional food depends mainly on how much work the individual does. The more active he or she is, the more food the body must catabolize and the higher the total metabolic rate will be. The **total metabolic rate (TMR)** is the total amount of energy used by the body per day (Figure 16-5).

When the number of calories in your food intake equals your TMR, your weight remains

TABLE 16-2

Major Vitamins

VITAMIN	DIETARY SOURCE	FUNCTIONS	SYMPTOMS OF DEFICIENCY
Vitamin A	Green and yellow vegetables, dairy products, and liver	Maintains epithelial tissue and produces visual pigments	Night blindness, dry eye possibly leading to blindness, and flaking skin
B-complex vitamins			
B_1 (thiamine)	Grains, meat, and legumes	Helps enzymes in the citric acid cycle	Nerve problems (beriberi), heart muscle weakness, and edema (B_1 deficiency common in alcoholism)
B_2 (riboflavin)	Green vegetables, organ meats, eggs, and dairy products	Helps enzymes in the citric acid cycle	Inflammation of skin and mucous membranes (including irritation around mouth and eyes)
B_3 (niacin)	Meat and grains	Helps enzymes in the citric acid cycle	Pellagra (scaly dermatitis and mental disturbances), nervous disorders, and diarrhea
B_5 (pantothenic acid)	Organ meat, eggs, and liver	Helps enzymes that connect fat and carbohydrate metabolism	Loss of coordination (rare)
B_6 (pyridoxine)	Vegetables, meats, and grains	Helps enzymes that catabolize amino acids	Convulsions, irritability, and anemia
B_{12} (cyanocobalamin)	Meat and dairy products	Involved in blood production and other processes	Pernicious anemia
Biotin	Vegetables, meat, and eggs	Helps enzymes in amino acid catabolism and fat and glycogen synthesis	Mental and muscle problems (rare)
Folic acid	Vegetables	Helps enzymes in amino acid catabolism and blood production	Digestive disorders, anemia, prenatal neural tube defects (NTDs)
Vitamin C (ascorbic acid)	Fruits and green vegetables	Helps in manufacture of collagen fibers	Scurvy and degeneration of skin, bone, and blood vessels
Vitamin D (calciferol)	Dairy products and fish liver oil	Helps in calcium absorption	Rickets and skeletal deformity
Vitamin E (tocopherol)	Green vegetables and seeds	Protects cell membranes from being catabolized	Muscle and reproductive disorders (rare)
Vitamins K_1, K_2	Intestinal bacteria (synthetic form is K_3)	Helps in blood clotting, bone metabolism	Blood clotting disorders, bone loss

FIGURE 16-5 Factors that determine the basal and total metabolic rates.

TABLE 16-3

Major Minerals

MINERAL	DIETARY SOURCE	FUNCTIONS	SYMPTOMS OF DEFICIENCY
Calcium (Ca)	Dairy products, legumes, and vegetables	Helps blood clotting, bone formation, and nerve and muscle function	Bone degeneration and nerve and muscle malfunction
Chlorine (Cl)	Salty foods	Helps in stomach acid production and acid-base balance	Acid-base imbalance
Cobalt (Co)	Meat	Helps vitamin B_{12} in blood cell production	Pernicious anemia
Copper (Cu)	Seafood, organ meats, and legumes	Involved in extracting energy from the citric acid cycle and in blood production	Fatigue and anemia
Iodine (I)	Seafood and iodized salt	Needed for thyroid hormone synthesis	Goiter (thyroid enlargement) and decrease of metabolic rate
Iron (Fe)	Meat, eggs, vegetables, and legumes	Involved in extracting energy from the citric acid cycle and needed for red blood cell production	Fatigue and anemia
Magnesium (Mg)	Vegetables and grains	Helps many enzymes	Nerve disorders, blood vessel dilation, and heart rhythm problems
Manganese (Mn)	Vegetables, legumes, and grains	Helps many enzymes	Muscle and nerve disorders
Phosphorus (P)	Dairy products and meat	Helps in bone formation and is used to make ATP, DNA, RNA, and phospholipids	Bone degeneration and metabolic problems
Potassium (K)	Seafood, milk, fruit, and meats	Helps muscle and nerve function	Muscle weakness, heart problems, and nerve problems
Sodium (Na)	Salty foods	Helps in muscle and nerve function and fluid balance	Weakness and digestive upset
Zinc (Zn)	Many foods	Helps many enzymes	Metabolic problems, diarrhea

constant (except for possible variations resulting from water retention or water loss). When your food intake provides more calories than your TMR, you gain weight; when your food intake provides fewer calories than your TMR, you lose weight. These weight control principles rarely fail to operate. Nature does not forget to count calories. Reducing diets make use of this knowledge. They contain fewer calories than the TMR of the individual eating the diet. See Appendix A for in-

formation on the *body mass index (BMI)* and its relationship to body weight.

BODY TEMPERATURE

Considering the fact that more than 60% of the energy released from food molecules during catabolism is converted to heat rather than being transferred to ATP, it is no wonder that maintaining a constant body temperature is a challenge. Main-

 Health and Well-Being

Vitamin Supplements for Athletes

Because a deficiency of vitamins **(avitaminosis)** can cause poor athletic performance, many athletes regularly consume vitamin supplements. However, research suggests that vitamin supplementation has little or no effect on athletic performance. A reasonably well-balanced diet supplies more

than enough vitamins for even the elite athlete. The use of vitamin supplements therefore has fueled some controversy among exercise experts. Opponents of vitamin supplements cite the cost and the possibility of liver damage associated with some forms of **hypervitaminosis,** whereas supporters cite the benefit of protecting against vitamin deficiency.

Research, Issues, & Trends

Measuring Energy

Physiologists studying metabolism must be able to express a quantity of energy in mathematical terms. The unit of energy measurement most often used is the calorie (cal). A **calorie** is the amount of energy needed to raise the temperature of 1 gram of water 1° C. Because physiologists often deal with very large amounts of energy, the larger unit, **kilocalorie** (kcal), or *Calorie* (notice the uppercase C), is used. There are 1,000 cal in 1 kcal, or Calorie. Nutritionists prefer to use **Calorie** when they express the amount of energy stored in a food.

---

taining homeostasis of body temperature, or **thermoregulation**, is the function of the hypothalamus. The hypothalamus operates a variety of negative-feedback mechanisms that keep body temperature in its normal range (36.2° to 37.6° C or 97° to 100° F).

The skin is often involved in negative-feedback loops that maintain body temperature. When the body is overheated, blood flow to the skin increases (Figure 16-6). Warm blood from the body's core can then be cooled by the skin, which acts as a radiator. At the skin, heat can be lost from blood by the following mechanisms:

1. Radiation—flow of heat waves away from the blood
2. Conduction—transfer of heat energy to the skin and then the external environment
3. Convection—transfer of heat energy to air that is continually flowing away from the skin
4. Evaporation—absorption of heat by water (sweat) vaporization

When necessary, heat can be conserved by reducing blood flow in the skin (see Figure 16-6).

A number of other mechanisms can be called on to help maintain the homeostasis of body temperature. Heat-generating muscle activities such as shivering and secretion of metabolism-regulating hormones are two of the body's processes that can be altered to adjust the body's temperature. The concept of using feedback control loops in homeostatic mechanisms was introduced in Chapter 1.

> ### ✓ QUICK CHECK
>
> 1. What is the overall job of vitamins in the body?
> 2. What is another name for the rate at which food is catabolized under resting conditions?
> 3. How does calories consumed relate to a person's body weight?
> 4. Can you describe the four main ways that heat leaves the body?

FIGURE 16-6   The skin as a thermoregulatory organ. A, When homeostasis requires that the body conserve heat, blood flow in the warm organs of the body's core increases. **B,** When heat must be lost to maintain the stability of the internal environment, flow of warm blood to the skin increases. Heat can be lost from the blood and skin by means of radiation, conduction, convection, and evaporation.

Food Science
George Washington Carver
(1864–1943)

At the dawn of the twentieth century, one figure loomed large in the world of food science—George Washington Carver. Born a slave on a Missouri plantation during the Civil War, Carver overcame great obstacles to become one of the most admired American scientists in history. Although talented in music and art, it was his knack for agriculture that led him to a long and successful career as a professor, researcher, and inventor in the agriculture department of Alabama's Tuskegee Institute. There, his work resulted in the creation of 325 products from peanuts, nearly 200 products from yams (sweet potatoes), and hundreds more from other plants native to the southern United States. Development of these new products helped poor farmers survive by allowing them to make money from a variety of crops that thrived on their land.

Today, breakthroughs continue in the world of agriculture and food science. Farmers and ranchers work closely with agricultural scientists and technicians to improve food crops and livestock—and ways of raising them. As did Carver, they strive to work in ways that benefit the land as well as the people. Of course, nutritionists, dietitians, chefs, and food preparers all play a role in getting these crops to our table in a healthy and appetizing way. Food scientists and other industrial scientists work to develop technologies and methods for preparing, preserving, storing, and packaging foods.

OUTLINE SUMMARY

DEFINITIONS
A. Nutrition — food, vitamins, and minerals that are ingested and assimilated into the body (see Figure 16-1)
B. Assimilation — process of getting food molecules into the cells of the body and chemically preparing them for use in the chemical reactions of the body
C. Metabolism — process of using food molecules as energy sources and as building blocks for our own molecules
D. Catabolism — breaks food molecules down, releasing their stored energy; oxygen used in catabolism
E. Anabolism — builds food molecules into complex substances

ROLE OF THE LIVER
A. Secretes bile, which breaks down large fat globules
B. Helps maintain normal blood glucose level
C. Helps metabolize carbohydrates, fats, and proteins; synthesizes several kinds of protein compounds
D. Removes toxins from the blood

NUTRIENT METABOLISM
A. Carbohydrates — preferred energy food of the body
   1. Three series of chemical reactions in glucose metabolism
      a. Glycolysis
         (1) Changes glucose to pyruvic acid
         (2) Anaerobic (uses no oxygen)
         (3) Yields small amount of energy, generating two ATPs
         (4) Occurs in cytoplasm
      b. Citric acid (Krebs) cycle
         (1) Changes pyruvic acid to carbon dioxide
         (2) Aerobic (requires oxygen)
         (3) Yields large amount of energy (mostly as high-energy electrons)
         (4) Occurs in mitochondria
      c. Electron transfer system
         (1) Transfers energy from high-energy electrons (from citric acid cycle) to ATP molecules
         (2) Located in mitochondria
   2. The mitochondrial part of the pathway (citric acid cycle and electron transport system) is aerobic (requires oxygen) and

generates up to 36 ATP molecules per original glucose molecule

3. Carbohydrates are primarily catabolized for energy (see Figure 16-2)
4. Adenosine triphosphate (ATP) — molecule in which energy obtained from breakdown of foods is stored; serves as a direct source of energy for cellular work (see Figure 16-3)
5. Storage of glucose
   a. Glucose that is not needed immediately for making ATP is stored as glycogen (a long chain of glucose subunits) in liver and muscle cells
   b. Glycogenesis — anabolic process of joining glucose molecules together in a chain to form glycogen (to store glucose for later use)
   c. Glycogenolysis — catabolic process of breaking apart glycogen chains, releasing individual glucose molecules for use in making ATP
6. Blood glucose (imprecisely, *blood sugar*) — normally stays between about 80 and 110 mg per 100 mL of blood during fasting; insulin accelerates the movement of glucose out of the blood into cells, therefore decreases blood glucose and increases glucose catabolism

B. Fats — catabolized to yield energy and anabolized to form adipose tissue (see Figure 16-4)

C. Proteins — primarily anabolized and secondarily catabolized

VITAMINS AND MINERALS

A. Vitamins — organic molecules that are needed in small amounts for normal metabolism (Table 16-2)
B. Minerals — inorganic molecules found naturally in the earth, required by the body for normal function (Table 16-3)

METABOLIC RATES

A. Basal metabolic rate (BMR) — rate of metabolism when a person is lying down but awake and not digesting food and when the environment is comfortably warm
B. Total metabolic rate (TMR) — the total amount of energy, expressed in calories, used by the body per day (see Figure 16-5)

BODY TEMPERATURE

A. Hypothalamus — regulates the homeostasis of body temperature (thermoregulation) through a variety of processes
B. Skin — can cool the body by losing heat from the blood through four processes: radiation, conduction, convection, evaporation (see Figure 16-6)

NEW WORDS

aerobic	calorie	glycogenesis	plasma protein
amino acid	carbohydrate loading	glycogenolysis	thermoregulation
anabolism	(*also called* glycogen	glycolysis	total metabolic rate
anaerobic	loading)	hypervitaminosis	(TMR)
assimilation	catabolism	insulin	vitamin
avitaminosis	citric acid cycle	kilocalorie	
basal metabolic rate	electron transport	metabolism	
(BMR)	system (ETS)	nutrition	

REVIEW QUESTIONS

1. Define *anabolism* and *catabolism*.
2. Explain the function of the liver.
3. Briefly explain the process of glycolysis.
4. Briefly explain the citric acid cycle.
5. What is the function of the electron transfer system?
6. Explain the ways in which energy stored in ATP is different than the energy stored in food molecules.
7. List the hormones that tend to increase the amount of sugar in the blood.
8. When does fat catabolism usually occur?
9. When does protein catabolism usually occur?
10. Explain what is meant by a nonessential amino acid.
11. Name three water-soluble and three fat-soluble vitamins.
12. Name three minerals needed by the body.
13. What is the function of vitamins and minerals in the body?
14. Differentiate between basal and total metabolic rate.
15. Name and explain three ways heat can be lost by the skin.

CRITICAL THINKING

16. Differentiate between absorption and assimilation.
17. Explain the advantage the body gains by having the blood go to the liver through the hepatic portal system.
18. Diagram the ATP-ADP cycle. Include where the energy is added and where it is released.
19. A man went on a 10-day vacation. His total metabolic rate was 2,600 calories a day. His calorie intake was 3,300 calories a day. He began his trip weighing 178 pounds. What did he weigh by the end of his vacation? (3,500 excess calories = 1 pound)

CHAPTER TEST

1. The process of _____ occurs when food molecules enter the cells and undergo chemical changes.
2. _____ is the term used to describe all the chemical processes that release energy from food.
3. _____ is the term used to describe all the chemical processes that build food molecules into larger compounds.
4. The plasma proteins _____ and _____ are made by the liver and are important in blood clot formation.

CHAPTER TEST—cont'd

5. The vitamins _____ and _____ can be stored in the liver.
6. The B vitamins are _____ soluble, whereas vitamins K and E are _____ soluble.
7. _____ is the total amount of energy used by the body per day.
8. _____ is the number of calories that must be used just to keep the body alive, awake, and comfortably warm.
9. To lose weight, your total caloric intake must be less than your _____.
10. One way heat can be lost by the skin is _____, which is the transfer of heat to the air that is continually flowing away from the skin.
11. One way heat can be lost by the skin is _____, which is the absorption of heat by water (sweat) vaporization.
12. _____ is the process used by the body as its second choice of energy metabolism. People with diabetes frequently must use this process.
13. In a healthy body, _____ is used almost exclusively for anabolism rather than catabolism.
14. _____ are amino acids needed by the body, but they can be made from other amino acids if they are not supplied by the diet.

Match each phrase in Column B with the correct corresponding term in Column A.

COLUMN A

15. _____ glycolysis
16. _____ citric acid cycle
17. _____ electron transfer system
18. _____ mitochondria cycle
19. _____ cytoplasm
20. _____ ATP
21. _____ glycogenesis
22. _____ ADP

COLUMN B

a. part of the cell in which glycolysis occurs
b. step in carbohydrate metabolism that does not require oxygen
c. process that converts high-energy molecules from citric acid to ATP
d. step in carbohydrate metabolism that requires oxygen
e. direct source of energy for the body
f. molecule produced when adenosine triphosphate loses a phosphate group
g. the part of the cell in which the citric acid cycle takes place
h. glucose anabolism

OBJECTIVES

AFTER YOU HAVE COMPLETED THIS CHAPTER, YOU SHOULD BE ABLE TO:

1. Identify the major organs of the urinary system and give the generalized function of each.
2. Name the parts of a nephron and describe the role each component plays in the formation of urine.
3. Explain the importance of filtration, tubular reabsorption, and tubular secretion in urine formation.
4. Discuss the mechanisms that control urine volume.
5. Discuss the normal amount and composition of urine.
6. Explain how the kidneys act as vital organs in maintaining homeostasis.

The Urinary System 17

As you continue to learn more about the structure and function of the body, the concept of **homeostasis** remains as a critically important and unifying theme. First introduced and emphasized in Chapter 1 (see pp. 12-14), the concept of homeostasis has served as the "glue" that has allowed you to "connect" information about specific cells, tissues, organs, and organ systems presented in every chapter of this text to an understanding of the body as a whole. Of course, by now you already know that homeostasis refers to the maintenance of relative constancy or stability of the internal environment of the body. And, because of metabolic activity occurring in every cell of the body and a host of both internal and external disturbances, you know as well that there are constant threats to both maintaining and restoring that stability. The constancy of body fluid volumes and the levels of many important chemicals required for normal metabolic activity in every cell of the body depend on normal urinary system functions. Therefore the **urinary system** plays a key and central role in maintaining homeostasis in the body as a whole. Producing and excreting urine from the body are only two of the most obvious functions of this critically important organ system. This chapter highlights the importance of these functions and also the many other important roles the urinary system plays in the maintenance of homeostasis and in healthy survival.

Unless the urinary system operates normally, the normal composition of blood cannot be maintained for long, and serious consequences soon follow. One function of the kidneys is to "clear" or clean the blood of the many waste products continually produced as a result of metabolism of foodstuffs in the body cells. As nutrients are

burned in the cells for energy, the wastes produced soon enter and must then be removed from the blood. Some of these waste products are cleared from the blood by the kidneys and must be quickly excreted in the urine or they rapidly accumulate to toxic levels—a condition called **uremia** (yoo-REE-mee-ah), or **uremic poisoning**. The kidneys also play vital roles in maintaining blood pressure, stimulating adequate RBC production, and in regulating electrolyte, water, blood pH levels, and acid-base balances in the body.

In this chapter, we discuss the structure and function of each organ of the urinary system. There are two kidneys, two ureters, one bladder, and one urethra (Figure 17-1). We also briefly mention disease conditions and abnormal functioning of urinary system organs characterized by disturbances in homeostasis.

To learn more about the urinary system, go to AnimationDirect on your CD-ROM.

KIDNEYS

Location

To locate the kidneys on your own body, stand erect and put your hands on your hips with your thumbs meeting over your backbone. When you are in this position, your kidneys lie above your thumbs on either side of your spinal column, but

FIGURE 17-1 **Urinary system. A,** Anterior view of urinary organs. **B,** Surface markings of the kidneys, eleventh and twelfth ribs, spinous processes of L1 to L4, and lower edge of pleura viewed from behind. **C,** Horizontal (transverse) section of the abdomen showing the retroperitoneal position of the kidneys. **D,** X-ray film of the urinary organs.

their placement is higher than you might think. Note in Figure 17-1 that the right kidney, which touches the liver, is lower than the left. Both are protected a bit by the lower rib cage and are located under the muscles of the back and *behind* the parietal peritoneum (the membrane that lines the abdominal cavity). Because of this *retroperitoneal* (reh-troh-pair-i-toh-NEE-al) location, a surgeon can operate on a kidney from behind without cutting through the parietal peritoneum, which covers the organ only on its anterior, or front, surface (see Figure 17-1, C). A heavy cushion of fat normally encases each kidney and helps hold it in place.

The right and left renal arteries emerge directly from the abdominal aorta at a level between L1 and L2. Both arteries are short but have a relatively large diameter. Normally a little more than 20% of the total blood pumped by the heart each minute enters the kidneys. The rate of blood flow through this organ is among the highest in the body. This is understandable because one of the main functions of the kidney is to remove waste products from the blood. Maintenance of a high

rate of blood flow and normal blood pressure in the kidneys is essential for the formation of urine.

Internal Structure

If you were to slice through a kidney from side to side and open it like the pages of a book (called a *coronal section*), you would see the structures shown in Figure 17-2. Identify each of the following parts:

1. **Renal cortex** (KOHR-teks)—the outer part of the kidney (the word *cortex* comes from the Latin word for "bark," so the cortex of an organ is its outer layer).
2. **Renal medulla** (meh-DUL-ah)—the inner portion of the kidney.
3. **Renal pyramids** (PEER-ah-midz)—the triangular divisions of the medulla of the kidney. Extensions of cortical tissue that dip down into the medulla between the renal pyramids are called *renal columns*.
4. **Renal papilla** (pah-PIL-ah) (pl. *papillae*)— narrow, innermost end of a pyramid.

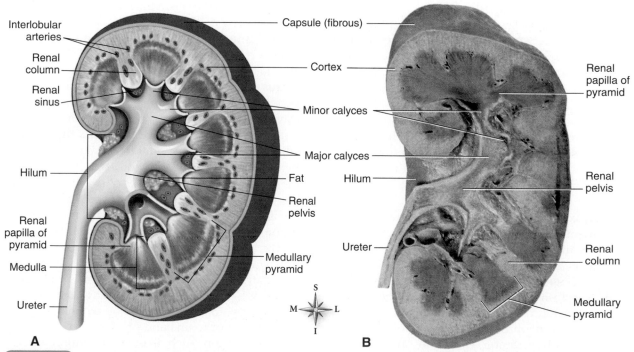

A   **B**

FIGURE 17-2 **Internal structure of the kidney. A,** Artist's rendering of a coronal section of the kidney. **B,** Photograph of coronal section of a preserved human kidney.

5. **Renal pelvis**—(also called the *kidney pelvis*) an expansion of the upper end of a ureter (the tube that drains urine into the bladder).
6. **Calyx** (KAY-liks) (pl. *calyces*)—a division of the renal pelvis (the papilla of a pyramid opens into each calyx).

Microscopic Structure

More than a million microscopic units called **nephrons** (NEF-ronz) make up each kidney's interior. The shape of a nephron is unique, unmistakable, and admirably suited to its function of producing urine. It looks a little like a tiny funnel with a very long stem, but it is an unusual stem in that it is highly convoluted (that is, it has many bends in it). The nephron is composed of two principle components: the *renal corpuscle* and the *renal tubule.* The renal corpuscle can be subdivided still further into two parts and the renal tubule into four regions or segments. Identify each part of the renal corpuscle and renal tubule described below in Figures 17-3 and 17-4.

1. **Renal corpuscle**
   a. **Bowman capsule**—the cup-shaped top of a nephron (the saclike Bowman capsule surrounds the glomerulus).
   b. **Glomerulus** (gloh-MER-yoo-lus) (pl. *glomeruli*)—a network of blood capillaries tucked into the Bowman capsule. (Note in Figure 17-3 that the small artery that delivers blood to the glomerulus [afferent arteriole] is larger in diameter than the blood vessel that drains blood from it [efferent arteriole] and that it is relatively short. This explains the high blood pressure that exists in the glomerular capillaries. This high pressure is required to filter wastes from the blood.)
2. **Renal tubule**
   a. **Proximal convoluted tubule**—the first segment of a renal tubule. (It is called *proximal* because it lies nearest the tubule's origin from the Bowman capsule, and it is called *convoluted* because it has several bends.)
   b. **Nephron loop** *(loop of Henle [HEN-lee])*—the extension of the proximal tubule. (Observe that the nephron loop consists of a straight descending limb, a hairpin loop, and a straight ascending limb.)
   c. **Distal convoluted tubule**—the part of the tubule distal to the ascending limb of the

nephron loop. (It is the extension of the ascending limb.)
   d. **Collecting tubule**—a straight (that is, not convoluted) part of a renal tubule. (Distal tubules of several nephrons join to form a single collecting tubule or duct.)

Look again at Figure 17-3. Note that the renal corpuscles (glomeruli surrounded by the Bowman capsule) and both proximal and distal convoluted tubules are located in the cortex of the kidney. The medulla contains the nephron loop and collecting tubules. Urine from the collecting tubules exits from the pyramid through the papilla and enters the calyx and renal pelvis before flowing into the ureter.

 To learn more about the nephron, go to AnimationDirect on your CD-ROM.

Function

The kidneys are vital organs. The function they perform, that of forming urine, is essential for homeostasis and maintenance of life. Early in the process of urine formation, fluid, electrolytes, and wastes from metabolism are *filtered* from the blood and enter the nephron. Additional wastes may be *secreted* into the tubules of the nephron as substances useful to the body are reabsorbed into the blood. Table 17-1 lists the components of normal versus abnormal urine. Normally the kidneys balance the amount of many substances entering and leaving the blood over time so that normal concentrations can be maintained. In short, the kidneys adjust their output to equal the intake of the body. By eliminating wastes and adjusting fluid balance, the kidneys play an essential part in maintaining homeostasis. Homeostasis cannot be maintained—nor can life itself—if the kidneys fail and the condition is not soon corrected. Nitrogenous waste products accumulate as a result of protein breakdown and quickly reach toxic levels if not excreted. If kidney function ceases because of injury or disease, life can be maintained by using an artificial kidney to cleanse the blood of wastes.

Excretion of toxins and of waste products containing nitrogen, such as urea and ammonia, represents only one of the important responsibilities of the kidney. The kidney also plays a key role in regulating the levels of many chemical substances

Location and components of the nephron. A, Magnified wedge cut from a renal pyramid. **B,** Schematic showing relationship of glomerulus to Bowman capsule and adjacent structures. **C,** Scanning electron micrograph showing several glomeruli and their associated blood vessels.

FIGURE 17-4 The nephron unit. Cross-sections from the four segments of the renal tubule are shown. The differences in appearance in tubular cells seen in a cross-section reflect the differing functions of each nephron segment.

in the blood such as chloride, sodium, potassium, and bicarbonate. The kidneys regulate the proper balance between body water content and salt by selectively retaining or excreting both substances as requirements demand. In addition, the cells of the *juxtaglomerular apparatus* (see Figure 17-4) function in blood pressure regulation. When blood pressure is low, these cells secrete a hormone (renin) that initiates constriction of blood vessels and thus raises blood pressure. The kidneys also play

an important role in maintaining adequate RBC numbers. They produce a hormone that stimulates production and normal maturation of RBCs in the bone marrow and then helps to prolong the life of mature RBCs in circulating blood. This fact helps explain why patients with chronic kidney function problems are often anemic. It is easy to understand why the kidneys are often considered to be the most important homeostatic organs in the body.

TABLE 17-1

Characteristics of Urine

	NORMAL CHARACTERISTICS	ABNORMAL CHARACTERISTICS
Color and Clarity	Normal urine should be clear; color varies with specific gravity Dilute urine: Transparent straw color Concentrated urine: Deep yellow amber (Occasionally, normal urine may be cloudy because of high dietary levels of fat or phosphate)	Abnormally colored urine may result from (1) pathological conditions, (2) certain foods, and (3) numerous drugs 　1. Pathological conditions (examples): 　　Kidney cancer (hemorrhage)—red (RBCs) 　　Bile duct obstruction (gallstones)—orange/yellow (bilirubin) 　　Pseudomonas infection—green (bacterial toxins) 　2. Foods (examples): 　　Beets—red 　　Rhubarb—brown 　　Carrots—dark yellow 　3. Drugs (examples): 　　Pyridium (urinary tract analgesic)—orange 　　Dilantin (anticonvulsant)—pink/red brown 　　Dyrenium (diuretic)—pale blue 　　Cloudy urine may result from (examples): 　　(1) bacteria—active infection of urinary system organs 　　(2) blood cells 　　　RBCs—hemorrhage from kidney cancer 　　　WBCs—pus from urinary tract infection (UTI) 　　(3) casts—various types of tubelike clumps (blood cell, epithelial, hyaline, waxy, etc.) that form in diseased renal tubes 　　(4) proteinuria—(protein—usually albumin) in urine 　　(5) crystals—usually uric acid or phosphate/calcium oxalate in concentrated urine
Compounds	Mineral ions (for example, Na^+, Cl^-, K^+) Nitrogenous wastes: ammonia, creatinine, urea, uric acid Urine pigment: urochrome (product of bilirubin metabolism)	Ketones—generally acetone Protein—generally albumin Glucose Crystals—generally uric acid and phosphate or calcium oxalate Pigments—abnormal levels of bilirubin metabolites
Odor	Slight aromatic Some foods produce a characteristic odor (asparagus) Ammonia-like odor on standing may result from decomposition in stored urine	Strong, sweet, fruity (acetone) odor—uncontrolled diabetes mellitus Foul odor—UTIs Musty odor—phenylketonuria Maple syrup odor—congenital defect in protein metabolism
pH	4.6 to 8.0 (average 6.0) Toward low normal: Some foods (meat & cranberries) and drugs (chlorothiazide diuretics) Toward high normal: Some foods (citrus fruits, dairy products) and drugs (bicarbonate antacids)	High in alkalosis (kidneys compensate by excreting excess base) Low in acidosis (kidneys compensate by excreting excess H^+)
Specific Gravity	Adult: 1.005 to 1.030 (usually 1.010 to 1.025) Elderly: values decrease with age Newborn: 1.001 to 1.020	Above normal limits: glycosuria, proteinuria, dehydration, high solute load (may result in precipitation of solutes and kidney stone formation) Below normal limits: chronic renal diseases (inability to concentrate urine), overhydration

Clinical Application

Artificial Kidney

The artificial kidney is a mechanical device that uses the principle of dialysis to remove or separate waste products from the blood. In the event of kidney failure, the process called **hemodialysis** can provide a reprieve from death for the patient. During a hemodialysis treatment, a semipermeable membrane is used to separate large (nondiffusible) particles such as blood cells from small (diffusible) ones such as urea and other wastes. Part *A* of the figure shows blood from the radial artery passing through a porous (semipermeable) cellophane tube that is housed in a tanklike container. The tube is surrounded by a bath, or dialysis solution, containing varying concentrations of electrolytes and other chemicals. The pores in the membrane are small and allow only very small molecules, such as urea, to escape into the surrounding fluid. Larger molecules and blood cells cannot escape and are returned through the tube to reenter the patient via a wrist or leg vein. By constantly replacing the bath solution in the di-

alysis tank with freshly mixed solution, levels of waste materials can be kept at low levels. As a result, wastes such as urea in the blood rapidly pass into the surrounding wash solution. For a patient with complete kidney failure, two or three hemodialysis treatments a week are required. New dialysis methods are now being developed, and dramatic advances in treatment are expected in the next few years.

Another technique used in the treatment of renal failure is called **continuous ambulatory peritoneal dialysis (CAPD).** In this procedure, 1 to 3 liters of sterile dialysis fluid is introduced directly into the peritoneal cavity through an opening in the abdominal wall (part *B* of the figure). Peritoneal membranes in the abdominal cavity transfer waste products from blood into the dialysis fluid, which is then drained back into a plastic container after about 2 hours. This technique is less expensive than hemodialysis and does not require the use of complex equipment.

A

B

Hemodialysis.

To learn more about the kidney, go to AnimationDirect on your CD-ROM.

✓ QUICK CHECK

1. What are the two main regions of the kidney?
2. Describe the structure of a nephron.
3. What is the role of filtration in the kidney?

FORMATION OF URINE

The kidney's two million or more nephrons form **urine** by a series of three processes: (1) filtration, (2) reabsorption, and (3) secretion (Figure 17-5).

Filtration

Urine formation begins with the process of **filtration,** which goes on continually in the renal corpuscles (Bowman capsules plus their encased

Formation of urine. Diagram shows examples of the steps in urine formation in successive parts of a nephron: filtration, reabsorption, and secretion.

glomeruli). Blood flowing through the glomeruli exerts pressure, and this glomerular blood pressure is high enough to push water and dissolved substances out of the glomeruli into the Bowman capsule. Briefly, glomerular blood pressure causes filtration through the glomerular-capsular membrane. If the glomerular blood pressure drops below a certain level, filtration and urine formation cease. Hemorrhage, for example, may cause a precipitous drop in blood pressure followed by *kidney failure.*

Glomerular filtration normally occurs at the rate of 125 milliliters (mL) per minute. As a result, about 180 liters (almost 190 quarts) of **glomerular filtrate** is produced by the kidneys every day.

By proceeding at a normal rate and without some type of intervention, glomerular filtration would result in draining away, as urine, all of our blood plasma in about an hour. Fortunately, as a result of normal kidney function, most of the fluid and nutrients that leave the blood by glomerular filtration—the first process in urine formation—are quickly reclaimed and returned to the blood by a second process called *tubular reabsorption.*

Reabsorption

Reabsorption is the movement of substances out of the renal tubules into the blood capillaries located around the tubules (peritubular capillaries). Water, glucose and other nutrients, and sodium and other ions are substances that are reabsorbed. Some ions may be transported from glomerular filtrate into the interstitial fluid by passing through the junctions holding adjacent tubular cells together. However, most substances that are reabsorbed from glomerular filtrate must pass through three barriers in their journey from glomerular filtrate to blood. First, the substances must pass through two plasma membranes. One membrane, called the *luminal membrane*, forms the epithelial surface of cells facing the interior or lumen of the tubule. This is the membrane that is in direct contact with the glomerular fluid passing through the tubule. After passing through the luminal membrane, the substances being reabsorbed must then traverse the interior of the tubular cell and exit through the plasma membrane of the cell that faces the interstitial fluid. Finally, substances in the interstitial fluid pass through the endothelial lining of the peritubular capillaries and enter the blood.

Reabsorption begins in the proximal convoluted tubules and continues in the nephron loop, distal convoluted tubules, and collecting tubules (see Figure 17-5). Different transport mechanisms exist for differing substances that must be moved from tubular fluid into the blood, and both active and passive transport mechanisms play important roles (see Chapter 3—Tables 3-2 and 3-3, pp. 45 and 47). Examples involving active transport mechanisms include functioning of membrane "carrier proteins" for certain nutrient molecules, ion pumps such as the coupled sodium-potassium membrane pump, and pinocytosis of small protein molecules, which are then digested to amino acids inside the tubule cell. Passive mechanisms include the action of osmosis important in the reabsorption of water and the mechanism for reabsorption of chloride ions.

Although water is reabsorbed from every segment of the renal tubule, most of the water in the 180 liters of glomerular filtrate produced each day is reabsorbed by osmosis from the proximal tubules. Chloride ions (Cl^-) passively move into the blood because they carry a negative electrical charge. Positively charged sodium ions that have been actively reabsorbed and moved into the blood "attract" the negatively charged chloride ions from the tubule fluid into the peritubular capillaries.

The nutrient glucose is actively transported, coupled with sodium, from the proximal tubules into the peritubular capillary blood. None of this valuable nutrient is wasted by being lost in the urine. However, exceptions occur. For example, in untreated diabetes mellitus, blood glucose concentration increases dramatically and large amounts of sugar pass into the tubular fluid. When the amount of glucose in tubular fluid increases above a certain level, called the **renal threshold** level for glucose, the kidney tubular cells are no longer able to reabsorb all of it, and the excess is excreted in the urine. Glucose in the urine—**glycosuria** (glye-koh-SOO-ree-ah)—is a well-known sign of poorly controlled diabetes mellitus.

Common table salt (NaCl) consumed in the diet or introduced by intravenous infusion of "normal saline" (0.9% NaCl) or other NaCl-containing fluids, provides the body with both sodium ions (Na$^+$) and chloride ions (Cl$^-$). For the most part, sodium ions are actively transported back into blood from the tubular fluid in all segments of the kidney tubule except the collecting ducts. The amount of sodium reabsorbed will depend largely on intake. In general the greater the amount of sodium intake, the less the amount reabsorbed and the greater the amount excreted in the urine. Also, the less sodium intake, the greater the reabsorption from kidney tubules and the less excreted in the urine.

Urine values of potassium ion (K$^+$) will vary greatly with diet. Some **diuretic** (dye-yoo-RET-ik) **drugs**, which stimulate the production of urine (see the Clinical Application: Diuretics box in Chapter 18, p. 421), are said to be "potassium wasting" because they increase *secretion* of potassium into tubular fluid and, ultimately, its excretion in the urine.

Secretion

Secretion is the process by which substances move into urine forming in the distal and collecting tubules from blood in the capillaries located around these tubules (peritubular capillaries). In this respect, secretion is reabsorption in reverse. Whereas reabsorption moves substances out of the urine into the blood, secretion moves substances out of the blood into the urine. Tubular secretion serves an important function by removing or "clearing" the blood of excess potassium and hydrogen ions, certain drugs including penicillin and phenobarbital, and numerous wastes such as urea, uric acid, and creatinine. Most substances that are secreted from peritubular blood enter the filtrate primarily in the proximal tubule and, to a lesser extent, the distal convoluted tubule and collecting ducts. The major exception to this "rule of thumb" is potassium ion, which is secreted primarily into the collecting ducts in an exchange with sodium. In the distal convoluted tubules and collecting ducts, sodium secretion is dependent on hormones also important in regulating urine volume, as discussed below. Ammonia is secreted passively by diffusion. Kidney tubule secretion plays a crucial role in maintaining the body's fluid, electrolyte, and acid-base balance, as discussed in Chapters 18 and 19.

In summary, the following processes occurring in successive portions of the nephron accomplish the function of urine formation (Table 17-2):

1. **Filtration**—of water and dissolved substances out of the blood in the glomeruli into the Bowman capsule

TABLE 17-2

Functions of Parts of Nephron in Urine Formation

PART OF NEPHRON	PROCESS IN URINE FORMATION	SUBSTANCES MOVED
Glomerulus	Filtration	Water and solutes (for example, sodium and other ions, glucose and other nutrients filtering out of glomeruli into Bowman capsules)
Proximal tubule	Reabsorption	Water and solutes (glucose, amino acids), Na$^+$
	Secretion	Nitrogenous wastes, some drugs
Nephron loop	Reabsorption	Sodium and chloride ions
Distal and collecting tubules	Reabsorption	Water, sodium, and chloride ions
	Secretion	Ammonia, potassium ions, hydrogen ions, and some drugs

2. **Reabsorption**—of water and dissolved substances out of kidney tubules back into blood (this prevents substances needed by the body from being lost in urine; usually, 97% to 99% of water filtered out of glomerular blood is retrieved from tubules)
3. **Secretion**—of hydrogen ions, potassium ions, and certain drugs

Control of Urine Volume

The body has ways to control the amount and composition of the urine that it excretes. It does this mainly by controlling the amount of water and dissolved substances that are reabsorbed by the convoluted tubules. For example, a hormone (antidiuretic hormone [ADH]) from the posterior pituitary gland decreases the amount of urine by making collecting tubules permeable to water. If no ADH is present, the tubules are practically impermeable to water, so little or no water is reabsorbed from them. When ADH is present in the blood, collecting tubules are permeable to water and water is reabsorbed from them. As a result, less water is lost from the body as urine, or more water is retained from the tubules whichever way you wish to say it. At any rate, for this reason ADH is accurately described as the "water-retaining hormone." You might also think of it as the "urine-decreasing hormone."

The hormone **aldosterone,** secreted by the adrenal cortex, plays an important part in controlling the kidney tubules' reabsorption of sodium. Primarily it stimulates the tubules to reabsorb sodium at a faster rate. Secondarily, aldosterone also increases tubular water reabsorption. As sodium is reabsorbed, water will follow it back into the blood by osmosis. The term *sodium- and water-retaining hormone* therefore is a descriptive nickname for aldosterone. In the absence of aldosterone, almost no sodium is reabsorbed from the collecting ducts. The result is rapid and catastrophic loss of sodium, resulting in death.

Another hormone, **atrial natriuretic hormone (ANH)**, secreted from the heart's atrial wall, has the opposite effect of aldosterone. ANH stimulates kidney tubules to secrete more sodium and thus lose more water. Thus ANH is a *salt- and water-losing hormone*. The body secretes ADH, aldosterone, and ANH in different amounts, depending on the homeostatic balance of body fluids at any particular moment.

Sometimes the kidneys do not excrete normal amounts of urine as a result of dehydration, kidney disease, cardiovascular disease, or stress. Here are some terms associated with abnormal amounts of urine:

1. **Anuria** (ah-NOO-ree-ah)—absence of urine
2. **Oliguria** (ohl-i-GYOO-ree-ah)—scanty amounts of urine
3. **Polyuria** (pol-ee-YOO-ree-ah)—an unusually large amount of urine

Because a change in urine volume or output is a significant indicator in many types of fluid alterations and diseases, measurement of both fluid intake and fluid output (urine volume) over a specified period of time, often abbreviated as **I & O,** is a common practice in clinical medicine. The normal adult urine output is about 1,500 to 1,600 mL per day.

Health and Well-Being

Proteinuria After Exercise

Proteinuria is the presence of plasma proteins in the urine. Proteinuria is probably the most important indicator of renal disease **(nephropathy)** because only damaged nephrons consistently allow plasma protein molecules to leave the blood. However, intense exercise causes temporary proteinuria in many individuals. Some exercise physiologists believed that intense athletic activities cause kidney damage, but subsequent research has ruled out that explanation. One current hypothesis is that hormonal changes during strenuous exercise increase the permeability of the nephron's filtration membrane, allowing some plasma proteins to enter the filtrate. Some postexercise proteinuria is usually considered normal.

QUICK CHECK
1. What are the three basic processes that occur in the nephron?
2. How do ADH and aldosterone affect urine output?
3. What is anuria? Polyuria?

URETERS

Urine drains out of the collecting tubules of each kidney into the renal pelvis and down the ureter into the urinary bladder (see Figures 17-1 and 17-7). The **renal pelvis** is the basinlike upper end of the ureter located inside the kidney. Ureters are narrow

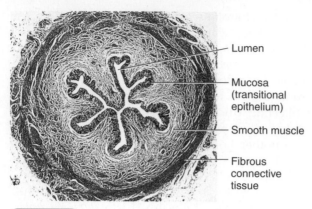

Lumen

Mucosa (transitional epithelium)

Smooth muscle

Fibrous connective tissue

FIGURE 17-6 **Ureter cross-section.** Note the many folds, covered by a specialized (transitional epithelium) mucous lining, which almost fill the lumen of the tube. A thick layer of smooth muscle can be seen surrounding the lumen. On its outer surface, the ureter is covered by a tough fibrous connective tissue coat.

tubes less than 6 millimeters (mm) (¼ inch) wide and 25 to 30 centimeters (cm) (10 to 12 inches) long. Mucous membranes line both ureters and each renal pelvis. Note in Figure 17-6 that the ureter has a thick, muscular wall. Contraction of the muscular coat produces peristaltic-type movements that as-

sist in moving urine down the ureters into the bladder. The lining membrane of the ureters is richly supplied with sensory nerve endings.

Attacks of **renal colic**—pain caused by the passage of a kidney stone—have been described in medical writings since antiquity. Kidney stones cause intense pain if they have sharp edges or are large enough to distend the walls or cut the lining of the ureters or urethra as they pass from the kidneys to the exterior of the body.

URINARY BLADDER

The empty urinary bladder lies in the pelvis just behind the pubic symphysis. When full of urine, it projects upward into the lower portion of the abdominal cavity. In women it sits in front of the uterus, whereas in men, it rests on the prostate (Figure 17-7).

Elastic fibers and involuntary muscle fibers in the wall of the urinary bladder make it well suited for expanding to hold variable amounts of urine and then contracting to empty itself. A specialized type of epithelial membrane lines the urinary bladder. The lining is loosely attached to the deeper muscular layer so that the bladder is very wrinkled and lies in folds called **rugae** when it is empty. When the bladder is filled, its inner surface is smooth. Note in Figure 17-7, *A*, that one triangular area on the back or posterior surface of the bladder is free of rugae. This area, called the **trigone,** is always smooth. There, the lining membrane is tightly fixed to the deeper muscle coat.

Ureter

Cut edge of peritoneum

Smooth muscle

Trigone

Opening of ureter

Opening of ureter

Rugae

Internal urinary sphincter

Prostate gland

External urinary sphincter

Prostatic urethra

Bulbourethral gland

A

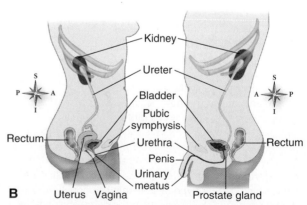

Kidney

Ureter

Bladder

Pubic symphysis

Urethra

Penis

Urinary meatus

Rectum

Rectum

B Uterus Vagina Prostate gland

FIGURE 17-7 **Structure and location of the urinary bladder. A,** Frontal view of a fully distended male bladder dissected to show the interior. Note the relationship of the prostate gland, which surrounds the urethra as it exits the bladder. This relationship is discussed in Chapter 20. **B,** Sagittal section of the female urinary system *(left)* and the male urinary system *(right)* showing relationship of the bladder to other anatomical structures.

The trigone extends between the openings of the two ureters above and the point of exit of the urethra below.

URETHRA

To leave the body, urine passes from the bladder, down the urethra, and out of its external opening, the **urinary meatus.** In other words, the urethra is the lowest part of the urinary tract. The same sheet of mucous membrane that lines each renal pelvis, the ureters, and the bladder extends down into the urethra, too; this is a structural feature worth noting because it accounts for the fact that an infection of the urethra may spread upward through the urinary tract. The urethra is a narrow tube; it is only about 4 cm (1½ inches) long in a woman, but it is about 20 cm (8 inches) long in a man. In a man, the urethra has two functions: (1) it is the terminal portion of the urinary tract, and (2) it is the passageway for movement of the reproductive fluid (semen) from the body. In a woman, the urethra is a part of only the urinary tract.

MICTURITION

The terms **micturition** (mik-too-RISH-un), **urination** (yoor-i-NAY-shun), and **voiding** refer to the passage of urine from the body or the emptying of the bladder.

Two **sphincters** (SFINK-terz), or rings of muscle tissue, guard the pathway leading from the bladder. When contracted, both sphincters function to seal off the bladder and allow urine to accumulate without leaking to the exterior. The *internal urethral sphincter* is formed of involuntary smooth muscle and is located, in both sexes, at the bladder exit circling around the bladder-urethral junction. The *external urethral sphincter* is voluntary and formed of striated muscle. In females this sphincter surrounds the middle third of the urethra below the neck of the bladder. In the male, it circles the urethra just below the prostate gland (see Figure 17-7, *A*).

The muscular wall of the bladder permits this organ to accommodate a considerable volume of urine with very little increase in pressure until a volume of 300 to 400 mL is reached. Then, as the bladder wall stretches, nervous impulses are transmitted to the second, third, and fourth sacral segments of the spinal cord, and an **emptying reflex** is initiated. The reflex causes contraction of the mus-

cle of the bladder wall and relaxation of the internal sphincter. Urine then enters the urethra. If the external sphincter, which is under voluntary control, is relaxed, micturition occurs. Voluntary contraction of the external sphincter suppresses the emptying reflex until the bladder is filled to capacity with urine and loss of control occurs. Contraction of this powerful sphincter also abruptly terminates urination voluntarily.

Higher centers in the brain also function in micturition by integrating bladder contraction and internal and external sphincter relaxation, with the cooperative contraction of pelvic and abdominal muscles. **Urinary retention** is a condition in which little or no urine is voided. The kidneys produce urine, but the bladder, for one reason or another (see Clinical Application: Prostatic Hypertropy box, p. 448), cannot completely empty itself, if at all. In these individuals the residual urine, a good culture medium for bacteria, is often the cause of repeated bladder infections, or **cystitis** (sis-TYE-tis). In some cases, surgery to remove an obstruction or intermittent or chronic **catheterization** may be necessary. In the procedure a hollow tube of *catheter* is inserted into the bladder through the urethra for withdrawal of urine. In **urinary suppression,** the kidneys do

Clinical Application

The Aging Kidney

As with other body organs, the kidneys undergo both age-related structural changes and decreasing functional capacity. Adults older than 35 years of age gradually lose functional nephron units, and kidney weight actually decreases. By approximately 80 to 85 years of age, most individuals will have experienced a 30% reduction in total kidney mass. In spite of a numerical reduction in actual kidney nephron units and a decrease in the metabolic activity of remaining tubular cells, most of these individuals continue to exhibit normal kidney function. This is possible because older persons generally have a lower overall lean body mass and therefore a reduced production of waste products that must be excreted from the body. However, the "margin of safety" is reduced, and any stress on the remaining functional nephrons, such as a systemic infection or a reduction in kidney blood flow, can produce almost immediate symptoms of kidney failure. Marginal kidney function in old age may make it difficult to excrete drugs that are easily cleared from the blood of younger persons, and dosages of many medications have to be adjusted accordingly for older patients.

not produce any urine, but the bladder retains the ability to empty itself.

Urinary incontinence (in-KON-ti-nens) is the involuntary leakage or voiding of urine of sufficient severity to be a health or social concern. Urinary incontinence is a widespread bladder control problem, especially for the elderly. Unfortunately, it is commonly hidden and not discussed with health care professionals. The condition is viewed by many as a social stigma and can lead to embarrassment, isolation, and depression that significantly affects lifestyle. For many elderly individuals, it often becomes an important precipitating factor in the decision to enter a nursing home.

Some cases of urinary incontinence, including those resulting from CNS disorders such as stroke, parkinsonism, and spinal cord injury or transection, are generally chronic and respond poorly or not at all to specific treatment interventions. Possible treatment in these cases using *stem cells* may become a treatment option in the future (see Clinical Application: Stem Cells box, p. 72). Currently, in these cases, management is generally nonspecific and involves helpful but expensive adult diapers and pads. Fortunately, many types of urinary incontinence are caused by reversible factors such as anatomical obstructions, bladder or sphincter weakness or irritability, or psychological factors that can often be effectively treated with surgery, drugs, or behavioral changes that may involve muscle exercises, fluid or dietary restrictions, or bladder training.

The term **overactive bladder** refers to the urge for frequent urination with or without incontinence. The amounts voided are generally small, and feelings of extreme urgency and pain are common. The condition is called *interstitial* (in-ter-STISH-al) *cystitis* and is treated with drugs to decrease nervous stimulation and with physical distention of the bladder with fluids to increase capacity.

✓ QUICK CHECK

1. Through what tube does urine leave the kidney?
2. What structural characteristics of the bladder allow it to expand to hold urine?
3. Through what structure does urine pass from the bladder to the outside of the body?
4. What is incontinence?

Clinical Application

Removal of Kidney Stones Using Ultrasound

Statistics suggest that approximately 1 in every 1,000 adults in the United States suffers from kidney stones, or **renal calculi** (KAL-kyoo-lye), at some point in his or her life. Although symptoms of excruciating pain are common, many kidney stones are small enough to pass out of the urinary system spontaneously. If this is possible, no therapy is required other than treatment for pain and antibiotics if the calculi are associated with infection. Larger stones, however, may obstruct the flow of urine and are much more serious and difficult to treat.

Until recently, only traditional surgical procedures were effective in removing relatively large stones that formed in the calyces and renal pelvis of the kidney. In addition to the risks that always accompany major medical procedures, surgical removal of stones from the kidneys frequently requires rather extensive hospital and home recovery periods, lasting 6 weeks or more.

A technique that uses ultrasound to pulverize the stones so that they can be flushed out of the urinary tract without surgery is used in hospitals across the United States. The specially designed ultrasound generator required for the procedure is called a **lithotriptor** (lith-oh-TRIP-tor). Using a lithotriptor, physicians break up the stones with ultrasound waves, in a process called **lithotripsy**, without making an incision. Recovery time is minimal; patient risk and costs are reduced. One of the original ultrasound lithotripsy techniques requires placement of the individual in a tub of water or in contact with a water cushion to transfer and focus the shock wave, which is generated outside the body and called an "extracorporeal shock wave," on the kidney stone. A number of other lithotripsy techniques are also in use. They use various types of controlled energy, such as pulsed dye lasers, high voltage spark, electromagnetic impulse generators, and direct contact pneumatic pressure probes to fragment kidney stones.

Fighting Infection
Alexander Fleming (1881–1955)

Unfortunately, the structure of the urinary tract puts it at risk for infection by bacteria and other microorganisms. Because it is open to the external environment, bacteria can enter easily. In women, the short length of the urethra and its location close to the anus may further increase the risk of bacteria getting to the urinary bladder.

A breakthrough in the treatment of urinary tract infections (UTIs) came in 1928 in the laboratory of Scots researcher Alexander Fleming. Some mold spores accidentally contaminated one of the dishes in which Fleming was growing bacteria. He marveled at the fact that no bacteria could grow near the mold growth. He isolated a substance from the mold responsible for this antibacterial effect and named it *penicillin*. Fleming subsequently showed that penicillin was effective against a variety of bacteria that cause serious infections in humans. Penicillin became the first "miracle drug" and rapidly became the tool of choice in fighting bacteria.

Although forms of penicillin and other antibiotics derived from natural sources are still the weapon of choice in battling many infections, the infectious bacteria are evolving into strains that resist common antibiotics. UTIs and other types of infections now require more powerful antibiotics and other special techniques to stop them. Some scientists fear that the era of simple antibiotic therapy may be nearing an end.

Many professions are involved directly in the fight against infection, and others continue in the quest to find newer and better treatments for UTIs and other infections that threaten human health.

OUTLINE SUMMARY

KIDNEYS

A. Location — under back muscles, behind parietal peritoneum, just above waistline; right kidney usually a little lower than left (see Figure 17-1)
B. Internal structure (see Figure 17-2)
  1. Cortex — outer layer of kidney substance
  2. Medulla — inner portion of kidney
  3. Pyramids — triangular divisions of medulla
  4. Papilla — narrow, innermost end of pyramid
  5. Pelvis — expansion of upper end of ureter; lies inside kidney
  6. Calyces — divisions of renal pelvis
C. Microscopic structure — nephrons are microscopic units of kidneys; consist of (see Figure 17-3):
  1. Renal corpuscle
    a. Bowman capsule — the cup-shaped top
    b. Glomerulus — network of blood capillaries surrounded by the Bowman capsule
  2. Renal tubule
    a. Proximal convoluted tubule — first segment

  b. Nephron loop — extension of proximal tubule; consists of descending limb, loop, and ascending limb
  c. Distal convoluted tubule — extension of ascending limb of the nephron loop
  d. Collecting tubule — straight extension of distal tubule
D. Functions
  1. Excretes toxins and nitrogenous wastes
  2. Regulates levels of many chemicals in blood
  3. Maintains water balance
  4. Helps regulate blood pressure via secretion of renin
  5. Hormone produced by juxtaglomerular apparatus cells stimulates RBC production and maturation

FORMATION OF URINE (See Figure 17-5)

A. Occurs by a series of three processes that take place in successive parts of nephron
  1. Filtration — goes on continually in renal corpuscles; glomerular blood pressure causes water and dissolved substances to filter out of glomeruli into the Bowman capsule; normal glomerular filtration rate 125 mL per minute

2. Reabsorption — movement of substances out of renal tubules into blood in peritubular capillaries; water, nutrients, and ions are reabsorbed; water is reabsorbed by osmosis from proximal tubules

3. Secretion — movement of substances into urine in the distal and collecting tubules from blood in peritubular capillaries; hydrogen ions, potassium ions, and certain drugs are secreted by active transport; ammonia is secreted by diffusion

B. Control of urine volume — mainly by posterior pituitary hormone's ADH, which decreases it

URETERS

A. Structure (see Figure 17-6) — narrow, long tubes with expanded upper end (renal pelvis) located inside kidney and lined with mucous membrane

B. Function — drain urine from renal pelvis to urinary bladder

URINARY BLADDER

A. Structure (see Figure 17-7)
1. Elastic muscular organ, capable of great expansion
2. Lined with mucous membrane arranged in rugae, as is stomach mucosa

B. Functions
1. Storage of urine before voiding
2. Voiding

URETHRA

A. Structure
1. Narrow tube from urinary bladder to exterior
2. Lined with mucous membrane

3. Opening of urethra to the exterior called *urinary meatus*

B. Functions
1. Passage of urine from bladder to exterior of the body
2. Passage of male reproductive fluid (semen) from the body

MICTURITION

A. Passage of urine from body (also called *urination* or *voiding*)

B. Regulatory sphincters
1. Internal urethral sphincter (involuntary)
2. External urethral sphincter (voluntary)

C. Bladder wall permits storage of urine with little increase in pressure

D. Emptying reflex
1. Initiated by stretch reflex in bladder wall
2. Bladder wall contracts
3. Internal sphincter relaxes
4. External sphincter relaxes, and urination occurs

E. Urinary retention — urine produced but not voided

F. Urinary suppression — no urine produced but bladder is normal

G. Urinary incontinence — urine is voided involuntarily; common bladder control problem in elderly people
1. May be caused by spinal injury or stroke
2. Retention of urine may cause cystitis

H. Cystitis — bladder infection

I. Overactive bladder — need for frequent urination
1. Called *interstitial cystitis*
2. Amounts voided are small
3. Extreme urgency and pain are common

NEW WORDS

aldosterone
anuria
atrial natriuretic
  hormone (ANH)
Bowman capsule
calyx
catheterization
continuous ambulatory
  peritoneal dialysis
  (CAPD)
cortex
cystitis

diuretic
glomerular filtrate
glomerulus
glycosuria
hemodialysis
nephron loop
incontinence
lithotripsy
lithotriptor
medulla
micturition
nephron

nephropathy
oliguria
overactive bladder
papilla
polyuria
proteinuria
pyramid
renal calculi
renal colic
renal corpuscle
renal pelvis
renal threshold

renal tubule
trigone
uremia (uremic
  poisoning)
urinary incontinence
urinary retention
urinary suppression
urinary system
urination
voiding

REVIEW QUESTIONS

1. Describe the location of the kidneys.
2. Name and describe the internal structures of the kidneys.
3. Define *filtration*, *reabsorption*, and *secretion* as they apply to kidney function.
4. Briefly explain the formation of urine.
5. Name several substances eliminated or regulated by the kidney.
6. Explain the function of the juxtaglomerular apparatus.
7. Describe the structure of the ureters.
8. Describe the structure of the bladder. What is the trigone?
9. Describe the structure of the urethra.
10. Briefly describe the process of micturition.
11. Differentiate between retention and suppression of urine.
12. What is incontinence? What can cause incontinence?

CRITICAL THINKING

13. Explain how salt and water balance are maintained by aldosterone and ADH.
14. Explain why proper blood pressure is necessary for proper kidney function?
15. If a person were doing strenuous work on a hot day and perspiring heavily, would there be a great deal of ADH in the blood or very little? Explain your answer.

CHAPTER TEST

1. The kidneys receive about _____% of the total amount of blood pumped by the heart each minute.

2. The renal corpuscle is made up of two structures: _____ and _____.

3. The two parts of the renal tubules that extend into the medulla of the kidney are the _____ and the _____.

4. The two parts of the renal tubules that are in the cortex of the kidney are the _____ and the _____.

5. The process of _____ is the movement of substances out of the renal tubules and into the blood capillaries.

6. The process of _____ causes substances in the blood to be pushed into the Bowman capsule as a result of blood pressure in the glomerulus.

7. The process of _____ is the movement of substances from the blood into the distal tubule or the collecting tube.

8. The hormone _____ is released from the posterior pituitary gland and reduces the amount of water lost in the urine.

9. The hormone _____ is made by the heart and stimulates the tubules to secrete sodium.

10. The hormone _____ is made in the adrenal cortex and causes the tubules to absorb sodium.

11. The involuntary muscle _____ is at the exit of the bladder.

12. _____ is a condition in which the bladder is able to empty itself but no urine is being produced by the kidneys.

13. _____ is a condition in which a person voids urine involuntarily.

14. _____ is a condition in which the bladder is full and the kidney is producing urine but the bladder is unable to empty itself.

CHAPTER TEST—cont'd

Match each descriptive phrase in Column B with its corresponding term in Column A.

COLUMN A

15. _____ cortex
16. _____ medulla
17. _____ pyramids
18. _____ renal pelvis
19. _____ urethra
20. _____ bladder
21. _____ ureter
22. _____ trigone
23. _____ Bowman capsule
24. _____ glomerulus
25. _____ nephron loop

COLUMN B

a. inner layer of the kidney
b. expansion of the ureter in the kidney
c. cup-shaped part of the nephron that catches the filtrate
d. tube leading from the bladder to outside the body
e. network of capillaries in the Bowman capsule
f. saclike structure used to hold urine until it is voided
g. outer part of the kidney
h. an area of the bladder that has openings for the two ureters and the urethra
i. the part of the renal tubules that is located between the proximal and distal tubules
j. tube connecting the kidney and bladder
k. the triangular divisions in the medulla of the kidney

OBJECTIVES

AFTER YOU HAVE COMPLETED THIS CHAPTER, YOU SHOULD BE ABLE TO:

1. List, describe, and compare the body fluid compartments and their subdivisions.
2. Discuss avenues by which water enters and leaves the body and the mechanisms that maintain fluid balance.
3. Discuss the nature and importance of electrolytes in body fluids and explain the aldosterone mechanism of extracellular fluid volume control.
4. Explain the interaction between capillary blood pressure and blood proteins.
5. Give examples of common fluid imbalances.

Fluid and Electrolyte Balance 18

ave you ever wondered why you sometimes excrete great volumes of urine and sometimes excrete almost none at all? Why sometimes you feel so thirsty that you can hardly get enough to drink and other times you want no liquids at all? These conditions and many more relate to one of the body's most important functions—that of maintaining its *fluid and electrolyte balance.*

The phrase **fluid balance** implies homeostasis, or relative constancy of body fluid levels—a condition required for healthy survival. It means that both the total volume and distribution of water in the body remain normal and relatively constant. Body "input" of water must be balanced by "output." If water in excess of requirements enters the body, it must be eliminated, and, if excess losses occur, prompt replacement is critical. Because fluid balance refers to normal homeostasis, *fluid imbalance* means that the total volume of water in the body or the amounts in one or more of its fluid compartments have increased or decreased beyond normal limits. **Electrolytes** are substances such as salts that dissolve or break apart in water solution. Health and sometimes even survival itself depend on maintaining proper balance of water and the electrolytes within it.

In this chapter you will find a discussion of body fluids and electrolytes, their normal values, the mechanisms that operate to keep them normal, and some of the more common types of fluid and electrolyte imbalances.

BODY FLUIDS

Of the hundreds of compounds present in your body, the most abundant is water. Medical reference tables often refer to "average" fluid volumes based on healthy, nonobese, young adults. In such tables, an average of 60% of the body weight of

STUDY TIPS

To make the study of fluid and electrolyte balance more efficient, we suggest these tips:

1. Review material in Chapter 2 related to dissociation, electrolytes, and ions (ions are charged particles—cations are positively charged ions, and anions are negatively charged ions).

2. Three factors must be controlled to maintain fluid and electrolyte balance: total amount of fluid, distribution of fluid to the various fluid compartments, and the concentration of various ions and other solutes.

3. Remember that plasma and interstitial fluid (IF) make up the extracellular fluid (ECF) compartments and that intracellular fluid (ICF) is located inside cells and constitutes the largest volume of fluid.

4. Use flash cards to review chapter terms, body fluid compartments, and the functional importance and location of specific electrolytes (in ECF, Na^+ is most abundant cation and Cl^- the most abundant anion—in ICF, K^+ is most abundant cation and HPO_4^- and protein molecules are the most important anions).

5. The capillary blood pressure and blood protein mechanism regulates the movement of water between the blood and interstitial fluid.

6. In your study group discuss the meaning of "where sodium goes, water soon follows"—review Figure 18-7.

7. Be sure to answer Quick Check questions; go over the questions in the back of the chapter, and write your own "possible test questions"—and answers—on flash cards for review. Exchange cards with others in your study group.

a male weighing 70 kilograms (kg) (154 pounds) will be water, nearly 40 liters (Figure 18-1); water weight for females is about 50%. The reason fluid volume values in reference tables are based on nonobese individuals is because adipose, or fat, tissue contains the least amount of water of any body tissue. The more fat there is in the body, the less the total water content is per pound of body weight. Therefore, regardless of age, obese

413

Plasma: (3L)

Interstitial and transcellular fluid (IF): (12L)

Intracellular fluid (ICF): (25L)

A

B

ICF

IF

Plasma

ICF

FIGURE 18-1 **Relative volumes of three body fluids.** Values represent fluid distribution in a young adult male.

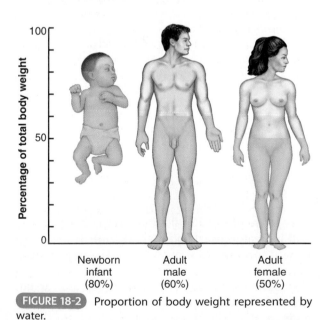

Percentage of total body weight

100

50

0

Newborn infant (80%)

Adult male (60%)

Adult female (50%)

FIGURE 18-2 Proportion of body weight represented by water.

individuals, with their high body fat content, have less body water per kilogram of weight than slender people. Although a nonobese male body typically consists of about 60% water, an obese male may consist of only 50% water, or even less. The female body typically contains slightly less water per pound of weight because it contains slightly more fat than the male body. Note in Figure 18-2 that age as well as gender influences the amount of water in the body. Infants have more water as a percent of total body weight than adults of either sex. In a newborn, water may account for up to 80% of total body weight. This is the reason fluid imbalances in infants, caused by diarrhea for example, can be so serious. The percentage of body water decreases rapidly during the first 10 years of life, and by adolescence, adult values are reached and gender differences, which account for about a 10% variation in body fluid volumes between the sexes, appear. In elderly individuals, the amount of water per pound of body weight decreases. One reason is that old age is often accompanied by a decrease in muscle mass (65% water) and an increase in fat (20% water).

BODY FLUID COMPARTMENTS

Physiologists divide all of the water in the body (*total body water*) into two major **fluid compartments.** Using this concept, total body water is subdivided into major compartments called *extracellular* and *intracellular* fluid compartments. Table 18-1 lists the differing volumes of each major body fluid compartment as a percentage of body weight in both the newborn and adults of both sexes.

Extracellular Fluid

Extracellular fluid (ECF) is body fluid found outside of cells. It can be subdivided into fluids found in separate spaces in the body: (1) **blood plasma**—the liquid part of whole blood found in the blood vessels; (2) **interstitial fluid (IF)**—fluid surrounding cells; and (3) **transcellular fluid**—a group of specialized extracellular fluids including lymph, cerebrospinal fluid, humors of the eye, and synovial fluid.

Intracellular Fluid

Intracellular fluid (ICF) is, as the name implies, body fluid found inside cells. It represents the largest volume of body fluid by far. Water has many functions in the body. Inside the cell it serves mainly as a solvent in which important chemical reactions can occur.

TABLE 18-1

Volumes of Body Fluid Compartments*

BODY FLUID	INFANT	ADULT MALE	ADULT FEMALE
Extracellular Fluid			
Plasma	4	4	4
Interstitial and trans-cellular fluid	26	16	11
Intracellular Fluid	45	40	35
Total	75	60	50

*Percentage of body weight.

> ### ✓ QUICK CHECK
> 1. What are the two main fluid compartments of the body?
> 2. What is meant by the term *fluid balance*?

MECHANISMS THAT MAINTAIN FLUID BALANCE

Under normal conditions, homeostasis of the total volume of water in the body is maintained or restored primarily by devices that adjust output (urine volume) to intake and secondarily by mechanisms that adjust fluid intake. There is no question about which of the two mechanisms is more important: the body's chief mechanism for maintaining fluid balance is that of adjusting its fluid output so that it equals its fluid intake.

Obviously, as long as output and intake are equal, the total amount of water in the body does not change. Figure 18-3 shows the three sources of fluid intake: the liquids we drink, the water in the foods we eat, and the water formed by catabolism of foods. Table 18-2 gives their normal volumes. However, these can vary a great deal and still be considered normal. Table 18-2 also indicates that fluid output from the body occurs through four organs: the kidneys, lungs, skin, and intestines. The fluid output that changes the most is that coming from the kidneys. The body maintains fluid balance mainly by changing the volume of urine excreted to match changes in the volume of fluid intake. Everyone knows this from experience. The more liquid one drinks, the more urine one excretes. Conversely, the less the fluid intake is, the less the urine volume will be. How changes in urine volume come about was discussed on p. 403. This would be a good time to review that page.

It is important to remember from your study of the urinary system that the rate of water and salt resorption from the renal tubules is the most important factor in determining urine volume. Urine volume is regulated chiefly by hormones secreted by the posterior lobe of the pituitary gland (antidiuretic hormone [ADH]) and the adrenal cortex (aldosterone). Atrial natriuretic hormone (ANH) from the atrial wall of the heart also affects urine volume. See p. 403 for a review of the hormonal control of urine volume.

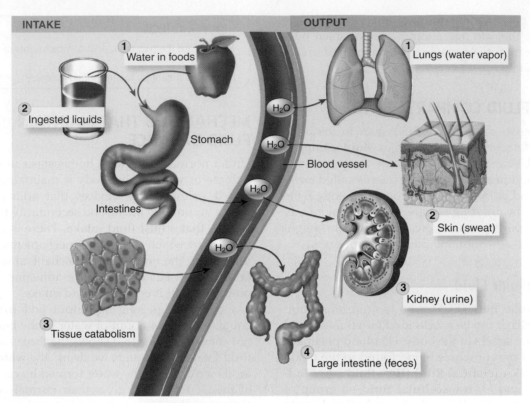

FIGURE 18-3 Sources of fluid intake and output.

TABLE 18-2			
Typical Normal Values for Each Portal of Water Entry and Exit (24 Hours)			
INTAKE	**AMOUNT***	**OUTPUT**	**AMOUNT***
Water in foods	700 mL	Lungs (water in expired air)	350 mL
Ingested liquids	1500 mL	Skin	
Water formed by catabolism	200 mL	By diffusion	350 mL
		By sweat	100 mL
		Kidneys (urine)	1400 mL
		Intestines (in feces)	200 mL
TOTALS	**2400 mL**		**2400 mL**

*Amounts vary widely.

A number of factors act as mechanisms for controlling plasma, IF, and ICF volumes. Our discussion here is limited to only three of these factors. Explanations of their effects on fluid volumes and some specific examples of how each factor works are provided. These main factors are the following:
1. Concentration of electrolytes in ECF
2. Capillary blood pressure
3. Concentration of proteins in blood

Regulation of Fluid Intake

Physiologists disagree about the exact detailed workings of the mechanism that controls and regulates fluid intake to compensate for factors that would otherwise lead to dehydration. In general the mechanism appears to operate in this way: When dehydration starts to develop—that is, when fluid loss from the body exceeds fluid intake—salivary secretion decreases, producing a "dry-mouth feeling" and the sensation of thirst. As a result, the individual then drinks water, thereby increasing fluid intake and compensating for previous fluid losses. This tends to restore fluid balance (Figure 18-4). If an individual takes nothing by mouth for days, can his or her fluid output decrease to zero? The answer—no—becomes obvious after reviewing the information in Table 18-2. Despite every effort of homeostatic mechanisms to compensate for zero intake, some output (loss) of fluid occurs as long as life continues. Water is continually lost from the body through expired air and diffusion through skin.

Although the body attempts to adjust fluid intake, factors that adjust fluid output, such as electrolytes and blood proteins, are far more important in maintaining homeostasis.

FIGURE 18-4 Homeostasis of the total volume of body water. A basic negative feedback loop mechanism for adjusting intake to compensate for excess output of body fluid is diagrammed (see also Figure 1-9 on p. 10).

> ✓ **QUICK CHECK**
>
> 1. Which does the body primarily adjust, fluid *intake* or fluid *output*?
> 2. What are the chief ways that fluid leaves the body?

Importance of Electrolytes in Body Fluids

Electrolytes Versus Nonelectrolytes

Recall from Chapter 2 that compounds such as ordinary table salt (sodium chloride [NaCl]) that have molecular bonds that permit them to break up, or **dissociate** (di-SOH-see-ayt), in water solution into separate particles (Na^+ and Cl^-) are called **electrolytes** (eh-LEK-troh-lytes). The name "electrolyte" is appropriate because electrolyte solutions are able to conduct an electrical current. The bonds that hold together the molecules of certain organic substances such as glucose do not permit the compound to break up, or dissociate, in water solution. Such compounds are called **nonelectrolytes** (non-eh-LEK-troh-lytes). Fluid balance is regulated largely by the compounds that do dissociate.

Ions

The dissociated particles of an electrolyte are called **ions** and carry either a positive or negative electrical charge. As a group, all positively charged ions, such as Na^+, are called **cations** and all negatively charged ions, such as Cl^-, are called **anions**. Each of the body fluid compartments contains differing levels of many important ions—both positively charged cations and negatively charged anions.

Important positively charged ions (cations) include sodium (Na^+), calcium (Ca^{++}), potassium (K^+), and magnesium (Mg^{++}). Important negatively charged ions (anions) include chloride (Cl^-), bicarbonate (HCO_3^-), phosphate (HPO_4^-), and many proteins. There are very important differences in the amounts of various anions and cations in ECF and IF. For example, Na^+ is the most common cation and Cl^- is the most common anion found in both subdivisions (blood plasma and interstitial fluid) of the extracellular fluid (ECF) compartment. Table 18-3 gives the levels of these electrolytes in blood plasma. In contrast, K^+ is the most common cation in the intracellular fluid (ICF) compartments, and phosphate ions (HPO_4^{--}) and

TABLE 18-3

Common Electrolytes Found in Blood Plasma*

POSITIVELY CHARGED IONS (CATIONS)	NEGATIVELY CHARGED IONS (ANIONS)
142 mEq Na^+	102 mEq Cl^-
4 mEq K^+	26 mEq HCO_3^-
5 mEq Ca^{++}	17 mEq protein
2 mEq Mg^{++}	6 mEq other
	2 mEq HPO_4^{--}
153 mEq/L plasma	153 mEq/L plasma

*mEq per liter (mEq/L) of plasma; values given represent midpoint of a normal range.

protein molecules, which carry a negative charge, are the most important anions. As elsewhere, structure determines function. In this instance, differences in the chemical structure of ECF and ICF help control water and electrolyte movement between them. Measurement of electrolyte levels in body fluids is a common practice in clinical medicine. The reason? Deviation from normal in electrolyte values is often an early indicator of failure in a homeostatic mechanism and the presence of disease.

Electrolyte Functions

A variety of electrolytes have important nutrient or regulatory roles in the body. Many ions are considered to be major, or important, "trace" elements in the body (see Chapter 2). Iron, for example, is required for hemoglobin production, and iodine must be available for synthesis of thyroid hormones. Electrolytes are also required for many cellular activities such as nerve conduction (K^+), acid-base balance (HCO_3^-), bone formation and blood clotting (Ca^{++}), and hydrochloric acid production in the stomach (Cl^-).

Fluid Volume Variation. Electrolytes also influence the movement of water among the three fluid compartments of the body. To help you remember how ECF electrolyte concentration affects fluid volumes, remember this one short sentence: where sodium goes, water soon follows. If, for example, the concentration of sodium in blood increases, the volume of blood soon increases. Intravenous administration of normal saline (0.9% NaCl) solution to treat acute blood loss is based on knowledge of this relationship between sodium and fluid movement. Administration of saline (salt) solution will increase blood levels of sodium and fluid will move out of the interstitial fluid and into

the plasma, thus increasing blood volume and stabilizing blood pressure. The result is temporary but may prove lifesaving if it provides the time required to obtain and administer blood. If the concentration of sodium in interstitial fluid spaces rises above normal, the volume of IF soon reaches abnormally high levels, too—this is one reason for the development of a condition called **edema** (eh-DEE-mah), which results in tissue swelling (see Clinical Application: Edema box). One of the most common areas in which swelling occurs is the subcutaneous tissues of the ankle and foot. The term **pitting edema** is used to describe depressions in swollen subcutaneous tissue that result from finger pressure exerted by an examiner. These depressions do not rapidly refill, as would be expected in normal tissue, thereby indicating the presence of edema (Figure 18-5).

Figure 18-6 traces one mechanism that tends to maintain fluid homeostasis. Aldosterone, secreted by the adrenal cortex, increases Na^+ reabsorption by the kidney tubules. Water reabsorption also increases, causing an increase in ECF volume. Begin in the upper right of the diagram and follow, in sequence, each of the informational steps. In summary:

1. Overall fluid balance requires that fluid output equal fluid intake.
2. The type of fluid output that changes most is urine volume.

FIGURE 18-5   Pitting edema. Note the finger tip–shaped depressions that do not rapidly refill after an examiner has exerted pressure.

Clinical Application

Edema

Edema (see Figure 18-5) may be defined as the presence of abnormally large amounts of fluid in the intercellular tissue spaces of the body. The condition is a classic example of fluid imbalance and may be caused by disturbances in any factor that governs the interchange between blood plasma and IF compartments. Examples include the following:

1. **Retention of electrolytes (especially Na⁺).** This can occur in the extracellular fluid as a result of increased aldosterone secretion or after serious kidney disease.
2. **An increase in capillary blood pressure.** Normally, fluid is drawn from the tissue spaces into the venous end of a tissue capillary because of the low venous pressure and the relatively high water-pulling force of the plasma proteins. This balance is upset by anything that increases the capillary hydrostatic pressure. The generalized venous congestion of heart failure is the most common cause of

widespread edema. In patients with this condition, blood cannot flow freely through the capillary beds, and therefore the pressure will increase until venous return of blood improves.

3. **A decrease in the concentration of plasma proteins.** Malnutrition, regardless of caloric intake, may result from a diet severely deficient in protein. In this type of malnutrition, especially in children, a condition called *kwashiorkor* (kwah-shee-OR-kor) may occur. In these individuals, low levels of plasma protein cause osmosis of water from the blood into the peritoneal space, and severe abdominal bloating and edema result. In addition to protein malnutrition, "leakage" into the interstitial spaces of proteins normally retained in the blood may occur as a result of increased capillary permeability caused by infection, burns, or shock.

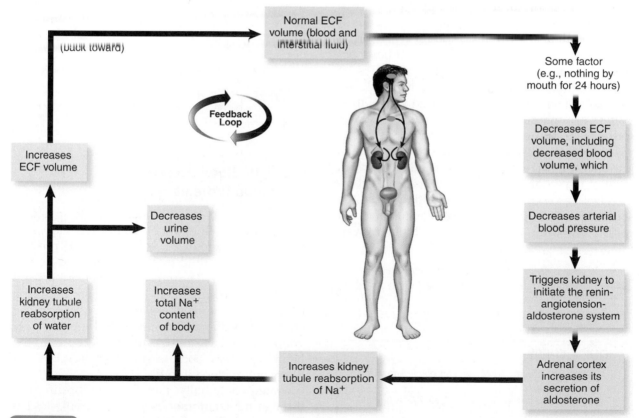

FIGURE 18-6   **Aldosterone mechanism.** Aldosterone restores normal extracellular fluid (ECF) volume when such levels decrease below normal. Excess aldosterone, however, leads to excess ECF volume—that is, excess blood volume (hypervolemia) and excess interstitial fluid volume (edema)—and also to an excess of the total Na⁺ content of the body.

3. Renal tubule regulation of salt and water is the most important factor in determining urine volume.

4. Aldosterone controls sodium reabsorption in the kidney.

5. The presence of sodium causes water to move (where sodium goes, water soon follows).

The flow chart diagram in Figure 18-6 explains, in a concise and brief way, the aldosterone mechanism that helps to restore normal ECF volume when it has decreased below normal. Try to construct a similar diagram to show the effect of ADH secretion on ECF volume.

Considerable daily variation in dietary sodium intake occurs. Therefore regulatory mechanisms are required to maintain homeostasis of blood sodium levels within a normal range. The milliequivalent (mEq) (see Table 18-3) is a unit of measurement related to reactivity. In a healthy individual, sodium excretion from the body by the kidney is about the same as intake. The kidney acts as the chief regulator of sodium levels in body fluids. It is important to know that many electrolytes such as sodium not only pass into and out of the body but also move back and forth between a number of body fluids during each 24-hour period. Figure 18-7 shows the large volumes of sodium-containing internal secretions produced each day. During a 24-hour period, more than 8 liters of fluid containing 1,000 to 1,300 mEq of sodium are poured into the digestive system as part of saliva, gastric secretions, bile, pancreatic juice, and IF secretions. This sodium, along with most of that contained in the diet, is almost completely reabsorbed in the large intestine. Very little sodium is lost in the feces. Precise regulation and control of sodium levels are required for survival.

> To learn more about the aldosterone regulation mechanism, go to AnimationDirect on your CD-ROM.

✔ **QUICK CHECK**

1. What is the difference between an *electrolyte* and a *nonelectrolyte*?
2. What are some of the major roles of ions in the body?
3. What hormones regulate ions in the body?

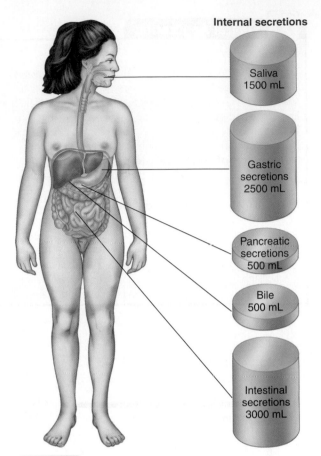

Internal secretions

Saliva 1500 mL

Gastric secretions 2500 mL

Pancreatic secretions 500 mL

Bile 500 mL

Intestinal secretions 3000 mL

FIGURE 18-7 Sodium-containing internal secretions. The total volume of these secretions may reach 8,000 mL or more in 24 hours.

Capillary Blood Pressure and Blood Proteins

Capillary blood pressure is a "water-pushing" force. It pushes fluid out of the blood in capillaries into the IF. Therefore, if capillary blood pressure increases, more fluid is pushed—filtered—out of blood into the IF. The effect of an increase in capillary blood pressure, then, is to transfer fluid from blood to IF. In turn, this *fluid shift*, as it is called, changes blood and IF volumes. It decreases blood volume by increasing IF volume. If, on the other hand, capillary blood pressure decreases, less fluid filters out of blood into IF.

Water continually moves in both directions through the membranous walls of capillaries (see Figure 18-1). The amount that moves out of capillary blood into IF depends largely on capillary

Clinical Application

Diuretics

The word **diuretic** (dye-yoo-RET-ik) is from the Greek word *diouretikos*, meaning "causing urine." By definition, a diuretic drug is a substance that promotes or stimulates the production of urine.

As a group, diuretics are among the most commonly used drugs in medicine. They are used because of their role in influencing water and electrolyte balance, especially sodium, in the body.

Diuretics have their effect on tubular function in the nephron, and the differing types of diuretics are often classified (1) according to their major site of action (proximal convoluted tubule, the Henle loop, distal convoluted tubule)

or (2) according to the effect the drug has on the concentration of sodium or other ions in tubular fluid.

Nursing implications for caregivers monitoring patients receiving diuretics, both in hospitals and in home health care environments, include keeping a careful record of repeated measurements of body weight over time and of fluid intake and output. These measurements are used in assessing the patient for signs and symptoms of electrolyte and water imbalance. For example, diuretic-induced dehydration resulting in a loss of only 6% of initial body weight will cause tingling in the extremities, stumbling gait, headache, fever, and an increase in both pulse and respiratory rates.

---

blood pressure, a water-pushing force. The amount that moves in the opposite direction (that is, into blood from IF) depends largely on the concentration of proteins in blood plasma. Plasma proteins act as a water-pulling or water-holding force. They *hold* water in the blood and also *pull* water into the blood from IF. If, for example, the concentration of proteins in blood decreases appreciably—as it does in some abnormal conditions such as dietary deficiency—less water moves into blood from IF. As a result, blood volume decreases and IF volume increases. Of the three main body fluids, IF volume varies the most. Plasma volume usually fluctuates only slightly and briefly. If a pronounced drop in its volume occurs, adequate circulation cannot be maintained.

 To learn more about fluid shift, go to AnimationDirect on your CD-ROM.

FLUID IMBALANCES

Fluid imbalances are common ailments. They take several forms and stem from a variety of causes, but they all share a common characteristic—that of abnormally low or abnormally high volumes of one or more body fluids.

Dehydration is the fluid imbalance seen most often. In this potentially dangerous condition, IF volume decreases first, but eventually, if treatment is not given, ICF and plasma volumes also decrease below normal levels. Either too small a fluid intake or too large a fluid output causes dehydration. Prolonged diarrhea or vomiting may result in dehydration because of the loss of body fluids. This is particularly true in infants, in whom the total fluid volume is much smaller than it is in adults. Loss of skin elasticity is a clinical sign of dehydration.

Overhydration can occur also but is much less common than dehydration. The grave danger of giving intravenous fluids too rapidly or in too-large amounts is **overhydration,** which can put too heavy a burden on the heart.

QUICK CHECK

1. How does an increase in capillary blood pressure cause fluid to move into the IF?
2. How do plasma proteins affect fluid balance?
3. What conditions might produce dehydration?

Science Application

The Constancy of the Body
Claude Bernard (1813–1877)

In 1834, a young Claude Bernard left his "boring" job as an apprentice apothecary (druggist) in Lyon, France, to make his fortune as a playwright in Paris. He found his plays were not appreciated in Paris. However, when he took a medical course in Paris, he found that many of the doctors did appreciate his research skills. Bernard went on to become one of the most important figures in the study of human physiology and experimental medicine. One of the most fundamental contributions he made to human physiology is the idea that the body is made up of cells living in an internal fluid environment.

Bernard stated that the internal fluid environment of the body is maintained in a relatively constant state—and that is what ensures the survival of the cells and therefore also ensures the survival of the whole body. Recall from Chapter 1 that we now call this concept *homeostasis* (see pp. 12-14). It was Bernard who showed that nearly every function of the body somehow relates to the success of keeping body fluids constant.

Today, nearly every health care professional uses concepts based on Bernard's original idea to assess the fluid and electrolyte balance of patients and possibly administer therapies to bring their fluids back into balance. Maintaining a healthy fluid and electrolyte balance is one of the key elements to successful patient care in the modern hospital and clinic.

OUTLINE SUMMARY

BODY FLUIDS
A. Water is the most abundant body compound
   1. References to "average" body water volume based on a healthy, nonobese, 70-kg male
   2. Water is 60% of body weight in males; 50% in females (see Table 18-1)
   3. Volume averages 40 liters in a 70-kg male (see Figure 18-1)
B. Variation in total body water is related to:
   1. Total body weight of individual
   2. Fat content of body — the more fat, the less water (adipose tissue is low in water content)
   3. Gender — female body has about 10% less water than male body (see Figure 18-2)
   4. Age — in a newborn infant, water may account for 80% of total body weight. In the elderly, water per pound of weight decreases (muscle tissue—high in water—replaced by fat, which is lower in water)

BODY FLUID COMPARTMENTS
A. Two major fluid compartments (see Table 18-1)
   1. Extracellular fluid (ECF)
      a. Types:
         (1) Plasma
         (2) Interstitial fluid (IF)
         (3) Transcellular fluid — lymph; joint fluids; cerebrospinal fluid; eye humors
      b. Called internal environment of body
      c. Surrounds cells and transports substances to and from them
   2. Intracellular fluid (ICF)
      a. Largest fluid compartment
      b. Located inside cells
      c. Serves as solvent to facilitate intracellular chemical reactions

MECHANISMS THAT MAINTAIN FLUID BALANCE
A. Fluid output, mainly urine volume, adjusts to fluid intake; antidiuretic hormone (ADH)

from posterior pituitary gland acts to increase kidney tubule reabsorption of sodium and water from tubular urine into blood, thereby tending to increase ECF (and total body fluid) by decreasing urine volume (see Figure 18-6)

B. ECF electrolyte concentration (mainly Na^+ concentration) influences ECF volume; an increase in ECF Na^+ tends to increase ECF volume by increasing movement of water out of ICF and by increasing ADH secretion, which decreases urine volume, and this, in turn, increases ECF volume

C. Capillary blood pressure pushes water out of blood, into IF; blood protein concentration pulls water into blood from IF; hence these two forces regulate plasma and IF volume under usual conditions

D. Importance of electrolytes in body fluids
   1. Nonelectrolytes — organic substances that do not break up, or dissociate, when placed in water solution (for example, glucose)
   2. Electrolytes — compounds that break up, or dissociate, in water solution into separate particles called ions (for example, ordinary table salt or sodium chloride)
   3. Ions — the dissociated particles of an electrolyte that carry an electrical charge (for example, sodium ion [Na^+])
      a. Positively charged ions (for example, potassium [K^+] and sodium [Na^+])
      b. Negatively charged particles (ions) (for example, chloride [Cl^-] and bicarbonate [HCO_3^-])
   4. Electrolyte composition of blood plasma (see Table 18-3)
   5. Sodium — most abundant and important positively charged ion of plasma
      a. Normal plasma level — 142 mEq/L
      b. Average daily intake (diet) — 100 mEq
      c. Chief method of regulation — kidney
      d. Aldosterone increases Na^+ reabsorption in kidney tubules (see Figure 18-6)
      e. Sodium-containing internal secretions (see Figure 18-7)

E. Capillary blood pressure and blood proteins

FLUID IMBALANCES

A. Dehydration — total volume of body fluids less than normal; IF volume shrinks first, and then if treatment is not given, ICF volume and plasma volume decrease; dehydration occurs when fluid output exceeds intake for an extended period

B. Overhydration — total volume of body fluids greater than normal; overhydration occurs when fluid intake exceeds output; various factors may cause this (for example, giving excessive amounts of intravenous fluids or giving them too rapidly may increase intake above output)

NEW WORDS

anion	edema	fluid compartment	overhydration
blood plasma	electrolyte	interstitial fluid (IF)	pitting edema
cation	extracellular fluid	intracellular fluid (ICF)	transcellular fluid
dissociate	(ECF)	ion	

REVIEW QUESTIONS

1. Name and give the location of the three main fluid compartments of the body. Which of these make up extracellular fluid?
2. What factors influence the percent of water in the body? Explain the effect of each factor.
3. List the three sources of water for the body.
4. List the four organs from which fluid output occurs.
5. Differentiate between an electrolyte and a nonelectrolyte.
6. Name three important negative ions.
7. Name three important positive ions.
8. Explain why the body is unable to reduce its fluid output to zero no matter how dehydrated it is.
9. Explain how aldosterone influences water movement between the kidney tubules and the blood.
10. Explain the role of capillary blood pressure in water movement between the plasma and interstitial fluid.
11. Explain the role of plasma proteins in water movement between the plasma and interstitial fluid.
12. Define dehydration and give a possible cause.
13. Define overhydration and give a possible cause.

CRITICAL THINKING

14. Name the three hormones that regulate the urine volume. State where each is made and what the specific effect on urine volume is.
15. Atrial natriuretic hormone has the opposite effect of aldosterone. Explain its effect on water movement between the kidney tubules and the blood.

CHAPTER TEST

1. The extracellular fluid compartment is composed of _____, _____, and _____.
2. The largest volume of water is in this fluid compartment: _____.

Fill in the blanks in questions 3, 4, and 5 with either "more" or "less" as appropriate.

3. In general, an obese person has _____ water per pound of body weight than a slim person.
4. In general, a man has _____ water per pound of body weight than a woman.
5. In general, an infant has _____ water per pound of body weight than an adult.
6. The body's chief mechanism for maintaining fluid balance is that of adjusting its _____.
7. The body has three sources of fluid intake: the liquids we drink, the water in the food we eat, and _____.

CHAPTER TEST—cont'd

8. The four organs from which fluid output occurs are the _____, _____, _____, and _____.

9. Urine volume is regulated by three hormones: ADH released from the pituitary gland, _____ released from the adrenal cortex, and _____ released from the heart.

10. When electrolytes dissociate in water, they form charged particles called _____.

11. The most abundant negatively charged particle in the blood is _____.

12. The most abundant positively charged particle in the blood is _____.

13. When the blood level of aldosterone increases:
    a. sodium is moved from the blood to the kidney tubules
    b. sodium is moved from the kidney tubules to the blood
    c. more urine is formed
    d. ANH is released

14. Aldosterone causes:
    a. an increase in intracellular fluid
    b. a decrease in intracellular fluid
    c. an increase in extracellular fluid
    d. a decrease in extracellular fluid

15. Increased capillary pressure:
    a. moves fluid from the intracellular to the extracellular compartment
    b. moves fluid from the plasma to the interstitial fluid
    c. moves fluid from the interstitial fluid to the plasma
    d. has no effect on fluid movement

16. Blood plasma proteins act to:
    a. move interstitial fluid into the plasma
    b. move plasma into the interstitial fluid
    c. move extracellular fluid into the intracellular fluid
    d. move interstitial fluid into the extracellular fluid

OBJECTIVES

**AFTER YOU HAVE COMPLETED THIS CHAPTER, YOU
SHOULD BE ABLE TO:**

1. Discuss the concept of pH and define the term *acid-base balance*.
2. Define the terms *buffer* and *buffer pair* and contrast strong and weak acids and bases.
3. Contrast the respiratory and urinary mechanisms of pH control.
4. Discuss compensatory mechanisms that may help return blood pH to near-normal levels in cases of pH imbalances.
5. Compare and contrast metabolic and respiratory types of pH imbalances.

Acid-Base Balance 19

Acid-base balance is one of the most important of the body's homeostatic mechanisms. Maintaining acid-base balance means keeping the concentration of hydrogen ions in body fluids relatively constant. Effective functioning of many important body proteins, such as cellular enzymes and hemoglobin, closely depends on maintaining precise regulation of hydrogen ion concentration. This is of vital importance. If the hydrogen ion concentration veers away from normal even slightly, serious illness or even death may occur. Healthy survival depends on the ability of the body to maintain, or quickly restore, the acid-base balance of its fluids if imbalances occur. Acid-base regulation requires a series of coordinated homeostatic mechanisms that involve the blood and other body fluids, the lungs, and the kidneys. Ultimately, all of these mechanisms are based on chemical processes. Recall that many important chemical principles related to the life process were covered in Chapter 2. You may wish to refer back to those principles of biochemistry as you study in this chapter how the body so precisely regulates its acid-base balance.

pH OF BODY FLUIDS

Water and all water solutions contain **hydrogen ions (H$^+$)** and **hydroxide ions (OH$^-$)**. The term **pH** followed by a number indicates a solution's hydrogen ion concentration and was first introduced in Chapter 2, pp. 25-26. The *pH scale* in Figure 19-1 is called a "negative logarithm scale." Using this type of scale, the pH of a solution is reported as a specific number (0 to 14), which is used to represent the negative logarithm (10^{-0} to 10^{-14}) of the number of grams of hydrogen ions (H$^+$) present in 1 liter of a solution. The differences in the concentration

of hydrogen ions in various solutions are huge. A solution with a pH of 0 has 1.0 gram of hydrogen ions (H$^+$) per liter (10^{-0}), whereas a solution with a pH of 14 contains only 0.00000000000001 (10^{-14}) grams of hydrogen ions (H$^+$) per liter. Sound complicated? Not really! When trying to remember what the letters in the term *pH* stand for, thinking **p** ("percentage" or "potential") and **H** ("hydrogen ion") might be helpful. Think of the pH scale as a convenient "shortcut" that makes it easy to express the acidity or basicity of a solution without writing a long complex number that contains multiple zeros. For example, when reporting the results of a urine pH test, its easier to report a pH of 8 rather than express the same test result as 0.00000001 (10^{-8}) grams of H^+ ions per liter of urine. In addition to being more convenient, using pH units to report or interpret test results that measure hydrogen ion concentration in body fluids greatly reduces the possibility of errors.

When using the pH scale (Figure 19-1), keep in mind that a pH of 7.0 means that a fluid is neutral in reaction. (See also Figure 2-5 on p. 23.) That is, neither acid nor alkaline. When such a solution *ionizes*, it produces equal amounts of acidic hydrogen (H^+) ions and basic hydroxide (OH^-) ions. Pure water, for example, is pH 7.0. A pH higher than 7.0 indicates an alkaline, or basic, solution and the more alkaline the solution is, the higher is its pH. A pH lower than 7.0 indicates an **acid solution**. The higher the hydrogen ion concentration is, the lower the pH is and the more acid the solution is. Remember, too, that in a negative logarithmic scale, each increase or decrease of one pH unit represents a tenfold difference in hydrogen ion concentration. Thus a relatively small change of only one pH unit results in a significant change in H^+ ion concentration. For example, if two urine samples are obtained from the same individual over a short period of time and they show a change from a pH of 7.0 in one sample to a pH of 8.0 in the second sample, the values indicate a change from neutral to basic urine, with a tenfold decrease in hydrogen ion concentration in the pH 8.0 sample.

With a pH of about 1.6, gastric juice is the most acidic substance in the body. Normally, the pH of arterial blood is about 7.45, and the pH of venous blood is about 7.35. Therefore arterial and venous blood are both slightly alkaline because both have a pH of slightly higher than 7.0. Venous blood, however, is less alkaline than arterial blood because venous blood's pH of about 7.35 is slightly lower than arterial blood's pH of 7.45. Deviations

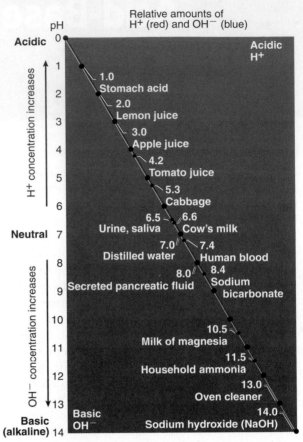

FIGURE 19-1 **The pH range.** The overall pH range is expressed numerically on what is called a *negative logarithmic scale* of 0 to 14 (10^{-0} to 10^{-14}). This means that a change of 1 pH unit represents a tenfold difference in actual concentration of hydrogen ions. As the concentration of H^+ increases, the solution becomes increasingly acidic and the pH value decreases. Decreases in H^+ concentration cause increases in pH values and indicate a more basic alkaline solution. A pH of 7 is neutral, a pH of 0 is very acidic, and a pH of 14 is very basic. See text for discussion.

in blood pH from a very narrow "range of normal" are called *pH imbalances* and are discussed later in the chapter.

✓ **QUICK CHECK**

1. Of what is pH a measurement?
2. What is meant by saying the pH of a solution is "neutral"?
3. What does it mean when a solution's pH increases?

MECHANISMS THAT CONTROL pH OF BODY FLUIDS

The body has three mechanisms for regulating the pH of its fluids. They are (1) the buffer mechanism, (2) the respiratory mechanism, and (3) the urinary mechanism. Together, they constitute the complex pH homeostatic mechanism—the machinery that normally keeps blood slightly alkaline, with a pH that stays remarkably constant. Its usual limits are very narrow, about 7.35 to 7.45.

The slightly lower pH of venous blood (7.36) compared with arterial blood (7.40) results primarily from carbon dioxide (CO_2) entering venous blood as a waste product of cellular metabolism. CO_2 is formed during the cellular breakdown of the nutrient glucose in the presence of oxygen. The process is called **aerobic** (air-OH-bik), or **cellular, respiration.** As CO_2 enters the blood, some of it combines with water (H_2O) and is converted into carbonic acid by **carbonic anhydrase,** an enzyme found in red blood cells. The following chemical equation represents this reaction. Before you read and study the paragraphs that follow, a quick review of Chapter 2, especially Table 2-2 on p. 22 and the discussion of acids, bases, and salts on pp. 25-26, will be particularly helpful.

$$CO_2 + H_2O \xrightarrow{\text{carbonic anhydrase}} H_2CO_3$$

The lungs remove the equivalent of more than 30 liters of carbonic acid each day from the venous blood by elimination of CO_2. This almost unbelievable quantity of acid is so well buffered that a liter of venous blood contains only about 1/100,000,000 grams more H^+ than does 1 liter of arterial blood. What incredible constancy! The pH homeostatic mechanism does indeed control effectively—astonishingly so.

Buffers

Buffers are chemical substances that prevent a sharp change in the pH of a fluid when an acid or base is added to it. Strong acids and bases, when added to blood, "dissociate" almost completely and release large quantities of H^+ or OH^- ions. If this should occur, the result would be drastic changes in blood pH. Survival itself depends on protecting the body from such drastic pH changes. The concept of dissociation was first discussed in Chapter 2 and explained more fully in Chapter 18, p. 417.

More acids than bases are usually added to body fluids. This is because catabolism, a process that goes on continually in every cell of the body, produces acids that enter blood as it flows through tissue capillaries. In addition to the acids produced by cellular breakdown of nutrients such as glucose and fats, some H^+ may be absorbed directly through the digestive tract. Almost immediately, one of the salts present in blood—a buffer, that is—reacts with these relatively strong acids to change them to weaker acids. The weaker acids decrease blood pH only slightly, whereas the stronger acids formed by catabolism would have decreased it greatly if they were not buffered.

Buffers consist of two kinds of substances and are therefore often called **buffer pairs.** One of the main blood buffer pairs is ordinary baking soda (sodium bicarbonate [$NaHCO_3$]) and carbonic acid (H_2CO_3).

Let us consider, as a specific example of buffer action, how the $NaHCO_3$–H_2CO_3 system works with a strong acid or base.

Addition of a strong acid, such as hydrochloric acid (HCl), to the $NaHCO_3$–H_2CO_3 buffer system would initiate the reaction shown in Figure 19-2. Note how this reaction between HCl and $NaHCO_3$ applies the principle of buffering. As a result of the buffering action of $NaHCO_3$, the weak acid, $H \cdot HCO_3$, replaces the very strong acid, HCl, and therefore the H^+ concentration of the blood increases much less than it would have if HCl were not buffered.

If, on the other hand, a strong base, such as sodium hydroxide (NaOH), were added to the same buffer system, the reaction shown in Figure 19-3 would take place. The H^+ of H_2CO_3 ($H \cdot HCO_3$), the weak acid of the buffer pair, combines with the OH^- of the strong base NaOH to form H_2O. Note what this accomplishes. It decreases the number of OH^- added to the solution, and this in turn prevents the drastic rise in pH that would occur without buffering.

Figure 19-2 shows how a buffer system works with a strong acid. Although useful in demonstrating the principles of buffer action, HCl or similar strong acids are never introduced directly into body fluids under normal circumstances. Instead,

FIGURE 19-2 **Buffering action of sodium bicarbonate.** Buffering of acid HCl by NaHCO₃. As a result of the buffer action, the strong acid (HCl) is replaced by a weaker acid (H • HCO₃). Note that HCl as a strong acid "dissociates" almost completely and releases more H⁺ than H_2CO_3. Buffering decreases the number of H⁺ in the system.

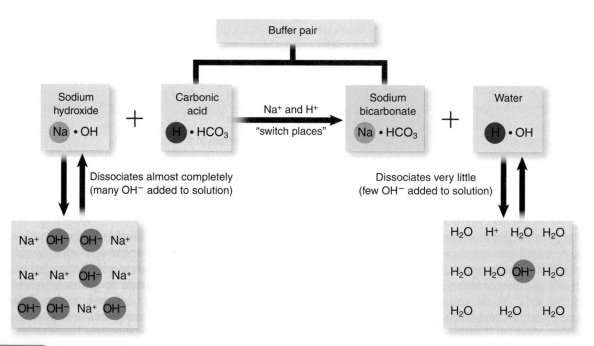

FIGURE 19-3 **Buffering action of carbonic acid.** Buffering of base NaOH by H_2CO_3. As a result of buffer action, the strong base (NaOH) is replaced by NaHCO₃ and H_2O. As a strong base, NaOH "dissociates" almost completely and releases large quantities of OH⁻. Dissociation of H_2O is minimal. Buffering decreases the number of OH⁻ in the system.

the NaCO$_3$ buffer system is most often called on to buffer a number of weaker acids produced during catabolism. Lactic acid is a good example. As a weak acid, it does not "dissociate" as completely as HCl. Incomplete dissociation of lactic acid results in fewer hydrogen ions being added to the blood and a less drastic lowering of blood pH than would occur if HCl were added in an equal amount. Without buffering, however, lactic acid build-up results in significant H$^+$ accumulation over time. The resulting decrease of pH can produce serious acidosis. Ordinary baking soda (sodium bicarbonate or NaHCO$_3$) is one of the main buffers of the normally occurring "fixed" acids in blood. Lactic acid is one of the most abundant of the "fixed" acids (acids that do not break down to form a gas). Figure 19-4 shows the compounds formed by buffering of lactic acid (a "fixed" acid), produced by normal catabolism of glucose in the absence of oxygen. The following changes in blood result from buffering of fixed acids in tissue capillaries:

1. The amount of H$_2$CO$_3$ in blood increases slightly because an acid (such as lactic acid) is converted to H$_2$CO$_3$.

2. The amount of bicarbonate in blood (mainly NaHCO$_3$) decreases because bicarbonate ions become part of the newly formed H$_2$CO$_3$. Normal arterial blood with a pH of 7.45 contains 20 times more NaHCO$_3$ than H$_2$CO$_3$. If this ratio decreases, blood pH decreases below 7.45.

3. The H$^+$ concentration of blood increases slightly. H$_2$CO$_3$ adds hydrogen ions to blood, but it adds fewer of them than lactic acid would have because it is a weaker acid than lactic acid. In other words, the buffering mechanisms do not totally prevent blood hydrogen ion concentration from increasing. It simply minimizes the increase.

4. Blood pH decreases slightly because of the small increase in blood concentration.

H$_2$CO$_3$ is the most abundant acid in body fluids because it is formed by the buffering of fixed acids and also because CO$_2$ forms it by combining with H$_2$O. Large amounts of CO$_2$, an end product of catabolism, continually pour into tissue capillary blood from cells. Much of the H$_2$CO$_3$ formed in blood diffuses into red blood cells where it is buffered by the potassium salt of hemoglobin. H$_2$CO$_3$ breaks down to form the gas CO$_2$ and water (H$_2$O).

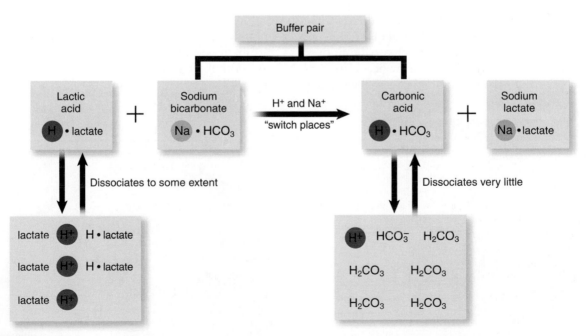

FIGURE 19-4 **Lactic acid buffered by sodium bicarbonate.** Lactic acid (H • lactate) and other "fixed" acids are buffered by NaHCO$_3$ in the blood. Carbonic acid (H • HCO$_3$ or H$_2$CO$_3$, a weaker acid than lactic acid) replaces lactic acid. As a result, fewer H$^+$ are added to blood than would be if lactic acid were not buffered.

This takes place in the blood as it moves through the lung capillaries. Read the next several paragraphs to find out how this affects blood pH.

> **QUICK CHECK**
> 1. What three mechanisms does the body have for regulating pH of body fluids?
> 2. What are buffers?

Respiratory Mechanism of pH Control

Respirations play a vital part in regulating H^+ concentrations and controlling body pH. With every expiration, CO_2 and H_2O leave the body in the expired air. The CO_2 has diffused out of the venous blood as it moves through the lung capillaries. Less CO_2 therefore remains in the arterial blood leaving the lung capillaries, so less of it is available for combining with water to form H_2CO_3. Hence the arterial blood contains less H_2CO_3 and fewer hydrogen ions and has a higher pH (7.45) than does the venous blood (pH 7.35).

Let us consider now how a change in respirations can change blood pH. Suppose you were to pinch your nose shut and hold your breath for a full minute or a little longer. Obviously, no CO_2 would leave your body by way of the expired air during that time, and the blood's CO_2 content would consequently increase. This would increase the amount of H_2CO_3 and the hydrogen-ion concentration of blood, which in turn would decrease blood pH.

Here then are two useful facts to remember: (1) Anything that causes an appreciable decrease in respirations will in time produce **acidosis.** (2) Conversely, anything that causes an excessive increase in respirations will in time produce **alkalosis.** Thus the respiratory control centers in the brain (see p. 343), by increasing or decreasing the rate and depth of respirations, can affect concentrations of CO_2 and H^+ in body fluids.

Urinary Mechanism of pH Control

Most people know that the kidneys are vital organs and that life soon ebbs away if they stop functioning. One reason for this is that the kidneys are the body's most effective regulators of blood pH. They can eliminate much larger amounts of acid than can the lungs and, if it becomes necessary, they can also excrete excess base. The lungs cannot. In short, the kidneys are the body's last and best defense against wide variations in blood pH. If they fail, homeostasis of pH—acid-base balance—will fail.

Because more acids than bases usually enter blood, more acids than bases are usually excreted by the kidneys. In other words, most of the time the kidneys acidify urine; that is, they excrete enough acid to give urine an acid pH, frequently as low as 4.8. (How does this compare with normal blood pH?) The distal tubules of the kidneys rid the blood of excess acid and at the same time conserve the base present in it by the two mechanisms illustrated by Figures 19-5 and 19-6. To

---

🩺 Clinical Application

Diabetic Ketoacidosis

An important part of home care for people with diabetes involves monitoring the level of glucose in the blood and, especially for patients taking insulin, carefully watching for the appearance of **ketone bodies** in the urine. Accumulation of these acidic substances in the blood results from the excessive metabolism of fats most often in uncontrolled type 1 diabetics. These individuals have trouble metabolizing carbohydrates and instead burn fat as a primary energy source. The accumulation of ketone bodies results in a condition called **diabetic ketoacidosis** that causes the blood to become dangerously acidic. The body attempts to correct or "compensate" for the acidosis by rapid breathing to "blow off" CO_2 and thus decrease blood carbonic acid levels. As blood levels of ketones increase, they "spill over" into the urine and can be detected by use of appropriate reagent strips.

Ketonuria. Using a reagent strip to check for the presence of ketone bodies in the urine of a diabetic patient.

FIGURE 19-5 Acidification of urine and conservation of base by distal renal tubule secretion of H⁺ ions.

FIGURE 19-6 Acidification of urine by tubule secretion of ammonia (NH_3). An amino acid (glutamine) moves into the tubule cell and loses an amino group (NH_2) to form ammonia, which is secreted into urine. In exchange, the tubule cell reabsorbs a basic salt (mainly $NaHCO_3$) into blood from urine.

understand these figures fully, you need to have some grasp of basic chemistry. If necessary, refer to Chapter 2 before proceeding. Then look at Figure 19-5 and find the CO_2 leaving the blood (as it flows through a kidney capillary) and entering one of the cells that helps form the wall of a distal kidney tubule. Note that in this cell the CO_2 combines with water to form H_2CO_3. This occurs rapidly because the cell contains carbonic anhydrase, an enzyme that accelerates this reaction. As soon as H_2CO_3 forms, some of it dissociates to yield hydrogen ions and bicarbonate ions. Note what happens to these ions. Hydrogen ions diffuse out of the tubule cell into the urine trickling down the tubule. There, it replaces one of the sodium ions (Na^+) in a salt (Na_2HPO_4) to form another salt (NaH_2PO_4), which leaves the body in the urine. Notice next that the Na^+ displaced from Na_2HPO_4 by the H^+ moves out of the tubular urine into a tubular cell. Here it combines with a bicarbonate (HCO_3^-) ion to form sodium bicarbonate, which then is reabsorbed by the paratubular capillaries into the blood. What this complex of reactions has accomplished is the adding of hydrogen ions to the urine—that is, acidify it—and to conserve $NaHCO_3$ by reabsorbing it into the blood.

Figure 19-6 illustrates another method of acidifying urine, as explained in the legend.

 To learn more about the urinary mechanism of pH control, go to AnimationDirect on your CD-ROM.

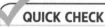 **QUICK CHECK**

1. How can breathing affect the pH of the blood?
2. By what mechanism can the kidney change the pH of the blood?

pH IMBALANCES

Acidosis and **alkalosis** are the two kinds of pH or acid-base imbalance. Although any pH value above 7.0 is considered chemically basic, in clinical medicine the term *acidosis* is used to describe an arterial blood pH of less than 7.35, and *alkalosis* is used to describe an arterial blood pH greater than 7.45. In acidosis the blood pH falls as H^+ ion concentration increases or bases are lost. Only rarely does it fall as low as 7.0 (neutrality), and almost never does it become even slightly acidic, because death usually

intervenes before the pH drops this much. In alkalosis, which develops less often than acidosis, the blood pH is higher than normal because of a loss of acids or an accumulation of bases.

From a clinical standpoint, disturbances in acid-base balance can be considered dependent on the relative quantities (ratio) of H_2CO_3 and $NaHCO_3$ in the blood. Components of this important buffer pair must be maintained at the proper ratio (20 times more $NaHCO_3$ than H_2CO_3) if acid-base balance is to remain normal. It is fortunate that the body can regulate both chemicals in the $NaHCO_3$–H_2CO_3 buffer system. Blood levels of $NaHCO_3$ can be regulated by the kidneys and H_2CO_3 levels by the respiratory system (lungs).

Metabolic and Respiratory Disturbances

Two types of disturbances, metabolic and respiratory, can alter the proper ratio of these components. Metabolic disturbances affect the bicarbonate ($NaHCO_3$) element of the buffer pair, and respiratory disturbances affect the H_2CO_3 element, as follows:

1. **Metabolic disturbances**
   a. **Metabolic acidosis** (bicarbonate deficit). Patients in metabolic acidosis with a bicarbonate deficit often suffer from renal disease, uncontrolled diabetes, or prolonged diarrhea or have ingested toxic chemicals such as antifreeze (ethylene glycol) or wood alcohol (methanol).
   b. **Metabolic alkalosis** (bicarbonate excess). The bicarbonate excess in metabolic alkalosis can result from diuretic therapy, loss of acid-containing gastric fluid caused by vomiting or suction, or from certain diseases such as Cushing syndrome.
2. **Respiratory disturbances**
   a. **Respiratory acidosis** (H_2CO_3 excess). The increase in H_2CO_3 characteristic of respiratory acidosis is caused most frequently by slow breathing (hypoventilation), which results in excess CO_2 in arterial blood. Causes include depression of the respiratory center by drugs or anesthesia or by pulmonary diseases such as emphysema and pneumonia. Serious respiratory acidosis also follows recovery from cardiac arrest.
   b. **Respiratory alkalosis** (H_2CO_3 deficit). Hyperventilation leads to a H_2CO_3 deficit caused by

excessive loss of CO_2 in expired air. The result is respiratory alkalosis. Anxiety (hyperventilation syndrome), overventilation of patients on ventilators, or hepatic coma can all reduce H_2CO_3 and CO_2 to dangerously low levels.

Vomiting and Metabolic Alkalosis

Vomiting, sometimes referred to as **emesis** (EM-eh-sis), is the forcible emptying or expulsion of gastric and occasionally intestinal contents through the mouth. A "vomiting center" in the brain regulates many coordinated (but primarily involuntary) steps involved (Figure 19-7, *A*). Severe vomiting such as the repeated vomiting associated with pyloric obstruction in infants can be life-threatening. One of the most frequent and serious complications of vomiting is metabolic alkalosis (see Figure 19-7, *B* [2]). The bicarbonate excess of metabolic alkalosis results because of the massive loss of chloride from the stomach as HCl. The loss of chloride causes an increase of bicarbonate in the extracellular fluid. As bicarbonate levels increase, the ratio of H_2CO_3 to $NaHCO_3$ may reach 1:40. The result is a condition called **uncompensated metabolic alkalosis** (see Figure 19-7, *B* [2]). Recall that the *ratio* of bicarbonate ion to carbonic acid in the blood is the key to acid-base balance. If the normal *ratio* can be maintained, the acid-base bal-

ance and pH will remain near normal despite changes (within limits) in the absolute amounts of either component of the buffer pair in the blood. In an attempt to "compensate" for the increasing bicarbonate load that results, the body reacts in two ways: (1) it slows respiration to retain more carbon dioxide in the body, thus increasing carbonic acid levels; and (2) it increases the elimination of bicarbonate in the urine. The result is a change in both the absolute amounts and in the *ratio* of carbonic acid to bicarbonate ion that helps restore blood pH toward a more normal and less dangerous level. The condition is then called **compensated metabolic alkalosis** (see Figure 19-7,

FIGURE 19-7 **Vomiting and metabolic alkalosis. A,** Note the many coordinated but primarily involuntary steps involved in vomiting. **B,** Diagram showing: (1) Metabolic balance before onset of metabolic alkalosis. (2) Uncompensated metabolic alkalosis showing increase in bicarbonate ions and change in carbonic acid: bicarbonate ion ratio (1:40). (3) Compensated metabolic alkalosis—new carbonic acid: bicarbonate ion ratio (1.25:30). (4) Excess bicarbonate ions replaced by chloride ions and metabolic balance is restored.

Clinical Application

Lactic Acidosis and Metformin

Metformin hydrochloride (Glucophage®, others) is one of the most widely used and effective of the oral antidiabetic drugs. It is used with diet and exercise to lower blood glucose levels in type 2 diabetes mellitus. A rare but very serious complication of metformin therapy is lactic acidosis. It is characterized by elevated blood lactate levels, electrolyte disturbances, and decreased blood pH. It is reported in only about 1 in 33,000 patients taking metformin over the course of a year. However, when it does occur, it can be fatal in nearly 50% of cases. Symptoms include a variety of gastrointestinal and respiratory complaints and feelings of weakness and muscle pain. Patients with kidney and liver disease are known to be at higher risk of developing lactic acidosis while taking the drug.

B [3]). Treatment is required to restore the normal carbonic acid and bicarbonate buffer pair ratio and return blood pH to normal. Administration of chloride-containing solutions such as normal saline provide the chloride ions needed to replace the excess bicarbonate ions that are then excreted in the urine (see Figure 19-7, *B* [4]). Following successful treatment, homeostatic balance is restored, blood pH returns to normal, and both the absolute amounts and the ratio of carbonic acid to bicarbonate ions is restored to normal levels maintained prior to onset of metabolic alkalosis (see Figure 19-7, *B* [1]).

Cardiac Arrest and Respiratory Acidosis

A cascade of rapid-fire catastrophic homeostatic failures follows cardiac arrest. One such failure involves almost immediate development of respiratory acidosis (carbonic acid excess) caused by retention of CO_2 in the body when respiration ceases and blood flow through the lung capillaries stops. Even if emergency CPR (cardiopulmonary resuscitation) measures can restore breathing and start the heart beating again, respiratory acidosis must be successfully treated and normal blood pH levels restored quickly in order to sustain life. As in other types of pH imbalances, absolute changes in the amount or ratio of the bicarbonate–carbonic acid buffer pair components is the first line of defense to prevent massive changes in blood pH. Then, the body initiates both respiratory and renal compensatory mechanisms to help deal with the carbonic acid excess in severe respiratory acidosis. The most important respiratory compensatory mechanism— increased breathing rate—does "blow off" some additional CO_2 but cannot significantly lower the very elevated carbonic acid build-up that follows cardiac arrest and remains after the blood buffers have been overwhelmed. Finally, renal compensatory mechanisms that stabilize blood pH and help control many forms of respiratory acidosis are initiated after cardiac arrest. They include (1) decreasing the elimination of bicarbonate ions (HCO_3^-) and (2) increasing the elimination of hydrogen ions (H^+) in acidic urine. Although helpful in controlling chronic forms of respiratory acidosis that develop slowly over time, these slow-acting homeostatic compensatory mechanisms are unable to adequately address the serious, acute-onset acidosis that follows cardiac arrest. Medical intervention is required. In the past, immediate intravenous (IV) infusion of bicarbonate- or lactate-containing solutions (lactate is converted to bicarbonate ions in the liver) was considered the emergency treatment of choice in treating respiratory acidosis after cardiac arrest, and these solutions are still used for that purpose. However, clinical studies have shown that aggressive treatment employing controlled ventilation to dramatically increase CO_2 elimination from the body may, in many cases, be more effective in restoring pH balance.

✓ QUICK CHECK

1. What is acidosis? What is alkalosis?
2. What factors may cause a metabolic disturbance in pH?
3. What situations may cause a respiratory disturbance in pH?
4. How does vomiting sometimes create an acid-base imbalance?

Science Application

The Body in Balance
Walter Bradford Cannon
(1871–1945)

Keeping the pH of the body stable is but one aspect of maintaining health. The American physiologist Walter Cannon gave us a name for the principle of balance, or constancy, of the internal fluid environment of the body—*homeostasis*. In 1932, his popular book *The Wisdom of the Body* finally gave a name to the concept first explained by Claude Bernard seven decades earlier (see p. 422). However, Cannon did more than name the concept. In his book, Cannon explained the incredibly complex set of mechanisms that allow our bodies to adjust to tremendous internal and external fluctuations that would otherwise kill us. Much of Cannon's thought came from

his groundbreaking discoveries in how the body copes with stress. In examining the fight-or-flight response, the effects of emotional stimuli, the mechanisms of cardiovascular shock, and in developing the "case study" approach to learning about human health and disease, Walter Cannon developed a clear understanding of the interactive nature of the organs of the body. It was Cannon who led scientists to look at their work in this new framework that explains the "big picture" of human body function.

Cannon's explanation of homeostasis revolutionized the way we look at the body—and how we look at patient care. As with fluid and electrolyte balance, knowledge of the mechanisms of acid-base balance is critical in direct patient care. Therefore many physicians, nurses, intravenous therapists, first responders (for example, emergency medical technicians and paramedics), and others need a basic knowledge of how the body maintains a constancy of pH in the blood.

OUTLINE SUMMARY

pH OF BODY FLUIDS
A. Definition of pH — a number that indicates the hydrogen ion (H^+) concentration of a fluid; pH 7.0 indicates neutrality, pH higher than 7.0 indicates alkalinity, and pH less than 7.0 indicates acidity (see Figure 19-1)
B. Normal arterial blood pH — about 7.45
C. Normal venous blood pH — about 7.35

MECHANISMS THAT CONTROL pH OF BODY FLUIDS
A. Buffers
   1. Definition — substances that prevent a sharp change in the pH of a fluid when an acid or base is added to it (see Figures 19-2 and 19-3)
   2. "Fixed" acids are buffered mainly by sodium bicarbonate ($NaHCO_3$)
   3. Changes in blood produced by buffering of "fixed" acids in the tissue capillaries
      a. Amount of carbonic acid (H_2CO_3) in blood increases slightly
      b. Amount of $NaHCO_3$ in blood decreases; ratio of amount of $NaHCO_3$ to the amount of H_2CO_3 does not normally change; normal ratio is 20:1
      c. H^+ concentration of blood increases slightly

   d. Blood pH decreases slightly below arterial level
B. Respiratory mechanism of pH control — respirations remove some CO_2 from blood as blood flows through lung capillaries, the amount of H_2CO_3 in blood is decreased and thereby its H^+ concentration is decreased, and this in turn increases blood pH from its venous to its arterial level
C. Urinary mechanism of pH control — being the body's most effective regulator of blood pH, kidneys usually acidify urine by the distal tubules secreting hydrogen ions and ammonia (NH_3) into the urine from blood in exchange for $NaHCO_3$ being reabsorbed into the blood

pH IMBALANCES
A. Acidosis and alkalosis — pH or acid-base imbalances
B. Disturbances in acid-base balance depend on relative quantities of $NaHCO_3$ and H_2CO_3 in the blood
C. Body can regulate both of the components of the $NaHCO_3$–H_2CO_3 buffer system
   1. Blood levels of $NaHCO_3$ regulated by kidneys
   2. H_2CO_3 levels regulated by lungs

D. Metabolic and respiratory disturbances — pH disturbances — can alter the normal 20:1 ratio of $NaHCO_3$ to H_2CO_3 in blood
   1. Metabolic disturbances affect the $NaHCO_3$ levels in blood
   2. Respiratory disturbances affect the H_2CO_3 levels in blood
E. Metabolic disturbances
   1. Metabolic acidosis — bicarbonate ($NaHCO_3$) deficit
   2. Metabolic alkalosis — bicarbonate ($NaHCO_3$) excess; complication of severe vomiting

F. Respiratory disturbances
   1. Respiratory acidosis (H_2CO_3 excess)
   2. Respiratory alkalosis (H_2CO_3 deficit)
G. In uncompensated metabolic acidosis, the normal ratio of $NaHCO_3$ to H_2CO_3 is changed; in compensated metabolic acidosis, the ratio remains close to 20:1, but the total amount of $NaHCO_3$ and H_2CO_3 changes
H. Cardiac arrest and respiratory acidosis

NEW WORDS

acid solution
acidosis (metabolic and respiratory) (compensated/ uncompensated)

aerobic (or cellular) respiration
alkaline solution
alkalosis (metabolic and respiratory)

(compensated/ uncompensated)
buffer
buffer pairs
carbonic anhydrase

emesis
hydrogen ion (H^+)
hydroxide ion (OH^-)
pH

REVIEW QUESTIONS

1. Explain the relationship between pH and the relative concentration of hydrogen and hydroxide ions in a solution.
2. Write out the chemical reaction that converts carbon dioxide and water to carbonic acid. What enzyme catalyzes this reaction?
3. What are buffers?
4. Explain how a buffer pair would react if more hydrogen ions were added to the blood.
5. Explain how a buffer pair would react if more hydroxide ions were added to the blood.
6. Explain the four changes that occur in the blood as the result of buffering fixed acids.
7. Explain the respiratory mechanism of pH control.
8. Explain how changes in the respiration rate affect blood pH.

9. Explain how the chemical reaction that occurs in the distal tubule of the kidney using NaH_2PO_4 removes hydrogen ions from the blood.
10. Define *acidosis* and *alkalosis*.
11. Explain metabolic disturbances of the buffer pair.
12. Explain respiratory disturbances of the buffer pair.

CRITICAL THINKING

13. Explain how excessive vomiting causes metabolic alkalosis and explain why normal saline can be used to correct it.
14. What is the proper ratio of $NaHCO_3$ and H_2CO_3 in a buffer pair? Explain how the body can use this ratio to correct uncompensated metabolic acidosis.

CHAPTER TEST

1. The enzyme that converts carbon dioxide and water into carbonic acid is _____.
2. _____ are chemical substances that prevent sharp changes in pH when an acid or base is added to it.
3. If a strong acid such as HCl were added to the buffer pair $NaHCO_3$ and H_2CO_3, the $NaHCO_3$ would become _____.
4. If a strong base such as NaOH were added to the buffer pair in question 3, the H_2CO_3 would become _____.
5. The part of the nephron that is important in regulation of blood pH is the _____.
6. When Na_2HPO_4 is used by the kidney to remove hydrogen ions from the blood, the end product that leaves the body in the urine is _____.
7. When ammonia is used by the kidney to remove hydrogen ions from the blood, the end product that leaves the body in the urine is _____.
8. The kidney is more effective in pH regulation than the lung because it can remove _____, which the lung cannot do.
9. The condition in which the blood pH is higher than normal is called _____.
10. The condition in which the blood pH is lower than normal is called _____.
11. For the buffer pair to function properly, the concentration of $NaHCO_3$ must be _____ times greater than the concentration of H_2CO_3.
12. Metabolic disturbances usually have an effect on the _____ part of the buffer pair.
13. Respiratory disturbances usually have an effect on the _____ part of the buffer pair.
14. Severe vomiting is a metabolic disturbance that can cause metabolic _____.
15. An acid solution has:
    a. a pH greater than 7.0
    b. a pH less than 7.0
    c. more hydroxide ions than hydrogen ions
    d. both a and c

16. An alkaline solution has:
    a. a pH greater than 7.0
    b. a pH less than 7.0
    c. more hydrogen ions than hydroxide ions
    d. both b and c
17. Which of the following statements is true?
    a. A solution with a pH of 5 has more hydrogen ions than a solution with a pH of 2
    b. A solution with a pH of 9 is a base
    c. The pH value increases as the number of hydrogen ions increase
    d. Both a and c are true
18. Arterial blood has a pH of 7.45, and venous blood has a pH of 7.35; therefore:
    a. arterial blood is slightly more acid than venous blood
    b. arterial blood is slightly more alkaline than venous blood
    c. venous blood is slightly more alkaline than arterial blood
    d. both a and c

For questions 19 through 24, fill in the blank with either "increases" or "decreases" as appropriate.
19. When a fixed acid is buffered in the blood, the amount of $NaHCO_3$ in the blood _____.
20. When a fixed acid is buffered in the blood, the amount of hydrogen ions in the blood _____.
21. When a fixed acid is buffered in the blood, the amount of H_2CO_3 in the blood _____.
22. When a fixed acid is buffered in the blood, the pH of the blood _____.
23. Anything that causes an excessive increase in the respiration rate _____ the pH of the blood.
24. Anything that causes an appreciable decrease in the respiration rate _____ the pH of the blood.

OBJECTIVES

AFTER YOU HAVE COMPLETED THIS CHAPTER, YOU
SHOULD BE ABLE TO:

1. List the essential and accessory organs of the male
   and female reproductive systems and give the general function of each.
2. Describe the gross and microscopic structure of the
   gonads in both sexes and explain the developmental steps in spermatogenesis and oogenesis.
3. Discuss the primary functions of the sex hormones
   and identify the cell type or structure responsible
   for their secretion.
4. Identify and describe the structures that constitute
   the external genitals in both sexes.
5. Identify and discuss the phases of the endometrial
   or menstrual cycle and correlate each phase with
   its occurrence in a typical 28-day cycle.

The Reproductive Systems

The offspring of many one-celled plants and bacteria come from a single parent. These organisms are said to be *asexual* because they do not produce specialized reproductive or sex cells called **gametes** (GAM-eets). In contrast, human beings, like all vertebrates, are said to reproduce *sexually* because they do produce these specialized sex cells. The gametes produced in the male reproductive system are called *sperm cells,* or simply **sperm,** whereas those produced in the female are called *egg cells,* or **ova.** In human beings, one sperm cell and one ovum come together during the process of fertilization to produce a cell called the **zygote** (ZYE-goht), which ultimately develops into the new individual. The zygote, which contains an intermingling of genetic messages from the sex cells of both parents, ultimately permits development of new human life. As with all sexually produced offspring, new human life results from the equal contribution of not one but two parent cells—the female ovum and male sperm.

This chapter deals with the structure and function of the reproductive system in men and women. We are truly "fearfully and wonderfully made." Almost any one of the body's organ systems might have inspired this statement, but of them all, perhaps the reproductive systems best deserve such praise. Their ultimate function is to transmit our genes into a new generation, ensuring that our genetic information continues after we are gone. Their awesome achievement is the creation of one of nature's most complex and beautiful structures—the human body. The topic of human development—a process extending from fertilization until death—is covered in Chapter 21.

COMMON STRUCTURAL AND FUNCTIONAL CHARACTERISTICS BETWEEN THE SEXES

Although the organs and specific functions of the male and female reproductive systems will be discussed separately, it is important to understand that a common general structure and function can be identified between the systems in both sexes and that both sexes contribute in uniquely important ways to overall reproductive success.

In both men and women, the organs of the reproductive system are adapted for the specific sequence of functions that permit development of sperm or ova followed by successful fertilization and then the normal development and birth of a baby. In addition, production of hormones that permit development of secondary sex characteristics, such as breast development in women and beard growth in men, occurs as a result of normal reproductive system activity.

As you study the specifics of each system, keep in mind that the male organs function to produce, store, and ultimately introduce mature sperm into the female reproductive tract and that the female system is designed to produce ova, receive the sperm, and permit fertilization. In addition, the highly developed and specialized reproductive system in women permits the fertilized ovum to develop and mature until birth. The complex and cyclic control of reproductive functions in both men and women is particularly crucial to overall reproductive success in humans. The production of sex hormones is required not only for development of the secondary sexual characteristics but also for normal reproductive functions in both sexes. This chapter ends with a table that compares the reproductive structures and functions in women and men.

> ✓ **QUICK CHECK**
> 1. What are gametes?
> 2. What is the ultimate function of the reproductive systems?

MALE REPRODUCTIVE SYSTEM

Structural Plan

You may recall from Chapter 17 (see p. 405) that in males the terminal portion of the urinary tract (urethra) has a dual function. It serves as a passageway for both urine and reproductive fluid (semen) from the body. It is because of this that, in reference to males, *urogenital system* is sometimes used in place of *reproductive system* to describe this important but very limited dual urinary and reproductive function. However, in this chapter we use the term *reproductive system* to better emphasize the primary function of the system structures in both males and females.

So many organs make up the male reproductive system that we need to look first at the structural plan of the system as a whole. Reproductive organs can be classified as *essential* or *accessory.*

Essential Organs

The **essential organs** of reproduction in men and women are called the **gonads.** The gonads of men consist of a pair of main sex glands called the *testes* (TES-teez). The testes produce the male sex cells, or **spermatozoa** (sper-mah-toh-ZOH-ah), and testosterone.

Accessory Organs

The **accessory organs** of reproduction in men consist of the following structures:

1. A series of passageways or ducts that carry the sperm from the testes to the exterior
2. Additional sex glands that provide secretions that protect and nurture sperm
3. The external reproductive organs called the *external genitals*

Table 20-1 lists the names of the essential and accessory organs of reproduction in men, and Figure 20-1 shows the location of most of them. The table and the illustration are included very early in the chapter to provide a preliminary but important overview. Refer back to this table and illustration frequently as you learn about each organ in the pages that follow.

Testes

Structure and Location

The paired **testes** are the gonads of men. They are located in the pouchlike **scrotum** (SKROH-tum), which is suspended outside of the body cavity below the penis (see Figure 20-1). This exposed location provides an environment about 1° C (3° F)

TABLE 20-1

Male Reproductive Organs

ESSENTIAL ORGANS	ACCESSORY ORGANS
Gonads: testes (right testis and left testis)	Ducts: epididymis (two), vas deferens (two), ejaculatory duct (two), and urethra Supportive sex glands: seminal vesicle (two), bulbourethral or Cowper's gland (two), and prostate gland External genitals: scrotum and penis

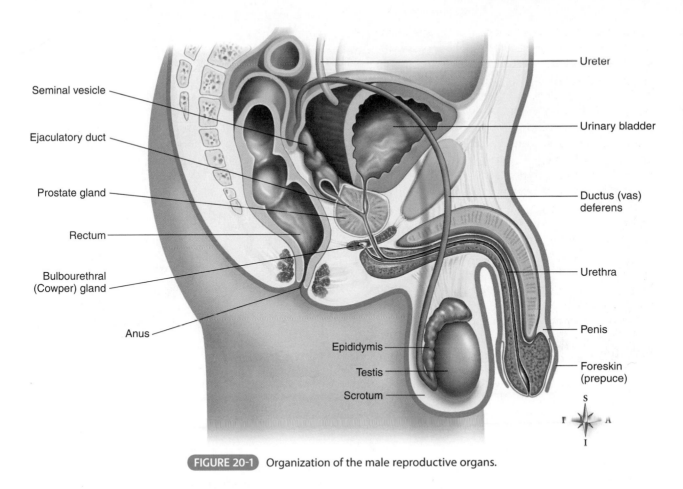

Seminal vesicle

Ejaculatory duct

Prostate gland

Rectum

Bulbourethral
(Cowper) gland

Anus

Epididymis

Testis

Scrotum

Ureter

Urinary bladder

Ductus (vas)
deferens

Urethra

Penis

Foreskin
(prepuce)

FIGURE 20-1 Organization of the male reproductive organs.

cooler than normal body temperature, an important requirement for the normal production and survival of sperm. Each testis is a small, oval gland about 3.8 centimeters (cm) (1.5 inches) long and 2.5 cm (1 inch) wide. The testis is shaped like an egg that has been flattened slightly from side to side. Note in Figure 20-2 that each testis is surrounded by a tough, whitish membrane called the **tunica** (TOO-nih-kah) **albuginea** (al-byoo-JIN-ee-ah). This membrane covers the testicle and then enters the gland to form the many septa that divide it into sections or lobules. As you can see in Figure 20-2, each lobule consists of a narrow but long and coiled **seminiferous** (seh-mih-NIF-er-us) **tubule.** These coiled structures form the bulk of the testicular tissue mass. Small, specialized cells lying near the septa that separate the lobules can be seen in Figure 20-3. These are the **interstitial** (in-ter-STISH-al) **cells** of the testes that secrete the male sex hormone **testosterone** (tes-TOS-teh-rohn).

Each seminiferous tubule is a long duct with a central lumen or passageway (see Figure 20-3). Sperm develop in the walls of the tubule and are

then released into the lumen and begin their journey to the exterior of the body (see Figure 20-5, *A*).

 To learn more about testes, go to AnimationDirect on your CD-ROM.

Testis Functions

Spermatogenesis. Sperm production is called **spermatogenesis** (sper-mah-toh-JEN-eh-sis). From puberty on, the seminiferous tubules continuously form spermatozoa (sperm). Although the number of sperm produced each day diminishes with increasing age, most men continue to produce significant numbers throughout life.

The testes prepare for sperm production before puberty by increasing the numbers of sperm precursor (stem) cells called **spermatogonia** (sper-mah-toh-GO-nee-ah). These cells are located near the outer edge of each seminiferous tubule (Figure 20-4, *A*). Before puberty, spermatogonia increase in number by the process of mitotic cell division, which was described in Chapter 3. Recall that

FIGURE 20-2   **Tubules of the testis and epididymis.** The ducts and tubules are exaggerated in size. In the photograph, the testicle is the darker sphere in the center.

FIGURE 20-3   **Testis tissue.** Several seminiferous tubules surrounded by septa containing interstitial cells are shown.

mitosis results in the division of a "parent" cell into two "daughter" cells, each identical to the parent and each containing a complete copy of the genetic material represented in the normal number of 46 chromosomes.

The hypothalamus is a small but functionally important structure located near the base of the brain. One of its many functions, in both males and females, is to secrete **gonadotropin releasing hormone (GnRH),** which then stimulates the anterior pituitary to secrete follicle stimulating hormone (FSH) and luteinizing hormone (LH) (see Chapter 10, pp. 231-232; see Figure 20-13). When a boy enters puberty, circulating levels of FSH cause spermatogonia to undergo a unique type of cell division that ultimately results in the formation of sperm. When the spermatogonium undergoes mitosis and cell division occurs under the influence of FSH, it produces two daughter cells. One of these cells remains as a spermatogonium and the other forms another, more specialized cell called a **primary spermatocyte** (SPER-mah-toh-syte). These primary spermatocytes then undergo a specialized type of division called **meiosis** (my-

OH-sis), which ultimately results in sperm formation. Note in Figure 20-4, *B*, that during meiosis, two cell divisions occur (not one as in mitosis) and four daughter cells (not two as in mitosis) are formed. The daughter cells are called **spermatids** (SPER-mah-tidz). Unlike the two daughter cells that result from mitosis, the four spermatids, which will develop into spermatozoa, have only half the genetic material and half of the chromosomes (23 instead of 46) of other body cells.

Look again at the diagram of meiosis in Figure 20-4, *B*. It shows that each primary spermatocyte ultimately produces four sperm cells. Note that, in the portion of a seminiferous tubule shown in Figure 20-4, *B*, spermatogonia are found at the outer surface of the tubule, primary and secondary spermatocytes lie deeper in the tubule wall, and mature but immotile sperm are seen about to enter the lumen of the tube and begin their journey through the reproductive ducts to the exterior of the body.

To learn more about spermatogenesis, go to AnimationDirect on your CD-ROM.

Spermatozoa. Spermatozoa are among the smallest and most highly specialized cells in the body (Figure 20-5, *A*). All of the characteristics that a

FIGURE 20-4 **Spermatogenesis. A,** Cross-section of tubule shows progressive meiotic cell types in the wall of a seminiferous tubule. **B,** Diagram of meiotic events and cell types leading to sperm formation.

A

B

FIGURE 20-5 **Human sperm. A,** Micrograph shows the heads and long, slender tails of several spermatozoa. **B,** Illustration shows the components of a mature sperm cell and an enlargement of a sperm head and midpiece.

baby will inherit from its father at fertilization are contained in the condensed nuclear (genetic) material found in each sperm head. However, this genetic information from the father can fuse with genetic material contained in the mother's ovum only if successful fertilization occurs. Ejaculation of sperm into the female vagina during sexual intercourse is only one step in the long journey that these sex cells must make before they can meet and fertilize an ovum. To accomplish their task, these

specialized packages of genetic information are equipped with tails for motility and are designed to penetrate the outer membrane of the ovum when contact occurs with it.

The structure of a mature sperm is diagrammed in Figure 20-5, *B*. Note the sperm head containing the nucleus with its genetic material from the father. The nucleus is covered by the **acrosome** (AK-roh-sohm)—a specialized structure containing enzymes that enable the sperm to break down the covering of the ovum and permit entry if contact occurs. In addition to the head with its covering of acrosome, each sperm has a midpiece and an elongated tail. Mitochondria in the midpiece synthesize adenosine triphosphate (ATP) to provide an energy source for the tail movements required to propel the sperm and allow them to "swim" for relatively long distances through the female reproductive ducts.

Production of Testosterone. In addition to spermatogenesis, the other function of the testes is to secrete the male hormone, testosterone. This function is carried out by the interstitial cells of the testes, not by their seminiferous tubules. At the time of puberty in the male, hypothalamic secretion of GnRH causes the anterior pituitary to secrete increasing amounts of LH, which stimulates the interstitial cells to secrete testosterone. Testosterone serves the following general functions:

1. Masculinization. The various characteristics that we think of as "male" develop because of testosterone's influence. For instance, when a young boy's voice changes, it is testosterone that brings this about.
2. Promotion and maintenance of the development of the male accessory organs (prostate gland, seminal vesicles, and so on).
3. Stimulation effect on protein anabolism. Testosterone thus is responsible for the greater muscular development and strength of the male.

A good way to remember testosterone's functions is to think of it as "the masculinizing hormone" and the "anabolic hormone."

QUICK CHECK
1. What is the name of the male gonads?
2. In what specific structures of the gonad are the sperm produced?
3. What hormone is produced in the male gonad?

Reproductive Ducts

The ducts through which sperm must pass after exiting from the testes until they reach the exterior of the body are important components of the accessory reproductive structures. The other two components included in the listing of accessory organs of reproduction in the male—the supportive sex glands and external genitals—are discussed separately.

Sperm are formed within the walls of the seminiferous tubules of the testes. When they exit from these tubules within the testis, they enter and then pass, in sequence, through the epididymis, ductus (vas) deferens, ejaculatory duct, and the urethra on their journey out of the body.

Epididymis

Each **epididymis** (ep-i-DID-i-mis) consists of a single and very tightly coiled tube about 6 meters (20 feet) in length. It is a comma-shaped structure (see Figure 20-2) that lies along the top and behind the testes inside the scrotum. Sperm mature and develop their ability to move or swim as they are temporarily stored in the epididymis. Specialized cells lining the epididymis secrete nutrients for developing sperm and also remove substantial amounts of excess testicular fluid as the developing sex cells enter and eventually pass through the lumen of this highly coiled tube.

Ductus (Vas) Deferens

The **ductus** (DUK-tus) **deferens** (DEF-er-enz), or vas deferens, is the tube that permits sperm to exit from the epididymis and pass from the scrotal sac upward into the abdominal cavity. Each ductus deferens is a thick, smooth, very muscular, and movable tube that can easily be felt or "palpated" through the thin skin of the scrotal wall. It passes through the inguinal canal into the abdominal cavity as part of the *spermatic cord,* a connective tissue sheath that also encloses blood vessels and nerves.

Ejaculatory Duct and Urethra

Once in the abdominal cavity, the ductus deferens extends over the top and down the posterior surface of the bladder, where it joins the duct from the seminal vesicle to form the **ejaculatory** (ee-JAK-yoo-lah-toh-ree) **duct.** Note in Figure 20-1 that the ejaculatory duct passes through the substance of the prostate gland and permits sperm to empty

Clinical Application

Cryptorchidism

Early in fetal life the testes are located in the abdominal cavity but normally descend into the scrotum about 2 months before birth. Occasionally a baby is born with undescended testes, a condition called **cryptorchidism** (krip-TOR-kih-diz-em), which is readily observed by palpation of the scrotum at delivery. The word *cryptorchidism* is from the Greek words *kryptikos* (hidden) and *orchis* (testis). Failure of the testes to descend may be caused by hormonal imbalances in the developing fetus or by a physical deficiency or obstruction. Regardless of cause, in the cryptorchid infant the testes remain "hidden" in the abdominal cavity. Because the higher temperature inside the body cavity inhibits spermatogenesis, measures must be taken to bring the testes down into the scrotum to prevent permanent sterility. Early treatment of this condition by surgery or by injection of testosterone, which stimulates the testes to descend, may result in normal testicular and sexual development.

Screening for cryptorchidism in newborn infant. Properly descended testicles can be palpated easily in the scrotal sac.

into the **urethra,** which eventually passes through the penis and opens to the exterior at the external urethral orifice.

To learn more about male reproductive ducts, go to AnimationDirect on your CD-ROM.

Accessory, or Supportive, Sex Glands

The term **semen** (SEE-men), or **seminal fluid,** is used to describe the mixture of sex cells, or sperm, produced by the testes and the secretions of the accessory, or supportive, sex glands. The accessory glands, which contribute more than 95% of the secretions to the gelatinous fluid part of the semen, include the two seminal vesicles, one prostate gland, and two bulbourethral (Cowper's) glands. In addition to the production of sperm, the seminiferous tubules of the testes contribute somewhat less than 5% of the seminal fluid volume. Usually 3 to 5 milliliters (mL) (about 1 teaspoon) of semen is ejaculated at one time, and each milliliter normally contains about 100 million sperm. Semen is alkaline and protects sperm from the acidic environment of the female reproductive tract.

Seminal Vesicles

The paired **seminal vesicles** are pouchlike glands that contribute about 60% of the seminal fluid volume. Their secretions are yellowish, thick, and rich in the sugar fructose. This fraction of the seminal fluid helps provide a source of energy for the highly motile sperm.

Prostate Gland

The **prostate gland** lies just below the bladder and is shaped like a doughnut. The urethra passes through the center of the prostate before traversing the penis to end at the external urinary orifice. The prostate secretes a thin, milk-colored fluid that constitutes about 30% of the total seminal fluid volume. This fraction of the ejaculate helps to activate the sperm and maintain their motility.

Bulbourethral Glands

Each of the two **bulbourethral** (BUL-boh-yoo-REE-thral) **glands** (also called *Cowper's glands*) resemble peas in size and shape. They are located just below the prostate gland and empty their secretions into the penile portion of the urethra. Because the bulbourethral secretion is often released just before most of the rest of the semen is ejaculated, it is sometimes called the "pre-ejaculate." The mucus-like secretions of these glands serve two protective functions: they (1) neutralize any residue of sperm damaging acidic urine in the terminal urethra and (2) lubricate the urethra to protect sperm from friction damage during **ejaculation.** The bulbourethral glands contribute less than 5% of the seminal fluid volume.

External Genitals

The penis (PEE-nis) and scrotum constitute the external reproductive organs, or **genitalia** (jen-i-TAIL-yah), of men. The **penis** (Figure 20-6) is the organ that, when made stiff and erect by the filling of its spongy or erectile tissue components with blood during sexual arousal, can enter and deposit sperm in the vagina during intercourse. The penis has three separate columns of erectile tissue in its shaft: one column of **corpus** (KOHR-pus) **spongiosum** (spun-jee-OH-sum), which surrounds the urethra, and two columns of **corpora** (KOHR-pohr-ah) **cavernosa** (kav-er-NO-sah), which lie above. The spongy nature of erectile tissue is apparent in Figure 20-6. At the distal end of the shaft of the penis is the enlarged **glans,** which is covered with highly sensitive skin. Over the sensitive skin of the glans is a doubly folded extension of the skin on the penis's shaft that forms a loose-fitting retractable collar called the **foreskin,** or **prepuce** (PREE-pus). If the foreskin fits too tightly about the glans, a **circumcision,** or surgical removal of the foreskin shortly after birth is usually performed to prevent

Clinical Application

Prostatic Hypertrophy

A noncancerous condition called **benign** (bee-NYNE) **prostatic hypertrophy** (hye-PER-troh-fee) **(BPH)** is a common problem in older men. The condition is characterized by an enlargement or hypertrophy of the prostate gland. That the urethra passes through the center of the prostate after exiting from the bladder is a matter of considerable clinical significance in this condition. As the prostate enlarges, it squeezes the urethra, frequently closing it so completely that urination becomes very difficult or even impossible. In some cases drugs (Avodart®, Flomax®, others) may be used to improve urine flow and reduce symptoms of BPH.

Surgical removal of part or all of the gland, a procedure called **prostatectomy** (pross-tah-TEK-toh-mee) is also a treatment option. **Prostate cancer** also causes hypertrophy of the gland and restricted or obstructed urine flow caused by malignant tumor growth. In addition to surgery, cancerous prostatic growths may also be treated using systemic chemotherapy, cryotherapy (freezing) of prostatic tissue, microwave (heat) therapy, hormonal therapy, inserting radioactive "seeds" directly into the tumor, and the use of various types of external-beam radiation. In addition to enlargement of the prostate, adult men often develop inflammation of the gland, a condition called **prostatitis** (pross-tah-TYE-tiss).

FIGURE 20-6 The penis. **A,** In this sagittal section of the penis viewed from above, the urethra is exposed throughout its length and can be seen exiting from the bladder and passing through the prostate gland before entering the penis to end at the external urethral orifice. **B,** Diagram showing partial separation of the penile erectile columns. The glans penis is the cup-shaped, expanded end of the corpus spongiosum. **C,** Photograph of a cross-section of the shaft of the penis. Note the urethra within the substance of the corpus spongiosum.

irritation. Although recommended by some authorities for other medical reasons such as reduction in the spread of AIDS and other sexually transmitted infections (STIs) later in life, most circumcisions are "elective" and are performed at the discretion of the parents for religious or cultural reasons. The external urethral orifice is the opening of the urethra at the tip of the glans.

The **scrotum** is a skin-covered pouch suspended from the groin. Internally, it is divided into two sacs by a septum; each sac contains a testis, epididymis, the lower part of the ductus deferens, and the beginning of the spermatic cords.

QUICK CHECK

1. What duct leads from the epididymis?
2. Which organs produce the fluid in semen?
3. What is the function of erectile tissues?

FEMALE REPRODUCTIVE SYSTEM

Structural Plan

The structural plan of the reproductive system in both sexes is similar in that organs are characterized as *essential* or *accessory*.

Essential Organs

The essential organs of reproduction in women, the gonads, are the paired *ovaries*. The female sex cells, or ova, and the hormones estrogen and progesterone are produced in the ovaries.

Accessory Organs

The accessory organs of reproduction in women consist of the following structures:
1. A series of ducts or modified duct structures that extend from near the ovaries to the exterior
2. Additional sex glands, including the mammary glands, which have an important reproductive function only in women
3. The external reproductive organs, or external genitals

Table 20-2 lists the names of the essential and accessory female organs of reproduction, and Figure 20-7 shows the location of most of them. Refer back to this table and illustration as you read about each structure in the pages that follow.

TABLE 20-2

Female Reproductive Organs

ESSENTIAL ORGANS	ACCESSORY ORGANS
Gonads: ovaries (right ovary and left ovary)	Ducts: uterine tubes (two), uterus, vagina Accessory sex glands: Bartholin's glands (two), breasts (two) External genitals: vulva

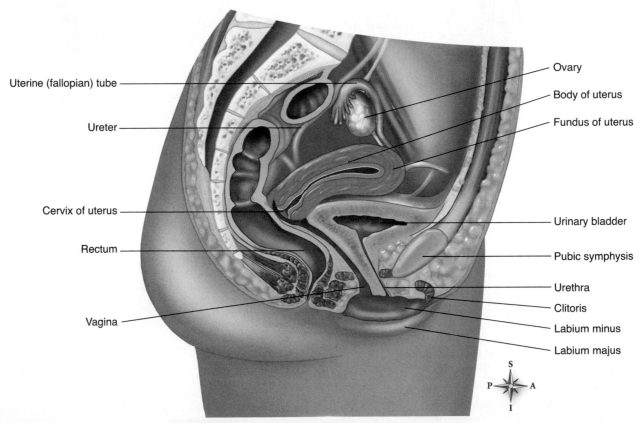

FIGURE 20-7 Organization of the female reproductive organs.

(Labels: Uterine (fallopian) tube, Ureter, Cervix of uterus, Rectum, Vagina, Ovary, Body of uterus, Fundus of uterus, Urinary bladder, Pubic symphysis, Urethra, Clitoris, Labium minus, Labium majus)

Ovaries

Structure and Location

The paired **ovaries** are the gonads of women. They have a puckered, uneven surface; each weighs about 3 grams. The ovaries resemble large almonds in size and shape and are attached to ligaments in the pelvic cavity on each side of the uterus.

Embedded in a connective tissue matrix just below the outer layer of each ovary in a newborn baby girl are about 1 million **ovarian follicles;** each contains an **oocyte,** an immature stage of the female sex cell. By the time a girl reaches puberty, however, further development has resulted in the formation of a reduced number (about 400,000) of what are now called **primary follicles.** Each primary follicle has a layer of **granulosa cells** around the oocyte. During the reproductive lifetime of most women, only about 350 to 500 of these primary follicles fully develop into **mature follicles,** which ovulate and release an ovum for potential fertilization. Follicles that do not mature degenerate and are reabsorbed into the ovarian tissue. A mature ovum in its sac is sometimes called a **graafian** (GRAH-fee-en) **follicle,** in honor of the Dutch anatomist who discovered the follicle some 300 years ago.

The progression of development from primary follicle to ovulation is shown in Figure 20-8. As the thickness of the granulosa cell layer around the oocyte increases, a hollow chamber called an **antrum** (AN-trum) appears, and a *secondary follicle* is formed. Development continues, and, after ovulation, the ruptured follicle is transformed into a hormone-secreting glandular structure called the **corpus** (KOHR-pus) **luteum** (LOO-tee-um), which is described later. Corpus luteum is from the Latin word meaning "yellow body," an appropriate name to describe the yellow appearance of this glandular structure.

> To learn more about the ovaries, go to AnimationDirect on your CD-ROM.

Ovary Functions

Oogenesis. The production of female gametes, or sex cells, is called **oogenesis** (oh-oh-JEN-eh-sis). The specialized type of cell division that results in sperm formation, meiosis, is also responsible for development of ova. During the developmental phases experienced by the female sex cell from its earliest stage to just after fertilization, two meiotic divisions occur. As a result of meiosis in the female

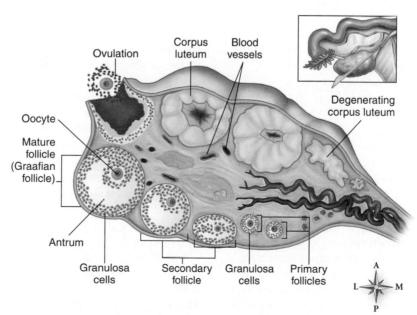

FIGURE 20-8 **Diagram of ovary and oogenesis.** Cross-section of mammalian ovary shows successive stages of ovarian (graafian) follicle and ovum development. Begin with the first stage (primary follicle) and follow around clockwise to the final state (degenerating corpus luteum).

sex cell, the number of chromosomes is reduced equally in each daughter cell to half the number (23) found in other body cells (46). However, the amount of cytoplasm is divided unequally. The result is formation of one large ovum and small daughter cells called *polar bodies* that degenerate.

The ovum, with its large supply of cytoplasm, is one of the body's largest cells and is uniquely designed to provide nutrients for rapid development of the embryo until implantation in the uterus occurs. At fertilization, the sex cells from both parents fuse, and the normal chromosome number (46) is achieved.

 To learn more about oogenesis, go to AnimationDirect on your CD-ROM.

Production of Estrogen and Progesterone. The second major function of the ovary, in addition to oogenesis, is secretion of the sex hormones, *estrogen* and *progesterone.* Hormone production in the ovary begins at puberty with the cyclic development and maturation of the ovum. The granulosa cells around the oocyte in the growing and mature follicle secrete estrogen. The corpus luteum, which develops after ovulation, chiefly secretes progesterone but also some estrogen.

Estrogen is the sex hormone that causes the development and maintenance of the female **secondary sex characteristics** and stimulates growth of the epithelial cells lining the uterus. Some of the actions of estrogen include the following:

1. Development and maturation of female reproductive organs, including the external genitals
2. Appearance of pubic hair and breast development
3. Development of female body contours by deposition of fat below the skin surface and in the breasts and hip region
4. Initiation of the first menstrual cycle

Progesterone is produced by the corpus luteum, which is a glandular structure that develops from a follicle that has just released an ovum. If stimulated by the appropriate anterior pituitary hormone, the corpus luteum produces progesterone for about 11 days after ovulation. Progesterone stimulates proliferation and vascularization of the epithelial lining of the uterus and acts with estrogen to initiate the menstrual cycle in girls entering puberty.

Reproductive Ducts

Uterine Tubes

The two **uterine tubes,** also called **fallopian** (fal-LOH-pee-an) **tubes** or **oviducts** (OH-vi-dukts), serve as ducts for the ovaries, even though they are not attached to them. The outer end of each tube terminates in an expanded, funnel-shaped structure that has fringelike projections called **fimbriae** (FIM-bree-ee) along its edge. This part of the tube curves over the top of each ovary (Figure 20-9) and opens into the abdominal cavity. The inner end of each uterine tube attaches to the uterus, and the cavity inside the tube opens into the cavity in the uterus. Each tube is about 10 cm (4 inches) in length.

After ovulation the discharged ovum first enters the abdominal cavity and then enters the uterine tube assisted by the wavelike movement of the fimbriae and the beating of the cilia on their surface. After it is in the tube, the ovum begins its journey to the uterus. Some ova never find their way into the oviduct and remain in the abdominal cavity where they are reabsorbed. In Chapter 21 the details of fertilization, which normally occurs in the outer one third of the uterine tube, will be discussed.

The mucosal lining of the uterine tubes is directly continuous with the lining of the abdominal cavity on one end and with the lining of the uterus and vagina on the other. This is of great clinical significance because infections of the vagina or uterus such as gonorrhea may pass into the abdominal cavity, where they may become life-threatening.

Uterus

The **uterus** (YOO-ter-us) is a small organ—only about the size of a pear—but it is extremely strong. It is almost all muscle, or **myometrium** (my-oh-MEE-tree-um), with only a small cavity inside. During pregnancy the uterus grows many times larger so that it becomes big enough to hold a baby and a considerable amount of fluid. The uterus is composed of two parts: an upper portion, the *body,*

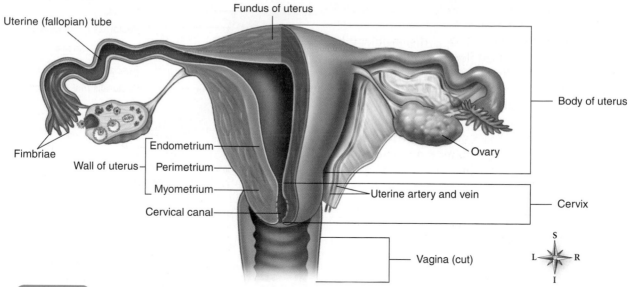

Fundus of uterus

Uterine (fallopian) tube

Body of uterus

Fimbriae

Endometrium

Ovary

Wall of uterus — Perimetrium

Myometrium

Uterine artery and vein

Cervical canal

Cervix

Vagina (cut)

FIGURE 20-9 The uterus. Sectioned view shows muscle layers of the uterus and its relationship to the ovaries and vagina.

and a lower narrow section, the **cervix.** Just above the level where the uterine tubes attach to the body of the uterus, it rounds out to form a bulging prominence called the **fundus** (see **Figure 20-9**). Except during pregnancy, the uterus lies in the pelvic cavity just behind the urinary bladder. By the end of pregnancy, it becomes large enough to extend up to the top of the abdominal cavity. It then pushes the liver against the underside of the diaphragm—a fact that explains a comment such as "I can't seem to take a deep breath since I've gotten so big," made by many women late in their pregnancies.

The uterus functions in three processes—menstruation, pregnancy, and labor. The corpus luteum stops secreting progesterone and decreases its secretion of estrogens about 11 days after ovulation. About 3 days later, when the progesterone and estrogen concentrations in the blood are at their lowest, menstruation starts. Small pieces of the mucous membrane lining of the uterus, or the **endometrium** (en-doh-MEE-tree-um), pull loose, leaving torn blood vessels underneath. Blood and bits of endometrium trickle out of the uterus into the vagina and out of the body. Immediately after menstruation the endometrium starts to repair itself. It again grows thick and becomes lavishly supplied with blood in preparation for pregnancy. If fertilization does not take place, the uterus again sheds the lining made ready for a pregnancy that

did not occur. Because these changes in the uterine lining continue to repeat themselves, they are spoken of as the **menstrual cycle** (see p. 455).

If fertilization occurs, pregnancy begins, and the endometrium remains intact. The events of pregnancy are discussed in Chapter 21.

Menstruation first occurs at puberty, often around the age of 11 to 12 years. Normally the cycle repeats about every 28 days or 13 times a year for some 30 to 40 years before it ceases at **menopause** (MEN-oh-pawz), when a woman is somewhere around the age of 50 years.

 Clinical Application

Ectopic Pregnancy

The term **ectopic** (ek-TOP-ik) **pregnancy** is used to describe a pregnancy resulting from the implantation of a fertilized ovum in any location other than the uterus. Occasionally, because the outer ends of the uterine tubes open into the pelvic cavity and are not actually connected to the ovaries, an ovum does not enter an oviduct but becomes fertilized and remains in the abdominal cavity. Although rare, if implantation occurs on the surface of an abdominal organ or on one of the mesenteries, development may continue to term. In such cases, delivery by caesarean section is required. Most ectopic pregnancies involve implantation in the uterine tube and are therefore called *tubal pregnancies*. They result in fetal death and, if not treated, tubal rupture.

Vagina

The **vagina** (vah-JYE-nah) is a distensible tube about 10 cm (4 inches) long, made mainly of smooth muscle and lined with mucous membrane. It lies in the pelvic cavity between the urinary bladder and the rectum (see Figure 20-7). As the part of the female reproductive tract that opens to the exterior, the vagina is the organ that sperm enter during their journey to meet an ovum, and it is also the organ from which a baby emerges to meet its new world.

 To learn more about female reproductive ducts, go to AnimationDirect on your CD-ROM.

Accessory, or Supportive, Sex Glands

Bartholin's Glands

One of the small **Bartholin's** (BAR-toh-linz), or **greater vestibular** (ves-TIB-yoo-lar), **glands** lies to the right of the vaginal outlet, and one lies to the left of it. Secretion of a mucus-like lubricating fluid is their function. Their ducts open into the space between the labia minora and the vaginal orifice called the **vestibule** (see Figure 20-11).

Breasts

The **breasts** lie over the pectoral muscles and are attached to them by connective tissue ligaments. Breast size is determined more by the amount of fat around the glandular (milk-secreting) tissue than by the amount of glandular tissue itself. Hence the size of the breast has little to do with its ability to secrete adequate amounts of milk after the birth of a baby.

Each breast consists of 15 to 20 divisions or lobes that are arranged radially (Figure 20-10). Each lobe consists of several lobules, and each lobule consists of milk-secreting glandular cells. The milk-secreting cells are arranged in grapelike clusters called *alveoli*. Small **lactiferous** (lak-TIF-er-us) **ducts** drain the alveoli and converge toward the nipple like the spokes of a wheel. Only one lactiferous duct leads from each lobe to an opening in the nipple. The colored area around the nipple is the **areola** (ah-REE-oh-lah).

Knowledge of the lymphatic drainage of the breast is important because cancerous cells from breast tumors often spread to other areas of the

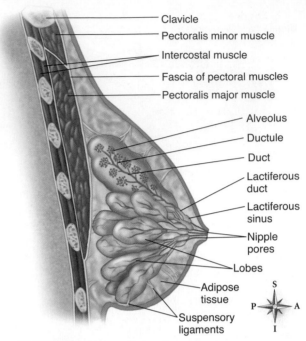

FIGURE 20-10 Lateral view of the breast. Sagittal section of a lactating breast. Notice how the glandular structures are anchored to the overlying skin and to the pectoral muscles by the suspensory ligaments of Cooper. Each lobule of glandular tissue is drained by a lactiferous duct that eventually opens through the nipple.

body through the lymphatic system. This lymphatic drainage is discussed in Chapter 13 (see Figure 13-5).

> **QUICK CHECK**
> 1. What is another name for the uterine tubes?
> 2. What three major functions does the uterus perform?
> 3. What substance is conducted through lactiferous ducts?

External Genitals

The **external genitalia,** or **vulva** (VUL-vah), of women consist of the following:
1. Mons pubis
2. Clitoris
3. Orifice of urethra
4. Labia minora (singular, *labium minus*) (small lips)
5. Hymen
6. Orifice, duct of Bartholin's gland

7. Orifice of vagina
8. Labia majora (singular, *labium majus*) (large lips)

The **mons pubis** is a skin-covered pad of fat over the symphysis pubis. Hair appears on this structure at puberty and persists throughout life. Extending downward from the elevated mons pubis are the **labia** (LAY-bee-ah) **majora** (mah-JO-rah), or "large lips." These elongated folds, which are composed mainly of fat and numerous glands, are covered with pigmented skin and hair on the outer surface and are smooth and free from hair on the inner surface. The **labia minora,** or "small lips," are located within the labia majora and are covered with modified skin. These two lips join anteriorly at the midline. The area between the labia minora is the vestibule (Figure 20-11). Several genital structures are located in the vestibule. The **clitoris** (KLIT-oh-ris), which is composed of erectile tissue, is located just behind the anterior junction of the labia minora. Situated between the clitoris above and the vaginal opening below is the orifice of the urethra. The vaginal orifice is sometimes partially closed by a membranous **hymen** (HYE-men). The ducts of Bar-tholin's glands open on either side of the vaginal orifice inside the labia minora.

The term **perineum** (pair-i-NEE-um) is used to describe the area between the vaginal opening and anus. This area is sometimes cut in a surgical procedure called an **episiotomy** (eh-piz-ee-OT-oh-mee) to prevent tearing of tissue during childbirth.

Menstrual Cycle

Phases and Events

The menstrual cycle consists of many changes in the uterus, ovaries, vagina, and breasts and in the anterior pituitary gland's secretion of hormones (Figure 20-12). In the majority of women, these changes occur with almost precise regularity throughout their reproductive years. The first indication of changes comes with the first menstrual period. The first **menses** (MEN-seez), or menstrual flow, is referred to as the **menarche** (meh-NAR-kee).

A typical menstrual cycle covers a period of about 28 days. The length of the cycle varies among women. Some women, for example, may have a regular cycle that covers about 24 days. The length

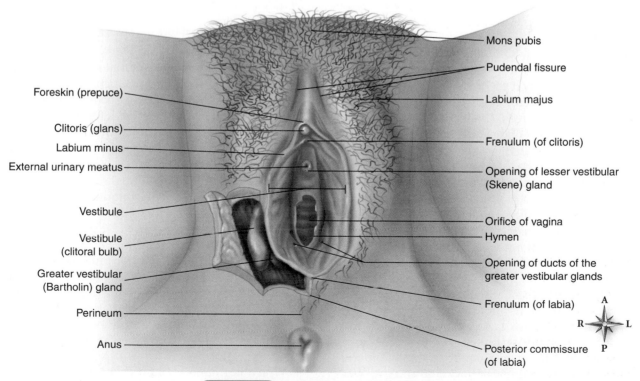

Foreskin (prepuce)
Clitoris (glans)
Labium minus
External urinary meatus
Vestibule
Vestibule (clitoral bulb)
Greater vestibular (Bartholin) gland
Perineum
Anus

Mons pubis
Pudendal fissure
Labium majus
Frenulum (of clitoris)
Opening of lesser vestibular (Skene) gland
Orifice of vagina
Hymen
Opening of ducts of the greater vestibular glands
Frenulum (of labia)
Posterior commissure (of labia)

A
R — L
P

FIGURE 20-11 External genitals of the female.

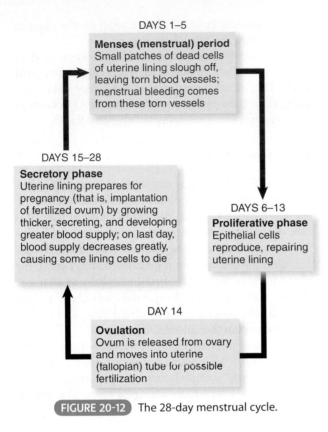

DAYS 1–5

Menses (menstrual) period
Small patches of dead cells of uterine lining slough off, leaving torn blood vessels; menstrual bleeding comes from these torn vessels

DAYS 15–28

Secretory phase
Uterine lining prepares for pregnancy (that is, implantation of fertilized ovum) by growing thicker, secreting, and developing greater blood supply; on last day, blood supply decreases greatly, causing some lining cells to die

DAYS 6–13

Proliferative phase
Epithelial cells reproduce, repairing uterine lining

DAY 14

Ovulation
Ovum is released from ovary and moves into uterine (fallopian) tube for possible fertilization

FIGURE 20-12 The 28-day menstrual cycle.

of the cycle also varies within one woman. Some women, for example, may have irregular cycles that range from 21 to 28 days, whereas others may have cycles that are 2 to 3 months long. Each cycle consists of three phases. The three periods of time in each cycle are called the **menses,** the **proliferative phase,** and the **secretory phase.** Refer often to Figure 20-13 as you read about the events occurring during each phase of the cycle in the hypothalamus and pituitary gland, the ovary, and in the uterus. Be sure that you do not overlook the event that occurs around day 14 of a 28-day cycle.

The menses is a period of 4 or 5 days characterized by menstrual bleeding. The first day of menstrual flow is considered day 1 of the menstrual cycle. The proliferative phase begins after the menstrual flow ends and lasts until ovulation. During this period the follicles mature, the uterine lining thickens (proliferates), and estrogen secretion increases to its highest level. The secretory phase of the menstrual cycle begins at ovulation and lasts until the next menses begins. It is during this phase of the menstrual cycle that the uterine lining reaches its greatest thickness and the ovary secretes its highest levels of progesterone.

As a general rule, during the 30 or 40 years that a woman has periods, only one ovum matures each month. However, there are exceptions to this rule. Some months, more than one matures, and some months, no ovum matures. Ovulation occurs 14 days before the next menses begins. In a 28-day cycle, this means that ovulation occurs around day 14 of the cycle, as shown in Figure 20-12. (Recall that the first day of the menses is considered the first day of the cycle.) In a 30-day cycle, however, ovulation would not occur on the 14th cycle day, but instead on the 16th. And in a 25-day cycle, ovulation would occur on the 11th cycle day.

The time of ovulation has great practical importance because the possibility of fertilization—the fusion of a sperm and egg—can occur only during a short period of time during each menstrual cycle. Although a few "super" sperm may remain viable for up to 5 days, most sperm retain their fertilizing power for only 24 to 72 hours after being deposited in the female reproductive tract following ejaculation. The oocyte remains viable and capable of being fertilized for only about 12 to 24 hours after ovulation. A woman's fertile period therefore lasts only a few days each month—from between 3 to 5 days prior to, and no later than 24 hours after, ovulation.

Control of Menstrual Cycle Changes

The anterior pituitary gland plays a critical role in regulating the cyclic changes that characterize the functions of the female reproductive system (see Chapter 10). As noted earlier, secretion of GnRH from the hypothalamus stimulates the anterior pituitary gland to secrete both FSH and LH. From day 1 to about day 7 of the menstrual cycle, GnRH selectively stimulates the anterior pituitary gland to secrete increasing amounts of FSH. A high blood concentration of FSH stimulates several immature ovarian follicles to start growing and secreting estrogen (see Figure 20-13). Working together, increasing levels of estrogen and GnRH in the blood stimulate the anterior pituitary gland to release increasing amounts of luteinizing hormone (LH). LH causes maturing of a follicle and its ovum, ovulation (rupturing of mature follicle with ejection of ovum), and luteinization (formation of a yellow body, the corpus luteum, from the ruptured follicle).

Which hormone—FSH or LH—would you call the "ovulating hormone"? Do you think ovulation

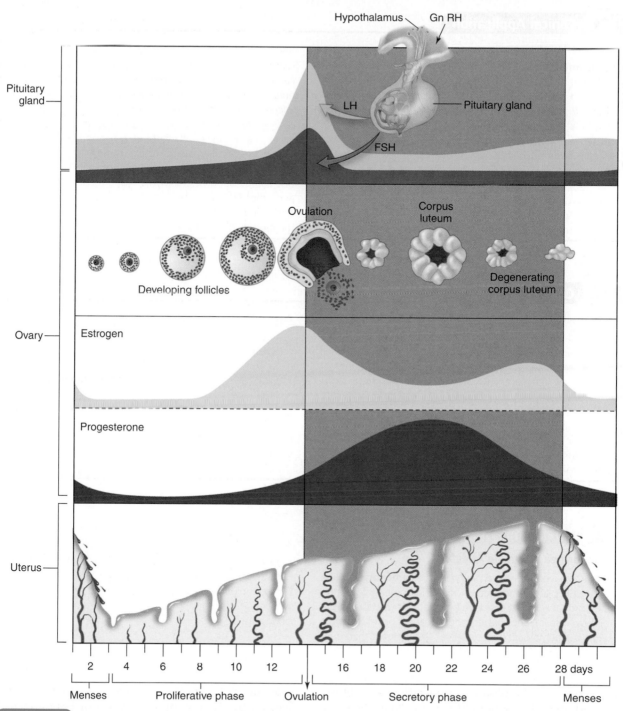

FIGURE 20-13 **The human menstrual cycle.** Diagram illustrates the interrelationship of pituitary, ovarian, and uterine functions throughout a usual 28-day cycle. A sharp increase in luteinizing hormone (LH) levels causes ovulation, whereas menstruation (sloughing off of the endometrial lining) is initiated by lower levels of progesterone.

Clinical Application

Pelvic Inflammatory Disease

Pelvic inflammatory disease (PID) is a common disorder that affects more than 800,000 women each year in the United States. It is characterized by pelvic pain, fever, and vaginal discharge. PID occurs as either an acute or a chronic inflammatory condition that can be caused by several different types of pathogens. Organisms that cause a number of *sexually transmitted infections (STIs)*, especially chlamydia (klah-MID-e-ah), continue as a common cause of PID. As the infection spreads upward from the vagina, it often involves the uterus, uterine tubes, ovaries, and other pelvic organs, often resulting in the development of scar tissue and adhesions. Some STIs that ultimately result in serious complica-tions, such as PID, do not initially cause symptoms and are said to be "asymptomatic." Chlamydia, the most common cause of PID, is often asymptomatic for extended periods of time. In addition, developing PID caused by the chlamydia infection may also remain asymptomatic until significant damage has occurred. In these cases, women may be un-aware that an infection is under way and causing serious problems. Infertility is one of the most commonly feared consequences of long-standing or chronic PID and is a seri-ous complication of chlamydia, gonorrhea (GON-o-RE-ah), and other STI infections. Direct laparoscopic examination is often used to determine the severity of the PID infection and the reproductive organs involved.

Clinical Application

Hysterectomy

The word **hysterectomy** (his-teh-REK-toh-mee) comes from the combination of two Greek words: *hystera*, meaning "uterus," and *ektome*, meaning "to cut out." By definition it is the surgical removal of the uterus. *Hysterectomy* is a term that is often misused, however, by incorrectly expanding its definition to include the removal of the ovaries or other re-productive structures. Only the uterus is removed in a hyster-ectomy. If the total uterus, including the cervix, is removed, the terms *total hysterectomy* or *panhysterectomy* may be used. If the cervical portion of the uterus is left in place and only the body of the organ is removed, the term *subtotal hysterectomy* is appropriate. The actual removal of the uterus may be performed through an incision made in the abdomi-nal wall—*abdominal hysterectomy*— or through the vagina— *vaginal hysterectomy*. The term **oophorectomy** (oh-off-eh-REK-toh-mee) is used to describe removal of the ovaries. Although the two surgical procedures may take place during the same operation—for a woman with uterine or ovarian cancer, for example—the terms used to describe them should not be used interchangeably.

Health and Well-Being

Amenorrhea in Female Athletes

Failure to have a menstrual period is called **amenorrhea** (ah-men-oh-REE-ah)**.** Amenorrhea occurs in some female ath-letes, probably resulting from a body fat composition that is too low to sustain normal reproductive function. Although it keeps the hematocrit (red blood cell level) higher than dur-ing menstruation, it is not considered a desirable condition. Besides infertility, amenorrhea may cause other problems. For example, the low blood levels of estrogen associated with long-term amenorrhea may cause osteoporosis (loss of bone mass).

could occur if the blood concentration of FSH re-mained low throughout the menstrual cycle? If you answered LH to the first question and no to the second, you answered both questions cor-rectly. Ovulation cannot occur if the blood level of FSH stays low because a high concentration of this hormone is essential to stimulation of ovarian fol-licle growth and maturation. With a low level of FSH, no follicles start to grow, and therefore none become ripe enough to ovulate. Ovulation is caused by the combined actions of FSH and LH. Birth control pills that contain estrogen substances suppress FSH secretion. This indirectly prevents ovulation.

Ovulation occurs, as we have said, because of the combined actions of the two anterior pitu-itary hormones, FSH and LH. The next question is, what causes menstruation? A brief answer is

TABLE 20-3

Analogous* Features of the Reproductive Systems

FEATURES	FEMALE	MALE
Essential organs	Ovaries	Testes
Sex cells	Ova (eggs)	Sperm
Hormones	Estrogen and progesterone	Testosterone
Hormone-producing cells	Granulosa cells and corpus luteum	Interstitial cells
Duct systems	Uterine (fallopian) tubes, uterus, and vagina	Ductus (vas) deferens, urethra, and epididymis
External genitals	Clitoris and vulva	Penis and scrotum

*Resembling or similar in some respects (function or appearance) but not in others (origin or development).

this: a sudden, sharp decrease in estrogen and progesterone secretion toward the end of the secretory phase causes the uterine lining to break down and another menstrual period to begin.

SUMMARY OF MALE AND FEMALE REPRODUCTIVE SYSTEMS

The reproductive systems in both sexes are centered around the production of highly specialized reproductive cells, or gametes (sperm and ova), as well as mechanisms that ensure union of these two cells; the fusion of these cells enables transfer of parental genetic information to the next genera-

tion. Table 20-3 compares several analogous components of the reproductive systems in both sexes. You can see that men and women have similar structures to accomplish complementary functions. In addition, the female reproductive system permits development and birth of the offspring— the first subject of the last chapter in this book.

✓ QUICK CHECK

1. Which female structure is made of erectile tissue?
2. What is another term for *menses*?
3. Which hormone reaches a high peak just before ovulation?

Science Application

Reproductive Sciences
William Masters (1915–2001) and Virginia Johnson (b. 1925)

The study of human reproduction, and especially sexual function, has many cultural implications. So it is no wonder that American researchers William Masters and Virginia Johnson encountered a great deal of controversy during their decades of pioneering work in the field of human sex and reproduction. They were the first to study human sexual physiology in the laboratory. William Masters was a gynecologist (physician specializing in women's health) and Virginia Johnson was a psychologist. In 1966, their book *Human Sexual Response* clearly explained the physiology of sex for the first time. Besides making discoveries in the physiology of human sex and reproduction, they also developed therapies for treating sex-related conditions, and they trained therapists from around the world. In addition to the broad fields of biology, medicine, psychology, and the behavioral sciences, the pioneering work of Masters and Johnson paved the way for advances in such diverse and specialized areas of knowledge as comparative neuroscience and social dynamics. Today, there are many opportunities to apply knowledge of reproductive science in a variety of professions.

OUTLINE SUMMARY

COMMON STRUCTURAL AND FUNCTIONAL CHARACTERISTICS BETWEEN THE SEXES

A. Common general structure and function can be identified between the systems in both sexes

B. Systems adapted for development of sperm or ova followed by successful fertilization, development, and birth of offspring

C. Sex hormones in both genders important in development of secondary sexual characteristics and normal reproductive system activity

MALE REPRODUCTIVE SYSTEM

A. Structural plan — organs classified as essential or accessory
  1. Essential organs of reproduction are the gonads (testes), which produce sex cells (sperm or spermatozoa)
  2. Accessory organs of reproduction
    a. Ducts — passageways that carry sperm from testes to exterior
    b. Sex glands — produce protective and nutrient solution for sperm
    c. External genitals

B. Testes — the gonads of men
  1. Structure and location (see Figure 20-2)
    a. Testes in scrotum — lower temperature
    b. Covered by tunica albuginea, which divides testis into lobules containing seminiferous tubules
    c. Interstitial cells produce testosterone
  2. Functions
    a. Spermatogenesis is process of sperm production (see Figure 20-4)
      (1) Sperm precursor cells called *spermatogonia*
      (2) Meiosis produces primary spermatocyte, which forms four spermatids with 23 chromosomes
      (3) Spermatozoa — highly specialized cells
        (a) Head contains genetic material
        (b) Acrosome contains enzymes to assist sperm in penetration of ovum
        (c) Mitochondria in midpiece provide energy for movement

    b. Production of testosterone by interstitial cells
      (1) Testosterone "masculinizes" and promotes development of male accessory organs
      (2) Promotes and maintains development of male accessory organs
      (3) Stimulates protein anabolism and development of muscle strength

C. Reproductive ducts — ducts through which sperm pass after exiting testes until they exit from the body
  1. Epididymis — single, coiled tube about 6 meters in length; lies along the top and behind the testis in the scrotum
    a. Sperm mature and develop the capacity for motility as they pass through epididymis
  2. Ductus (vas) deferens — receives sperm from the epididymis and transports them from scrotal sac through the abdominal cavity
    a. Passes through inguinal canal
    b. Joins duct of seminal vesicle to form the ejaculatory duct

D. Accessory, or supportive, sex glands — semen: mixture of sperm and secretions of accessory sex glands. Averages 3 to 5 mL per ejaculation, with each milliliter containing about 100 million sperm
  1. Seminal vesicles
    a. Pouchlike glands that produce about 60% of seminal fluid volume
    b. Secretion is yellowish, thick, and rich in fructose to provide energy needed by sperm for motility
  2. Prostate gland
    a. Shaped like a doughnut and located below bladder
    b. Urethra passes through the gland
    c. Secretion represents 30% of seminal fluid volume — is thin and milk-colored
    d. Activates sperm and is needed for ongoing sperm motility
  3. Bulbourethral (Cowper's) glands
    a. Resemble peas in size and shape
    b. Secrete mucus-like fluid constituting less than 5% of seminal fluid volume

E. External genitals
  1. Penis and scrotum called *genitalia*
  2. Penis has three columns of erectile tissue — two dorsal columns called *corpora cavernosa* and one ventral column surrounding urethra called *corpus spongiosum*
  3. Glans penis covered by foreskin (prepuce)
  4. Surgical removal of foreskin called *circumcision*

FEMALE REPRODUCTIVE SYSTEM

A. Structural plan — organs classified as essential or accessory
  1. Essential organs are gonads (ovaries), which produce sex cells (ova)
  2. Accessory organs of reproduction
    a. Ducts or modified ducts — including oviducts, uterus, and vagina
    b. Sex glands — including the breasts
    c. External genitals
B. Ovaries
  1. Structure and location
    a. Paired glands weighing about 3 grams each
    b. Resemble large almonds
    c. Attached to ligaments in pelvic cavity on each side of uterus
    d. Microscopic structure (see Figure 20-8)
      (1) Ovarian follicles — contain an oocyte, which is an immature sex cell (about 1 million at birth)
      (2) Primary follicles — about 400,000 at puberty are covered with granulosa cells
      (3) About 350 to 500 mature follicles ovulate during the reproductive lifetime of most women — sometimes called *graafian follicles*
      (4) Secondary follicles have a hollow chamber called the *antrum*
      (5) Corpus luteum forms after ovulation
  2. Functions
    a. Oogenesis — this meiotic cell division produces daughter cells with equal chromosome numbers (23) but unequal cytoplasm. Ovum is large; polar bodies are small and degenerate
    b. Production of estrogen and progesterone
      (1) Granulosa cells surrounding the oocyte in the mature and growing follicles produce estrogen
      (2) Corpus luteum produces progesterone
      (3) Estrogen causes development and maintenance of secondary sex characteristics
      (4) Progesterone stimulates secretory activity of uterine epithelium and assists estrogen in initiating menses
C. Reproductive ducts
  1. Uterine (fallopian) tubes (oviducts)
    a. Extend about 10 cm from uterus into abdominal cavity
    b. Expanded distal end surrounded by fimbriae
    c. Mucosal lining of tube is directly continuous with lining of abdominal cavity
  2. Uterus — composed of body, fundus, and cervix (see Figure 20-9)
    a. Lies in pelvic cavity just behind urinary bladder
    b. Myometrium is muscle layer
    c. Endometrium lost in menstruation
    d. Menopause — end of repetitive menstrual cycles (about 45 to 50 years of age)
  3. Vagina
    a. Distensible tube about 10 cm long
    b. Located between urinary bladder and rectum in the pelvis
    c. Receives penis during sexual intercourse and is birth canal for normal delivery of baby at end of term of pregnancy
D. Accessory, or supportive, sex glands
  1. Bartholin's (greater vestibular) glands
    a. Secrete mucus-like lubricating fluid
    b. Ducts open between labia minora
  2. Breasts (see Figure 20-10)
    a. Located over pectoral muscles of thorax
    b. Size determined by fat quantity more than amount of glandular (milk-secreting) tissue
    c. Lactiferous ducts drain at nipple, which is surrounded by pigmented areola
    d. Lymphatic drainage important in spread of cancer cells to other body areas
E. External genitals (see Figure 20-11)
  1. Vulva includes mons pubis, clitoris, orifice of urethra, Bartholin's gland, vagina, labia minora and majora, and hymen

2. Perineum — area between vaginal opening and anus
   a. Surgical cut during childbirth called *episiotomy*
F. Menstrual cycle — involves many changes in the uterus, ovaries, vagina, and breasts (see Figures 20-12 and 20-13)
   1. Length — about 28 days, varies from month to month among individuals and in the same individual
   2. Phases
      a. Menses — about the first 4 or 5 days of the cycle, varies somewhat; characterized by sloughing of bits of endometrium (uterine lining) with bleeding
      b. Proliferative phase — days between the end of menses and secretory phase; varies in length; the shorter the cycle, the shorter the proliferative phase; the longer the cycle, the longer the proliferative phase; examples: in 28-day cycle, proliferative phase ends on day 13, but in 26-day cycle, it ends on the 11th day and in 32-day cycle, it ends on day 17; characterized by repair of endometrium
      c. Secretory phase — days between ovulation and beginning of next menses; secretory about 14 days before next menses; characterized by further thickening of endometrium and secretion by its glands in preparation for implantation of fertilized ovum; combined actions of the anterior pituitary hormones FSH and LH cause ovulation; sudden sharp decrease in estrogens and progesterone bring on menstruation if pregnancy does not occur.

SUMMARY OF MALE AND FEMALE REPRODUCTIVE SYSTEMS

A. In men and women the organs of the reproductive system are adapted for the specific sequence of functions that permit development of sperm or ova after the successful fertilization and then the normal development and birth of offspring
B. The male organs produce, store, and ultimately introduce mature sperm into the female reproductive tract
C. The female system produces ova, receives the sperm, and permits fertilization followed by fetal development and birth, with lactation afterward
D. Production of sex hormones is required for development of secondary sex characteristics and for normal reproductive functions in both sexes

NEW WORDS

acrosome	ejaculation	meiosis	progesterone
amenorrhea	ejaculatory duct	menarche	prostate gland
antrum	endometrium	menopause	prostatectomy
areola	epididymis	menses	prostatic hypertrophy
Bartholin's (greater vestibular) gland	episiotomy	menstrual cycle	prostatitis
	estrogen	mons pubis	scrotum
benign prostatic hypertrophy (BPH)	external genitalia	myometrium	semen (seminal fluid)
	fimbriae	oocyte	seminal vesicle
bulbourethral gland	gametes	oogenesis	seminiferous tubule
circumcision	gonad	oophorectomy	spermatid
clitoris	gonadotropin releasing hormone (GnRH)	ova	spermatogenesis
corpora cavernosa		ovulation	spermatogonia
corpus luteum	graafian follicle	pelvic inflammatory disease (PID)	spermatozoa (sperm)
corpus spongiosum	hymen		testes
cryptorchidism	hysterectomy	perineum	tunica albuginea
ductus deferens (also known as *vas deferens*)	interstitial cell	prepuce (also called *foreskin*)	vagina
	labia (majora/minora)		vestibule
ectopic pregnancy	lactiferous duct	primary spermatocyte	zygote

REVIEW QUESTIONS

1. Describe the structure and location of the testes.
2. Describe the structure of the spermatozoa.
3. List the functions of testosterone.
4. List and briefly describe the reproductive ducts of the male reproductive system.
5. List and briefly describe the glands of the male reproductive system. What does each gland contribute to seminal fluid?
6. Describe the structure and location of the ovaries.
7. Explain the development of an ovarian follicle from the primary follicle to the corpus luteum.
8. List the functions of estrogen.
9. List the functions of progesterone.
10. Describe the structure of the uterine tubes.
11. Describe the structure of the uterus.
12. Describe the structure of the vagina.
13. Describe the structure of the breasts.
14. Explain what occurs during the proliferative phase of the reproductive cycle.
15. Explain what occurs during the secretory phase of the reproductive cycle.
16. Name the four hormones involved in the regulation of the reproductive cycle. Where is each produced, and what is the function of each?

CRITICAL THINKING

17. Differentiate between spermatogenesis and oogenesis. How do these differences relate to the role of the male and female in reproduction?
18. Why are the testes located outside the body cavity in the scrotum?
19. What is unique about the chromosome content of the gametes? Why is this important?

CHAPTER TEST

1. The essential organs of the male reproductive system are the _____.
2. The pouchlike sac where the male gonads are located is called the _____.
3. The membrane that covers the testicle and also divides the interior into lobes is called the _____.
4. The _____ is a long duct in the testicle where sperm develop.
5. The _____ are the cells in the testes that secrete testosterone.
6. The primary spermatocyte develops from a cell called the _____.
7. The primary spermatocyte forms sperm cells by undergoing a specialized type of cell division called _____.
8. The sperm cell contains an _____, which contains an enzyme that can digest the covering of the ovum.
9. The _____ is a reproductive duct that consists of a tightly coiled tube that lies along the top and behind the testes.
10. The _____ is a reproductive duct that permits the sperm to move out of the scrotum upward into the abdominal cavity.
11. The _____ is a gland that secretes a thin, milk-colored fluid that makes up about 20% of the seminal fluid.
12. The _____ are a pair of glands that produce a thick, yellowish, fructose-rich fluid that makes up about 60% of the seminal fluid.

Continued on following page.

CHAPTER TEST—cont'd

13. The penis is composed of three columns of erectile tissue: one is called the corpus spongiosum, and the other two are called the _____.

14. The essential organs of the female reproductive system are the _____.

15. Another name for a mature ovarian follicle is a _____ follicle.

16. The process that produces the female gamete is called _____.

17. Meiosis in the female produces one large ovum and three small daughter cells called _____, which degenerate.

18. The _____ are the reproductive tubes connecting the ovary and the uterus.

19. The muscle layer of the uterus is called the _____.

20. The uterus is composed of two parts: the upper part, called the body, and the narrow lower part, called the _____.

21. The innermost layer of the uterus, which is shed during menstruation, is called the _____.

22. The _____ is the part of the female reproductive system that opens to the exterior.

23. The _____ glands are glands that secrete a mucus-like lubricating fluid into the vestibule.

24. The milk-secreting glandular cells of the breast are arranged in grapelike structures called _____. These drain into _____ ducts that converge toward the nipple.

CHAPTER TEST—cont'd

Match each phrase in Column B with the correct corresponding term in Column A.

COLUMN A

25. _____ FSH
26. _____ menstruation
27. _____ corpus luteum
28. _____ estrogen
29. _____ secretory phase
30. _____ progesterone
31. _____ LH
32. _____ proliferative phase
33. _____ ovulation

COLUMN B

a. what the egg follicle becomes after ovulation
b. ovarian hormone that reaches its highest concentration in the proliferative phase
c. caused by the rapid drop of blood levels of estrogen and progesterone
d. phase of the reproductive cycle that begins after ovulation
e. ovarian hormone that reaches its highest concentration during the secretory phase
f. term used to describe the egg being released from the ovary
g. the uterine wall begins to thicken during this phase of the reproductive cycle
h. pituitary hormone that stimulates the formation of an egg follicle
i. pituitary hormone that can be called the ovulating hormone

OBJECTIVES

AFTER YOU HAVE COMPLETED THIS CHAPTER, YOU SHOULD BE ABLE TO:

1. Discuss the concept of development as a biological process characterized by continuous modification and change.
2. Discuss the major developmental changes characteristic of the prenatal stage of life from fertilization to birth.
3. Discuss the three stages of labor that characterize a normal vaginal birth.
4. Identify the three primary germ layers and several derivatives in the adult body that develop from each layer.
5. List and discuss the major developmental changes characteristic of the four postnatal periods of life.
6. Discuss the effects of aging on the major body organ systems.

Growth and Development 21

Many of your fondest and most vivid memories are probably associated with your birthdays. The day of birth is an important milestone of life. Most people continue to remember their birthday in some special way each year; birthdays serve as pleasant and convenient reference points to mark periods of transition or change in our lives. The actual day of birth marks the end of one phase of life called the **prenatal period** and the beginning of a second called the **postnatal period.** The prenatal period begins at conception and ends at birth; the postnatal period begins at birth and continues until death. Although important periods in our lives such as childhood and adolescence are often remembered as a series of individual and isolated events, they are in reality part of an ongoing and continuous process. In reviewing the many changes that occur during the cycle of life from conception to death, it is often convenient to isolate certain periods such as infancy or adulthood for study. It is important to remember, however, that life is not a series of stop-and-start events or individual and isolated periods of time. Instead, it is a biological process that is characterized by continuous modification and change.

This chapter discusses some of the events and changes that occur in the development of a human from conception to death. Study of development during the prenatal period is followed by a discussion of the birth process and a review of changes that occur during infancy and adulthood. Finally, some important changes that occur in the individual organ systems of the body as a result of aging are discussed.

PRENATAL PERIOD

The *prenatal stage of development* begins at the time of conception, or **fertilization** (that is, at the moment the female ovum and the male sperm cells unite) (Figure 21-1). The period of prenatal development continues until the birth of the child about

Cytoplasm   Ovum   Nucleus   Sperm cell

FIGURE 21-1 **Fertilization.** Fertilization is a specific biological event. It occurs when the male and female sex cells fuse. After union between a sperm cell and the ovum has occurred, the cycle of life begins. The scanning electron micrograph shows spermatozoa attaching themselves to the surface of an ovum. Only one will penetrate and fertilize the ovum.

39 weeks later. The science of the development of the offspring before birth is called **embryology** (em-bree-OL-oh-jee). It is a story of biological marvels, describing the means by which a new human life is started and the steps by which a single microscopic cell is transformed into a complex human being.

Fertilization to Implantation

After ovulation the discharged ovum first enters the abdominal cavity and then finds its way into a uterine (fallopian) tube. Sperm cells "swim" up the uterine tubes toward the ovum. Look at the relationship of the ovary, the two uterine tubes,

and the uterus in Figure 21-2. Recall from Chapter 20 that each uterine tube extends outward from the uterus for about 10 centimeters (cm). It then ends in the abdominal cavity near the ovary, as you can see in Figure 21-2, in an opening surrounded by fringelike processes, the *fimbriae*.

Sperm cells that are deposited in the vagina must enter and "swim" through the uterus and through the uterine tube to meet the ovum. Fertilization most often occurs in the outer one third of the oviduct, as shown in Figure 21-2. The fertilized ovum, or **zygote** (ZYE-goht), is genetically complete; it represents a new single-celled offspring. Time and nourishment are all that is needed for expression of characteristics such as sex, body build, and skin color that were determined at the time of fertilization. As you can see in the figure, the zygote immediately begins mitotic division, and in about 3 days a solid mass of cells called a **morula** (MOR-yoo-lah) is formed (see Figure 21-2). The cells of the morula continue to divide, and by the time the developing embryo reaches the uterus, it is a hollow ball of cells called a **blastocyst** (BLAS-toh-sist).

During the 10 days from the time of fertilization to the time when the blastocyst completes **implantation** in the uterine lining, few nutrients from the mother are available. The rapid cell division taking place up to the blastocyst stage occurs with no significant increase in total mass compared with the zygote (Figure 21-3). One of the specializations of the ovum is its incredible store of nutrients that help support this embryonic development until implantation has occurred.

Note in Figure 21-4 that the blastocyst consists of an outer layer of cells and an inner cell mass. As the blastocyst develops, it forms a structure with two cavities, the **yolk sac** and **amniotic** (am-nee-OT-ik) **cavity.** The yolk sac is most important in animals, such as birds, that depend heavily on yolk as the sole source of nutrients for the developing embryo. In these animals the yolk sac digests the yolk and provides the resulting nutrients to the embryo. Because uterine fluids provide nutrients to the developing embryo in humans until the placenta develops, the function of the yolk sac is not a nutritive one. Instead, it has other functions, including production of blood cells.

The amniotic cavity becomes a fluid-filled, shock-absorbing sac, sometimes called the *bag of waters*, in which the embryo floats during development. The **chorion** (KOH-ree-on), shown in

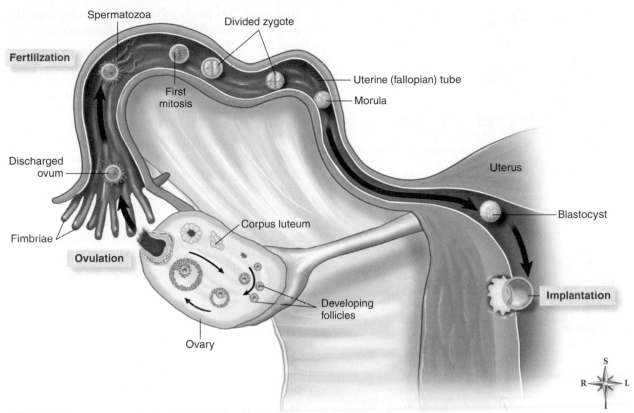

FIGURE 21-2 **Fertilization and implantation.** At ovulation, an ovum is released from the ovary and begins its journey through the uterine tube. While in the tube, the ovum is fertilized by a sperm to form the single-celled zygote. After a few days of rapid mitotic division, a ball of cells called a *morula* is formed. After the morula develops into a hollow ball called a *blastocyst*, implantation occurs.

FIGURE 21-3 **Early stages of human development. A,** Fertilized ovum or zygote. **B** to **D,** Early cell divisions produce more and more cells. The solid mass of cells shown in **D** forms the morula—an early stage in embryonic development.

Figures 21-4 and 21-5, develops into an important fetal membrane in the **placenta** (plah-SEN-tah). The **chorionic villi,** shown in Figure 21-5, connect the blood vessels of the chorion to the rest of the placenta. The placenta (see Figure 21-5) anchors the developing fetus to the uterus and pro-vides a "bridge" for the exchange of nutrients and waste products between mother and baby.

The *placenta* is a unique structure that has a temporary but very important series of functions during pregnancy. It is composed of tissues from mother and child and functions not only as a (see Figure 21-5).

structural "anchor" and nutritive bridge but also as an excretory, respiratory, and endocrine organ (see Figure 21-5).

Placental tissue normally separates the maternal blood, which fills the lacunae of the placenta, from the fetal blood so that no intermixing occurs. The very thin layer of placental tissue that separates maternal and fetal blood also serves as an effective "barrier" that can protect the developing baby from many harmful substances that may enter the mother's bloodstream. Unfortunately, toxic substances, such as alcohol and some infectious organisms, may nonetheless penetrate this protective placental barrier and injure the developing baby. The virus responsible for German measles (rubella), for example, can easily pass through the placenta and cause tragic developmental defects in the fetus.

 To learn more about fertilization and implantation, go to AnimationDirect on your CD-ROM.

Periods of Development

The length of pregnancy (about 39 weeks)—called the *gestation period*—is divided into three 3-month segments called *trimesters*. A number of terms are

FIGURE 21-4 **Implantation and early development.** The hollow blastocyst implants itself in the uterine lining about 10 days after ovulation. Until the placenta is functional, nutrients are obtained by diffusion from uterine fluids. Notice the developing chorion and how the blastocyst eventually forms a yolk sac and amniotic cavity.

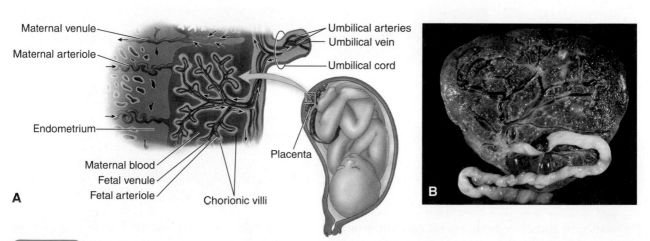

FIGURE 21-5 **The placenta.** Relationship of uterus, developing infant, and placenta. The close placement of the fetal blood supply and the maternal blood in the lacunae of the placenta permits diffusion of nutrients and other substances. It also forms a thin barrier to prevent diffusion of most harmful substances. No mixing of fetal and maternal blood occurs. **A,** Diagram showing a cross-section of the placental structure. **B,** Photograph of a normal, full-term placenta (fetal side) showing the branching of the placental blood vessels.

Research, Issues, & Trends

In Vitro Fertilization

The Latin term *in vitro* means, literally, "within a glass." In the case of in vitro fertilization, it refers to the glass laboratory dish where an ovum and sperm are mixed and where fertilization occurs.

In the classic technique, the ovum is obtained from the mother by first inserting a fiberoptic viewing instrument called a **laparoscope** through a very small incision in the woman's abdomen. After it is in the abdominal cavity, the device allows the physician to view the ovary and then puncture and "suck up" an ovum from a mature follicle. Over the years refinements to this technique have been made, and less invasive procedures are currently being used. After fertilization in a laboratory dish and about 2.5 days' growth in a temperature-controlled environment, the developing zygote, which by then has reached the 8- or 16-cell stage, is returned by the physician to the mother's uterus. If implantation is successful, growth will continue and the subsequent pregnancy will progress. In the most successful fertility clinics in the United States, a normal term birth will occur in about 30% of in vitro fertilization attempts.

FIGURE 21-6   Human embryos and fetuses. **A,** At 35 days. **B,** At 49 days. **C,** At the end of the first trimester. **D,** At 4 months.

used to describe development during these periods, known as the first, second, and third trimesters of pregnancy.

During the first trimester or 3 months of pregnancy, many terms are used. *Zygote* describes the ovum just after fertilization by a sperm cell. After about 3 days of constant cell division, the solid mass of cells, identified earlier as the *morula*, enters the uterus. Continued development transforms the morula into the hollow *blastocyst*, which then implants into the uterine wall.

The **embryonic phase** of development extends from the third week after fertilization until the end of week 8 of **gestation**. During this period in the first trimester, the term **embryo** is used to describe the developing offspring. The period of development extending from week 9 to week 39 is termed the **fetal phase**. During this period, the term *embryo* is replaced by **fetus**.

By day 35 of gestation (Figure 21-6, *A*), the heart is beating and, although the embryo is only 8 millimeters (mm) (about ⅜ inch) long, the eyes and *limb buds*, which ultimately form the arms and legs, are clearly visible. Figure 21-6, *C*, shows the stage of development of the fetus at the end of the first trimester of gestation. Body size is about 7 to 8 cm

Research, Issues, & Trends

How Long Does Pregnancy Last?

This seems like a silly question to most of us; the answer is 9 months, isn't it? Actually, the length of gestation (the amount of time one is pregnant) is defined in different ways in different situations and can vary from one pregnancy to another. The average gestation in humans is 266 days, starting at the day of conception. But physicians instead usually count from the beginning of the woman's last menstrual period, for an average of 280 days. But these are only averages. What is normal in one case can be different from what is normal in another case. In practice, any pregnancy of less than 37 weeks (259 days) is said to be premature, and any lasting more than 42 weeks (294 days) is said to be postmature. So, as with many statistics regarding human function, what is "normal" can be spoken of only in generalities and averages.

(3.2 inches) long. The facial features of the fetus are apparent, the limbs are complete, and gender can be identified. By month 4 (see Figure 21-6, *D*) all organ systems are complete and in place.

Formation of the Primary Germ Layers

At the very beginning of the embryonic stage, all of the cells are **stem cells.** Stem cells are unspecialized cells that reproduce to form specific lines of specialized cells. At this stage, they have their highest "stemness" or potency—that is, they are capable of producing many different kinds of cells in the body. Some stem cells, such as the hematopoietic stem cells found in adult bone marrow, remain throughout development and maturity.

Adult stem cells are found in the skin, many glands, muscles, nerve tissue, bone, and the gastrointestinal (GI) tract. Adult stem cells replace the specialized cells in a tissue and thus ensure stable, functional populations of the cell types needed for survival.

Early in the first trimester of pregnancy, three layers of stem cells develop that embryologists call the **primary germ layers** (Table 21-1). Each layer gives rise to definite structures such as the skin, nervous tissue, muscles, or digestive organs. Table 21-1 lists a number of structures derived from each primary germ layer called, respectively, **endoderm** (EN-doh-derm), or inside layer; **ectoderm** (EK-toh-derm), or outside layer; and **mesoderm** (MEZ-oh-derm), or middle layer.

Science Application

Embryology
Rita Levi-Montalcini (b. 1909)

Rita Levi-Montalcini had just finished a medical degree in her native Italy when in 1938 the Fascist government under Mussolini barred all "non-Aryans" from working in academic and professional careers. Being Jewish, Levi-Montalcini was forced to move to Belgium to work. But when Belgium was about to be invaded by the Nazis, she decided to return home to Italy and work in secret. Her home laboratory was very crude, but in it she made some important discoveries about how the nervous system develops during embryonic development. After World War II, she was invited to Washington University in St. Louis to work. There, she discovered the existence of *nerve growth factor (NGF)*, for which she later won the 1986 Nobel Prize. Her discovery of a chemical that regulates the growth of new nerves during early brain development has led to many different paths of investigation. For example, by learning more about growth regulators, we now know more about how the nervous system develops, as well as other tissues, organs, and systems of the body.

Today, many professions make use of the discoveries of embryology—the study of early development. Not only are these discoveries important for health professionals such as obstetricians, obstetric nurses, and others involved in prenatal health care, they are also important in understanding adult medicine more fully. In fact, even gerontology (study of aging) and geriatrics (treatment of the aged) have benefited from embryological research. How? By providing insights on how tissue development is regulated in the embryo, scientists can better understand how to possibly stimulate damaged tissue in older adults to repair or regenerate themselves.

TABLE 21-1

Primary Germ Layer Derivatives

ECTODERM	MESODERM	ENDODERM
Epidermis of skin	Dermis of skin	Lining of gastrointestinal tract
Tooth enamel	Circulatory system	Lining of lungs
Lens and cornea of eye	Many glands	Lining of hepatic and pancreatic ducts
Outer ear	Kidneys	Kidney ducts and bladder
Nasal cavity	Gonads	Anterior pituitary gland (adenohypophysis)
Facial bones	Muscle	Thymus gland
Skeletal muscles in head	Bones (except facial)	Thyroid gland
Brain and spinal cord		Parathyroid gland
Sensory neurons		Tonsils
		Adrenal medulla

Histogenesis and Organogenesis

The process of how the primary germ layers develop into many different kinds of tissues is called **histogenesis** (his-toh-JEN-eh-sis). The way in which those tissues arrange themselves into organs is called **organogenesis** (or-gah-no-JEN-eh-sis). The fascinating story of histogenesis and organogenesis in human development is long and complicated; its telling belongs to the science of *embryology*. But for the beginning student of anatomy and physiology, it seems sufficient to appreciate that human development begins when two sex cells unite to form a single-celled zygote and that the offspring's body evolves by a series of processes that consist of cell differentiation, multiplication, growth, and rearrangement, all of which

take place in a definite, orderly sequence (Figure 21-7). Development of structure and function go hand in hand, and from 4 months of gestation, when every organ system is complete and in place, until term (about 280 days), fetal development is mainly a matter of growth. Figure 21-8, *A*, shows the normal intrauterine placement of a fetus just before birth in a full-term pregnancy.

Birth Defects

Developmental problems present at birth are often called **birth defects.** Such abnormalities may be structural or functional, perhaps even involving behavior and personality. Birth defects may be caused by genetic factors such as abnormal genes or inheritance of an abnormal number of

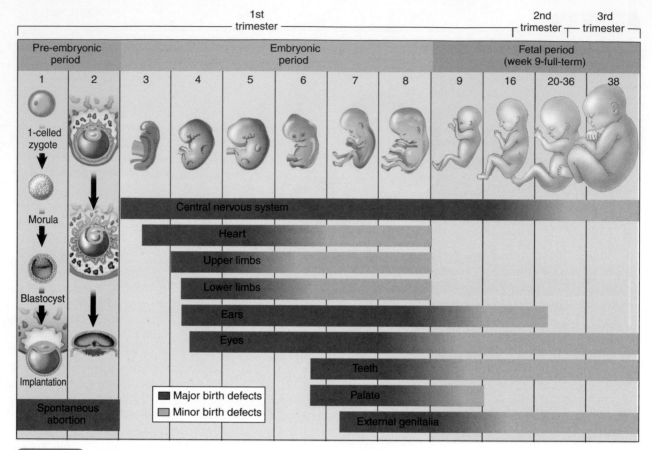

FIGURE 21-7 **Critical periods of neonatal development.** The red areas show when teratogens are most likely to cause major birth defects, and the yellow areas show when minor defects are more likely to arise. Numbers refer to weeks of gestation.

chromosomes. Birth defects also may be caused by exposure to environmental factors called **teratogens** (TAYR-ah-toh-jenz). Teratogens include radiation (for example, x rays), chemicals (for example, drugs, cigarettes, or alcohol), and infections in the mother (for example, herpes or rubella). Some teratogens are also mutagens because they do their damage by changing the genetic code in cells of the developing embryo. Nutritional deficiencies during pregnancy also can lead to birth defects.

As Figure 21-7 shows, the period during the first trimester when the tissues are beginning to differentiate and the organs are just starting to develop is the time that teratogens are most likely to cause damage. In fact, teratogens can cause spontaneous abortion (miscarriage) if significant damage occurs during the pre-embryonic stage.

QUICK CHECK

1. What is the postnatal period? The prenatal period?
2. What is a zygote? How is it different from a morula or blastocyst?
3. What are germ layers?
4. What is meant by the term *organogenesis*?

BIRTH, OR PARTURITION

The process of birth, or **parturition** (pahr-too-RI-shun), is the point of transition between the prenatal and postnatal periods of life. As pregnancy draws to a close, the uterus becomes "irritable" and, ultimately, muscular contractions begin and cause the cervix to dilate or open, thus permitting the fetus to move from the uterus through the vagina, or "birth canal," to the exterior. The process

1 The relation of the fetus to the mother.

Placenta
Pubic symphysis
Urinary bladder
Urethra
Vagina
Cervix
Rectum

2 The fetus moves into the opening of the birth canal, and the cervix begins to dilate.

Placenta
Umbilical cord
Amniotic sac
Vagina
Cervix

3 Dilation of the cervix is complete. Rupture in amniotic sac widens.

Ruptured amniotic sac

4 The fetus is expelled from the uterus.

Placenta

5 The placenta is expelled.

Uterus
Placenta (maternal side)
Placenta (fetal side)
Umbilical cord

A
S   I
P

FIGURE 21-8   Parturition.

normally begins with the fetus taking a head-down position against the cervix (see Figure 21-8, *A*). When contractions occur, the amniotic sac, or "bag of waters," ruptures, and labor begins.

Stages of Labor

Labor is the process that results in the birth of a baby. It has three stages (see Figure 21-8, *B* to *E*):

1. Stage 1—period from onset of uterine contractions until dilation of the cervix is complete
2. Stage 2—period from the time of maximal cervical dilation until the baby exits through the vagina
3. Stage 3—process of expulsion of the placenta through the vagina

The time required for normal vaginal birth varies widely and may be influenced by many variables, including whether the woman has previously had a child. In most cases, stage 1 of labor lasts from 6 to 24 hours, and stage 2 lasts from a few minutes to an hour. Delivery of the placenta (stage 3) normally occurs within 15 minutes after the birth of the baby.

 To learn more about the three stages of birth, go to AnimationDirect on your CD-ROM.

QUICK CHECK

1. What is meant by the term *parturition?*
2. What are the three stages of labor?

POSTNATAL PERIOD

The **postnatal period** begins at birth and lasts until death. Although it is often divided into major periods for study, we need to understand and appreciate that growth and development are continuous processes that occur throughout the life cycle. Gradual changes in the physical appearance of the body as a whole and in the relative proportions of the head, trunk, and limbs are quite noticeable between birth and adolescence. Note in Figure 21-9 the obvious changes in the size of bones and in the proportionate sizes between different bones and body areas. The head, for example, becomes proportionately smaller. Whereas the infant head is approximately one fourth of the total height of the body, the adult head is only about one eighth of the total height. The facial bones also show several changes between infancy and adulthood. In an infant the face is one eighth of the skull surface, but in an adult the face is half of the skull surface. Another change in proportion involves the trunk and lower extremities. The legs become

---

 Research, Issues, & Trends

Freezing Umbilical Cord Blood

The concept of development of blood cells from red bone marrow, a process called **hematopoiesis,** was introduced in Chapter 11. Ultimately, the presence of "stem cells" is required for bone marrow to produce blood cells. The fact that umbilical cord blood is rich in these stem cells has great clinical significance.

In the past, if the stem cells in the bone marrow of a child were destroyed as a result of leukemia or by chemotherapy, death would result unless a bone marrow transplant was possible. Infusion of stored umbilical cord blood obtained from the child at the time of birth is an attractive alternative. The blood is rich in stem cells and can be obtained without risk; this procedure is much more cost-effective than a bone marrow transplant.

Removing and freezing umbilical cord blood at the time of birth may become a type of biological insurance against some types of leukemia that may affect a child later in life. Cord blood is readily available at birth and is a better source of stem cells than is bone marrow.

When the umbilical cord is cut after birth, the blood that remains in the cord is simply drained into a sterile bag (*see* photo), frozen, and then stored in liquid nitrogen in one of about a dozen cord-blood centers in the United States.

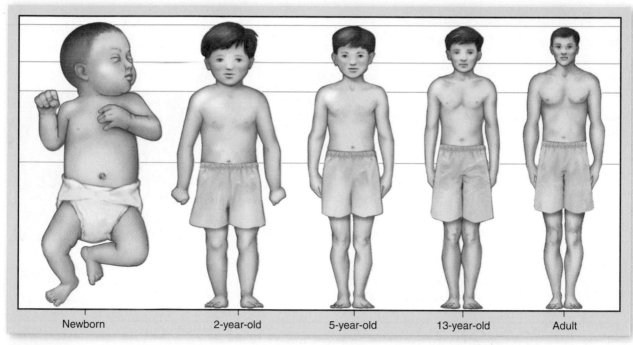

| Newborn | 2-year-old | 5-year-old | 13-year-old | Adult |

FIGURE 21-9 Changes in the proportions of body parts from birth to maturity. Note the dramatic differences in head proportion.

proportionately longer and the trunk proportionately shorter. In addition, the thoracic and abdominal contours change, roughly speaking, from round to elliptical.

Such changes are good examples of the ever-changing and ongoing nature of growth and development. It is unfortunate that many of the changes that occur in the later years of life do not result in increased function. These degenerative changes are certainly important, however, and are discussed later in this chapter. The following are

the most common postnatal periods: (1) infancy, (2) childhood, (3) adolescence and adulthood, and (4) older adulthood.

Infancy

The period of **infancy** begins abruptly at birth and lasts about 18 months. The first 4 weeks of infancy are often referred to as the **neonatal** (nee-oh-NAY-tal) **period** (Figure 21-10). The baby is referred to as a **neonate.** Dramatic changes occur at a rapid rate

 Health and Well-Being

Quickening

Pregnant women usually notice fetal movement for the first time between weeks 16 and 18 of pregnancy. The term **quickening** has been used for generations to describe these first recognizable movements of the fetus. From an occasional "kick" during months 4 and 5 of pregnancy, the frequency of fetal movements steadily increases as gestation progresses. The frequency of fetal movements is an excellent indicator of the unborn baby's health.

Recent studies have shown that simply by recording the number of fetal movements each day after week 28 of preg-

nancy, a woman can provide her physician with extremely useful information about the health of her unborn child. Ten or more movements during a daily measurement period are considered normal.

Educating pregnant women about fetal movements and how to monitor their frequency is but one example of expanded interest in prenatal home care. Assisting pregnant women with making informed judgments about nutrition, exercise, lifestyle adjustments, and birthing options before they enter the hospital for delivery of their babies is an important and growing part of home health care services.

Antenatal Diagnosis and Treatment

Advances in **antenatal** (from the Latin *ante*, "before," *natus*, "birth") **medicine** now permit extensive diagnosis and treatment of disease in the fetus much like that in any other patient. This new dimension in medicine began with techniques by which Rh-positive babies could be given transfusions before birth.

Current procedures using images provided by ultrasound equipment (Figures A and B) allow physicians to prepare for and perform, before the birth of a baby, corrective surgical procedures such as bladder repair. These procedures also allow physicians to monitor the progress of other types of treatment on a developing fetus. Figure *A* shows placement of the ultrasound transducer on the abdominal wall. The resulting image (see Figure *B*), called an **ultrasonogram**, shows a 21-week embryo.

FIGURE 21-10 The neonate infant. The umbilical cord has been cut.

during this short but critical period. **Neonatology** (nee-oh-nay-TOL-oh-jee) is the medical and nursing specialty concerned with the diagnosis and treatment of disorders of the newborn. Advances in this area have resulted in dramatically reduced infant mortality.

Many of the changes that occur in the cardiovascular and respiratory systems at birth are necessary for survival. Whereas the fetus totally depends on the mother for life support, the newborn infant must become totally self-supporting in terms of blood circulation and respiration immediately after birth. A baby's first breath is deep and forceful. The stimulus to breathe results primarily from the increasing amounts of carbon dioxide (CO_2) that accumulate in the blood after the umbilical cord is cut following delivery.

Many developmental changes occur between the end of the neonatal period and 18 months of age. Birth weight doubles during the first 4 months and then triples by 1 year. The baby also increases in length by 50% by the 12th month. The "baby fat" that accumulated under the skin during the first year begins to decrease, and the plump infant becomes leaner.

Early in infancy the baby has only one spinal curvature (Figure 21-11, *A*). The lumbar curvature appears between 12 and 18 months, and the once-helpless infant becomes a toddler who can stand (see Figure 21-11, *B*). One of the most striking changes to occur during infancy is the rapid development of the nervous and muscular systems. This permits the infant to follow a moving object with the eyes (2 months); lift the head and raise the chest (3 months); sit when well supported (4 months); crawl (10 months); stand alone (12 months); and run, although a bit stiffly (18 months).

Childhood

Childhood extends from the end of infancy to sexual maturity or puberty—12 to 14 years in girls and 14 to 16 years in boys. Overall, growth during early childhood continues at a rather rapid pace,

FIGURE 21-11 Spinal curvatures. **A,** Normal rounded curvature of the vertebral column in an infant. **B,** Normal vertebral curvature in a toddler. The dark shadow emphasizes the distinct lumbar curvature that develops with the ability to walk. (See Figure 6-12 on p. 120 to compare to the adult curvatures.)

Research, Issues, & Trends

Fetal Alcohol Syndrome

Consumption of alcohol by a woman during her pregnancy can have tragic effects on a developing fetus. Educational efforts to inform pregnant women about the dangers of alcohol use are now receiving national attention. Even very limited consumption of alcohol during pregnancy poses significant hazards to the developing baby because alcohol can easily cross the placental barrier and enter the fetal bloodstream.

When alcohol enters the fetal blood, the potential result, called **fetal alcohol syndrome (FAS),** can cause tragic congenital abnormalities such as "small head," or **microcephaly** (my-kroh-SEF-ah-lee), low birth weight, developmental disabilities such as mental retardation, and even fetal death.

but month-to-month gains become less consistent. By the age of 6 the child appears more like a pre-adolescent than an infant or toddler. The child becomes less chubby, the potbelly becomes flatter, and the face loses its babyish look. The nervous and muscular systems continue to develop rapidly during the middle years of childhood; by 10 years of age, the child has developed numerous motor and coordination skills.

The *deciduous teeth,* which began to appear at about 6 months of age, are lost during childhood, beginning at about 6 years of age. The permanent teeth, with the possible exception of the third molars (or wisdom teeth), all erupt by age 14.

Adolescence and Adulthood

The average age range of **adolescence** varies, but generally the teenage years (13 to 19) are called the adolescent years. This period is marked by rapid and intense physical growth, which ultimately results in sexual maturity. Many of the developmental changes that occur during this period are controlled by the secretion of sex hormones and are classified as **secondary sex characteristics.** Breast development is often the first sign of approaching puberty in girls, beginning about age 10. Most girls begin to menstruate at 12 to 13 years of age, which is about 3 years earlier than a century ago. In boys the first sign of puberty is often enlargement of the testicles, which begins between 10 and 13 years of age. Both sexes show a spurt in height during adolescence (Figure 21-12). In girls the spurt in height begins between the ages of 10 and 12 and is nearly complete by 14 or 15 years. In boys the period of rapid growth begins between 12 and 13 and is generally complete by 16.

Many developmental changes that began early in childhood are not completed until the early or middle years of **adulthood.** Examples include the

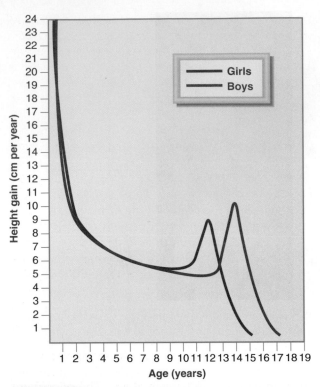

FIGURE 21-12 **Growth in height.** The figure shows typical patterns of gain in height to adulthood for girls and boys. Notice the rapid gain in height during the first few years, a period of slower growth, then another burst of growth during adolescence—finally ending at the beginning of adulthood.

FIGURE 21-13 **Some biological changes associated with maturity and aging.** *Insets* show proportion of remaining function in the organs of a person in late adulthood compared with that of a 20-year-old. These are average numbers, so many individuals experience far different situations.

maturation of bone, resulting in the full closure of the growth plates, and changes in the size and placement of other body components such as the sinuses. Many body traits do not become apparent for years after birth. Normal balding patterns, for example, are determined at the time of fertilization by heredity but do not appear until maturity. As a general rule, adulthood is characterized by maintenance of existing body tissues. With the passage of years the ongoing effort of maintenance and repair of body tissues becomes more and more difficult. As a result, degeneration begins. It is the process of aging, and it culminates in death.

Older Adulthood

Most body systems are in peak condition and function at a high level of efficiency during the early years of adulthood. As a person grows older, a gradual but certain decline takes place in the functioning of every major organ system in the

body. The study of aging is called **gerontology.** The remainder of this chapter deals with a number of the more common degenerative changes that frequently characterize **senescence** (seh-NES-ens), or **older adulthood.** Many of the biological changes associated with advancing age are shown in Figure 21-13. The illustration highlights the proportion of remaining function in a number of organs in older adulthood when compared with a 20-year-old person.

✓ **QUICK CHECK**
1. How do the proportions of the human body change during postnatal development?
2. What is the neonatal period of development? Senescence?
3. During which phase of development do the deciduous teeth appear?
4. What biological changes happen during puberty?

EFFECTS OF AGING

Aging is an imperfectly understood process. Although advanced age brings with it the higher risk of many disorders, it also brings some biological advantages. We explore just a few of the changes associated with aging here.

Integumentary System (Skin)

With advancing age the skin becomes dry, thin, and inelastic. It "sags" on the body because of increased wrinkling and skinfolds. Pigmentation changes and the thinning or loss of hair are also common problems associated with the aging process.

Skeletal System

In older adulthood, bones undergo changes in texture, degree of calcification, and shape. Instead of clean-cut margins, older bones develop indistinct and shaggy-appearing margins with spurs—a process called *lipping*. This type of degenerative change restricts movement because of the piling up of bone tissue around the joints. With advancing age, changes in calcification may result in reduction of bone size and in bones that are porous and subject to fracture. The lower cervical and thoracic vertebrae are the sites of frequent fractures. The result is curvature of the spine and the shortened stature so typical of late adulthood. Degenerative joint diseases such as **osteoarthritis** (OS-tee-oh-ar-THRY-tis) are also common in elderly adults.

However, many of the aging effects seen in the skeleton can be lessened by physical activity—especially if exercise starts earlier in life. Loss of bone mass and reduced mobility can be avoided or reduced by an ongoing program of physical activity coupled with good nutrition.

Central Nervous System

Advancing age brings with it the risk of *dementia* (de-MEN-sha)—the loss of memory and other functions of conscious thinking—and other degenerative conditions that affect the central nervous system. For most of us, however, our memories remain mostly intact and have helped us develop a mature ability to reason and make decisions. Although some elderly individuals suffer

from depression, especially when they become ill or separated from family, the average elderly person is happier than during early and middle adulthood.

Special Senses

The sense organs, as a group, all show a gradual decline in performance and capacity as a person ages. Most people are farsighted by age 65 because eye lenses become hardened and lose elasticity; the lenses cannot become curved to accommodate for near vision. This hardening of the lens is called **presbyopia** (pres-bee-OH-pee-ah), which means "old eye." Many individuals first notice the change at about 40 or 45 years of age, when it becomes difficult to do close-up work or read without holding printed material at arm's length. This explains the increased need, with advancing age, for bifocals (glasses that incorporate two lenses) to assist the eye in accommodating for near and distant vision. Loss of transparency of the lens or its covering capsule is another common age-related eye change. If the lens actually becomes cloudy and significantly impairs vision, it is called a **cataract** (KAT-ah-rakt) and must be removed surgically. The incidence of **glaucoma** (glaw-KOH-mah), the most serious age-related eye disorder, increases with age. Glaucoma causes an increase in the pressure within the eyeball and, unless treated, often results in blindness. The risk of retinal degeneration or detachment also increases with age.

In many elderly people a very significant loss of hair cells in the organ of Corti (inner ear) causes a serious decline in the ability to hear certain frequencies. In addition, the eardrum and attached ossicles become more fixed and less able to transmit mechanical sound waves. Some degree of hearing impairment is universally present in the older adult.

The senses of smell and taste are also decreased. The resulting loss of appetite may be caused partly by the replacement of taste buds with connective tissue cells. Only about 40% of the taste buds present at age 30 remain in an individual at age 75.

Cardiovascular System

Degenerative heart and blood vessel disease is one of the most common and serious effects of aging. Fatty deposits build up in blood vessel walls and narrow the passageway for the movement of blood, much as the build-up of scale in a water pipe decreases flow and pressure. The resulting condition, called **atherosclerosis** (ath-er-oh-skleh-ROH-sis), often leads to eventual blockage of the coronary arteries and a "heart attack" (myocardial infarction [MI]). If fatty accumulations or other substances in blood vessels calcify, actual hardening of the arteries, or **arteriosclerosis** (ar-tee-ree-oh-skleh-ROH-sis), occurs. Rupture of a hardened vessel in the brain (stroke or cerebrovascular accident [CVA]) is a frequent cause of serious disability or death in the older adult. **Hypertension (HTN),** or high blood pressure, is also more common.

Respiratory System

In older adulthood the costal cartilages that connect the ribs to the sternum become hardened or calcified. This makes it difficult for the rib cage to expand and contract as it normally does during inspiration and expiration. In time the ribs gradually become "fixed" to the sternum, and chest movements become difficult. When this occurs, the rib cage remains in a more expanded position, respiratory efficiency decreases, and a condition called "barrel chest" results. With advancing years a generalized atrophy or wasting of muscle tissue takes place as the contractile muscle cells are replaced by connective tissue. This loss of muscle cells decreases the strength of the muscles associated with inspiration and expiration.

Urinary System

The number of nephron units in the kidney decreases by almost 50% between the ages of 30 and 75. Also, because less blood flows through the kidneys as an individual ages, there is a reduction in overall function and excretory capacity or the ability to produce urine. In the bladder, significant age-related problems often occur because of diminished muscle tone. Muscle atrophy (wasting) in the bladder wall results in decreased capacity and inability to empty or void completely.

QUICK CHECK

1. What are some changes that occur in the skeleton as one ages? Are they avoidable?
2. How does one's eyesight change during late adulthood?
3. What changes in the cardiovascular system occur in older adults?
4. How is kidney function affected during old age?

Research, Issues, & Trends

Extending the Human Life Span

When reviewing a previous edition of this textbook, a colleague of ours said that ending with the depressing topic of "degeneration associated with aging" was not appropriate to the overall upbeat tone of our book. At first we thought our ending was better than the most obvious and technically accurate ending: "then you die." But it occurred to us that we could take this opportunity to point out one of the most remarkable and important areas of achievement in modern medical research—extending the length, and improving the quality, of life.

In the past few decades, the increased availability of better food, safer surroundings, and advanced medical care has extended quality living for many around the world. But even simple changes in lifestyle, regardless of modern medical wonders, can keep the effects of aging from creeping up too soon. Perhaps the three most important "low-tech" methods for improving the quality of life as you age are healthy diet, exercise, and stress management. A well-balanced diet is not available to some individuals, but it is available to most of us. We are learning more every day about what kind of diet is best, even to the point of being able to manage specific diseases through diet. Exercise performed on a regular basis, even if light or moderate, can not only keep our skeletal and muscular systems more fit but also decrease aging's effects on the nervous system, endocrine system, digestive system, immune system—the list seems endless. And last, even ancient and simple techniques of stress management such as meditation have been shown to help reduce the effects of aging and the diseases that often accompany aging, such as heart disease and strokes.

So to end this chapter, and this book, we say: you can stay young much longer if you *eat right*, *exercise*, and *relax*. And keep studying human structure and function so you'll know that you are doing it right!

OUTLINE SUMMARY

PRENATAL PERIOD

A. Prenatal period begins at conception and continues until birth (about 39 weeks)

B. Science of fetal growth and development called *embryology*

C. Fertilization to implantation requires about 10 days
   1. Fertilization normally occurs in outer third of oviduct (see Figure 21-2)
   2. Fertilized ovum called a *zygote*; zygote is genetically complete — all that is needed for expression of hereditary traits is time and nourishment
   3. After 3 days of cell division, the zygote has developed into a solid cell mass called a *morula*
   4. Continued cell divisions of the morula produce a hollow ball of cells called a *blastocyst*
   5. Blastocyst implants in the uterine wall about 10 days after fertilization
   6. Blastocyst forms the amniotic cavity and chorion of the placenta (see Figure 21-4)
   7. Placenta provides for exchange of nutrients between the mother and fetus

D. Periods of development
   1. Length of pregnancy, or gestation period, is about 39 weeks
   2. Embryonic phase extends from the third week after fertilization to the end of week 8 of gestation
   3. Fetal phase extends from week 8 to week 39 of gestation
   4. All organ systems are formed and functioning by month 4 of gestation (see Figure 21-6)

E. Stem cells — unspecialized cells that reproduce to form specific lines of specialized cells

F. Three primary germ layers appear in the developing embryo after implantation of the blastocyst (see Table 21-1):
   1. Endoderm — inside layer
   2. Ectoderm — outside layer
   3. Mesoderm — middle layer

G. Histogenesis and organogenesis
   1. Formation of new organs (organogenesis) and tissues (histogenesis) occurs from specific development of the primary germ layers
   2. Each primary germ layer gives rise to definite structures such as the skin and muscles
   3. Growth processes include cell differentiation, multiplication, growth, and rearrangement
   4. From 4 months of gestation until delivery, the development of the baby is mainly a matter of growth

H. Birth defects
   1. Any structural or functional abnormality present at birth
   2. May be caused by genetic factors
      a. Abnormal genes
      b. Abnormal number of chromosomes
   3. May be caused by environmental factors
      a. Environmental factors are called *teratogens*
      b. Include radiation, chemicals, and infections
      c. Especially harmful during the first trimester (see Figure 21-7)

BIRTH, OR PARTURITION

A. Process of birth called *parturition* (see Figure 21-8)
   1. At the end of week 39 of gestation, the uterus becomes "irritable"
   2. Fetus takes head-down position against the cervix
   3. Muscular contractions begin, and labor is initiated
   4. Amniotic sac ("bag of waters") ruptures
   5. Cervix dilates
   6. Fetus moves through vagina to exterior

B. Stages of labor
   1. Stage 1 — period from onset of uterine contractions until dilation of the cervix is complete
   2. Stage 2 — period from the time of maximal cervical dilation until the baby exits through the vagina
   3. Stage 3 — process of expulsion of the placenta through the vagina

POSTNATAL PERIOD

A. Postnatal period begins at birth and lasts until death

B. Divisions of postnatal period into isolated time frames can be misleading; life is a continuous process; growth and development are continuous

C. Obvious changes in the physical appearance of the body — in whole and in proportion — occur between birth and maturity (see Figure 21-9)

D. Divisions of postnatal period
   1. Infancy
   2. Childhood
   3. Adolescence and adulthood
   4. Older adulthood

E. Infancy
   1. First 4 weeks called *neonatal period* (see Figure 21-10)
   2. Neonatology — medical and nursing specialty concerned with the diagnosis and treatment of disorders of the newborn
   3. Many cardiovascular changes occur at the time of birth; fetus is totally dependent on mother, whereas the newborn must immediately become totally self-supporting (in respect to respiration and circulation)
   4. Respiratory changes at birth include a deep and forceful first breath
   5. Developmental changes between the neonatal period and 18 months include:
      a. Doubling of birth weight by 4 months and tripling by 1 year
      b. Fifty-percent increase in body length by 12 months
      c. Development of normal spinal curvature by 15 months (see Figure 21-11)
      d. Ability to raise head by 3 months
      e. Ability to crawl by 10 months
      f. Ability to stand alone by 12 months
      g. Ability to run by 18 months

F. Childhood
   1. Extends from end of infancy to puberty — 13 years in girls and 15 in boys
   2. Overall rate of growth remains rapid but decelerates
   3. Continuing development of motor and coordination skills
   4. Loss of deciduous (baby) teeth and eruption of permanent teeth

G. Adolescence and adulthood
   1. Average age range of adolescence varies; usually considered to be from 13 to 19 years
   2. Period of rapid growth resulting in sexual maturity (adolescence)
   3. Appearance of secondary sex characteristics regulated by secretion of sex hormones
   4. Growth spurt typical of adolescence; begins in girls at about 10 and in boys at about 12 (see Figure 21-12)
   5. Growth plates fully close in adult; other structures such as the sinuses assume adult placement
   6. Adulthood characterized by maintenance of existing body tissues
   7. Degeneration of body tissue begins in adulthood

H. Older adulthood (see Figure 21-13)
   1. Degenerative changes characterize older adulthood (also called *senescence*)
   2. Every organ system of the body undergoes degenerative changes
   3. Senescence culminates in death

EFFECTS OF AGING

A. Integumentary system (skin)
   1. With age, skin "sags" and becomes thin, dry, wrinkled
   2. Pigmentation problems are common
   3. Frequently thinning or loss of hair occurs

B. Skeletal system
   1. Aging causes changes in the texture, calcification, and shape of bones
   2. Bone spurs develop around joints
   3. Bones become porous and fracture easily
   4. Degenerative joint diseases such as osteoarthritis are common
   5. Physical activity can reduce loss of bone mass and mobility

C. Central nervous system
   1. Increased risk of dementia
   2. Mature reasoning ability

D. Special senses
   1. All sense organs show a gradual decline in performance with age
   2. Eye lenses become hard and cannot accommodate for near vision; result is farsightedness in many people by age 45 (presbyopia, or "old eye")

3. Loss of transparency of lens or cornea is common (cataract)
4. Glaucoma (increase in pressure in eyeball) is often the cause of blindness in older adulthood
5. Increased risk of retinal degeneration or detachment
6. Loss of hair cells in inner ear produces frequency deafness in many older people
7. Decreased transmission of sound waves caused by loss of elasticity of eardrum and fixing of the bony ear ossicles is common in older adulthood
8. Some degree of hearing impairment is universally present in the aged
9. Smell and taste may be reduced — only about 40% of the taste buds present at age 30 remain at age 75

E. Cardiovascular system
1. Degenerative heart and blood vessel disease is among the most common and serious effects of aging
2. Fat deposits in blood vessels (atherosclerosis) decrease blood flow to the heart and may cause complete blockage of the coronary arteries
3. Hardening of arteries (arteriosclerosis) may result in rupture of blood vessels, especially in the brain (stroke)
4. Hypertension or high blood pressure is common in older adulthood

F. Respiratory system
1. Calcification of costal cartilages causes rib cage to remain in expanded position — barrel chest
2. Wasting of respiratory muscles decreases respiratory efficiency
3. Respiratory membrane thickens; movement of oxygen from alveoli to blood is slowed

G. Urinary system
1. Nephron units decrease in number by 50% between ages 30 and 75
2. Blood flow to kidney decreases and therefore ability to form urine decreases
3. Bladder problems such as inability to void completely are caused by muscle wasting in the bladder wall.

NEW WORDS

adolescence	embryology	implantation	presbyopia
adulthood	embryonic phase	infancy	primary germ layer
amniotic cavity	endoderm	laparoscope	secondary sex
antenatal medicine	fertilization	mesoderm	characteristic
arteriosclerosis	fetal alcohol syndrome	microcephaly	stem cell
atherosclerosis	(FAS)	morula	quickening
birth defect	fetal phase	neonatal period	senescence
blastocyst	fetus	neonate	teratogen
cataract	gerontology	neonatology	ultrasonogram
childhood	gestation	older adulthood	yolk sac
chorion	glaucoma	organogenesis	zygote
chorionic villi	hematopoiesis	osteoarthritis	
ectoderm	histogenesis	parturition	
embryo	hypertension (HTN)	postnatal period	

REVIEW QUESTIONS

1. Explain what occurs between ovulation and the implantation of the fertilized egg into the uterus.
2. Explain the function of the chorion and placenta.
3. Name the three primary germ layers, and name three structures that develop from each layer.
4. Define *histogenesis* and *organogenesis*.
5. Describe and give the approximate length of the three stages of labor.
6. What is the stimulus for the baby's first breath?
7. Name three developmental changes that occur during infancy.
8. Briefly explain what developmental changes occur during childhood.
9. Briefly explain what developmental changes occur during adolescence.
10. Briefly explain what developmental changes occur during adulthood.
11. Explain the effects of aging on the skeletal system.
12. Explain the effects of aging on the respiratory system.
13. Explain the effects of aging on the cardiovascular system.
14. Explain the effects of aging on vision.

CRITICAL THINKING

15. Where do the nutrients used by the zygote from fertilization to implantation come from?
16. Explain the evolution of the function of the yolk sac.
17. What hormones are produced by the placenta? What is their function?

CHAPTER TEST

1. The fertilized ovum is called a _____.
2. After about 3 days of mitosis, the fertilized ovum forms a solid mass of cells called the _____.
3. Mitosis continues, and by the time the developing egg reaches the uterus, it has become a solid ball of cells called the _____.
4. The _____ anchors the developing fetus to the uterus and provides a bridge for exchanging of substances between mother and baby.
5. The _____ period lasts about 39 weeks and is divided into trimesters.
6. The three primary germ layers are the _____, _____, and the _____.
7. The process by which the primary germ layers develop into tissues is called _____.
8. The process by which tissues develop into organs is called _____.
9. The process of birth is called _____.
10. The first 4 weeks of infancy is referred to as the _____ period.
11. _____ is a degenerative joint disease that is common in older adults.
12. _____ is another name for "hardening of the arteries."
13. _____ means "old eye" and causes older adults to be farsighted.
14. If the lens of the eye becomes cloudy and impairs vision, the condition is called a _____.
15. _____ causes an increase in pressure within the eyeball.

Match each phrase in Column B with the correct corresponding term in Column A.

COLUMN A

16. _____ infancy
17. _____ childhood
18. _____ adolescence
19. _____ adulthood
20. _____ older adulthood

COLUMN B

a. period in which the deciduous teeth are lost
b. period in which closure of the bone growth plates occurs
c. period that begins at birth
d. senescence
e. period during which the secondary sex characteristics usually begin to develop

Appendix A

Body Mass Index

Are you a healthy weight? One way that researchers and health professionals use to determine whether you are overweight is called the *body mass index (BMI)*. Here is how to calculate your BMI:

1. Multiply your height (m*) by itself (that is, square it).
2. Divide your weight (kg*) by your answer in step 1.

An even easier way is to use the diagram shown here. Simply find your weight along the bottom of the graph and go straight up from that point to the horizontal line that is closest to your height. That

---

*kg is kilograms (to find your weight in kilograms, divide your weight in pounds by 2.2); m is meters (to find your height in meters, divide your height in inches by 39.4).

point is at your BMI. If it is in the 18.5 to 25 range, you are a healthy weight, according to current research. If it is in the 25 to 30 range, you are considered to be "overweight" and at a greater than normal risk for health problems such as heart disease, diabetes, and certain types of cancer. In the range higher than 30, you are considered to be "obese" and at a very high risk for health problems.

The use of BMI is not universal and it has its critics among health professionals. Because it does not take into account the proportion of lean tissue (muscle) and fat in a person's body, it's not a complete picture of a person's health risks. However, for many it continues to be useful as a quick and easy "snapshot" that may serve as an important warning sign for overweight people.

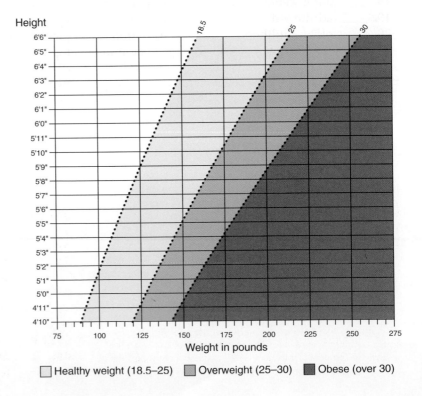

Body mass index chart. (Adapted from the Report of the Dietary Guidelines Advisory Committee on the Dietary Guidelines for Americans, 2000.)

Common Medical Abbreviations, Prefixes, and Suffixes

ABBREVIATIONS AND ACRONYMS

aa	of each
ā.c̄.	before meals
ad lib.	as much as desired
alb.	albumin
am	before noon
amt.	amount
ante	before
aq.	water
AV.	average
AZT ♦	azidothymidine
Ba	barium
b.i.d.	twice a day
b.m.	bowel movement
BMR	basal metabolic rate
BP	blood pressure
BRP	bathroom privileges
BUN	blood urea nitrogen
c̄	with
CBC	complete blood cell count
cc ♦	cubic centimeter
CCU	coronary care unit
CHF	congestive heart failure
CNS	central nervous system
Co	cobalt
CVA	cerebrovascular accident, stroke
D&C	dilation and curettage
d/c ♦	discontinue
DOA	dead on arrival
Dx	diagnosis
ECG	electrocardiogram
EDC	expected date of confinement
EEG	electroencephalogram
EENT	ear, eye, nose, throat
EKG	electrocardiogram
ER	emergency room
FUO	fever of undetermined origin
GI	gastrointestinal
GP	general practitioner
GU	genitourinary
h.	hour
Hb	hemoglobin
HCT	hematocrit
h.s.	at bedtime
H_2O	water
ICU	intensive care unit
IU ♦♦	International Unit
KUB	kidney, ureter, and bladder
MI	myocardial infarction
non rep.	do not repeat
NPO	nothing by mouth
NSAID	nonsteroidal anti-inflammatory drug
OR	operating room
p.c.	after meals
per	by
PH	past history
PI	previous illness
pm	after noon
p.r.n.	as needed
q.	every
q.d. ♦	every day
q.h.	every hour
q.i.d.	four times a day
q.n.s.	quantity not sufficient
q.o.d. ♦♦	every other day
q.s.	quantity required or sufficient
RBC	red blood cell
Rx	prescription
s̄	without
sp. gr.	specific gravity
SQ ♦	subcutaneous
ss. ♦	one half or sliding scale
SSRI ♦	serotonin-specific reuptake inhibitor
stat.	at once, immediately
T & A	tonsillectomy and adenoidectomy

ALERT! Items marked with ♦ are subject to health-threatening errors of interpretation and should no longer be used in clinical settings even though they are still often used in nonclinical or research settings. Items with ♦♦ are banned from use in clinical settings by The Joint Commission (TJC), formerly The Joint Commission on Accreditation of Healthcare Organizations (JCAHO).

T.B.	tuberculosis
t.i.d.	three times a day
TPR	temperature, pulse, respiration
TUR	transurethral resection
WBC	white blood cell

retro-	backward, back
semi-	half
sub-	under, beneath
super-	above, over
supra-	above, on the upper side
syn-	with, together
trans-	across, beyond
ultra-	excessive

PREFIXES

A prefix is a word part used at the *beginning* of a term and describes or alters the meaning of the word part(s) that follows the prefix. For example, *an-* means "without," so *anuria* means "without urine," or the condition of having no urine output.

a-	without
ab-	away from
ad-	to, toward
adeno-	glandular
amphi-	on both sides
an-	without
ante-	before, forward
anti-	against
bi-	two, double, twice
circum-	around, about
contra-	opposite, against
de-	away from, from
di-	double
dia-	across, through
dis-	separate from, apart
dys-	difficult
e-	out, away
ecto-	outside
en-	in
endo-	in, inside
epi-	on
eu-	well
ex-	from, out of, away from
exo-	outside
extra-	outside, beyond; in addition
hemi-	half
hyper-	over, excessive, above
hypo-	under, deficient
infra-	underneath, below
inter-	between, among
intra-	within, on the side
intro-	into, within
iso-	equal, like
para-	beside
peri-	around, beyond
post-	after, behind
pre-	before, in front of
pro-	before, in front of
re-	again

SUFFIXES

A suffix is a word part used at the *end* of a term and describes or alters the meaning of the word part(s) that comes before the suffix. For example, *-ectomy* means "cut out," so *appendectomy* means "appendix cut out," or the procedure of surgically removing the appendix.

-algia	pain, painful
-asis	condition
-blast	young cell
-cele	swelling
-centesis	puncture for aspiration
-cide	killer
-cyte	cell
-ectomy	cut out
-emia	blood
-genesis	production, development
-itis	inflammation
-kin	in motion, action
-logy	study of
-megaly	enlargement
-odynia	pain
-oid	resembling
-oma	tumor
-osis	condition
-opathy	disease
-penia	abnormal reduction
-pexy	fixation
-phagia	eating, swallowing
-phasia	speaking condition
-phobia	fear
-plasty	plastic surgery
-plegia	paralysis
-poiesis	formation
-ptosis	downward displacement
-rhaphy	suture
-scope	instrument for examination
-scopy	examination
-stomy	creation of an opening
-tomy	incision
-uria	urine

Chapter Test Answers

Chapter 1
1. anatomy
2. physiology
3. theory, law
4. chemical, cell, tissue, organ, organ system
5. prone, supine
6. transverse
7. frontal
8. sagittal
9. midsagittal
10. axial
11. appendicular
12. c
13. b
14. d
15. d
16. b
17. e
18. d
19. a
20. c
21. b

Chapter 2
1. matter
2. atoms
3. protons
4. energy
5. compounds
6. covalent
7. ion
8. electrolyte
9. organic
10. solvent
11. dehydration synthesis
12. acids
13. buffers

14. d
15. f
16. g
17. e
18. a
19. c
20. b
21. c
22. a
23. d
24. b
25. c

Chapter 3
1. phospholipid, cholesterol
2. organelle
3. active transport, passive transport
4. pinocytosis
5. DNA, mRNA
6. translation
7. transcription
8. gene
9. genome
10. epithelial, muscle, nerve, connective
11. a
12. c
13. a
14. b
15. c
16. d
17. g
18. c
19. e
20. i
21. b
22. a

23. d
24. f
25. h

Chapter 4
1. gastrointestinal tract
2. skeletal, striated
3. smooth, visceral
4. nerve impulses
5. hair, nails, glands, sense organs
6. thymus
7. urethra
8. testes, ovaries
9. cartilage, ligament
10. f
11. k
12. a
13. i
14. b
15. g
16. c
17. j
18. d
19. e
20. h

Chapter 5
1. cutaneous, serous, mucous
2. basement membrane
3. parietal pleura
4. visceral peritoneum
5. synovial membrane
6. stratum corneum, stratum germinativum
7. keratin
8. dermal papillae
9. eccrine

10. apocrine
11. sebum
12. protection, sensation, temperature regulation
13. c
14. d
15. a
16. b
17. b
18. d
19. a
20. c

Chapter 6

1. articular cartilage
2. medullary cavity
3. trabeculae
4. haversian systems
5. lacunae
6. osteoclasts
7. osteoblasts
8. endochondral ossification
9. epiphyseal plate
10. axial, appendicular
11. synarthroses, amphiarthroses, diarthroses
12. ligaments
13. c
14. b
15. a
16. d
17. c
18. b
19. a
20. b
21. d
22. d
23. c
24. d
25. c
26. c
27. d
28. b
29. a
30. d
31. a
32. c
33. a
34. b
35. a

Chapter 7

1. muscle fiber
2. heart
3. insertion
4. origin
5. actin
6. myosin
7. sarcomere
8. movement, posture, heat production
9. ATP
10. lactic acid
11. motor unit
12. threshold stimulus
13. isotonic
14. isometric
15. abduction
16. extension
17. supination
18. b
19. d
20. a
21. b
22. d
23. d
24. a
25. c or b
26. c
27. d
28. a
29. c
30. d
31. b

Chapter 8

1. peripheral nervous system
2. central nervous system
3. nerve
4. neurons, glia
5. reflex arc
6. nerve impulse
7. positive, negative
8. sodium
9. synapse
10. neurotransmitters
11. dura mater, arachnoid layer, pia mater
12. 12, 31
13. dermatomes
14. parasympathetic nervous system

15. sympathetic nervous system
16. acetylcholine, norepinephrine
17. acetylcholine, acetylcholine
18. cardiac muscle, smooth muscle, glandular epithelial
19. g
20. c
21. e
22. a
23. b
24. f
25. d
26. d
27. a
28. h
29. f
30. b
31. g
32. e
33. c

Chapter 9

1. chemoreceptors, proprioceptors
2. organ of Corti
3. crista ampullaris
4. taste
5. sweet, sour, bitter, salty, umami, metallic
6. papillae
7. olfactory receptors
8. e
9. i
10. j
11. b
12. a
13. g
14. c
15. f
16. h
17. d
18. k
19. f
20. g
21. a
22. b
23. e
24. c
25. d

Chapter 10
1. exocrine
2. endocrine, hormones
3. protein, steroid
4. target organ
5. cyclic AMP (cAMP)
6. on the cell membrane, in the nucleus
7. prostaglandins
8. posterior pituitary (neurohypophysis)
9. anterior pituitary (adenohypophysis)
10. posterior pituitary gland, hypothalamus
11. d
12. b
13. c
14. b
15. b
16. a
17. d
18. f
19. i
20. a
21. e
22. c
23. h
24. g
25. b

Chapter 11
1. plasma
2. albumin, globulin, fibrinogen
3. serum
4. red blood cells (erythrocytes), white blood cells (leukocytes), platelets (thrombocytes)
5. myeloid, lymphatic
6. hemoglobin
7. anemia
8. polycythemia
9. neutrophils
10. B lymphocytes
11. calcium
12. fibrinogen, fibrin
13. K
14. thrombus
15. embolus

16. antigen
17. A and B, no (none)
18. B, anti-A
19. Type O, Rh-negative
20. Type AB, Rh-positive
21. erythroblastosis fetalis

Chapter 12
1. ventricles
2. atria
3. myocardium
4. interventricular septum
5. endocardium
6. epicardium
7. systole
8. diastole
9. tricuspid (right atrioventricular)
10. stroke volume
11. sinoatrial node
12. Purkinje fibers
13. QRS complex
14. P wave
15. veins
16. arteries
17. capillaries
18. tunica intima
19. tunica adventitia
20. pulmonary circulation
21. foramen ovale, ductus arteriosus
22. blood viscosity, heart rate
23. a. 7
    b. 2
    c. 3
    d. 6
    e. 10
    f. 8
    g. 9
    h. 5
    i. 1
    j. 4

Chapter 13
1. lymph
2. thoracic duct
3. right lymphatic duct
4. cisterna chyli
5. lymph nodes
6. afferent, efferent

7. T lymphocytes (T cells), thymosin
8. palatine, pharyngeal, lingual
9. spleen
10. inflammation
11. complement fixation
12. monocytes
13. c
14. b
15. d
16. a
17. B
18. B
19. T
20. B
21. T
22. T
23. B
24. T
25. B

Chapter 14
1. air distributor, gas exchanger
2. nose, pharynx, larynx
3. trachea, bronchial tree, lungs
4. respiratory membrane
5. respiratory mucosa
6. paranasal sinuses
7. lacrimal
8. conchae
9. pharynx
10. larynx
11. trachea
12. primary bronchi, secondary bronchi, bronchioles, alveolar ducts
13. surfactant
14. 3, 2
15. internal respiration
16. external respiration
17. diaphragm
18. oxyhemoglobin
19. bicarbonate, carbaminohemoglobin
20. medulla
21. stretch receptors
22. chemoreceptors
23. tidal

24. tidal, expiratory reserve, inspiratory reserve
25. residual

Chapter 15
1. digestion, absorption
2. muscularis
3. submucosa
4. mucosa
5. serosa
6. uvula, soft palate
7. crown, neck, root
8. parotid, submandibular, sublingual
9. esophagus
10. fundus, body, pylorus
11. duodenum, jejunum, ileum
12. villi
13. lacteal
14. common hepatic duct, cystic duct
15. transverse colon
16. sigmoid colon
17. mesentery, greater omentum
18. absorption
19. e
20. i
21. j
22. k
23. b
24. l
25. f
26. g
27. d
28. c
29. a
30. h

Chapter 16
1. assimilation
2. catabolism
3. anabolism
4. prothrombin, fibrinogen
5. A, D
6. water, fat
7. total metabolic rate
8. basal metabolic rate
9. total metabolic rate
10. convection
11. evaporation
12. fat metabolism

13. protein
14. nonessential amino acids
15. b
16. d
17. c
18. g
19. a
20. e
21. h
22. f

Chapter 17
1. 20
2. Bowman capsule, glomerulus
3. Henle loop, collecting tubule
4. proximal convoluted tubule, distal convoluted tubule
5. reabsorption
6. filtration
7. secretion
8. antidiuretic hormone
9. atrial natriuretic hormone
10. aldosterone
11. internal urethral sphincter
12. suppression
13. urinary incontinence
14. retention
15. g
16. a
17. k
18. b
19. d
20. f
21. j
22. h
23. c
24. e
25. i

Chapter 18
1. interstitial fluid, plasma, and transcellular fluid
2. intracellular fluid
3. less
4. more
5. more
6. fluid output
7. water from catabolism
8. kidneys, skin, lungs, intestines

9. aldosterone, atrial natriuretic hormone
10. ions
11. chloride
12. sodium
13. b
14. c
15. b
16. a

Chapter 19
1. carbonic anhydrase
2. buffers
3. H_2CO_3
4. $NaHCO_3$
5. distal tubule
6. NaH_2PO_4
7. NH_4Cl
8. base
9. alkalosis
10. acidosis
11. 20
12. $NaHCO_3$ (bicarbonate)
13. H_2CO_3
14. alkalosis
15. b
16. a
17. b
18. b
19. decreases
20. increases
21. increases
22. decreases
23. increases
24. decreases

Chapter 20
1. testes
2. scrotum
3. tunica albuginea
4. seminiferous tubule
5. interstitial cells
6. spermatogonium
7. meiosis or spermatogenesis
8. acrosome
9. epididymis
10. ductus deferens (vas deferens)
11. prostate gland
12. seminal vesicles
13. corpora cavernosa

14. ovaries
15. graafian
16. oogenesis
17. polar bodies
18. uterine tubes (oviducts, fallopian tubes)
19. myometrium
20. cervix
21. endometrium
22. vagina
23. greater vestibular
24. alveoli, lactiferous
25. h
26. c
27. a

28. b
29. d
30. e
31. i
32. g
33. f

Chapter 21
1. zygote
2. morula
3. blastocyst
4. placenta
5. gestation
6. ectoderm, mesoderm, endoderm

7. histogenesis
8. organogenesis
9. parturition
10. neonatal
11. osteoarthritis
12. arteriosclerosis
13. presbyopia
14. cataract
15. glaucoma
16. c
17. a
18. e
19. b
20. d

Illustration/Photo Credits

CHAPTER 1

1-2, 1-4, 1-6, 1-7, Barbara Cousins; 1-3, Copyright Kevin Patton, Lion Den, Inc., Weldon Spring, MO; 1-5, Rolin Graphics; Science Application box, Joe Kulka (art), National Library of Medicine (photo).

CHAPTER 2

2-1, From Sugimoto Y et al: Chemical identification of individual surface atoms by atomic force microscopy, *Nature* 466:64-67, 2007; Science Application box, Joe Kulka.

CHAPTER 3

3-3A, Courtesy Charles Flickinger, University of Virginia; 3-3B, Lennart Nilsson, Albert Bonniers Forlag, Stockholm, Sweden; 3-10, 3-11B, 3-12B, 3-13B, 3-14B, Barbara Cousins; 3-11A, 3-12A, 3-13A, 3-14A, 3-20, Courtesy Gartner LP, Hiatt JL: *Color textbook of histology*, ed 3, 2007, Saunders; 3-15, Courtesy Stanley Erlandsen, from Gartner LP, Hiatt JL: *Color atlas of histology*, St Louis, 1992, Mosby; 3-16, 3-17, 3-18, 3-19, 3-21, 3-23, 3-24, Dennis Strete; 3-22, Edward Reschke; Tables 3-2, 3-3, Network Graphics; Science Application box, Joe Kulka.

CHAPTER 4

4-3, 4-7, Barbara Cousins; Science Application box, CNRI/Photo Researchers.

CHAPTER 5

5-3, Edward Reschke; 5-4, Habif, TP: *Clinical Dermatology*, ed 4, St Louis, Mosby, 2004; 5-7A, From Goldman L, Ausiello D: *Cecil textbook of medicine*, ed 23, Philadelphia, 2008, Saunders; 5-7B, From Noble J: *Textbook of primary care medicine*, ed 3, Philadelphia, 2001, Mosby; 5-7C, From Townsend C, Beauchamp RD, Evers BM, Mattox K: *Sabiston textbook of surgery*, ed 18, Philadelphia, 2008, Saunders; 5-7D, From Rakel R: *Textbook of family medicine*, ed 7, Philadelphia, 2007, Saunders; 5-8, Barbara Cousins; 5-9, Courtesy Dr. Richard L Judd, Dwight D Ponsell, from *Mosby's first responder*, ed 2, 1988, Mosby; Clinical Application box: Pressure Ulcers, From Potter P, Perry A: *Fundamentals of nursing*, ed 7, St Louis, 2009, Mosby; Science Application box, Joe Kulka.

CHAPTER 6

6-4, From Gartner LP, Hiatt JL: *Color textbook of histology*, ed 3, Philadelphia, 2007, Saunders; 6-5, Dennis Strete; 6-6, Adapted from McCance K, Huether S: *Pathophysiology*, ed 4, St Louis, 2002, Mosby; 6-8, Network Graphics; 6-10, 6-13, 6-16 (drawing), 6-18 (drawing), 6-23, Barbara Cousins; 6-14, From Hockenberry MJ, Wilson D: *Wong's essentials of pediatric nursing*, ed 8, St Louis, 2009, Mosby; 6-16C, 6-17, 6-18B, D, Courtesy Vidic B, Suarez FR: *Photographic atlas of the human body*, St Louis, 1984, Mosby; 6-20, Yvonne Wylie Walston; Clinical Application box: Epiphyseal Fracture, JM Booher, GA Thibodeau, from *Athletic injury assessment*, ed 4, New York, 2001, McGraw Hill; Clinical Application box: Palpable Bony Landmarks, Terry Cockerham, Synapse Media Production; Clinical Application box: Total Hip Replacement, ST Canale, from *Campbell's operative orthopaedics*, ed 9, St Louis, 1998, Mosby; The Knee Joint box (photo), from Cummings N, Stanley-Croop S, Higgs P: *Perspectives in athletic training*, St Louis, 2009, Mosby; Science Application box, Joe Kulka.

CHAPTER 7

7-3B, Courtesy Dr. HE Huxley; 7-5, Courtesy Dr. Paul C Letourneau, Department of Anatomy, Medical School, University of Minnesota, Minneapolis; 7-7A, C, 7-8A, C, Rolin Graphics; 7-10, 7-11, 7-12, John V Hagen; Science Application box, Joe Kulka; Clinical Application box: Muscle Injury, Courtesy Rob Williams, from Booher JM, Thibodeau GA: *Athletic injury assessment*, ed 2, St Louis, 1989, Mosby.

CHAPTER 8

8-2C, Dennis Strete; 8-4, Courtesy Dr. Richard Kessel, Professor of Biological Sciences, University of Iowa, Iowa City; 8-9B, 8-10 (photo), 8-11 (photo), Courtesy Vidic B, Suarez FR: *Photographic atlas of the human body*, St Louis, 1984, Mosby; Clinical Application box: Herpes Zoster (photo), Courtesy TP Habif: *Clinical dermatology*, ed 2, 1990 Mosby; Science Application box, Joe Kulka; Clinical Application box: Lumbar Puncture, From Forbes CD, Jackson WD: *Color atlas and text of clinical medicine*, ed 3, London, 2003, Mosby.

CHAPTER 9

Clinical Application box: Color Blindness, From *Ishihara's tests for colour deficiency*, Tokyo, Japan, 1973, Kanehara Trading Co, Copyright Isshinkai Foundation; Science Application box, Joe Kulka.

CHAPTER 10

Clinical Application box: Thyroid Hormone Abnormalities, **A**, Seidel HM, Ball JW, Dains JE, Benedict GW: *Mosby's guide to physical examination*, ed 5, St Louis, 2002, Mosby; **B**, Swartz MH: *Textbook of physical diagnosis,* ed 4, Philadelphia, 2002, Saunders; Clinical Application box: Adrenal Hormone Abnormalities, Courtesy Gower Medical Publishers; Science Application box, Joe Kulka.

CHAPTER 11

11-1, 11-5, 11-7, Barbara Cousins; 11-2, Courtesy Bevelander G, Ramalay JA: *Essentials of histology,* ed 8, St Louis, 1979, Mosby; 11-3**D**, Zakus SM: *Clinical procedures for medical assistants,* ed 3, St Louis, 1995, Mosby; 11-4, Dennis Strete; 11-6**B**, Copyright Dennis Kunkel Microscopy, Inc.; 11-7 (photos), Belcher AE: *Blood disorders,* St Louis, 1993, Mosby; Science Application box, Joe Kulka.

CHAPTER 12

12-8, Barbara Cousins; Science Application box, Joe Kulka.

CHAPTER 13

13-5, Courtesy Ballinger P, Frank ED: *Merrill's atlas of radiographic positions & radiologic procedures,* vol 1, ed 10, St Louis, 2002, Mosby; 13-11, Courtesy Emma Shelton; 13-14, Courtesy James T Barrett; Science Application box, Joe Kulka.

CHAPTER 14

14-1, Barbara Cousins; 14-5**C**, Custom Medical Stock Photo, Chicago, IL; 14-6 (photo), Courtesy Stanley Erlandsen, from Gartner LP, Hiatt JL: *Color atlas of histology*, St Louis, 1992, Mosby; 14-7, Network Graphics; Research, Issues, & Trends box: Lung Volume Reduction Surgery, Courtesy Andrew P Evan, University of Indiana; Science Application box, Joe Kulka.

CHAPTER 15

15-5**C**, From Zitelli BJ, Davis HW: *Atlas of pediatric physical diagnosis,* ed 5, Philadelphia, 2007, Mosby; 15-11, Courtesy Vidic B, Suarez RF: *Photographic atlas of the human body,* St Louis, 1984, Mosby; 15-12**B**, Mettler FA: *Essentials of radiology,* ed 2, Philadelphia, 2004, Elsevier; 15-15, Barbara Cousins; Clinical Application box: Malocclusion, Thibodeau GA, Patton KT: *Anatomy & physiology,* ed 5, St Louis, 2003,

Mosby; Clinical Application box: Gallstones and Weight Loss, Courtesy Thompson JM, Wilson SF: *Health assessment for nursing practice*, St Louis, 1996, Mosby; Science Application box, Joe Kulka.

CHAPTER 16

Science Application box, Joe Kulka.

CHAPTER 17

17-1**B**, 17-2**B**, Abrahams P, Hutchings RT, Marks SC: *McMinn's color atlas of human anatomy,* ed 5, St Louis, 2003, Mosby; 17-3**C**, Courtesy Andrew P Evan, Indiana University School of Medicine; 17-6, Stevens A, Lowe J: *Human histology,* ed 3, Philadelphia, 2005, Elsevier; Clinical Application box: Dialysis, Lewis S: *Medical-surgical nursing,* ed 7, St Louis, 2007, Mosby; Science Application box, Joe Kulka.

CHAPTER 18

18-4 (photo), Copyright Kevin Patton, Lion Den Inc., Weldon Spring, MO; 18-5, From Bloom A, Ireland J: *Color atlas of diabetes,* ed 2, St Louis, 1992, Mosby; Science Application box, Joe Kulka.

CHAPTER 19

Science Application box, Joe Kulka.

CHAPTER 20

20-2**A**, Lennart Nilsson, Albert Bonniers Forlag AB, Stockholm, Sweden; 20-4**A**, courtesy Stanley Erlandsen (from *Color atlas of histology,* St. Louis, 1992, Mosby); 20-5**A**, Carolyn Coulam and John A McIntyre; 20-6**C**, Barbara Cousins; Science Application box, Joe Kulka.

CHAPTER 21

21-1 (micrograph), 21-6, Lennart Nilsson, Albert Bonniers Forlag AB, Stockholm, Sweden; 21-3, Courtesy Lucinda L Veeck, Jones Institute for Reproductive Medicine, Norfolk, VA; 21-5**B**, From Cotran R, Kumar V, Collins T: *Robbins pathologic basis of disease,* ed 6, Philadelphia, 1999, Saunders; 21-9, Barbara Cousins; 21-10, Courtesy Marjorie M Pyle for Lifecircle, Costa Mesa, CA; 21-11**A**, From Hockenberry MJ, Wilson D: *Wong's essentials of pediatric nursing,* ed 8, St Louis, 2009, Mosby; 21-11**B**, Copyright Kevin Patton, Lion Den Inc., Weldon Spring, MO; 21-12, Mahan LK, Escott-Stump S: *Krause's food, nutrition, and diet therapy,* ed 11, St Louis, 2004, Elsevier; Research, Issues, & Trends box: Freezing Umbilical Cord Blood, Courtesy Craig Borck, *St Paul Pioneer Press*; Antenatal Diagnosis and Treatment box, **B, C,** Copyright Kevin Patton, Lion Den Inc., Weldon Spring, MO; Science Application box, Joe Kulka.

A

abdomen (AB-doe-men) body area between the diaphragm and pelvis

abdominal cavity (ab-DOM-i-nal KAV-i-tee) the cavity containing the abdominal organs

abdominal muscles (ab-DOM-i-nal MUS-elz) muscles supporting the anterior aspect of the abdomen

abdominal quadrants (ab-DOM-i-nal KWOD-rants) health professionals divide the abdomen (through the navel) into four areas to help locate specific organs

abdominal regions (ab-DOM-i-nal REE-junz) anatomists have divided the abdomen into nine regions to identify the location of organs

abdominopelvic cavity (ab-DOM-i-no-PEL-vik KAV-i-tee) term used to describe the single cavity containing the abdominal and pelvic organs

abduct (ab-DUKT) move away from the center or midline; see **abduction**

abduction (ab-DUK-shun) moving away from the midline of the body; opposite motion of adduction

absorption (ab-SORP-shun) passage of a substance through a membrane, such as skin or mucosa, into blood

accessory organ (ak-SES-oh-ree OR-gan) an organ that assists other organs in accomplishing their functions

acetabulum (ass-eh-TAB-yoo-lum) socket in the hip bone (os coxa or innominate bone) into which the head of the femur fits

acetylcholine (ass-ee-til-KOH-leen) chemical neurotransmitter

acid (ASS-id) any substance that, when dissolved in water, contributes to an excess of H⁻ ions (i.e., a *low* pH)

acid-base balance (ASS-id base BAL-ans) maintaining the concentration of hydrogen ions in body fluids

acidosis (ass-i-DOH-sis) condition in which there is an excessive proportion of acid in the blood (and thus an abnormally low blood pH); opposite of alkalosis

acne (AK-nee) a bacterial infection of the skin characterized by red pustules formed when hair follicles become infected

acquired immunity (ah-KWIRED i-MYOO-ni-tee) immunity that is obtained after birth through the use of injections or exposure to a harmful agent

acquired immunodeficiency syndrome (AIDS) (ah-KWIRED i-myoo-no-deh-FISH-en-see SIN-drohm) disease in which the HIV virus attacks the T cells, thereby compromising the body's immune system

acromegaly (ak-roh-MEG-ah-lee) condition caused by hypersecretion of growth hormone after puberty, resulting in enlargement of facial features (e.g., jaw, nose), fingers, and toes

acrosome (AK-roh-sohm) specialized structure on the sperm containing enzymes that break down the covering of the ovum to allow entry

actin (AK-tin) contractile protein found in the thin myofilaments of skeletal muscle

action potential (AK-shun poh-TEN-shal) nerve impulse

active transport (AK-tiv TRANS-port) movement of a substance into and out of a living cell requiring the use of cellular energy

Addison disease (AD-i-son di-ZEEZ) disease of the adrenal gland resulting in low blood sugar, weight loss, and weakness

adaptive immunity (ah-DAP-tiv i-MYOO-ni-tee) another name for **specific immunity**

adduct (ad-DUKT) move toward the center or midline; see **adduction**

adduction (ah-DUK-shun) moving toward the midline of the body, opposite motion of abduction

adductor muscle (ad-DUK-tor MUS-el) any of a group of muscles of the leg that each originate on the pelvic bone and insert on the femur (along the inside thigh) and draw the leg toward the midline of the body (adduction)

adenohypophysis (ad-eh-no-hye-POF-i-sis) anterior pituitary gland, which has the structure of an endocrine gland

adenoid (AD-eh-noyd) literally, glandlike; adenoids, or pharyngeal tonsils, are paired lymphoid structures in the nasopharynx

adenosine diphosphate (ADP) (ah-DEN-oh-seen dye-FOS-fayt) molecule similar to adenosine triphosphate but containing only two phosphate groups

adenosine triphosphate (ATP) (ah-DEN-oh-seen try-FOS-fayt) chemical compound that provides energy for use by body cells

adipose (AD-i-pohs) fat tissue

adolescence (ad-oh-LESS-ens) period between puberty and adulthood

adrenal cortex (ah-DREE-nal KOHR-teks) outer portion of adrenal gland that secretes hormones called *corticoids*

adrenal gland (ah-DREE-nal) glands that rest on the top of the kidneys, made up of the cortex and medulla

adrenal medulla (ah-DREE-nal meh-DUL-ah) inner portion of adrenal gland that secretes epinephrine and norepinephrine

adrenergic fiber (ad-ren-ER-jik FYE-ber) axon whose terminal releases norepinephrine and epinephrine

adrenocorticotropic hormone (ACTH) (ah-dree-no-kor-teh-koh-TROH-pic HOR-mohn) hormone that stimulates the adrenal cortex to secrete larger amounts of hormones

adulthood (ah-DULT-hood) period after adolescence

aerobic respiration (air-OH-bik res-pi-RAY-shun) the stage of cellular respiration requiring oxygen

aerobic training (air-OH-bik TRAIN-ing) continuous vigorous exercise requiring the body to increase its consumption of oxygen and develop the muscles' ability to sustain activity over a long period

afferent (AF-fer-ent) carrying or conveying toward the center (e.g., an afferent neuron carries nerve impulses toward the central nervous system)

afferent lymph vessel (AF-fer-ent limf VESS-el) any small lymphatic vessel that carries lymphatic fluid toward a lymph node; compare to **efferent lymph vessel**

afferent neuron (AF-fer-ent NOO-ron) neuron that carries impulses toward the central nervous system from the periphery; sensory neuron

agglutinate (ah-GLOO-tin-ayt) antibodies causing antigens to clump or stick together

aging process (AJ-ing PROS-es) the gradual degenerative changes that occur after young adulthood as a person ages

AIDS see **acquired immunodeficiency syndrome**

AIDS-related complex (ARC) (AIDS ree-LAY-ted KOM-pleks) a more mild form of AIDS that produces fever, weight loss, and swollen lymph nodes

albumin (al-BYOO-min) one of several types of proteins normally found in blood plasma; helps thicken the blood

aldosterone (AL-deh-steh-rohn *or* al-DAH-stair-ohn) hormone that stimulates the kidney to retain sodium ions and water

alimentary canal (al-i-MEN-tar-ee kah-NAL) the digestive tract as a whole

alkaline (AL-kah-lin) base; any substance that, when dissolved in water, contributes to an excess of OH⁻ ions (thus creating a high pH)

alkalosis (al-kah-LOH-sis) condition in which there is an excessive proportion of alkali (base) in the blood, causing an abnormally high blood pH; opposite of acidosis

allergy (AL-er-jee) hypersensitivity of the immune system to relatively harmless environmental antigens

all or none when stimulated, a muscle fiber will contract fully or not at all; whether a contraction occurs depends on whether the stimulus reaches the required threshold

alpha cell (AL-fah sell) pancreatic cell that secretes glucagon

alveolar duct (al-VEE-oh-lar dukt) airway that branches from the smallest bronchioles; alveolar sacs arise from alveolar ducts

alveolar sac (al-VEE-oh-lar sak) each alveolar duct ends in several sacs that resemble a cluster of grapes

alveolus (al-VEE-oh-lus) (*pl.,* alveoli) literally, a small cavity; alveoli of lungs are microscopic saclike dilations of terminal bronchioles

amenorrhea (ah-men-oh-REE-ah) absence of normal menstruation

amino acid (ah-MEE-no ASS-id) category of chemical units from which protein molecules are built; *essential amino acids* are those that must be in the diet but *nonessential amino acids* can be missing from the diet because they can be made by the body

amniotic cavity (am-nee-OT-ik KAV-i-tee) cavity within the blastocyst that will become a fluid-filled sac in which the embryo will float during development

amphiarthrosis (am-fee-ar-THROH-sis) slightly movable joint such as the joint joining the two pubic bones

amylase (AM-i-lays) enzyme that digests carbohydrates

anabolic steroid (an-ah-BOL-ik STAYR-oyd) a lipid molecule of the steroid variety that acts as a hormone to stimulate anabolism (specifically protein synthesis) in body tissues such as muscle (e.g., testosterone)

anabolism (ah-NAB-oh-liz-em) cells making complex molecules (e.g., hormones) from simpler compounds (e.g., amino acids); opposite of catabolism

anaerobic (an-air-OH-bik) metabolic process that does not require the presence of oxygen

anal canal (AY-nal kah-NAL) terminal portion of the rectum

anaphase (AN-ah-fayz) stage of mitosis; duplicate chromosomes move to poles of dividing cell

anaphylactic shock (an-ah-fi-LAK-tik shock) shock resulting from a severe allergic reaction; may be fatal

anatomical position (an-ah-TOM-i-kal poh-ZISH-un) the reference position for the body, which gives meaning to directional terms

anatomy (ah-NAT-oh-mee) the study of the structure of an organism and the relationships of its parts

androgen (AN-droh-jen) male sex hormone

anemia (ah-NEE-mee-ah) deficient number of red blood cells or deficient hemoglobin

anesthesia (an-es-THEE-zhah) loss of sensation

angina pectoris (an-JYE-nah PECK-tor-is) severe chest pain resulting when the myocardium is deprived of sufficient oxygen

angioplasty (AN-jee-oh-plas-tee) medical procedure in which vessels occluded by arteriosclerosis ("hardening of arteries") are opened (i.e., the channel for blood flow is widened)

angstrom (ANG-strom) unit of length equivalent to 0.0000000001 m (1/10,000,000,000 of a meter or about 1/250,000,000 of an inch)

anion (AN-eye-on) negatively charged particle

anorexia nervosa (an-oh-REK-see-ah ner-VO-sah) a behavior involving an irrational fear of being overweight, resulting in severe weight loss caused by self-starvation

antagonist muscle (an-TAG-oh-nist MUSS-el) those having opposing actions; for example, muscles that flex the upper arm are antagonists to muscles that extend it

antebrachial (an-tee-BRAY-kee-al) refers to the forearm

antecubital (an-tee-KYOO-bi-tal) refers to the elbow

antenatal medicine (an-tee-NAY-tal MED-i-sin) prenatal medicine

anterior (an-TEER-ee-or) front or ventral; opposite of posterior or dorsal

antibody (AN-ti-bod-ee) substance produced by the body that destroys or inactivates a specific substance (antigen) that has entered the body

antibody-mediated immunity (AN-ti-bod-ee MEE-dee-ayt-ed i-MYOO-ni-tee) immunity that is produced when antibodies make antigens unable to harm the body

antidiuretic hormone (ADH) (an-tee-dye-yoo-RET-ik HOR-mohn) hormone produced in the posterior pituitary gland to regulate the balance of water in the body by accelerating the reabsorption of water

antigen (AN-ti-jen) substance that, when introduced into the body, causes formation of antibodies against it

antioxidant (an-tee-awk-seh-dant) chemical substance that prevents oxidizers such as free radicals from damaging chemical structures of the body

antrum (AN-trum) cavity

anuria (ah-NOO-ree-ah) absence of urine

anus (AY-nus) distal end or outlet of the rectum

aorta (ay-OR-tah) main and largest artery in the body

aortic body (ay-OR-tik BOD-ee) small cluster of chemosensitive cells that respond to carbon dioxide and oxygen levels

aortic semilunar valve (ay-OR-tic sem-i-LOO-nar valve) valve between the aorta and left ventricle that prevents blood from flowing back into the ventricle

apex (AY-peks) pointed end of a conical structure

aplastic anemia (ay-PLAS-tik ah-NEE-mee-ah) blood disorder characterized by a low red blood cell count; caused by destruction of myeloid tissue in the bone marrow

apnea (AP-nee-ah) temporary cessation of breathing

apocrine (AP-oh-krin) sweat glands located in the axilla and genital regions; these glands enlarge and begin to function at puberty

apoptosis (ap-op-TOH-sis) programmed cell death by means of several biochemical processes built into each cell; apoptosis clears space for newer cells, as in early embryonic development or in tissue repair

appendage (ah-PEN-dij) something that is attached

appendicitis (ah-pen-di-SYE-tis) inflammation of the vermiform appendix

appendicular (ah-pen-DIK-yoo-lar) refers to the upper and lower extremities of the body

appendicular skeleton (ah-pen-DIK-yoo-lar SKEL-eh-ton) the bones of the upper and lower extremities of the body

aqueous humor (AY-kwee-us HYOO-mor) watery fluid that fills the anterior chamber of the eye, in front of the lens

aqueous solution (AY-kwee-us) liquid mixture in which water is the solvent; for example, saltwater is an aqueous solution because water is the solvent

arachnoid mater (ah-RAK-noyd MAH-ter) delicate, weblike middle membrane covering the brain; the meninges

areola (ah-REE-oh-lah) small space; the pigmented ring around the nipple

areolar (ah-REE-oh-lar) a type of connective tissue consisting of fibers and a variety of cells embedded in a loose matrix of soft, sticky gel

arrector pili (ah-REK-tor PYE-lye) smooth muscles of the skin, which are attached to hair follicles; when contraction occurs, the hair stands up, resulting in "goose flesh"

arteriole (ar-TEER-ee-ohl) small branch of an artery

arteriosclerosis (ar-tee-ree-oh-skleh-ROH-sis) hardening of arteries; materials such as lipids (as in atherosclerosis) accumulate in arterial walls, often becoming hardened as calcium is deposited

artery (AR-ter-ee) vessel carrying blood away from the heart

articular cartilage (ar-TIK-yoo-lar KAR-ti-lij) cartilage covering the joint ends of bones

articulation (ar-tik-yoo-LAY-shun) joint

artificial kidney (ar-ti-FISH-al KID-nee) mechanical device that removes wastes from the blood that would normally be removed by the kidney

artificial pacemaker (ar-ti-FISH-al PAYS-may-ker) an electrical device that is implanted into the heart to treat a heart block

asexual (a-SEKS-yoo-al) one-celled plants and bacteria that do not produce specialized sex cells

assimilation (ah-sim-i-LAY-shun) when food molecules enter the cell and undergo chemical changes

association area (ah-so-shee-AY-shun AIR-ee-ah) region of the cerebral cortex of the brain that functions to put together or associate information from many parts of the brain to help make sense of or analyze the information

astrocyte (ASS-troh-syte) a glial cell

atherosclerosis (ath-er-oh-skleh-ROH-sis) hardening of the arteries; lipid deposits lining the inside of the arteries

atom (AT-om) smallest particle of a pure substance (element) that still has the chemical properties of that substance; composed of protons, electrons, and neutrons (subatomic particles)

atomic mass (ah-TOM-ik mas) combined total number of protons and neutrons in an atom

atomic number (ah-TOM-ik NUM-ber) total number of protons in an atom's nucleus; atoms of each element have a characteristic atomic number

atrial natriuretic hormone (ANH) (AY-tree-al nah-tree-yoo-RET-ik HOR-mohn) hormone secreted by the heart cells that regulates fluid and electrolyte homeostasis

atrioventricular (AV) node (ay-tree-oh-ven-TRIK-yoo-lar) see **AV node**

atrioventricular (AV) valves (ay-tree-oh-ven-TRIK-yoo-lar valvz) two valves that separate the atrial chambers from the ventricles

atrium (AY-tree-um) chamber or cavity; for example, atrium of each side of the heart

atrophy (AT-roh-fee) wasting away of tissue; decrease in size of a part; sometimes referred to as *disuse atrophy*

auditory tube (AW-di-toh-ree) tube that connects the throat with the middle ear to equalize air pressure on both sides of the tympanum (eardrum); also called **eustachian tube**

auricle (AW-ri-kul) part of the ear attached to the side of the head; earlike appendage of each atrium of the heart

autonomic effector (aw-toh-NOM-ik ef-FEK-tor) tissues to which autonomic neurons conduct impulses

autonomic nervous system (ANS) (aw-toh-NOM-ik NER-vus SIS-tem) division of the human nervous system that regulates involuntary actions

autonomic neuron (aw-toe-NOM-ik NOO-ron) motor neurons that make up the autonomic nervous system

AV bundle (A V BUN-dul) fibers in the heart that relay a nerve impulse from the AV node to the ventricles; also known as the *bundle of His*

AV node a small mass of specialized cardiac muscle tissue; part of the conduction system of the heart; see **atrioventricular (AV) node**

avitaminosis (ay-vye-tah-mi-NO-sis) vitamin deficiency

axial (AK-see-al) refers to the head, neck, and torso, or trunk of the body

axial skeleton (AK-see-al SKEL-eh-ton) the bones of the head, neck, and torso

axilla (AK-sil-ah) refers to the armpit

axon (AK-son) nerve cell process that transmits impulses away from the cell body

B

B cell a lymphocyte; activated B cells develop into plasma cells, which secrete antibodies into the blood; also called *B lymphocyte*

Bartholin gland (BAR-tuh-lin) either of two glands, each located to the side of the vaginal outlet that secretes mucus-like lubricating fluid; also known as *greater vestibular gland*

basal cell carcinoma (BAY-sal sell car-sin-OH-mah) one of the most common forms of skin cancer, usually occurring on upper face, with low potential for metastasizing

basal ganglion (BAY-sal GANG-lee-on) also known as *basal nucleus*; see **cerebral nucleus**

basal metabolic rate (BMR) (BAY-sal met-ah-BOL-ik) number of calories of heat that must be produced per hour by catabolism to keep the body alive, awake, and comfortably warm

basal nucleus (BAY-sal NOO-klee-us) see **cerebral nucleus**

base 1. A chemical that, when dissolved in water, reduces the relative concentration of H^+ ions in the whole solution (sometimes by adding OH^- ions); 2. In the context of nucleic acids (DNA and RNA), *base or nitrogen base* refers to one part of a nucleotide (sugar, phosphate, and base) that is the basic building block of nucleic acid molecules; possible bases include adenine, thymine, guanine, cytosine, and uracil

basement membrane the connective tissue layer of the serous membrane that holds and supports the epithelial cells

basophil (BAY-soh-fil) white blood cell that stains readily with basic dyes

benign prostatic hypertrophy (bee-NYNE pros-TAT-ik hye-PER-troh-fee) a noncancerous enlargement of the prostate in older men

benign tumor (bee-NYNE TOO-mer) a relatively harmless neoplasm

beta cell (BAY-tah) pancreatic islet cell that secretes insulin

bicarbonate loading (bye-KAR-boh-nayte) ingesting large amounts of sodium bicarbonate to counteract the effects of lactic acid build-up, thereby reducing fatigue; however, there are potentially dangerous side effects

biceps brachii (BYE-seps BRAY-kee-eye) the primary flexor of the forearm

biceps femoris (BYE-seps FEM-oh-ris) powerful flexor of the lower leg

bicuspid (bye-KUSS-ped) tooth type with a large flat surface and two or three grinding cusps; also called *premolars*

bicuspid valve (bye-KUSS-ped) one of the two AV valves; located between the left atrium and ventricle and sometimes called the **mitral valve**

bile substance that reduces large fat globules into smaller droplets of fat that are more easily broken down

bile duct structure formed by the union of the common hepatic and cystic ducts; drains bile into the small intestine

biochemistry (bye-oh-KEM-iss-tree) scientific field that studies the chemical properties and processes of living organisms

biological filtration (bye-oh-LOJ-eh-kal fil-TRAY-shun) process in which cells alter the contents of the filtered fluid

birth defect (birth DEE-fekt) any abnormality, whether caused by genetic or environmental factors, that exists at birth; see **teratogen**

blackhead sebum that accumulates, darkens, and enlarges some of the ducts of the sebaceous glands; also known as a *comedo*

bladder (BLAD-der) a sac, usually referring to the urinary bladder

blastocyst (BLAS-toh-sist) postmorula stage of developing embryo that implants in uterine wall; hollow ball of cells plus an inner cell mass

blister (BLIS-ter) a baglike fluid-filled elevation of the skin caused by an irritant such as heat, friction, or a chemical

blood-brain barrier two-ply wall formed by the wall of a capillary and the surrounding extensions of a glial cell called an *astrocyte*; functions to prevent harmful chemicals from entering vital brain tissue

blood doping (blud DOH-ping) reinfusion of red blood cells (RBCs) (or drugs that increase RBC production) into an athlete prior to competition in an attempt to increase performance levels or stamina by increasing the oxygen-carrying capacity of the blood

blood pressure pressure of blood exerted on walls of the blood vessels; expressed as systolic pressure over diastolic pressure (e.g., 120/80 mm Hg)

blood pressure gradient (GRAY-dee-ent) the difference between two blood pressures in the body

blood type any of the different types of blood that are identified by specific antigens in red blood cells (A, B, AB, O, and Rh-negative or Rh-positive)

body unified and complex assembly of structurally and functionally interactive components

body composition percentages of the body made of lean tissue and fat tissue

bolus (BOW-lus) a small, rounded mass of masticated food to be swallowed

bone highly specialized connective tissue whose matrix is hard and calcified

bone marrow (MAIR-oh) soft material that fills cavities of the bones; red bone marrow is vital to blood cell formation, yellow bone marrow is inactive fatty tissue

bony labyrinth (BONE-ee LAB-i-rinth) the fluid-filled complex maze of three spaces (the vestibule, semicircular canals, and cochlea) in the temporal bone

Bowman capsule (BOH-men KAP-sul) the cup-shaped top of a nephron that surrounds the glomerulus

brachial (BRAY-kee-al) pertaining to the arm

breast anterior aspect of the chest; in females, also an accessory sex organ

bronchi (BRONG-kye) (*sing.*, bronchus) the branches of the trachea

bronchiole (BRONG-kee-ole) small branch of a bronchus

buccal (BUK-al) pertaining to the cheek

buffer (BUF-er) compound that combines with an acid or with a base to form a weaker acid or base, thereby lessening the change in hydrogen-ion concentration that would occur without the buffer

buffer pair (BUF-er) two kinds of chemical substances that together prevent a sharp change in the pH of a fluid; for example, sodium bicarbonate ($NaHCO_3$) and carbonic acid (H_2CO_3)

buffy coat thin layer of white blood cells (WBCs) and platelets located between red blood cells (RBCs) and plasma in a centrifuged sample of blood

bulbourethral gland (BUL-boh-yoo-REE-thral) small gland located just below the prostate gland whose mucus-like secretions lubricate the terminal portion of the urethra and contribute less than 5% of the seminal fluid volume; also known as *Cowper's gland*

bundle of His (BUN-dul of his) see **AV bundle**

burn an injury to tissues resulting from contact with heat, chemicals, electricity, friction, or radiant and electromagnetic energy; classified into four categories, depending on the number of tissue layers involved

bursa (BER-sah) (*pl.*, bursae) small, cushion-like sac found alongside joints, cushioning moving bones

bursitis (ber-SYE-tis) inflammation of a bursa

C

calcaneus (kal-KAY-nee-us) heel bone; largest tarsal in the foot

calcitonin (CT) (kal-si-TOH-nin) a hormone secreted by the thyroid that decreases calcium in the blood

calorie (c) (KAL-or-ree) heat unit; the amount of heat needed to raise the temperature of 1 gram of water 1° C

Calorie (C) (KAL-or-ree) heat unit; kilocalorie; the amount of heat needed to raise the temperature of 1 kilogram of water 1° C

calyx (KAY-liks) cup-shaped division of the renal pelvis

canaliculus (kan-ah-LIK-yoo-lus) (*pl.* canaliculi) an extremely narrow tubular passage or channel in compact bone

canine tooth (KAY-nyne) the tooth with the longest crown and the longest root, which is located lateral to the second incisor; also called *cuspids* or *eye teeth*

capillary (KAP-i-lair-ee) tiny vessels that connect arterioles and venules

capillary blood pressure (KAP-i-lair-ee) the blood pressure found in the capillary vessels

capsule (KAP-sul) found in diarthrotic joints; holds the bones of joints together while allowing movement; made of fibrous connective tissue lined with a smooth, slippery synovial membrane

carbaminohemoglobin (karb-am-ee-no-hee-moh-GLOH-bin) the compound formed by the union of carbon dioxide with hemoglobin

carbohydrate (kar-boh-HYE-drayt) organic compounds containing carbon, hydrogen, and oxygen in certain specific proportions (C, H, O in a 1:2:1 ratio); for example, sugars, starches, and cellulose

carbohydrate loading (kar-boh-HYE-drayt) the method used by athletes to increase the stores of muscle glycogen, allowing more sustained aerobic exercise

carbonic anhydrase (kar-BON-ik an-HYE-drays) the enzyme that converts carbon dioxide into carbonic acid

cardiac (KAR-dee-ak) refers to the heart

cardiac cycle (KAR-dee-ak) each complete heartbeat, including contraction and relaxation of the atria and ventricles

cardiac muscle (KAR-dee-ak) the specialized muscle that makes up the heart

cardiac output (KAR-dee-ak) volume of blood pumped by one ventricle per minute

cardiac sphincter (KAR-dee-ak SFINK-ter) a ring of muscle between the stomach and esophagus that prevents food from re-entering the esophagus when the stomach contracts; also called **gastroesophageal sphincter**

cardiac vein (KAR-dee-ak) any vein that carries blood from the myocardial capillary beds to the coronary sinus

cardiopulmonary resuscitation (CPR) (kar-dee-oh-PUL-moh-nair-ree ree-sus-i-TAY-shun) combined external cardiac (heart) massage and artificial respiration

cardiovascular (kar-dee-oh-VAS-kyoo-lar) pertaining to the heart and blood vessels

caries (KAIR-eez) decay of teeth or of bone; often called **dental caries**

carotid body (kah-ROT-id) chemoreceptor located in the carotid artery that detects changes in oxygen, carbon dioxide, and blood acid levels

carpal (KAR-pal) pertaining to the wrist

carpal tunnel syndrome (KAR-pul TUN-el SIN-drohm) muscle weakness, pain, and tingling in the radial side (thumb side) of the wrist, hand, and fingers—perhaps radiating to the forearm and shoulder; caused by compression of the median nerve within the carpal tunnel (a passage along the ventral concavity of the wrist)

cartilage (KAR-ti-lij) a specialized, fibrous connective tissue that has the consistency of a firm plastic or gristlelike gel

catabolism (kah-TAB-oh-liz-em) breakdown of food compounds or cytoplasm into simpler compounds; opposite of anabolism, the other phase of metabolism

catalyst (KAT-ah-list) chemical that speeds up reactions without being changed itself

cataract (KAT-ah-rakt) opacity of the lens of the eye

catecholamines (kat-eh-KOHL-ah-meenz) norepinephrine and epinephrine

catheterization (kath-eh-ter-i-ZAY-shun) passage of a flexible tube (catheter) into the bladder through the urethra for the withdrawal of urine (urinary catheterization)

cation (KAT-eye-on) positively charged particle

cavity (KAV-i-tee) hollow place or space in a tooth; see **dental caries**

cecum (SEE-kum) blind pouch; the pouch at the proximal end of the large intestine

cell the basic biological and structural unit of the body consisting of a nucleus surrounded by cytoplasm and enclosed by a membrane

cell body the main part of a neuron from which the dendrites and axons extend

cell-mediated immunity (sell MEE-dee-ayt-ed i-MYOO-ni-tee) resistance to disease organisms resulting from the actions of cells; chiefly sensitized T cells

cellular respiration (SELL-yoo-lar res-pi-RAY-shun) enzymes in the mitochondrial wall and matrix using oxygen to break down glucose and other nutrients to release energy needed for cellular work

centimeter (SEN-ti-mee-ter) 1/100 of a meter; approximately 2.5 cm equals 1 inch

central nervous system (CNS) (SEN-tral NER-vus SIS-tem) the brain and spinal cord

central venous pressure (SEN-tral VEE-nus PRESH-ur) venous blood pressure within the right atrium that influences the pressure in the large peripheral veins

centriole (SEN-tree-ol) one of a pair of tiny cylinders in the centrosome of a cell; believed to be involved with the spindle fibers formed during mitosis

centromere (SEN-troh-meer) a beadlike structure that attaches one chromatid to another during the early stages of mitosis

centrosome (SEN-troh-sohm) area of the cytoplasm near the nucleus that coordinates the building and breaking up of microtubules in the cell; contains centrioles

cephalic (seh-FAL-ik) refers to the head

cerebellum (sair-eh-BELL-um) the second largest part of the human brain that plays an essential role in the production of normal movements

cerebral cortex (seh-REE-bral KOHR-teks) a thin layer of gray matter made up of neuron dendrites and cell bodies that compose the surface of the cerebrum

cerebral nucleus (seh-REE-bral NOO-klee-us) any of a group of islands of gray matter located in the base of the cerebrum that are responsible for automatic movements and postures; also called *basal nucleus*; historically known as *basal ganglion*

cerebrospinal fluid (CSF) (seh-ree-broh-SPY-nal FLOO-id) fluid that fills the subarachnoid space in the brain and spinal cord and in the cerebral ventricles

cerebrovascular accident (CVA) (seh-ree-broh-VAS-kyoo-lar AK-si-dent) a hemorrhage or cessation of blood flow through cerebral blood vessels resulting in destruction of neurons; commonly called a *stroke*

cerebrum (seh-REE-brum) the largest and uppermost part of the human brain that controls consciousness, memory, sensations, emotions, and voluntary movements

cerumen (seh-ROO-men) ear wax

ceruminous gland (seh-ROO-mi-nus) gland that produces a waxy substance called cerumen (ear wax)

cervical (SER-vi-kal) refers to the neck

cervix (SER-viks) neck; any necklike structure

chemoreceptor (kee-moh-ree-SEP-tor) any receptor that responds to chemicals, such as those responsible for taste and smell

chest thorax

childhood (CHILD-hood) from infancy to puberty

cholecystectomy (kohl-eh-sis-TEK-toh-mee) the surgical removal of the gallbladder

cholecystokinin (CCK) (koh-lee-sis-toh-KYE-nin) hormone secreted from the intestinal mucosa of the duodenum that stimulates the contraction of the gallbladder, resulting in bile flowing into the duodenum

cholesterol (koh-LESS-ter-ol) steroid lipid found in all body cell membranes and in animal fat present in food

cholinergic fiber (koh-lin-ER-jik FYE-ber) axon whose terminals release acetylcholine

chondrocyte (KON-droh-syte) cartilage cell

chordae tendineae (KOHR-dee ten-DIN-ee) group of stringlike structures that attach the AV valves to the wall of the heart

chorion (KOH-ree-on) develops into an important fetal membrane in the placenta

chorionic gonadotropin (koh-ree-ON-ik goh-na-doh-TROH-pin) hormone secreted by the developing placenta during pregnancy and that have a gonad-stimulating effect

chorionic villus (koh-ree-ON-ik VIL-lus) (*pl.* villi) tiny fingerlike projections connect the placental blood vessels of the uterine wall

choroid (KOH-royd) middle layer of the eyeball that contains a dark pigment to prevent the scattering of incoming light rays

choroid plexus (KOH-royd PLEK-sus) a network of brain capillaries that are involved with the production of cerebrospinal fluid

chromatid (KROH-mah-tid) either of two replicated chromatin (DNA) strands within a chromosome of a cell ready to divide

chromatin granule (KROH-mah-tin GRAN-yool) easily stained substance in the nucleus of cells made up of DNA strands wound around spools of protein; condenses into chromosomes during mitosis

chromosome (KROH-moh-sohm) DNA molecule that has coiled to form a compact mass during mitosis or meiosis; each chromosome is composed of regions called *genes*, each of which transmits hereditary information

chyme (kyme) partially digested food mixture leaving the stomach

cilia (SIL-ee-ah) (*sing.,* cilium) hairlike projections of cells

circulatory system (SER-kyoo-lah-tor-ee SIS-tem) the system that supplies transportation for cells of the body

circumcision (ser-kum-SIH-zhun) surgical removal of the foreskin or prepuce

circumduct (sir-kum-DUKT) move the distal end in a circular path; see **circumduction**

circumduction (ser-kum-DUK-shun) the process of moving the distal end of a body part in a circular path; see **circumduct**

cisterna chyli (sis-TER-nah KYE-lye) an enlarged pouch on the thoracic duct that serves as a storage area for lymph moving toward its point of entry into the venous system

citric acid cycle (SIT-rik) the second series of chemical reactions in the process of glucose metabolism; an aerobic process; also called *Krebs cycle*

clavicle (KLAV-i-kul) collarbone; connects the upper extremity to the axial skeleton

cleavage furrow (KLEEV-ij FUR-oh) depression in the parent cell surface during cell division; appears at the end of anaphase and begins to divide the cell into two daughter cells

clitoris (KLIT-oh-ris) erectile tissue located at the anterior corner of the vestibule of the vagina

clone (klohn) any of a family of many identical cells descended from a single "parent" cell

cochlea (KOHK-lee-ah) snail shell or structure of similar shape

cochlear duct (KOHK-lee-ar) membranous tube within the bony cochlea

collagen (KAHL-ah-jen) principal organic constituent of connective tissue

collecting tubule (koh-LEK-ting TOO-byool) a straight part of a renal tubule formed by distal tubules of several nephrons joining together

colloid (KOL-oyd) dissolved particles with diameters of 1 to 100 millimicrons (1 millimicron equals about 1/25,000,000 of an inch)

colon (KOH-lon) part of the large intestine

colostomy (koh-LAH-stoh-mee) surgical procedure in which an artificial anus is created on the abdominal wall by cutting the colon and bringing the cut end or ends out to the surface to form an opening called a *stoma*

columnar (koh-LUM-nar) shape in which cells are taller than they are wide

combining site antigen-binding site; any of the antigen receptor regions on antibody molecule; shape of each combining site is complementary to shape of a specific antigen

compact bone (kom-PAKT) dense bone

compensated metabolic acidosis (KOM-pen-say-ted met-ah-BOL-ik ass-i-DOH-sis) condition in which metabolic acidosis has occurred and the body is able to make adjustments to return the blood pH to near normal levels

complement (KOM-pleh-ment) any of several inactive enzymes normally present in blood, which, when activated, kill foreign cells by dissolving them

complementary base pairing bonding purines and pyridines in DNA; adenine always binds with thymine, and cytosine always binds with guanine

complement cascade (kass-KAYD) rapid-fire series of chemical reactions involving proteins called *complements* (normally present in blood plasma), which are triggered by certain antibody-antigen reactions (and other stimuli), and resulting in the formation of tiny protein rings that create holes in a foreign cell and thus cause its destruction

complement fixation (fik-SAY-shun) highly specialized antigen-antibody complexes are formed to destroy a foreign cell

compound substance whose molecules have more than one kind of element in them

concave (KON-kayv) a rounded, somewhat depressed surface

concentric contraction (kon-SENT-rik kon-TRAK-shen) type of isotonic muscle contraction in which a muscle's length decreases

concentric lamella (kon-SEN-trik lah-MEL-ah) (*pl.* lamellae) ring of calcified matrix surrounding the Haversian canal

conchae (KONG-kee) shell-shaped structure; for example, bony projections into the nasal cavity

conduction (kon-DUK-shun) transfer of heat energy to the skin and then the external environment

cone receptor cell located in the retina that is stimulated by bright light

conjunctiva (kon-junk-TI-vah) mucous membrane that lines the eyelids and covers the sclera (white portion)

connective tissue (koh-NEK-tiv) most abundant and widely distributed tissue in the body; has numerous functions

connective tissue membrane (ko-NEK-tiv) one of the two major types of body membranes; composed exclusively of various types of connective tissue

constipation (kon-sti-PAY-shun) retention of feces

contact dermatitis (KON-takt der-mah-TYE-tis) a local skin inflammation lasting a few hours or days after being exposed to an antigen

continuous ambulatory peritoneal dialysis (CAPD) (kon-TIN-yoo-us AM-byoo-lah-tor-ee pair-i-toh-NEE-al dye-AL-i-sis) an alternative form of treatment for renal failure rather than the more complex and expensive hemodialysis

contractile unit (kon-TRAK-til YOO-nit) the sarcomere, the basic functional unit of skeletal muscle

contractility (kon-TRAK-til-i-tee) the ability to contract a muscle

contraction (kon-TRAK-shun) ability of muscle cells to shorten or contract

convection (kon-VEK-shun) transfer of heat energy to air that is flowing away from the skin

convex (KON-veks) a rounded, somewhat elevated surface

cornea (KOR-nee-ah) transparent, anterior portion of the sclera

coronal (koh-ROH-nal) literally "like a crown"; a coronal plane divides the body or an organ into anterior and posterior regions

coronary artery (KOHR-oh-nair-ee AR-ter-ee) the first artery to branch off the aorta; supplies blood to the myocardium (heart muscle)

coronary bypass surgery (KOHR-oh-nair-ee BYE-pass SER-jer-ee) surgery to relieve severely restricted coronary blood flow; veins are taken from other parts of the body to bypass the partial blockage

coronary circulation (KOHR-oh-nair-ee ser-kyoo-LAY-shun) delivery of oxygen and removal of waste product from the myocardium (heart muscle)

coronary embolism (KOHR-oh-nair-ee EM-boh-liz-em) blocking of a coronary blood vessel by a clot

coronary heart disease (KOHR-oh-nair-ee) disease (blockage or other deformity) of the vessels that supply the myocardium (heart muscle); one of the leading causes of death among adults in the United States

coronary sinus (KOHR-oh-nair-ee SYE-nus) area that receives deoxygenated blood from the coronary veins and empties into the right atrium

coronary thrombosis (KOHR-oh-nair-ee throm-BOH-sis) formation of a blood clot in a coronary blood vessel

corpora cavernosa (KOHR-pohr-ah kav-er-NO-sah) two columns of erectile tissue found in the shaft of the penis

corpus callosum (KOHR-pus kah-LOH-sum) where the right and left cerebral hemispheres are joined

corpus luteum (KOHR-pus LOO-tee-um) a hormone-secreting glandular structure transformed after ovulation from a ruptured follicle; it secretes chiefly progesterone, with some estrogen secreted as well

corpus spongiosum (KOHR-pus spun-jee-OH-sum) a column of erectile tissue surrounding the urethra in the penis

cortex (KOHR-teks) outer part of an internal organ; for example, the outer part of the cerebrum and of the kidneys

corticoid (KOHR-ti-koyd) category of hormones secreted by any of the three cell layers of the adrenal cortex

cortisol (KOHR-ti-sol) hormone secreted by the adrenal cortex to stimulate the availability of glucose in the blood; in large amounts, cortisol can depress immune functions, as when it is used as a drug treatment; see **hydrocortisone**

cotransport (koh-TRANS-port) active transport process in which two substances are moved together across a cell membrane; for example, sodium and glucose may be transported together across a membrane

covalent bond (koh-VAY-lent) chemical bond formed when atoms share electrons by overlapping their energy levels (electron shells)

coxal bone (KOKS-al) the pelvic bone or hipbone (also known as the *os coxae* or the *innominate bone*); formed by fusion of three distinct bones (ilium, ischium, and pubis) during skeletal development

cranial (KRAY-nee-al) toward the head

cranial cavity (KRAY-nee-al KAV-i-tee) space inside the skull that contains the brain

cranial nerve (KRAY-nee-al) any of 12 pairs of nerves that attach to the undersurface of the brain and conduct impulses between the brain and structures in the head, neck, and thorax

craniosacral (kray-nee-oh-SAY-kral) pertaining to parasympathetic nerves

cranium (KRAY-nee-um) bony vault made up of eight bones that encase the brain

crenation (kreh-NAY-shun) abnormal notching in an erythrocyte resulting from shrinkage after suspension in a hypertonic solution

cretinism (KREE-tin-iz-em) dwarfism caused by hyposecretion of the thyroid gland

crista ampullaris (KRIS-tah am-pyoo-LAIR-is) a specialized receptor located within the semicircular canals that detects head movements

crown topmost part of an organ or other structure

cruciate ligament (KRU-shee-ayt LIG-a-ment) either of two crossed ligaments inside the knee joint cavity that connect the tibia to the femur; the *anterior cruciate ligament (ACL)* and the *posterior cruciate ligament (PCL)*

crural (KROOR-al) refers to the leg

cryptorchidism (krip-TOR-kih-diz-em) undescended testicles

cubital (KYOO-bi-tal) refers to the elbow or to the forearm

cuboid (KYOO-boyd) resembling a cube

cuboidal (KYOO-boyd-al) cell shape resembling a cube

Cushing syndrome (KOOSH-ing SIN-drohm) condition caused by the hypersecretion of glucocorticoids from the adrenal cortex

cuspid (KUSS-ped) tooth that serves to pierce or tear food being eaten; also called **canine tooth**

cutaneous (kyoo-TAYN-ee-us) pertaining to the skin

cutaneous membrane (kyoo-TAYN-ee-us) primary organ of the integumentary system; the skin

cuticle (KYOO-ti-kul) skinfold covering the root of the nail

cyanosis (SYE-ah-NO-sis) bluish appearance of the skin caused by deficient oxygenation of the blood

cyclic AMP (cAMP) (SIK-lik A M P) adenosine monophosphate, one of several second messengers that delivers information inside the cell and thus regulates the cell's activity

cystic duct (SIS-tik) joins with the common hepatic duct to form the common bile duct

cystitis (sis-TYE-tis) inflammation of the urinary bladder

cytoplasm (SYE-toh-plaz-em) the gel-like substance of a cell exclusive of the nucleus and other organelles

cytoskeleton (sye-toh-SKEL-e-ton) cell's internal supporting, moving framework

D

deciduous (deh-SID-yoo-us) temporary; shedding at a certain stage of growth; for example, deciduous teeth that are commonly referred to as baby teeth

deep farther away from the body's surface

deglutition (deg-loo-TISH-un) swallowing

dehydration (dee-hye-DRAY-shun) excessive loss of body water; the most common fluid imbalance; an abnormally low volume of one or more body fluids

dehydration synthesis (dee-hye-DRAY-shun SIN-theh-sis) chemical reaction in which large molecules are formed by removing water from smaller molecules and joining them together

deltoid (DEL-toyd) triangular; for example, the deltoid muscle

dendrite (DEN-dryte) branching or treelike; a nerve cell process that transmits impulses toward the body

dense bone bone with an outer layer that is hard and dense

dental caries (KAIR-eez) decay of teeth; see **cavity**

deoxyribonucleic acid (DNA) (dee-OK-see-rye-boh-noo-KLEE-ik) genetic material of the cell that carries the chemical "blueprint" of the body

depolarization (dee-poh-lar-i-ZAY-shun) the electrical activity that triggers a contraction of the heart muscle

dermal-epidermal junction (DER-mal-EP-i-dermal JUNK-shun) junction between the thin epidermal layer of the skin and the dermal layer providing support for the epidermis

dermal papillae (DER-mal pah-PIL-ee) upper region of the dermis that forms part of the dermal-epidermal junction and forms the ridges and grooves of fingerprints

dermatome (DER-mah-tohmz) any of the skin surface areas supplied by a single spinal nerve

dermis (DER-mis) the deeper of the two major layers of the skin, composed of dense fibrous connective tissue interspersed with glands, nerve endings, and blood vessels; sometimes called the *true skin*

developmental process changes and functions occurring during a human's early years as the body becomes more efficient and more effective

diabetes insipidus (dye-ah-BEE-teez in-SIP-i-dus) condition resulting from hyposecretion of ADH in which large volumes of urine are formed and, if left untreated, may cause serious health problems

diabetes mellitus (dye-ah-BEE-teez MELL-i-tus) a condition resulting when the pancreatic islets secrete too little insulin, resulting in increased levels of blood glucose

diabetic ketoacidosis see **ketoacidosis**

dialysis (dye-AL-i-sis) separation of smaller (diffusible) particles from larger (nondiffusible) particles through a semipermeable membrane

diaphragm (DYE-ah-fram) membrane or partition that separates one thing from another; the flat muscular sheet that separates the thorax and abdomen and is a major muscle of respiration

diaphysis (dye-AF-i-sis) shaft of a long bone

diarrhea (dye-ah-REE-ah) defecation of liquid feces

diarthrosis (dye-ar-THROH-sis) (pl. diarthroses) freely movable joint

diastole (dye-ASS-toh-lee) relaxation of the heart, interposed between its contractions; opposite of systole

diastolic pressure (dye-ah-STOL-ik PRESH-ur) blood pressure in arteries during diastole (relaxation) of the heart

diencephalon (dye-en-SEF-ah-lon) "between" brain; parts of the brain between the cerebral hemispheres and the mesencephalon or midbrain

differential WBC count (dif-er-EN-shal) proportion of each type of WBC reported as a percentage of the total WBC count

differentiate (dif-er-EN-shee-ayt) a process by which daughter cells become different in structure and function (by using different genes from the genome all cells of the body share), as when some of the original cells of early developmental stages differentiate to become muscle cells and other cells become nerve cells, and so on (*differentiation* is another form of this term)

diffusion (di-FYOO-shun) spreading; for example, scattering of dissolved particles

digestion (di-JEST-chun) the breakdown of food materials either mechanically (i.e., chewing) or chemically (i.e., digestive enzymes)

digestive system (di-JEST-tiv) organs that work together to ensure proper digestion and absorption of nutrients

digital (DIJ-i-tal) refers to fingers and toes

diploë (DIP-lo-EE) region of cancellous (spongy) bone within the wall of a flat bone of the cranium

discharging chambers (dis-CHARJ-ing CHAM-berz) the two lower chambers of the heart called *ventricles*

dissection (di-SEK-shun) cutting technique used to separate body parts for study

dissociate (dis-SOH-see-ayt) when a compound breaks apart in solution

dissociation (dis-soh-see-AY-shun) separation of ions as they dissolve in water

distal (DIS-tal) toward the end of a structure; opposite of proximal

distal convoluted tubule (DIS-tal KON-vo-looted TOO-byool) the part of the tubule distal to the ascending limb of the nephron loop in the kidney

disuse atrophy (DIS-yoos AT-ro-fee) when prolonged inactivity results in the muscles getting smaller in size

diuretic (dye-yoo-RET-ik) a substance that promotes or stimulates the production of urine; diuretic drugs are among the most commonly used drugs in medicine

DNA replication (DNA rep-li-KAY-shun) the unique ability of DNA molecules to make copies of themselves

dopamine (DOH-pah-meen) chemical neurotransmitter

dorsal (DOR-sal) referring to the back; opposite of ventral; in humans, the posterior is dorsal

dorsal body cavity (DOR-sal BOD-ee KAV-i-tee) includes the cranial and spinal cavities

dorsiflexion (dor-si-FLEK-shun) when the top of the foot is elevated (brought toward the front of the lower leg) with the toes pointing upward

double helix (HE-lix) shape of DNA molecules; a double spiral

ductless gland (DUKT-less) specialized gland that secretes hormones directly into the blood

ductus arteriosus (DUK-tus ar-teer-ee-OH-sus) connects the aorta and the pulmonary artery, allowing most blood to bypass the fetus' developing lungs

ductus deferens (DUK-tus DEF-er-enz) a thick, smooth, muscular tube that allows sperm to exit from the epididymis and pass from the scrotal sac into the abdominal cavity; also known as the **vas deferens**

ductus venosus (DUK-tus veh-NOH-sus) a continuation of the umbilical vein that shunts blood returning from the placenta past the fetus's developing liver directly into the inferior vena cava

duodenal papillae (doo-o-DEE-nal pah-PIL-ee) ducts located in the middle third of the duodenum that empty pancreatic digestive juices and bile from the liver into the small intestine; there are two ducts the major duodenal papillae and the minor papillae

duodenum (doo-oh-DEE-num) the first subdivision of the small intestine where most chemical digestion occurs

dura mater (DOO-rah MAH-ter) literally "strong or hard mother"; outermost layer of the meninges

dust cells macrophages that ingest particulate matter in the small air sacs of the lungs

dwarfism (DWARF-iz-em) condition of abnormally small stature, sometimes resulting from hyposecretion of growth hormone

dyspnea (DISP-nee-ah) difficult or labored breathing

E

eardrum (EAR-drum) the tympanic membrane that separates the external ear and middle ear

eccentric contraction (ek-SENT-rik kon-TRAK-shun) type of isotonic muscle contraction in which a muscle's length increases under a load

eccrine (EK-rin) small sweat glands distributed over the total body surface

ectoderm (EK-toh-derm) the innermost of the primary germ layers that develops early in the first trimester of pregnancy

ectopic pregnancy (ek-TOP-ik PREG-nan-see) a pregnancy in which the fertilized ovum implants some place other than in the uterus

edema (eh-DEE-mah) excessive fluid in the tissues

effector (ef-FEK-tor) responding organ; for example, voluntary and involuntary muscle, the heart, and glands

efferent (EF-fer-ent) carrying from, as neurons that transmit impulses from the central nervous system to the periphery; opposite of afferent

efferent lymph vessel (EE-fer-ent limf VESS-el) any of the small lymphatic vessels that carry lymphatic fluid away from a lymph node; compare to *afferent lymph vessel*

efferent neuron (EF-fer-ent NOO-ron) neuron that transmits impulses from the central nervous system to the periphery; opposite (in direction) of *afferent neuron*; see **efferent**

ejaculation (ee-jak-yoo-LAY-shun) sudden discharge of semen from the body

ejaculatory duct (ee-JAK-yoo-lah-toh-ree dukt) duct formed by the joining of the ductus deferens and the duct from the seminal vesicle that allows sperm to enter the urethra

elastin (e-LAS-tin) protein found in elastic fiber

electrocardiogram (ECG) (ee-lek-troh-KAR-dee-oh-gram) graphic record of the heart's action potentials

electrocardiograph (ee-lek-troh-KAR-dee-oh-graf) machine that produces electrocardiograms, graphic records of the heart's electrical activity (voltage fluctuations)

electrolyte (eh-LEK-troh-lyte) substance that ionizes (dissociates to form ions) in solution, rendering the solution capable of conducting an electric current

electrolyte balance (eh-LEK-troh-lyte BAL-ans) homeostasis of electrolytes

electron (eh-LEK-tron) negatively charged particle orbiting the nucleus of an atom

electron transport system (ETS) (eh-LEK-tron TRANS-port SIS-tem) cellular process within mitochondria that transfers energy from high-energy electrons from glycolysis and the citric acid cycle to ATP molecules so that the energy is available to do work in the cell

element pure substance, composed of only one type of atom

embolism (EM-boh-liz-em) obstruction of a blood vessel by foreign matter carried in the bloodstream

embolus (EM-boh-lus) a blood clot or other substance (bubble of air) that is moving in the blood and may block a blood vessel

embryo (EM-bree-oh) animal in early stages of intrauterine development; in humans, the first 3 months after conception

embryology (em-bree-OL-oh-jee) study of the development of an individual from conception to birth

embryonic phase (em-bree-ON-ik faze) the period extending from fertilization until the end of the eighth week of gestation; during this phase the term *embryo* is used

emesis (EM-eh-sis) vomiting

emptying reflex (EMP-tee-ing REE-fleks) the reflex that causes the contraction of the bladder wall and relaxation of the internal sphincter to allow urine to enter the urethra, which is followed by urination if the external sphincter is voluntarily relaxed

emulsify (eh-MUL-seh-fye) in digestion, when bile breaks up fats

endocarditis (en-doh-kar-DYE-tis) inflammation of the lining of the heart

endocardium (en-doh-KAR-dee-um) thin layer of very smooth tissue lining each chamber of the heart

endochondral ossification (en-doh-KON-dral os-i-fi-KAY-shun) the process in which most bones are formed from cartilage models

endocrine (EN-doh-krin) secreting into the blood or tissue fluid rather than into a duct; opposite of exocrine

endocrine gland (EN-doh-krin) any of the ductless glands that are part of the endocrine system and secrete hormones into intercellular spaces, where they diffuse into the bloodstream

endocrine system (EN-doh-krin SIS-tem) the series of ductless glands that are found in the body

endoderm (EN-doh-derm) the outermost layer of the primary germ layers that develops early in the first trimester of pregnancy

endolymph (EN-doh-limf) thick, clear fluid that fills the membranous labyrinth of the inner ear

endometrium (en-doh-MEE-tree-um) mucous membrane lining the uterus

endoneurium (en-doh-NOO-ree-um) the thin wrapping of fibrous connective tissue that surrounds each axon in a nerve

endoplasmic reticulum (ER) (en-doh-PLAS-mik reh-TIK-yoo-lum) network of tubules and vesicles in cytoplasm

endorphin (en-DOR-fin) any of a group of chemicals in the central nervous system that influence pain perception; a natural painkiller

endosteum (en-DOS-tee-um) a fibrous membrane that lines the medullary cavity

endothelium (en-doh-THEE-lee-um) squamous epithelial cells that line the inner surface of the entire circulatory system and the vessels of the lymphatic system

endurance training continuous vigorous exercise requiring the body to increase its consumption of oxygen and developing the muscles' ability to sustain activity over a prolonged period

energy level limited region surrounding the nucleus of an atom at a certain distance containing electrons; also called a *shell*

enkephalin (en-KEF-ah-lin) peptide chemical in the central nervous system that acts as a natural painkiller

enzyme (EN-zyme) a functional protein acting as a biochemical catalyst, allowing chemical reactions to take place in a suitable time frame

eosinophil (ee-oh-SIN-oh-filz) white blood cell that is readily stained by eosin

epicardium (ep-i-KAR-dee-um) the inner layer of the pericardium that covers the surface of the heart; also called the *visceral pericardium*

epidermis (ep-i-DER-mis) "false" skin; outermost layer of the skin

epididymis (ep-i-DID-i-mis) tightly coiled tube that lies along the top and behind the testes where sperm mature and develop the ability to swim

epigastric region (ep-i-GAS-trik REE-jun) superior, center region of nine regions of the abdominopelvic cavity, as identified by a "tic-tac-toe" grid laid out over the abdominopelvic area; found just inferior to the sternum

epiglottis (ep-i-GLOT-is) lidlike cartilage over-hanging the entrance to the larynx

epinephrine (ep-i-NEF-rin) adrenaline; secretion of the adrenal medulla

epineurium (ep-i-NOO-ree-um) a tough fibrous sheath that covers the whole nerve

epiphyseal fracture (ep-i-FEEZ-ee-al FRAK-cher) when the epiphyseal plate is separated from the epiphysis or diaphysis; can disrupt the normal growth of the bone

epiphyseal plate (ep-i-FEEZ-ee-al) the cartilage plate that is between the epiphysis and the diaphysis and allows growth to occur; some-times referred to as a *growth plate*

epiphysis (eh-PIF-i-sis) (*pl.* epiphyses) ends of a long bone

episiotomy (eh-piz-ee-OT-oh-mee) a surgical procedure used during birth to prevent a lacer-ation of the mother's perineum or the vagina

epithelial membrane (ep-i-THEE-lee-al) mem-brane composed of epithelial tissue with an underlying layer of specialized connective tissue

epithelial tissue (ep-i-THEE-lee-al) covers the body and its parts; lines various parts of the body; forms continuous sheets that contain no blood vessels; classified according to shape and arrangement

erythroblastosis fetalis (eh-rith-roh-blas-TOH-sis feh-TAL-is) a disease that may develop when an Rh-negative mother has anti-Rh anti-bodies and gives birth to an Rh-positive baby and the antibodies react with the Rh-positive cells of the baby

erythrocyte (eh-RITH-roh-syte) red blood cell

esophagus (eh-SOF-ah-gus) the muscular, mucus-lined tube that connects the pharynx with the stomach; also known as the *foodpipe*

essential organ (ee-SEN-shal OR-gan) any repro-ductive organ that must be present for repro-duction to occur and is known as a **gonad**

estrogen (ES-troh-jen) sex hormone secreted by the ovary that causes the development and maintenance of the female secondary sex char-acteristics and stimulates growth of the epithe-lial cells lining the uterus

eupnea (YOOP-nee-ah) normal respiration

eustachian tube (yoo-STAY-shun) see **auditory tube**

evaporation (ee-vap-oh-RAY-shun) heat being lost from the skin by sweat being vaporized

eversion (ee-VER-zhen) foot movement that turns the ankle so that the sole faces out to the side

exhalation (eks-hah-LAY-shun) moving air out of the lungs; also known as **expiration**

exocrine (EK-so-krin) secreting into a duct; opposite of endocrine

exocrine gland (EK-so-krin) glands that secrete their products into ducts that empty onto a surface or into a cavity; for example, sweat glands

experimental control any procedure within a sci-entific experiment that ensures that the test sit-uation itself is not affecting the outcome of the experiment

experimentation performing an experiment, which is usually a test of a tentative explana-tion of nature called a **hypothesis**

expiration (eks-pi-RAY-shun) moving air out of the lungs; also known as **exhalation**

expiratory center (eks-PYE-rah-tor-ee) one of the two most important respiratory control centers, located in the medulla

expiratory muscle (eks-PYE-rah-tor-ee) any of the muscles that allow more forceful expiration to increase the rate and depth of ventilation; the internal intercostals and the abdominal muscles

expiratory reserve volume (ERV) (eks-PYE-rah-tor-ee) the amount of air that can be forcibly exhaled after expiring the tidal volume (TV)

extend (eks-TEND) straighten a bend; see **extension**

extension (ek-STEN-shun) increasing the angle between two bones at a joint

external auditory canal (eks-TER-nal AW-di-toh-ree) a curved tube (approximately 2.5 cm) extending from the auricle into the temporal bone, ending at the tympanic membrane

external ear (eks-TER-nal) the outer part of the ear that is made up of the auricle and the external auditory canal

external genitalia (eks-TER-nal jen-i-TAIL-yah) external reproductive organs

external intercostal (eks-TER-nal in-ter-KOS-talz) any of the inspiratory muscles between the ribs that enlarge the thorax, causing the lungs to expand and air to rush in

external nares (eks-TER-nal NAY-reez) nostrils

external oblique (eks-TER-nal oh-BLEEK) the outermost layer of the anterolateral abdominal wall

external otitis (eks-TER-nal oh-TYE-tis) a common infection of the external ear; also known as *swimmer's ear*

external respiration (eks-TER-nal res-pi-RAY-shun) the exchange of gases between air in the lungs and in the blood

extracellular fluid (ECF) (eks-trah-SELL-yoo-lar) the water found outside of cells located in two compartments between cells (interstitial fluid) and in the blood (plasma)

F

facial (FAY-shal) referring to the face

fallen arch condition in which the tendons and ligaments of the foot weaken, allowing the normally curved arch to flatten out

fallopian tube (fal-LOH-pee-an) either of the pair of tubes that conduct the ovum from the ovary to the uterus; also called **uterine tubes**

false rib (fawls) member of the eighth, ninth, and tenth pairs of ribs that are attached to the cartilage of the seventh ribs rather than the sternum

fascia (FAY-shah) general name for the fibrous connective tissue masses located throughout the body, surrounding various organs

fascicle (FAS-i-kul) small bundle of fibers, as in a small bundle of nerve fibers or muscle fibers

fasciculus (fah-SIK-yoo-lus) little bundle

fat one of the three basic food types; primarily a source of energy

fatigue (fah-TEEG) loss of muscle power; weakness

fat tissue adipose tissue; specialized to store lipids

feces (FEE-seez) waste material discharged from the intestines

feedback control loop a highly complex and integrated communication control network, classified as negative or positive; negative feedback loops are the most important and most numerous homeostatic control mechanisms

femoral (FEM-or-al) referring to the thigh

femur (FEE-mur) the thigh bone, which is the longest bone in the body

fertilization (FER-ti-li-ZAY-shun) the moment the female's ovum and the male's sperm cell unite

fetal alcohol syndrome (FAS) (FEE-tal AL-koh-hol SIN-drohm) a condition that may cause congenital abnormalities in a baby that results from a woman consuming alcohol during pregnancy

fetal phase (FEE-tal fayz) period extending from the eighth to the thirty-ninth week of gestation; during this phase the term *fetus* is used

fetus (FEE-tus) unborn young, especially in the later stages; in human beings, from the third month of the intrauterine period until birth

fiber (FYE-ber) threadlike structure; for example, collagen fiber, nerve fiber, or muscle fiber

fibrin (FYE-brin) insoluble protein in clotted blood

fibrinogen (fye-BRIN-oh-jen) soluble blood protein that is converted to insoluble fibrin during clotting

fibrous connective tissue (FYE-brus koh-NEK-tiv) strong, nonstretchable, white collagen fibers that compose tendons

fibula (FIB-yoo-lah) the slender non–weight-bearing bone located on the lateral aspect of the leg

fight-or-flight response the changes produced by increased sympathetic impulses allowing the body to deal with any type of stress

filtration (fil-TRAY-shun) movement of water and solutes through a membrane by a higher hydrostatic pressure on one side

fimbriae (FIM-bree-ee) fringe

first-degree burn minor burn with only minimal discomfort and no blistering; epidermis may peel but no dermal injury occurs

flagellum (flah-JEL-um) (*pl.,* flagella) single projection extending from the cell surface; only example in humans is the "tail" of the male sperm

flat bone one of the four types of bone; the frontal bone is an example of a flat bone

flat feet condition in which the tendons and ligaments of the foot weaken, allowing the normally curved arch to flatten out

flex (fleks) bend; see **flexion**

flexion (FLEK-shun) act of bending; decreasing the angle between two bones at the joint

floating rib member of the eleventh and twelfth pairs of ribs, which are attached only to the thoracic vertebrae

fluid balance (FLOO-id BAL-ans) homeostasis of fluids; the volumes of interstitial fluid, intracellular fluid, and plasma and total volume of water remain relatively constant

fluid compartment any of the areas in the body where the fluid is located; for example, interstitial fluid or intracellular fluid

follicle (FOL-li-kul) a pocketlike structure, such as the cylindrical pocket from which a hair grows

follicle-stimulating hormone (FSH) (FOL-li-kul STIM-yoo-lay-ting HOR-mohn) hormone present in males and females; in males, FSH stimulates the production of sperm; in females, FSH stimulates the ovarian follicles to mature and follicle cells to secrete estrogen

fontanels (FON-tah-nelz) "soft spots" on the infant's head; unossified areas in the infant skull

foramen (foh-RAY-men) small opening; for example, the vertebral foramen, which allows the spinal cord to pass through the vertebral canal

foramen ovale (foh-RAY-men oh-VAL-ee) shunts blood from the right atrium directly into the left atrium, allowing most blood to bypass the baby's developing lungs

foreskin (FORE-skin) a loose-fitting retractable casing located over the glans of the penis; also known as the **prepuce**

fourth-degree burn a full-thickness burn that destroys both dermis and epidermis and also extends below the subcutaneous tissue to damage underlying tissues such as muscles or bone

fovea centralis (FOH-vee-ah sen-TRAL-iss) small depression in the macula lutea where cones are most densely packed; vision is sharpest where light rays focus on the fovea

fractal geometry (FRAK-tul jee-OM-eh-tree) the study of surfaces with a seemingly infinite area, such as the lining of the small intestine

free nerve endings specialized receptors in the skin that respond to pain

free radical (free RAD-i-kel) an atom or molecule with one or more unpaired electrons, making it highly reactive and therefore potentially damaging to other molecules in the body

frenulum (FREN-yoo-lum) the thin membrane that attaches the tongue to the floor of the mouth

frontal (FRON-tal) lengthwise plane running from side to side, dividing the body into anterior and posterior portions

frontal muscle (FRON-tal MUSS-el) one of the muscles of facial expression; it moves the eyebrows and furrows the skin of the forehead

frontal sinusitis (FRON-tal sye-nyoo-SYE-tis) inflammation in the frontal sinus

full-thickness burn burn that (1) destroys epidermis, dermis, and subcutaneous tissue (see **third-degree burn**); and (2) extends below skin and subcutaneous tissue to reach muscle and bone (see **fourth-degree burn**)

G

gallstones (GAWL-stohnz) solid concretions or stones, often composed of cholesterol or bile salts, found in the gallbladder

gametes (GAM-eets) either of the two sex cells, sperm cells (spermatozoa) from the male or eggs (ova) from the female

ganglia (GANG-lee-ah) a region of gray (unmyelinated) nerve tissue (usually this term is used only for gray matter regions in the PNS)

gastric gland (GAS-trik) any of the many tiny glands in the stomach lining that secrete enzymes, mucus, and hydrochloric acid

gastrocnemius (GAS-trok-NEE-mee-us) superficial muscle of the calf of the leg, connected (along with the soleus muscle) to the calcaneus bone of the foot by way of the Achilles (calcaneal) tendon; its action is to dorsiflex the foot, bending the toes upward

gastroesophageal reflux disease (GAS-troh-eh-soff-eh-jee-al REE-fluks) also known as GERD, a set of symptoms resulting from a hiatal hernia that allows stomach (gastric) contents to flow back (reflux) into the esophagus; symptoms include heartburn or chest pain and coughing or choking during or just after a meal

gastroesophageal sphincter (GAS-troh-eh-soff-eh-jee-al SFINK-ter) a ring of smooth muscle around the opening of the stomach at the lower end of the esophagus that acts as a valve to allow food to enter the stomach but prevents stomach contents from moving back into the esophagus; also called **cardiac sphincter** or **lower esophageal sphincter (LES)**

gastrointestinal (GI) tract (GAS-troh-in-TESS-tih-nul) principal tubelike structure of the digestive system extending from mouth to anus; sometimes called the **alimentary canal**

gene (jean) one of many segments of a chromosome (DNA molecule); each gene contains the genetic code for synthesizing a protein molecule such as an enzyme or hormone

genitalia (jen-i-TAIL-yah) external reproductive organs

genome (JEE-nohm) entire set of chromosomes in a cell; the human genome refers to the entire set of human chromosomes

genomics (jeh-NO-miks) field of endeavor involving the analysis of the genetic code contained in the human or other species' genome

gerontology (jair-on-TAHL-oh-jee) study of the aging process

gestation (jes-TAY-shun) the length of pregnancy, approximately 9 months in humans

ghrelin (GRAY-lin) hormone secreted by epithelial cells lining the stomach; boosts appetite, slows metabolism, and reduces fat burning; may be involved in the development of obesity

gigantism (jye-GAN-tiz-em) a condition produced by hypersecretion of growth hormone during the early years of life; results in a child who grows to gigantic size

gingivitis (jin-ji-VYE-tis) inflammation of the gum (gingiva), often caused by poor oral hygiene

gland secreting structure

glandular epithelium (GLAN-dyoo-lar ep-i-THEE-lee-um) cells that are specialized for secreting activity

glans the distal end of the shaft of the penis

glaucoma (glaw-KOH-mah) disorder characterized by elevated pressure in the eye

glia (GLEE-ah) supporting cells of nervous tissue; also called *neuroglia*

glioma (glee-OH-mah) one of the most common types of brain tumors

globulin (GLOB-yoo-lin) a type of plasma protein that includes antibodies

glomerular filtrate (gloh-MER-yoo-lar) water and dissolved substances forced out of the blood in the glomerular capillaries and into Bowman capsule

glomerulus (gloh-MER-yoo-lus) compact cluster; for example, capillaries in the kidneys

glottis (GLOT-iss) the space between the vocal cords

glucagon (GLOO-kah-gon) hormone secreted by alpha cells of the pancreatic islets

glucocorticoid (GC) (gloo-koh-KOHR-ti-koyd) category of hormones that influences food metabolism; secreted by the adrenal cortex

gluconeogenesis (gloo-koh-nee-oh-JEN-eh-sis) formulation of glucose or glycogen from protein or fat compounds

glucose (GLOO-kohs) monosaccharide or simple sugar; the principal blood sugar

gluteal (GLOO-tee-al) of or near the buttocks

gluteus maximus (GLOO-tee-us MAX-i-mus) major extensor of the thigh and also supports the torso in an erect position

glycerol (GLIS-er-ol) product of fat digestion

glycogen (GLYE-koh-jen) polysaccharide made up of a chain of glucose (monosaccharide) molecules; animal starch

glycogenesis (glye-koh-JEN-eh-sis) formation of glycogen from glucose or from other monosaccharides, fructose, or galactose

glycogen loading (GLYE-koh-jen) see **carbohydrate loading**

glycogenolysis (glye-koh-jeh-NOL-i-sis) hydrolysis of glycogen to glucose 6-phosphate or to glucose

glycolysis (glye-KOHL-i-sis) the first series of chemical reactions in glucose metabolism; changes glucose to pyruvic acid in a series of anaerobic reactions

glycosuria (glye-koh-SOO-ree-ah) glucose in the urine; a sign of diabetes mellitus

goblet cell (GOB-let) specialized cell found in simple columnar epithelium that produces mucus

goiter (GOY-ter) enlargement of the thyroid gland

Golgi apparatus (GOL-jee ap-ah-RAH-tus) small sacs stacked on one another near the nucleus that makes carbohydrate compounds, combines them with protein molecules, and packages the product in a globule

Golgi tendon receptors (GOL-jee TEN-don ree-SEP-torz) sensors that are responsible for proprioception

gonads (GO-nadz) sex glands in which reproductive cells are formed

G protein a protein molecule usually embedded in a cell's plasma membrane that plays an important role in getting a signal from a receptor (also in the plasma membrane) to the inside of the cell

graafian follicle (GRAH-fee-en FOL-li-kul) a mature ovum in its sac

gradient (GRAY-dee-ent) a slope or difference between two levels; for example, blood pressure gradient a difference between the blood pressure in two different vessels

gram the unit of measure in the metric system on which mass is based (approximately 454 grams equals 1 pound)

granulosa cell (gran-yoo-LO-sah sell) cell layer surrounding the oocyte

gray matter tissue comprising cell bodies and unmyelinated axons and dendrites

greater omentum (oh-MEN-tum) a pouchlike extension of the visceral peritoneum

greater vestibular gland (ves-TIB-yoo-lar) either of the glands located on each side of the vaginal outlet; secretes mucuslike lubricating fluid; also known as **Bartholin gland**

growth hormone (HOR-mohn) hormone secreted by the anterior pituitary gland that controls the rate of skeletal and visceral growth

gustatory cell (GUS-tah-tor-ee) cells of taste; chemoreceptors

gyrus (JYE-rus) convoluted ridge

H

hair follicle (hair FOL-li-kul) a small tube where hair growth occurs

hair papilla (pah-PIL-ah) a small, cap-shaped cluster of cells located at the base of the follicle where hair growth begins

hamstring muscle (HAM-string MUSS-el) any of the powerful flexors of the hip; the hamstring group is made up of the semimembranosus, semitendinosus, and biceps femoris muscles

hard palate (PAL-let) hard, bony, anterior portion of roof of mouth formed by parts of palatine and maxillary bones

Haversian canal (ha-VER-shun) the canal in the Haversian system that contains a blood vessel; also called *central canal*

Haversian system (hah-VER-shun) the circular arrangements of calcified matrix and cells that give bone its characteristic appearance

heart block a blockage of impulse conduction from atria to ventricles so that the heart beats at a slower than normal rate

heartburn burning sensation characterized by pain and a feeling of fullness beneath the sternum; caused by the esophageal mucosa being irritated by stomach acid

Heimlich maneuver (HIME-lik mah-NOO-ver) lifesaving technique used to free the trachea of objects blocking the airway

hematocrit (hee-MAT-oh-krit) volume percent of blood cells in whole blood

hematopoiesis (hee-MA-toh-poy-EE-sis) blood cell formation

hematopoietic tissue (hee-MAH-toh-poy-EE-tik) specialized connective tissue that is responsible for the formation of blood cells and lymphatic system cells; found in red bone marrow, spleen, tonsils, and lymph nodes

heme (HEEM) iron-containing component of hemoglobin molecule

hemodialysis (hee-moh-dye-AL-i-sis) use of dialysis to separate waste products from the blood

hemoglobin (hee-moh-GLOH-bin) iron-containing protein in red blood cells

hemorrhagic anemia (HEM-oh-raj-ick ah-NEE-mee-ah) condition characterized by low oxygen-carrying capacity of blood; caused by decreased red blood cell (RBC) life span and/or increased rate of RBC destruction

heparin (HEP-ah-rin) substance obtained from the liver; inhibits blood clotting

hepatic colic flexure (heh-PAT-ik KOL-ik FLEK-sher) the bend between the ascending colon and the transverse colon; also called *right colic flexure*

hepatic duct (heh-PAT-ik) any of the small tubes that drain bile out of the liver

hepatic portal circulation (heh-PAT-ik POR-tal ser-kyoo-LAY-shun) the route of blood flow through the liver

hepatic portal vein (heh-PAT-ik POR-tal) delivers blood directly from the gastrointestinal tract to the liver

hepatitis (hep-ah-TYE-tis) inflammation of the liver due to viral or bacterial infection, injury, damage from alcohol, drugs, or other toxins, or other factors

herpes zoster (HER-peez ZOS-ter) "shingles," viral infection that affects the skin of a single dermatome

hiatal hernia (hye-AY-tal HER-nee-ah) a bulging out (hernia) of the stomach through the opening (hiatus) of the diaphragm through which the esophagus normally passes; this condition may prevent the valve between the esophagus and stomach from closing, thus allowing stomach contents to flow back into the esophagus; see **gastroesophageal reflux disease**

hiccup (HIK-up) involuntary spasmodic contraction of the diaphragm

hip the joint connecting the legs to the trunk; pelvic girdle

histogenesis (his-toh-JEN-eh-sis) formation of tissues from primary germ layers of embryo

homeostasis (hoh-mee-oh-STAY-sis) relative uniformity of the normal body's internal environment

homeostatic mechanism (hoh-mee-oh-STAT-ik MEK-ah-niz-em) a system that maintains a constant environment enabling body cells to function effectively

hormone (HOR-mohn) substance secreted by an endocrine gland

human immunodeficiency virus (HYOO-man i-myoo-no-deh-FISH-en-see VYE-rus) (HIV) the retrovirus that causes acquired immunodeficiency syndrome (AIDS)

humerus (HYOO-mer-us) the second longest bone in the body; the long bone of the arm

humoral immunity (HYOO-mor-al i-MYOO-ni-tee) see **antibody-mediated immunity**

hybridomas (hye-brid-OH-mahz) fused or hybrid cells that continue to produce the same antibody as the original lymphocyte

hydrocephalus (hye-droh-SEF-ah-lus) abnormal accumulation of cerebrospinal fluid; "water on the brain"

hydrocortisone (hye-droh-KOHR-ti-zohn) a hormone secreted by the adrenal cortex; cortisol; compound F

hydrogen ion (HYE-droh-jen eye-on) found in water and water solutions; produces an acidic solution; H^+

hydrolysis (hye-DROL-i-sis) chemical reaction in which water is added to a large molecule, causing it to break apart into smaller molecules

hydrostatic pressure (hye-droh-STAT-ik) the force of a fluid pushing against some surface

hydroxide ion (hye-DROK-side EYE-on) found in water and water solutions; produces an alkaline solution; H^-

hymen (HYE-men) Greek for "membrane"; mucous membrane that may partially or entirely occlude the vaginal outlet

hyperacidity (hye-per-ah-SID-i-tee) excessive secretion of acid; an important factor in the formation of ulcers

hypercalcemia (hye-per-kal-SEE-mee-ah) a condition in which there is harmful excess of calcium in the blood

hyperglycemia (hye-per-glye-SEE-mee-ah) higher than normal blood glucose concentration

hyperopia (hye-per-OH-pee-ah) farsightedness

hypersecretion (hye-per-seh-KREE-shun) too much of a substance is being secreted

hypertension (hye-per-TEN-shun) abnormally high blood pressure

hyperthyroidism (hye-per-THYE-royd-iz-em) oversecretion of thyroid hormones that increases metabolic rate, resulting in loss of weight, increased appetite, and nervous irritability

hypertonic (hye-per-TON-ik) a solution containing a higher level of salt (NaCl) than is found in a living red blood cell (above 0.9% NaCl)

hypertrophy (hye-PER-troh-fee) increased size of a part caused by an increase in the size of its cells

hyperventilation (hye-per-ven-ti-LAY-shun) very rapid deep respirations

hypervitaminosis (hye-per-vye-tah-mi-NO-sis) condition caused by excess amounts of vitamins; usually associated with the use of vitamin supplements

hypochondriac regions (hy-poh-KON-dree-ak) far left and right superior corner regions of nine regions of the abdominopelvic cavity, as identified by a "tic-tac-toe" grid laid out over the abdominopelvic area; located partly beneath the cartilage of the lower rib cage

hypodermis (hye-poh-DER-mis) the loose, ordinary (areolar) tissue just under the skin and superficial to the muscles; also called **subcutaneous tissue** or *superficial fascia*

hypogastric region (hye-poh-GAS-trik) inferior, center region of nine regions of the abdominopelvic cavity, as identified by a "tic-tac-toe" grid laid out over the abdominopelvic area; located approximately in the central pelvic area

hypoglycemia (hye-poh-glye-SEE-mee-ah) lower-than-normal blood glucose concentration

hyposecretion (hye-poh-seh-KREE-shun) too little of a substance is being secreted

hypothalamus (hye-poh-THAL-ah-muss) vital neuroendocrine and autonomic control center beneath the thalamus

hypothermia (hye-poh-THER-mee-ah) subnormal core body temperature below 37° C

hypothesis (hye-POTH-eh-sis) (*pl.*, hypotheses) a proposed explanation of an observed phenomenon

hypothyroidism (hye-poh-THY-royd-iz-em) undersecretion of thyroid hormones; early in life results in cretinism; later in life results in myxedema

hypotonic (hye-poh-TON-ik) a solution containing a lower level of salt (NaCl) than is found in a living red blood cell (below 0.9% NaCl)

hypoventilation (hye-poh-ven-ti-LAY-shun) slow and shallow respirations

hypovitaminosis (hye-poh-VYTE-ah-min-oh-sis) condition of having too few vitamin molecules in the body for normal function

hypoxia (hye-POCK-see-ah) abnormally low concentration of oxygen in the blood or tissue fluids

hysterectomy (his-teh-REK-toh-mee) surgical removal of the uterus

I

ileocecal valve (il-ee-oh-SEE-kal) the sphincter-like structure between the end of the small intestine and the beginning of the large intestine

ileum (IL-ee-um) the distal portion of the small intestine

iliac crest (IL-ee-ak) the superior edge of the ilium

iliac regions (IL-ee-ak) far left and right inferior corner regions of nine regions of the abdominopelvic cavity, as identified by a "tic-tac-toe" grid laid out over the abdominopelvic area; located in the right and left pelvic areas

iliopsoas (il-ee-op-SO-us) a flexor of the thigh and an important stabilizing muscle for posture

ilium (IL-ee-um) one of the three separate bones that forms the os coxa

immune system (i-MYOON) the body's defense system against disease

immunization (i-myoo-ni-ZAY-shun) deliberate artificial exposure to disease to produce acquired immunity

implantation (im-plan-TAY-shun) when a fertilized ovum implants in the uterus

inborn immunity (IN-born i-MYOO-ni-tee) immunity to disease that is inherited

incisor (in-SYE-zor) one of the four front teeth in each dental arch; each incisor has a crown that is chisel shaped and has a sharp cutting edge for biting off pieces of tough food; prominent in plant-eating animals

incontinence (in-KON-ti-nens) when an individual voids urine involuntarily

incus (IN-kus) the anvil; the middle ear bone that is shaped like an anvil

infancy (IN-fan-see) from birth to about 18 months of age

infant respiratory distress syndrome (IRDS) (IN-fant RES-per-ah-toh-ree di-STRESS SIN-drohm) leading cause of death in premature babies, due to a lack of surfactant in the alveolar air sacs

inferior lower; opposite of superior

inferior vena cava (VEE-nah KAY-vah) one of two large veins carrying blood into the right atrium

inflammatory response (in-FLAM-ah-toh-ree) nonspecific immune process produced in response to injury and resulting in redness, pain, heat, and swelling and promoting movement of white blood cells to the affected area

inguinal (ING-gwi-nal) of the groin

inhalation (in-huh-LAY-shun) inspiration or breathing in; opposite of exhalation or expiration

inherited immunity (in-HAIR-i-ted i-MYOO-ni-tee) inborn immunity

inhibiting hormone (in-HIB-i-ting HOR-mohn) hormone produced by the hypothalamus that slows the release of anterior pituitary hormones

innate immunity (in-AYT i-MYOON-i-tee) see **nonspecific immunity**

inorganic compound (in-or-GAN-ik) compound whose molecules do not contain carbon-carbon or carbon-hydrogen bonds

INR (International Normalized Ratio) a mathematical calculation reported as a number (normal 0.8 to 1.2) used to standardize the results of anticoagulation testing

insertion (in-SER-shun) attachment of a muscle to the bone that it moves when contraction occurs (as distinguished from its origin)

inspiration (in-spi-RAY-shun) moving air into the lungs; same as inhalation, opposite of exhalation or expiration

inspiratory center (in-SPY-rah-tor-ee) one of the two most important control centers located in the medulla; the other is the expiratory center

inspiratory muscle (in-SPY-rah-tor-ee MUSS-el) the muscles that increase the size of the thorax, including the diaphragm and external intercostals, and allow air to rush into the lungs

inspiratory reserve volume (IRV) (in-SPY-rah-tor-ee) the amount of air that can be forcibly inspired over and above a normal respiration

insulin (IN-suh-lin) hormone secreted by the pancreatic islets

integument (in-TEG-yoo-ment) the skin

integumentary system (in-teg-yoo-MEN-tar-ee) the skin; the largest and most important organ in the body

intercalated disk (in-TER-kah-lay-ted) any of the disklike cell connections that exist between cardiac muscle fibers

intercostal muscles (in-ter-KOS-tal MUSS-els) the respiratory muscles located between the ribs

interferon (in-ter-FEER-on) small proteins produced by the immune system that inhibit virus multiplication

internal oblique (in-TER-nal oh-BLEEK) the middle layer of the anterolateral abdominal walls

internal respiration (in-TER-nal res-pi-RAY-shun) the exchange of gases that occurs between the blood and cells of the body

interneuron (in-ter-NOO-ron) nerve that conducts impulses from sensory neurons to motor neurons; sometimes called a *central* or *connecting neuron*

interphase (IN-ter-fayz) the phase immediately before the visible stages of cell division when the DNA of each chromosome replicates itself

interstitial cell (in-ter-STISH-al) small specialized cells in the testes that secrete the male sex hormone, testosterone

interstitial cell-stimulating hormone (ICSH) (in-ter-STISH-al sell STIM-yoo-lay-ting HOR-mohn) name by which luteinizing hormone (as produced in males) was previously known; causes testes to develop and secrete testosterone

interstitial fluid (in-ter-STISH-al) fluid located in the microscopic spaces between the cells

intestinal gland (in-TES-ti-nal) any of thousands of glands found in the mucous membrane of the mucosa of the small intestines; secretes intestinal digestive juice

intracellular fluid (ICF) (in-tra-SELL-yoo-lar) a fluid located within the cells; largest fluid compartment

inversion (in-VER-zhen) foot movement that turns the ankle so that the sole faces inward toward the midline of the body

in vitro (in VEE-troh) refers to the glass laboratory container in which a mature ovum is fertilized by a sperm

involuntary muscle smooth muscles that are not under conscious control and are found in hollow organs such as the stomach and small intestine

involution (in-vo-LOO-shun) return of an organ to its normal size after an enlargement; also retrograde or degenerative change

I&O abbreviation used in clinical medicine to indicate the measurement of fluid intake and urine output over a period of time

ion (EYE-on) electrically charged atom or group of atoms

ion pump (EYE-on) a specialized cellular component that moves ions from an area of low concentration to an area of high concentration

ionic bond (eye-ON-ik) chemical bond formed by the positive-negative attraction between two ions

iris (EYE-ris) colored portion of the eye

iron deficiency anemia (EYE-ern deh-FISH-en-see ah-NEE-mee-ah) condition in which there are inadequate levels of iron in the diet so that less hemoglobin is produced; results in extreme fatigue

ischium (IS-kee-um) one of three separate bones that form the os coxa

isometric contraction (eye-so-MET-rik kon-TRAK-shen) type of muscle contraction in which muscle does not shorten

isotonic contraction (eye-so-TON-ik kon-TRAK-shen) of the same tension or pressure

J

jaundice (JAWN-dis) abnormal yellowing of skin, mucous membranes, and white of eyes

jejunum (jeh-JOO-num) the middle third of the small intestine

joints (joynts) articulation

K

Kaposi sarcoma (KS) (KAH-poh-see sar-KOH-mah) a malignant neoplasm (cancer) of the skin characterized by purplish spots

keratin (KER-ah-tin) protein substance found in hair, nails, outer skin cells, and horny tissues

keratotomy (kair-ah-TOT-ah-mee) superficial incisions made on the surface of the cornea, usually to correct vision

ketoacidosis (kee-toh-ass-i-DOH-sis) a condition of abnormally low blood pH (acidity) caused by the presence of an abnormally large number of ketone bodies or "keto acids" that are produced when fats are converted to forms of glucose to be used for cellular respiration; often occurs in diabetes mellitus, when it is more specifically called **diabetic ketoacidosis**; see also **acidosis**

ketone body (KEE-tohn) any of the acidic products of lipid metabolism that may accumulate in blood of individuals with uncontrolled type 1 diabetes

kidney (KID-nee) organ that cleanses the blood of waste products continually produced by metabolism

kilocalorie (Kcal) (KIL-oh-kal-oh-ree) 1,000 calories; see **Calorie**

kinesthesia (kin-es-THEE-zee-ah) "muscle sense"; that is, sense of position and movement of body parts

Krause end bulb (KROWZ) skin receptor that detects sensations of cold

Kupffer cell (KOOP-fer sell) macrophage found in spaces between liver cells

L

labia majora (LAY-bee-ah mah-JO-rah) (*sing.,* labium majus) "large lips" of the vulva

labia minora (LAY-bee-ah mi-NO-rah) (*sing.,* labium minus) "small lips" of the vulva

labor the process that results in the birth of the baby

lacrimal gland (LAK-ri-mal) the glands that produce tears, located in the upper lateral portion of the orbit

lacrimal sacs (LAK-ri-mal sakz) pouches that collect tears from the eye, and then drain them toward the nose

lacteal (LAK-tee-al) a lymphatic vessel located in each villus of the intestine; serves to absorb fat materials from the chyme passing through the small intestine

lactiferous duct (lak-TIF-er-us) the duct that drains the grapelike cluster of milk-secreting glands in the breast

lacuna (lah-KOO-nah) (*pl.,* lacunae) space or cavity; for example, lacunae in bone contain bone cells

lambdoidal suture (LAM-doyd-al SOO-chur) the immovable joint formed by the parietal and occipital bones

lamella (lah-MEL-ah) thin layer, as of bone

lanugo (lah-NOO-go) the extremely fine and soft hair found on a newborn infant

laparoscope (LAP-ah-roh-skope) specialized optical viewing tube

large intestine (in-TESS-tin) part of GI tract that includes cecum; ascending, transverse, descending, and sigmoid colons; rectum; and anal canal

laryngopharynx (lah-ring-go-FAIR-inks) the lowest part of the pharynx

larynx (LAIR-inks) the voice box, located just below the pharynx; the largest piece of cartilage making up the larynx is the thyroid cartilage, commonly known as the Adam's apple

LASIK (laser-assisted in situ keratomileusis) (LAY-zer ah-SIS-ted in SYE-too kair-at-oh-mill-YOO-sis) refractory eye surgery using a microkeratome to cut a corneal cap, which is replaced after an excimer laser is used to vaporize and reshape underlying corneal tissue

lateral (LAT-er-al) of or toward the side; opposite of medial

latissimus dorsi (lah-TIS-i-muss DOR-sye) an extensor of the upper arm

law a scientific law is a theory, or explanation of a scientific principle, with an extraordinarily high degree of confidence of scientists based on experimentation

lens (lenz) the refracting mechanism of the eye that is located directly behind the pupil

leptin (LEHP-tin) hormone, secreted by fat-storing cells, that regulates how hungry or full we feel and how fat is metabolized by the body

leukemia (loo-KEE-mee-ah) blood cancer characterized by an increase in white blood cells

leukocyte (LOO-koh-syte) white blood cells

leukocytosis (loo-koh-sye-TOH-sis) abnormally high white blood cell numbers in the blood

leukopenia (loo-koh-PEE-nee-ah) abnormally low white blood cell numbers in the blood

levodopa (LEV-oh-doh-pah) also called L-*dopa* (el DOH-pah), this chemical is manufactured by the brain cells and then converted to the neurotransmitter dopamine; it has been used to treat disorders involving dopamine deficiencies such as in Parkinson disease

ligament (LIG-ah-ment) bond or band connecting two objects; in anatomy a band of white fibrous tissue connecting bones

limbic system (LIM-bik) a collection of various small regions of the brain that act together to produce emotion and emotional response; sometimes called "the emotional brain"

lipase (LYE-payse) fat-digesting enzymes

lipid organic molecule usually composed of glycerol and fatty acid units; types include triglycerides, phospholipids, and cholesterol; a fat, wax, or oil

lithotripsy (li-thoh-TRIP-see) use of ultrasound waves to break up kidney stones without making an incision

lithotriptor (LITH-oh-trip-tor) a specialized ultrasound generator that is used to pulverize kidney stones

liver glycogenolysis (LIV-er glye-koh-jeh-NOL-i-sis) chemical process by which liver glycogen is converted to glucose

lock-and-key model concept that explains how molecules react when they fit together in a complementary way in the same manner that a key fits into a lock to cause the lock to open or close; the analogy is often used to explain the action of hormones, enzymes, and other biological molecules

longitudinal arch (lon-ji-TOO-di-nal) two arches, the medial and lateral, that extend lengthwise in the foot

lower respiratory tract (RES-pih-rah-tor-ee) division of respiratory tract that is within the thorax and is composed of the trachea, all segments of the bronchial tree, and the lungs

lumbar (LUM-bar) lower back, between the ribs and pelvis

lumbar puncture (LUM-bar PUNK-chur) when some cerebrospinal fluid is withdrawn from the subarachnoid space in the lumbar region of the spinal cord

lumbar regions (LUM-bar) the far left and right middle regions of nine regions of the abdominopelvic cavity, as identified by a "tic-tac-toe" grid laid out over the abdominopelvic area; located at approximately the same level as the lumbar vertebrae

lumen (LOO-men) the hollow space within a tube

lung organ of respiration; the right lung has three lobes and the left lung has two lobes

lunula (LOO-nyoo-lah) crescent-shaped white area under the proximal nail bed

luteinization (loo-tee-in-eye-ZAY-shun) the formation of a golden body (corpus luteum) in the ruptured follicle

luteinizing hormone (LH) (LOO-tee-in-EYE-zing HOR-mohn) acts in conjunction with follicle-stimulating hormone (FSH) to stimulate follicle and ovum maturation and release of estrogen and ovulation; known as the *ovulating hormone*; in males, causes testes to develop and secrete testosterone

lymph (limf) specialized fluid, formed in the tissue spaces, that returns excess fluid and protein molecules to the blood

lymphatic capillary (lim-FAT-ik CAP-i-lair-ee) any of the tiny, blind-ended lymph-collecting tubes distributed in the tissue spaces

lymphatic duct (lim-FAT-ik) terminal vessel into which lymphatic vessels empty lymph; the duct then empties the lymph into the circulatory system

lymphatic system (lim-FAT-ik) a system that plays a critical role in the functioning of the immune system; moves fluids and large molecules from the tissue spaces and fat-related nutrients from the digestive system to the blood

lymphatic tissue (lim-FAT-ik) tissue that is responsible for manufacturing lymphocytes and monocytes; found mostly in the lymph nodes, thymus, and spleen

lymphatic vessels (lim-FAT-ik) vessels that carry lymph to its eventual return to the circulatory system

lymph node (limf) performs biological filtration of lymph on its way to the circulatory system

lymphocyte (LIM-foh-syte) type of white blood cell; see **B cell** and **T cell**

lyse (lize) disintegration of a cell

lysosome (LYE-so-sohm) membranous organelles containing various enzymes that can dissolve most cellular compounds; hence called *digestive bags* or *suicide bags* of cells

M

macrophages (MAK-roh-fay-jez) phagocytic cells in the immune system

malignant (mah-LIG-nant) cancerous growth

malleus (MAL-ee-us) hammer; the tiny middle ear bone that is shaped like a hammer

malocclusion (MAL-oh-cloo-zhun) abnormal contact between the teeth of the upper jaw and lower jaw

mammary glands (MAM-er-ee) breasts; classified as external accessory sex organs in females

masseter (mas-EET-er) large muscle of the cheek, used to lift the lower jaw (mandible) and thus provide chewing movement

mastication (mas-ti-KAY-shun) chewing

matrix (MAY-triks) the intracellular substance of a tissue; for example, the matrix of bone is calcified, whereas that of blood is liquid

matter any substance that occupies space and has mass

mature follicle (mah-CHUR FOL-li-kul) see **graafian follicle**

maximum oxygen consumption (VO$_{2max}$) the maximum amount of oxygen taken up by the lungs, transported to the tissues, and used to do work

mechanoreceptor (mek-an-oh-ree-SEP-tor) receptors that are mechanical in nature; for example, equilibrium and balance sensors in the ears

medial (MEE-dee-al) of or toward the middle; opposite of lateral

mediastinum (mee-dee-ass-TI-num) a subdivision in the midportion of the thoracic cavity

medulla (meh-DUL-ah) Latin for "marrow"; hence the inner portion of an organ in contrast to the outer portion or cortex

medullary cavity (MED-yoo-lair-ee KAV-i-tee) hollow area inside the diaphysis of the bone that contains yellow bone marrow

medulla oblongata (meh-DUL-ah ob-long-GAH-tah) the lowest part of the brainstem; an enlarged extension of the spinal cord; the vital centers are located within this area

meiosis (my-OH-sis) nuclear division in which the number of chromosomes is reduced to half the original number; produces gametes

Meissner corpuscle (MYZ-ner KOR-pus-ul) a sensory receptor located in the skin close to the surface that detects light touch

melanin (MEL-ah-nin) brown skin pigment

melanocyte (MEL-ah-no-syte) specialized cells in the pigment layer that produce melanin

melanoma (mel-ah-NO-mah) a malignant neoplasm (cancer) of the pigment-producing cells of the skin (melanocytes); also called *malignant melanoma*

melatonin (mel-ah-TOH-nin) important hormone produced by the pineal gland that is believed to regulate the onset of puberty and the menstrual cycle; also referred to as the *third eye* because it responds to levels of light and is thought to be involved with the body's internal clock

membrane thin layer or sheet

membranous labyrinth (MEM-brah-nus LAB-i-rinth) a membranous sac that follows the shape of the bony labyrinth and is filled with endolymph

memory cell cell that remains in reserve in the lymph nodes until its ability to secrete antibodies is needed

menarche (meh-NAR-kee) beginning of the menstrual function

meninges (meh-NIN-jeez) fluid-containing membranes surrounding the brain and spinal cord

meniscus (meh-NIS-kus) (*pl.,* menisci) articular cartilage disk

menopause (MEN-oh-pawz) termination of menstrual cycles

menses (MEN-seez) menstrual flow

menstrual cycle (MEN-stroo-al) the cyclical changes in the uterine lining

mesentery (MEZ-en-tair-ee) a large double fold of peritoneal tissue that anchors the loops of the digestive tract to the posterior wall of the abdominal cavity

mesoderm (MEZ-oh-derm) the middle layer of the primary germ layers

messenger RNA (mRNA) a duplicate copy of a gene sequence on the DNA that passes from the nucleus to the cytoplasm

metabolic acidosis (met-ah-BOL-ik ass-i-DOH-sis) a disturbance affecting the bicarbonate element of the bicarbonate-carbonic acid buffer pair; bicarbonate deficit

metabolic alkalosis (met-ah-BOL-ik al-kah-LOH-sis) disturbance affecting the bicarbonate element of the bicarbonate-carbonic acid buffer pair; bicarbonate excess

metabolism (meh-TAB-oh-liz-em) complex process by which food is used by a living organism

metacarpal (met-ah-KAR-pal) the part of the hand between the wrist and fingers

metaphase (MET-ah-fayz) second stage of mitosis, during which the nuclear envelope and nucleolus disappear

metatarsal arch (met-ah-TAR-sal) the arch that extends across the ball of the foot; also called the **transverse arch**

meter (MEE-ter) a measure of length in the metric system; equal to about 39.5 inches

microcephaly (my-kroh-SEF-ah-lee) a congenital abnormality in which an infant is born with a small head

microfilaments (my-kroh-FIL-ah-ments) smallest types of fibers in the cytoskeleton of the cell; "cellular muscles"

microglia (my-KROG-lee-ah) one type of connective tissue found in the brain and spinal cord

micron (MY-kron) 1/1000 millimeter; 1/25,000 inch

microtubule (my-kroh-TOOB-yool) thick cell fiber (compared to microfilament); hollow tube responsible for movement of substances within the cell or movement of the cell itself

microvilli (my-kroh-VIL-eye) (*sing.*, microvillus) small, moving cell extensions that form the brushlike border made up of epithelial cells found on each villus in the small intestine; increase the surface area for absorption of nutrients

micturition (mik-too-RISH-un) urination, voiding

midbrain (MID-brain) one of the three parts of the brainstem

middle ear a tiny and very thin epithelium-lined cavity in the temporal bone that houses the ossicles; in the middle ear, sound waves are amplified

midsagittal (mid-SAJ-i-tal) a cut or plane that divides the body or any of its parts into two equal halves

mineralocorticoid (MC) (min-er-al-oh-KOHR-ti-koyd) hormone that influences mineral salt metabolism; secreted by adrenal cortex; aldosterone is the chief mineralocorticoid

minerals inorganic elements or salts found naturally in the earth that are vital to the proper functioning of the body

mitochondria (my-toh-KON-dree-ah) threadlike structures

mitosis (my-TOH-sis) indirect cell division involving complex changes in the nucleus

mitral valve (MY-tral) also known as the **bicuspid valve**; located between the left atrium and ventricle

molecular motor (mo-LEK-yoo-lar) small structures in the cell made up of one or two molecules and that act as mechanisms of movement

molecule (MOL-eh-kyool) particle of matter composed of one or more smaller units called **atoms**

monoclonal antibody (mon-oh-KLONE-al AN-ti-bod-ee) specific antibody produced from a population of identical cells

monocyte (MON-oh-syte) a phagocyte

mons pubis (monz PYOO-bis) skin-covered pad of fat over the symphysis pubis in the female

morula (MOR-yoo-lah) a solid mass of cells formed by the divisions of a fertilized egg

motor neuron (NOO-ron) transmits nerve impulses from the brain and spinal cord to muscles and glandular epithelial tissues

motor unit a single motor neuron with the muscle cells it innervates

mucocutaneous junction (myoo-koh-kyoo-TAY-nee-us JUNK-shun) the transitional area where the skin and mucous membrane meet

mucosa (myoo-KOH-sah) mucous membrane

mucous membrane (MYOO-kus) epithelial membranes that line body surfaces opening directly to the exterior and secrete a thick, slippery material called **mucus**

mucus (MYOO-kus) thick, slippery material that is secreted by the mucous membrane and that keeps the membrane moist

multiple sclerosis (MS) (skleh-ROH-sis) the most common primary disease of the central nervous system; a myelin disorder

muscle fiber the specialized contractile cells of muscle tissue that are grouped together and arranged in a highly organized way

muscular system the muscles of the body

muscularis (mus-kyoo-LAIR-is) two layers of muscle surrounding the digestive tube that produce wavelike, rhythmic contractions, called **peristalsis**, which move food material along the digestive tract

myelin (MY-eh-lin) lipoid substance found in the myelin sheath around some nerve fibers

myelinated fiber (MY-eh-li-nay-ted) axons outside the central nervous system that are surrounded by a segmented wrapping of myelin

myeloid (MY-eh-loyd) tissue pertaining to bone marrow

myocardial infarction (MI) (my-oh-KAR-dee-al in-FARK-shun) death of cardiac muscle cells resulting from inadequate blood supply as in coronary thrombosis

myocardium (my-oh-KAR-dee-um) muscle of the heart

myofilaments (my-oh-FIL-ah-ments) ultramicroscopic, threadlike structures found in myofibrils

myoglobin (my-oh-GLO-bin) large protein molecule in the cytoplasm of muscle cells that attracts oxygen and holds it temporarily

myometrium (my-oh-MEE-tree-um) muscle layer in the uterus

myopia (my-OH-pee-ah) nearsightedness

myosin (MY-oh-sin) contractile protein found in the thick filaments of skeletal muscle

myxedema (mik-seh-DEE-mah) condition caused by deficiency of thyroid hormone in adults

N

nail body the visible part of the nail

nail root the part of the nail that is hidden by the cuticle

nanometer (NAN-oh-mee-ter) a measure of length in the metric system; one billionth of a meter

nares (NAY-reez) nostrils

nasal cavity (NAY-zal KAV-i-tee) the moist, warm cavities lined by mucosa located just beyond the nostrils; olfactory receptors are located in the mucosa

nasal septum (NAY-zal SEP-tum) a partition that separates the right and left nasal cavities

nasopharynx (nay-zoh-FAIR-inks) the uppermost portion of the tube just behind the nasal cavities

neck (of tooth) narrow portion of tooth that joins crown of tooth to the root

negative feedback see **negative feedback loop**

negative feedback loop homeostatic control system in which information feeding back to the control center causes the level of a variable to be changed in the direction opposite to that of the initial stimulus; see also **feedback control loop**

neonatal period (nee-oh-NAY-tal) developmental stage that occurs during the first 4 weeks after birth

neonate (NEE-oh-NAYT) a newborn infant

neonatology (nee-oh-nay-TOL-oh-jee) diagnosis and treatment of disorders of the newborn infant

neoplasm (NEE-oh-plaz-em) an abnormal mass of proliferating cells that may be either benign or malignant

nephritis (neh-FRY-tis) kidney disease; inflammation of the nephrons

nephron (NEF-ron) anatomical and functional unit of the kidney, consisting of the renal corpuscle and the renal tubule

nephron loop extension of the proximal tubule of the kidney; also known as *loop of Henle* or *Henle loop*

nephropathy (neh-FROP-ah-thee) kidney disease

nerve collection of nerve fibers

nerve impulse signals that carry information along the nerves

nervous tissue consists of neurons and glia that provide rapid communication and control of body function

neurilemma (noo-ri-LEM-mah) nerve sheath

neurohypophysis (noo-roh-hye-POF-i-sis) posterior pituitary gland

neuromuscular junction (noo-roh-MUSS-kyoo-lar JUNK-shun) the point of contact between the nerve endings and muscle fibers

neuron (NOO-ron) nerve cell, including its processes (axons and dendrites)

neurotransmitter (noo-roh-trans-MIT-ter) chemicals by which neurons communicate

neutron (NOO-tron) electrically neutral particle within the nucleus of an atom

neutrophil (NOO-troh-fil) white blood cell that stains readily with neutral dyes

Nobel Prize international award created by the late Alfred Nobel and awarded each year to up to three recipients in each of several categories such as chemistry, physics, and medicine or physiology (each Nobel laureate [prizewinner] receives a diploma, a medal, and a cash prize at a ceremony in Stockholm, Sweden)

nodes of Ranvier (rahn-vee-AY) indentations that are found between adjacent Schwann cells

nonelectrolyte (non-eh-LEK-troh-lyte) compound that does not dissociate into ions in solution; for example, glucose

nonspecific immunity (non-spih-SIH-fik i-MYOON-i-tee) the protective mechanisms that provide immediate, generic protection against any bacteria, toxin, or other injurious particle; also called **innate immunity**

nonsteroid hormone (non-STAYR-oyd HOR-mohn) general type of hormone that does have the lipid steroid structure (derived from cholesterol) but is instead a protein or protein derivative; also sometimes called *protein hormone*

norepinephrine (nor-ep-i-NEF-rin) hormone secreted by adrenal medulla; released by sympathetic nervous system

nose respiratory organ

nosocomial infection (no-zoh-KOAM-ee-al) infection that begins in the hospital or clinic

nuclear envelope (NOO-klee-ar) membrane that surrounds the cell nucleus

nucleic acid (noo-KLEE-ik ASS-id) the two major nucleic acids are ribonucleic acid, abundant in the cytoplasm, and deoxyribonucleic acid, found in the nucleus; made up of units called *nucleotides,* each of which includes a phosphate, a five-carbon sugar, and a nitrogen base

nucleolus (noo-KLEE-oh-lus) critical to protein formation because it "programs" the formation of ribosomes in the nucleus

nucleoplasm (NOO-klee-oh-plaz-em) a special type of cytoplasm found in the nucleus

nucleotide (NOO-klee-oh-tide) chemical subunit made up of three types of chemical groups (sugar, phosphate, nitrogen base) that can act alone or to make up a larger molecule (nucleic acid, such as RNA or DNA)

nucleus (NOO-klee-us) spherical structure within a cell; a group of neuron cell bodies in the brain or spinal cord; central core of the atom, made up of protons and (sometimes) neutrons

nutrition food, vitamins, and minerals that are ingested and assimilated into the body

O

older adulthood see **senescence**

olecranon fossa (oh-LEK-rah-nahn FOS-ah) a large depression on the posterior surface of the humerus

olecranon process (oh-LEK-rah-non PROSS-es) the large bony process of the ulna; commonly referred to as the tip of the elbow

olfaction (ohl-FAK-shun) sense of smell

olfactory receptor (ol-FAK-tor-ee) chemical receptors responsible for the sense of smell;

located in the epithelial tissue in the upper part of the nasal cavity

oligodendrocyte (ohl-i-go-DEN-droh-syte) a cell that holds nerve fibers together and produces the myelin sheath around axons in the central nervous system

oliguria (ohl-i-GYOO-ree-ah) scanty amounts of urine

oocyte (OH-oh-syte) immature stage of the female sex cell

oogenesis (oh-oh-JEN-eh-sis) production of female gametes

oophorectomy (oh-off-eh-REK-toh-mee) surgical procedure to remove the ovaries

opposition moving the thumb to touch the tips of the fingers; the movement used to hold a pencil to write

optic disc (OP-tic) the area in the retina where the optic nerve fibers exit and there are no rods or cones; also known as a *blind spot*

oral cavity mouth

orbicularis oculi (or-bik-yoo-LAIR-is OK-yoo-lie) facial muscle that causes a squint

orbicularis oris (or-bik-yoo-LAIR-is OH-ris) facial muscle that puckers the lips

organ group of several tissue types that performs a special function

organelle (or-gah-NELL) cell organ; for example, the ribosome

organism an individual, living thing

organ of Corti (KOHR-tye) the organ of hearing located in the cochlea and filled with endolymph; also called *Corti organ* or *spiral organ*

organic compound (or-GAN-ik) compound whose large molecules contain carbon and that include C—C bonds and/or C—H bonds

organogenesis (or-gah-no-JEN-eh-sis) formation of organs from the primary germ layers of the embryo

origin (OR-i-jin) the attachment of a muscle to the bone that does not move when contraction occurs, as distinguished from insertion

oropharynx (oh-roh-FAIR-inks) the portion of the pharynx that is located behind the mouth

osmosis (os-MOH-sis) movement of a fluid through a semipermeable membrane

ossicle (OS-si-kul) little bone; for example, the auditory ossicles found in the ears

osteoarthritis (os-tee-oh-ar-THRY-tis) degenerative joint disease; a noninflammatory disorder of a joint characterized by degeneration of articular cartilage

osteoblast (OS-tee-oh-blast) bone-forming cell

osteoclast (OS-tee-oh-klast) bone-absorbing cell

osteocyte (OS-tee-oh-syte) bone cell

osteon (OS-tee-on) structural unit of compact bone tissue made up of concentric layers (lamellae) of hard bone matrix and bone cells (osteocytes); also called **Haversian system**

osteoporosis (os-tee-oh-poh-ROH-sis) a bone disease in which there is an excessive loss of calcified matrix and collagenous fibers from bone

otitis media (oh-TYE-tis MEE-dee-ah) a middle ear infection

ova (OH-vah) (*sing.,* ovum) female sex cells

oval window a small, membrane-covered opening that separates the middle and inner ear

ovarian follicle (oh-VAIR-ee-an FOL-li-kul) pockets in the ovaries that contain developing oocytes

ovary (O-var-ee) either of paired female gonads that produce ova (sex cells)

overactive bladder refers to frequent urination characterized by urgency and pain

overhydration (oh-ver-hye-DRAY-shun) too large a fluid input that can put a burden on the heart

oviduct (OH-vi-dukt) uterine or fallopian tube

ovulation (ov-yoo-LAY-shun) release of an egg (ovum) from the ovary

oxygen concentrator a device used in health care that increases the proportion of oxygen gas in the air of the room in which it is placed—it is sometimes used in respiratory and other conditions that produce hypoxia (low oxygen concentration in the blood)

oxygen debt continued increased metabolism that occurs in a cell to remove excess lactic acid that resulted from exercise

oxygen therapy administration of oxygen gas to individuals suffering from hypoxia (low oxygen concentration in the blood)

oxyhemoglobin (ahk-see-hee-moh-GLOH-bin) hemoglobin combined with oxygen

oxytocin (ahk-see-TOH-sin) hormone secreted by the posterior pituitary gland before and after delivering a baby; thought to initiate and maintain labor, it also causes the release of breast milk into ducts for the baby to suck

P

pacemaker (PASE-may-ker) see **sinoatrial (SA) node**

pacinian corpuscle (pah-SIN-ee-an KOR-pus-ul) a receptor found deep in the dermis that detects pressure on the skin surface

palate (PAL-let) the roof of the mouth; made up of the hard (anterior portion of the mouth) and soft (posterior portion of the mouth) palates

palmar (PAHL-mar) palm of the hand

pancreas (PAN-kree-as) endocrine gland located in the abdominal cavity; contains pancreatic islets that secrete glucagon and insulin

pancreatic islet (pan-kree-AT-ik eye-LET) endocrine portion of the pancreas; made up of small groupings of alpha and beta cells among others; also known as *islet of Langerhans*

papilla (pah-PIL-ah) (*pl.,* papillae) small, nipple-shaped elevations

paralysis (pah-RAL-i-sis) loss of the power of motion, especially voluntary motion

paranasal sinus (pair-ah-NAY-sal SYE-nus) four pairs of sinuses that have openings into the nose

parasympathetic nervous system (PNS) (par-ah-sim-pah-THET-ik) part of the autonomic nervous system; ganglia are connected to the brainstem and the sacral segments of the spinal cord; controls many visceral effectors under normal conditions

parathyroid gland (PAIR-ah-THY-royd) any of the endocrine glands located in the neck on the posterior aspect of the thyroid gland; secretes parathyroid hormone

parathyroid hormone (PTH) (PAIR-ah-THY-royd HOR-mohn) hormone produced by the parathyroid gland that increases the concentration of calcium in the blood

parietal (pah-RYE-i-tal) of the walls of an organ or cavity

parietal pericardium (pah-RYE-i-tal pair-i-KAR-dee-um) pericardium surrounding the heart like a loose-fitting sack to allow the heart enough room to beat

parietal portion (pah-RYE-i-tal) serous membrane that lines the walls of a body cavity

Parkinson disease (PARK-in-son) a chronic disease of the nervous system characterized by a set of signs called *parkinsonism* that results from a deficiency of the neurotransmitter dopamine in certain regions of the brain that normally inhibit overstimulation of skeletal muscles; parkinsonism is characterized by muscle rigidity and trembling of the head and extremities, forward tilt of the body, and shuffling manner of walking

parotid gland (pah-ROT-id) largest of the salivary glands located just below and in front of each ear at the angle of the jaw

partial pressure pressure exerted by any one gas in a mixture of gases or in a liquid; symbol used to designate partial pressure is the capital letter P preceding the chemical symbol for the gas

partial-thickness burn term used to describe both minor burn injury (see **first-degree burn**) and more severe burns that injure both epidermis and dermis (see **second-degree burn**)

parturition (pahr-too-RI-shun) act of giving birth

patella (pah-TEL-ah) small, shallow pan; the kneecap

pectoral girdle (PEK-toe-ral GIR-dul) shoulder girdle; the scapula and clavicle

pectoralis major (pek-teh-RAH-liss MAY-jor) major flexor of the upper arm

pedal (PEED-al) foot

pelvic cavity (PEL-vik KAV-i-tee) the lower portion of the ventral cavity; the distal portion of the abdominopelvic cavity

pelvic girdle (PEL-vik GIR-dul) connects the legs to the trunk; hip bones

pelvic inflammatory disease (PID) inflammatory disease of the female reproductive and other pelvic organs caused by a number of different pathogens, including those responsible for many STDs (sexually transmitted diseases) such as gonorrhea

pelvis (PEL-vis) basin or funnel-shaped structure

penis (PEE-nis) forms part of the male genitalia; when sexually aroused, becomes stiff to enable it to enter and deposit sperm in the vagina

pepsinogen (pep-SIN-oh-jen) component of gastric juice that is converted into pepsin by hydrochloric acid

peptide bond (PEP-tyde) covalent bond linking amino acids within a protein molecule

pericarditis (pair-i-kar-DYE-tis) when the pericardium becomes inflamed

pericardium (pair-i-KAR-dee-um) membrane that surrounds the heart

perilymph (PAIR-i-limf) a watery fluid that fills the bony labyrinth of the ear

perineal (pair-i-NEE-al) refers to the area between the anus and genitals; the perineum

perineum (pair-i-NEE-um) see **perineal**

perineurium (pair-i-NOO-ree-um) connective tissue that encircles a bundle of nerve fibers within a nerve

periodontitis (pair-ee-oh-don-TYE-tis) inflammation of the periodontal membrane (periodontal ligament) that anchors teeth to jaw bone; common cause of tooth loss among adults

periosteum (pair-ee-OS-tee-um) tough, connective tissue covering the bone

peripheral (peh-RIF-er-al) pertaining to an outside surface

peripheral nervous system (PNS) (peh-RIF-er-al) the nerves connecting the brain and spinal cord to other parts of the body

peripheral resistance (peh-RIF-er-al) resistance (blocked effort) to blood flow encountered in the peripheral arteries (arteries that branch off the aorta and pulmonary arteries)

peristalsis (pair-i-STAL-sis) wavelike, rhythmic contractions of the stomach and intestines that move food material along the digestive tract

peritoneal space (pair-i-toh-NEE-al) small, fluid-filled space between the visceral and parietal layers that allows the layers to slide over each other freely in the abdominopelvic cavity

peritoneum (pair-i-toh-NEE-um) large, moist, slippery sheet of serous membrane that lines the abdominopelvic cavity (parietal layer) and its organs (visceral layer)

peritonitis (pair-i-toh-NYE-tis) inflammation of the serous membranes in the abdominopelvic cavity; sometimes a serious complication of an infected appendix

permeable membrane (PER-mee-ah-bul) a membrane that allows passage of substances

pernicious anemia (per-NISH-us ah-NEE-mee-ah) deficiency of red blood cells resulting from a lack of vitamin B_{12}

peroneal muscle (per-oh-NEE-al) any of a group of plantar flexors and evertors of the foot; the peroneus longus forms a support arch for the foot

peroneus group (per-on-EE-uss) see **peroneal muscles**

perspiration (per-spih-RAY-shun) transparent, watery liquid released by glands in the skin that eliminates ammonia and uric acid and helps maintain body temperature; also known as **sweat**

pH (pee-AYCH) mathematical expression of relative H^+ concentration (acidity); pH value higher than 7 is basic, pH value less than 7 is acidic, pH value equal to 7 is neutral

phagocyte (FAG-oh-syte) white blood cell that engulfs microbes and digests them

phagocytosis (fag-oh-sye-TOH-sis) ingestion and digestion of particles by a cell

phalanges (fah-LAN-jeez) (*sing.,* phalanx) the bones that make up the fingers and toes

pharyngeal tonsil (fah-RIN-jee-al TAHN-sil) tonsil located in the nasopharynx on its posterior wall; when enlarged, referred to as *adenoids*

pharynx (FAIR-inks) organ of the digestive and respiratory system; commonly called the *throat*

phospholipid (fos-foh-LIP-id) phosphate-containing fat molecule found in cell membranes; one end of the molecule is water-soluble and the other end is lipid-soluble

photopigment (foh-toh-PIG-ment) any of the chemicals in retinal cells that are sensitive to light

photoreceptor cell (FOH-toh-ree-sep-tor) specialized nerve cell stimulated by light; for example, rods and cones of the retina

phrenic nerve (FREN-ik) the nerve that stimulates the diaphragm to contract

physiology (fiz-ee-OL-oh-jee) the study of body function

pia mater (PEE-ah MAH-ter) the vascular innermost covering (meninx) of the brain and spinal cord

pigment layer the layer of the epidermis that contains the melanocytes that produce melanin to give skin its color

pineal gland (PIN-ee-al) endocrine gland located in the third ventricle of the brain; produces melatonin

pinocytosis (pin-oh-sye-TOH-sis) the active transport mechanism used to transfer fluids or dissolved substances into cells

pituitary gland (pi-TOO-i-tair-ee) endocrine gland located in the skull; made up of the adenohypophysis and the neurohypophysis

placenta (plah-SEN-tah) anchors the developing fetus to the uterus and provides a "bridge" for the exchange of nutrients and waste products between the mother and developing baby

plantar (PLAN-tar) pertaining to the sole of the foot

plantar flexion (PLAN-tar FLEK-shun) action of the bottom of the foot being directed downward; this motion allows a person to stand on his or her tiptoes

plasma (PLAZ-mah) the liquid part of the blood

plasma cell (PLAZ-mah sell) type of lymphocyte (B lymphocyte) white blood cell that secretes huge amounts of antibody into the blood

plasma membrane (PLAZ-mah) membrane that separates the contents of a cell from the tissue fluid; encloses the cytoplasm and forms the outer boundary of the cell

plasma protein (PLAZ-mah PROH-teen) any of several proteins normally found in the plasma; includes albumins, globulins, and fibrinogen

platelet plug (PLAYT-let) a temporary accumulation of platelets (thrombocytes) at the site of an injury; it precedes the formation of a blood clot

pleura (PLOOR-ah) the serous membrane in the thoracic cavity

pleural cavity (PLOOR-al KAV-i-tee) a subdivision of the thorax

pleural space (PLOOR-al) the space between the visceral and parietal pleurae filled with just enough fluid to allow them to glide effortlessly with each breath

pleurisy (PLOOR-i-see) inflammation of the pleura

plica (PLYE-kah) (*pl.,* plicae) multiple circular folds

pneumocystotis (noo-moh-sis-TOE-tis) a protozoan infection; most likely to invade the body when the immune system has been compromised

pneumothorax (noo-moh-THOH-raks) accumulation of air in the pleural space, causing collapse of the lung

polycythemia (pol-ee-sye-THEE-mee-ah) an excessive number of red blood cells

polyuria (pol-ee-YOO-ree-ah) unusually large amounts of urine

pons (ponz) the part of the brainstem between the medulla oblongata and the midbrain

popliteal (pop-li-TEE-al) behind the knee

pore pinpoint-size opening on the skin that serves as an outlet of a small duct from the eccrine sweat glands

positive feedback see **positive feedback loop**

positive feedback loop homeostatic control system in which information feeding back to the control center causes the level of a variable to be pushed further in the direction of the original deviation, causing an amplification of the original stimulus; ordinarily this mechanism is used by the body to amplify a process and quickly finish it, as in labor contractions and blood clotting; see **feedback control loop**

posterior (pos-TEER-ee-or) located behind; opposite of anterior

posterior pituitary gland (pos-TEER-ee-or pi-TOO-i-tair-ee) neurohypophysis; hormones produced are ADH and oxytocin

posterior root ganglion (pos-TEER-ee-or root GANG-lee-un) ganglion located near the spinal cord; where the neuron cell body of the dendrites of the sensory neuron is located

postganglionic neuron (post-gang-lee-ON-ik NOO-ron) autonomic neuron that conducts nerve impulses from a ganglion to cardiac or smooth muscle or glandular epithelial tissue

postnatal period (POST-nay-tal) the period beginning after birth and ending at death

postsynaptic neuron (post-si-NAP-tik NOO-ron) a neuron situated distal to a synapse

posture (POS-chur) position of the body

precapillary sphincter (pree-CAP-pi-lair-ee SFINK-ter) smooth muscle cells that guard the entrance to the capillary

preganglionic neuron (pree-gang-lee-ON-ik NOO-ron) autonomic neuron that conducts nerve impulses between the spinal cord and a ganglion

prenatal period (PREE-nay-tal) the period beginning after conception and lasting until birth

prepuce (PREE-pus) loose-fitting, retractable, double fold of skin covering the glans penis, also known as the **foreskin**

presbyopia (pres-bee-OH-pee-ah) farsightedness of old age

presynaptic neuron (pree-si-NAP-tik NOO-ron) a neuron situated proximal to a synapse

primary bronchi (BRAHN-kye) first branches of the trachea (right and left primary bronchi)

primary follicle (FOL-li-kulz) the type of ovarian follicle present at puberty; covered with granulosa cells

primary germ layer any of the three layers of specialized cells that give rise to definite structures as the embryo develops

primary spermatocyte (SPER-mah-toh-syte) specialized cell that undergoes meiosis to ultimately form sperm

prime mover the muscle responsible for producing a particular movement

product any substance formed as a result of a chemical reaction

progesterone (proh-JES-ter-ohn) hormone produced by the corpus luteum; stimulates secretion of the uterine lining; with estrogen, helps to initiate the menstrual cycle in girls entering puberty

prolactin (proh-LAK-tin) hormone secreted by the anterior pituitary gland during pregnancy to stimulate the breast development needed for lactation

proliferative phase (proh-LIF-eh-rah-tiv) phase of menstrual cycle that begins after the menstrual flow ends and lasts until ovulation

pronate (PROH-nayt) to turn the palm downward

pronation (proh-NAY-shen) see **pronate**

prone term used to describe the body lying in a horizontal position facing downward

prophase (PROH-fayz) first stage of mitosis during which chromosomes become visible

proprioceptor (proh-pree-oh-SEP-tor) receptor located in the muscles, tendons, and joints; allows the body to recognize its position

prostaglandin (PG) (pross-tah-GLAN-din) any of a group of naturally occurring fatty acids that regulate body functions within a local area; also called *tissue hormones*

prostatectomy (pross-tah-TEK-toh-mee) surgical removal of part or all of the prostate gland

prostate gland (PROSS-tayt) gland that lies just below the bladder; secretes a fluid that constitutes about 30% of the seminal fluid volume; helps activate sperm and helps them maintain motility

prostatitis (pross-tah-TYE-tiss) inflammation of the prostate gland

protease (PROH-tee-ayse) protein-digesting enzyme

protein (PROH-teen) one of the basic nutrients needed by the body; a nitrogen-containing organic compound composed of a folded strand of amino acids

proteinuria (proh-teen-YOO-ree-ah) presence of abnormally high amounts of plasma protein in the urine; usually an indicator of kidney disease

proteome (PROH-tee-ohm) the entire group of proteins encoded by the genome; see **genome**

proteomics (proh-tee-OH-miks) the endeavor that involves the analysis of the proteins encoded by the genome, with the ultimate goal of understanding the role of each protein in the body

prothrombin (proh-THROM-bin) a protein present in normal blood that is required for blood clotting

prothrombin activator (proh-THROM-bin AK-tiv-ayt-or) a protein formed by clotting factors from damaged tissue cells and platelets; converts prothrombin into thrombin, a step essential to forming a blood clot

proton (PROH-ton) positively charged particle within the nucleus of an atom

proximal (PROK-si-mal) next or nearest; located nearest the center of the body or the point of attachment of a structure

proximal convoluted tubule (PROK-si-mal kon-voh-LOO-ted TOOB-yool) the first segment of a renal tubule

pseudo (SOO-doh) false

pubis (PYOO-bis) joint in the midline between the two pubic bones

pulmonary artery (PUL-moh-nair-ee AR-ter-ee) artery that carries deoxygenated blood from the right ventricle to the lungs

pulmonary circulation (PUL-moh-nair-ee ser-kyoo-LAY-shun) venous blood flow from the right atrium to the lung and returning to the left atrium

pulmonary semilunar valve (PUL-moh-nair-ee sem-i-LOO-nar) valve located at the beginning of the pulmonary artery

pulmonary vein (PUL-moh-nair-ee vane) any vein that carries oxygenated blood from the lungs to the left atrium

pulmonary ventilation (PUL-moh-nair-ee ven-ti-LAY-shun) breathing; process that moves air in and out of the lungs

pulse (puls) alternating expansion and recoil of the arterial walls produced by the alternate contraction and relaxation of the ventricles; travels as a wave away from the heart

pupil (PYOO-pil) the opening in the center of the iris that regulates the amount of light entering the eye

Purkinje fiber (pur-KIN-jee FYE-ber) conductive cardiac muscle cell located in the walls of the ventricles; relays impulses from the AV node to the ventricles, causing them to contract

P wave deflection on an ECG that occurs with depolarization of the atria

pyloric sphincter (pye-LOR-ik SFINK-ter) sphincter that prevents food from leaving the stomach and entering the duodenum

pylorus (pye-LOR-us) the small narrow section of the stomach that joins the first part of the small intestine

pyramid (PEER-ah-midz) any of the triangular-shaped divisions of the medulla of the kidney; also called *renal pyramids*

Q

QRS complex (Q R S KOM-pleks) deflection on an ECG that occurs as a result of depolarization of the ventricles

quadriceps femoris (KWOD-reh-seps feh-MOR-is) extensor of the lower leg

quickening (KWIK-en-ing) moment when a pregnant woman first feels recognizable movements of the fetus

R

radiation (ray-dee-AY-shun) flow of heat waves away from the blood

radiography (ray-dee-OG-rah-fee) imaging technique using x rays that pass through certain tissues more easily than others, allowing an image of tissues to form on a photographic plate; invented by Wilhelm Röntgen in 1895

radiopaque material (ray-dee-oh-PAYK) substance that does not permit passage of x rays, such as barium sulfate

radius (RAY-dee-us) one of the two bones in the forearm; located on the thumb side of the forearm

reabsorption (ree-ab-SORP-shun) process of absorbing again that occurs in the kidneys

reactant (ree-AK-tant) any substance entering (and being changed by) a chemical reaction

receiving chamber (ree-SEE-ving CHAME-ber) either atrium of the heart; receives blood from the superior and inferior vena cava (right) or pulmonary veins (left)

receptor (ree-SEP-tor) peripheral beginning of a sensory neuron's dendrite

rectum (REK-tum) distal portion of the large intestine

rectus abdominis (REK-tus ab-DOM-i-nis) muscle that runs down the middle of the abdomen; protects the abdominal viscera and flexes the spinal column

reflex (REE-fleks) involuntary action

reflex arc (REE-fleks ark) allows an impulse to travel in only one direction

reflux (REE-fluhks) backflow, as in flow of stomach contents back into esophagus

refraction (ree-FRAK-shun) bending of a ray of light as it passes from a medium of one density to one of a different density

releasing hormone (ree-LEE-sing HOR-mohn) hormone produced by the hypothalamus gland that causes the anterior pituitary gland to release its hormones

renal calculus (REE-nal KAL-kyoo-lus) (*pl.*, calculi) kidney stones

renal colic (REE-nal KOL-ik) pain caused by the passage of a kidney stone

renal corpuscle (REE-nal KOR-pus-ul) the part of the nephron located in the cortex of the kidney

renal pelvis (REE-nal PEL-vis) basinlike upper end of the ureter that is located inside the kidney

renal threshold (REE-nal THRESH-hold) when the amount of a substance that is normally fully reabsorbed from tubular fluid (such as glucose) increases above this "threshold" level, the kidney tubules are unable to reabsorb all of it and the substances "spill over" into the urine

renal tubule (REE-nal TOOB-yool) one of the two principal parts of the nephron

repolarization (ree-poh-lah-ri-ZAY-shun) phase that begins just before the relaxation phase of cardiac muscle activity

reproductive system produces hormones that permit the development of sexual characteristics and the propagation of the species

residual volume (RV) (reh-ZID-yoo-al) the air that remains in the lungs after the most forceful expiration

respiratory acidosis (RES-pih-rah-tor-ee ass-i-DOH-sis) a respiratory disturbance that results in a carbonic acid excess

respiratory alkalosis (RES-pih-rah-tor-ee al-kah-LOH-sis) a respiratory disturbance that results in a carbonic acid deficit

respiratory arrest (RES-pih-rah-tor-ee ah-REST) cessation of breathing without resumption

respiratory control centers (RES-pih-rah-tor-ee) centers located in the medulla and pons that stimulate the muscles of respiration

respiratory membrane (RES-pih-rah-tor-ee) the single layer of cells that makes up the wall of the alveoli

respiratory mucosa (RES-pih-rah-tor-ee myoo-KOH-sah) mucus-covered membrane that lines the tubes of the respiratory tree

respiratory muscle (RES-pih-rah-tor-ee MUSS-el) any of the muscles that are responsible for the changing shape of the thoracic cavity that allows air to move in and out of the lungs

respiratory system (re-SPY-rah-tor-ee) the organs that allow the exchange of oxygen from the air with the carbon dioxide from the blood

respiratory therapist (RES-pih-rah-tor-ee THAYR-ah-pist) health professional who helps patients increase respiratory function or overcome or cope with the effects of respiratory conditions

respiratory tract (RES-pih-rah-tor-ee trakt) the two divisions of the respiratory system are the upper and lower respiratory tracts

reticular formation (reh-TIK-yoo-lar for-MAY-shun) located in the medulla where bits of gray and white matter mix intricately

reticular tissue (reh-TIK-yoo-lar) meshwork of netlike tissue that forms the framework of the spleen, lymph nodes, and bone marrow

retina (RET-i-nah) innermost layer of the eyeball; contains rods and cones and continues posteriorly with the optic nerve

retroperitoneal (reh-troh-pair-i-toh-NEE-al) area outside of the peritoneum

Rh-negative (R H NEG-ah-tiv) red blood cells that do not contain the antigen called Rh factor

RhoGAM (RO-gam) an injection of a special protein given to an Rh-negative woman who is pregnant to prevent her body from forming anti-Rh antibodies, which may harm an Rh-positive baby in a subsequent pregnancy

Rh-positive (R H POZ-i-tiv) red blood cells that contain an antigen called Rh factor

ribonucleic acid (RNA) (rye-boh-noo-KLAY-ik ASS-id) a nucleic acid found in the cytoplasm that is crucial to protein synthesis

ribosomal RNA (rRNA) (rye-boh-SOHM-al R-N-A) a form of RNA that makes up most of the structures (subunits) of the ribosome organelle of the cell

ribosome (RYE-boh-sohm) organelle in the cytoplasm of cells that synthesizes proteins; also known as a *protein factory*

right lymphatic duct (lim-FAT-ik dukt) short vessel into which lymphatic vessels from the right upper quadrant of the body empty lymph; the duct then empties the lymph into the circulatory system at the right subclavian vein; compare to **thoracic duct**

rod receptor located in the retina that is responsible for night vision

rotation (roh-TAY-shun) movement around a longitudinal axis; for example, shaking your head "no"

rugae (ROO-gee) (*sing.*, ruga [ROO-gah]) wrinkles or folds

"rule of nines" a frequently used method to determine the extent of a burn injury; the body is divided into 11 areas of 9% each and 1% to the perineum to help estimate the amount of skin surface burned in an adult

S

sagittal (SAJ-i-tal) a longitudinal section extending from front to back, dividing body or body part into right and left subdivisions

salivary amylase (SAL-i-vair-ee AM-eh-lays) digestive enzyme found in the saliva that begins the chemical digestion of carbohydrates

saltatory conduction (SAL-tah-tor-ee kon-DUK-shun) when a nerve impulse encounters myelin and "jumps" from one node of Ranvier to the next

sarcomere (SAR-koh-meer) contractile unit of muscle; length of a myofibril between two Z bands

scapula (SKAP-yoo-lah) shoulder blade

Schwann cells (shwon) large nucleated cells that form myelin

scientific method any logical and systematic approach to discovering principles of nature, often involving testing of tentative explanations called *hypotheses*

sclera (SKLEH-rah) white outer coat of the eyeball

scrotum (SKROH-tum) pouchlike sac that contains the testes

sebaceous gland (seh-BAY-shus) oil-producing gland found in the skin

sebum (SEE-bum) secretion of sebaceous glands

secondary bronchi (BRAHN-kye) smaller bronchial branches resulting from division of primary bronchi

secondary sexual characteristics sexual characteristics that appear at the onset of puberty

second-degree burn a partial-thickness burn injury that is more severe than a first-degree burn and often involves damage to the dermis

second messenger chemical that provides communication within a hormone's target cell; for example, cyclic AMP

secretory phase phase of menstrual cycle that begins at ovulation and lasts until the next menses begins

sella turcica (SEL-lah TER-sih-kah) small depression of the sphenoid bone that contains the pituitary gland

semen (SEE-men) male reproductive fluid; also called **seminal fluid**

semicircular canal (sem-i-SIR-kyoo-lar kah-NAL) any of the curved, fluid-filled tubes located in the inner ear; contain a specialized receptor called *crista ampullaris* that generates a nerve impulse on movement of the head

semilunar (SL) valve (sem-i-LOO-nar) valve located between either the ventricular chamber or the large artery that carries blood away from the heart; SL valves also found in the veins

seminal fluid (SEM-i-nal FLOO-id) semen

seminal vesicle (SEM-i-nal VES-i-kul) paired, pouchlike gland that contributes about 60% of the seminal fluid volume; rich in fructose, which is a source of energy for sperm

seminiferous tubule (seh-mih-NIF-er-us TOOB-yool) long, coiled structure that forms the bulk of the testicular mass

senescence (seh-NES-ens) older adulthood; aging

sensory neuron (SEN-sor-ee NOO-ron) neuron that transmits impulses to the spinal cord and brain from all parts of the body

serosa (seh-ROH-sah) outermost covering of the digestive tract; composed of the parietal pleura in the abdominal cavity

serotonin (sair-oh-TOH-nin) a neurotransmitter that belongs to a group of compounds called **catecholamines**

serous membrane (SEE-rus) a two-layered epithelial membrane that lines body cavities and covers the surfaces of organs

serum (SEER-um) blood plasma minus its clotting factors, still contains antibodies

shingles (SHING-ulz) see **herpes zoster**

sickle cell anemia (SIK-ul sell ah-NEE-mee-ah) severe, possibly fatal, hereditary disease caused by an abnormal type of hemoglobin

sickle cell trait (SIK-ul sell trayt) when only one defective gene is inherited and only a small amount of hemoglobin that is less soluble than usual is produced

sigmoid colon (SIG-moyd KOH-lon) S-shaped segment of the large intestine that terminates in the rectum

signal transduction (tranz-DUK-shen) term that refers to the whole process of getting a chemical signal (such as a hormone or neurotransmitter) to the inside of a cell; in a way, signal transduction is really "signal translation" by the cell

sinoatrial (SA) node (sye-no-AY-tree-al) the heart's pacemaker; where the impulse conduction of the heart normally starts; located in the wall of the right atrium near the opening of the superior vena cava

sinus (SYE-nus) a space or cavity inside some of the cranial bones

sinusitis (sye-nyoo-SYE-tis) sinus infections

skeletal muscle (SKEL-eh-tal MUSS-el) also known as **voluntary muscle**; muscle under willed or voluntary control

skeletal system (SKEL-eh-tal) the bones, cartilage, and ligaments that provide the body with a rigid framework for support and protection

sliding filament theory (SLY-ding FILL-ah-ment THEE-ree) concept in muscle physiology describing the contraction of a muscle fiber in terms of the sliding of microscopic protein filaments past each other within the myofibrils in a manner that shortens the myofibrils and thus the entire muscle

small intestine (in-TEST-in) part of GI tract that includes duodenum, jejunum, and ileum

smooth muscle (MUSS-el) muscle that is not under conscious control; also known as *involuntary* or *visceral muscle*; forms the walls of blood vessels and hollow organs

sodium-potassium pump (SO-dee-um poh-TAS-ee-um) a system of coupled ion pumps that actively transports sodium ions out of a cell and potassium ions into the cell at the same time; found in all living cells

soft palate (PAL-let) soft, muscular posterior portion of the roof of the mouth

solute (SOL-yoot) substance that dissolves into another substance; for example, in saltwater the salt is the solute dissolved in water

solvent (SOL-vent) substance in which other substances are dissolved; for example, in saltwater the water is the solvent for salt

somatic nervous system (so-MAH-tik NER-vus SIS-tem) the motor neurons that control the voluntary actions of skeletal muscles

specific immunity (i-MYOON-i-tee) the protective mechanisms that provide specific protection against certain types of bacteria or toxins

sperm the male spermatozoon; sex cell

spermatids (SPER-mah-tidz) the resulting daughter cells from the primary spermatocyte undergoing meiosis; these cells have only half the genetic material and half the chromosomes of other body cells

spermatogenesis (sper-mah-toh-JEN-eh-sis) the production of sperm cells

spermatogonia (sper-mah-toh-GO-nee-ah) sperm precursor cells

spermatozoa (sper-mah-toh-ZOh-ah) (*sing.,* spermatozoon) sperm cells

sphincter (SFINK-ter) ring-shaped muscle

sphygmomanometer (sfig-moh-mah-NAH-meh-ter) device for measuring blood pressure in the arteries of a limb

spinal cavity (SPY-nal KAV-i-tee) the space inside the spinal column through which the spinal cord passes

spinal nerve (SPY-nal) nerve that connects the spinal cord to peripheral structures such as the skin and skeletal muscles

spinal tract (SPY-nal trakt) any of the white columns of the spinal cord that provide two-way conduction paths to and from the brain; ascending tract carries information to the brain, whereas descending tracts conduct impulses from the brain

spindle fiber (SPIN-dul FYE-ber) a network of tubules formed in the cytoplasm between the centrioles as they are moving away from each other

spirometer (spih-ROM-eh-ter) an instrument used to measure the amount of air exchanged in breathing

spleen largest lymphoid organ; filters blood, destroys worn-out red blood cells, salvages iron from hemoglobin, and serves as a blood reservoir

splenectomy (spleh-NEK-toh-mee) surgical removal of the spleen

splenic colic flexure (SPLEEN-ik KOH-lik FLEK-shur) point at which the descending colon turns downward on the left side of the abdomen; left colic flexure

spongy bone (SPUN-jee) porous bone in the end of the long bone; may be filled with marrow; also called *cancellous bone* or *trabecular bone*

squamous (SKWAY-muss) scalelike

squamous cell carcinoma (SKWAY-muss sell car-sih-NO-mah) malignant tumor of the epidermis; slow-growing cancer that is capable of metastasizing; the most common type of skin cancer

squamous suture (SKWAY-muss SOO-chur) the immovable joint between the temporal bone and the sphenoid bone

stapes (STAY-peez) tiny, stirrup-shaped bone in the middle ear

staph (staff) a short form of the term *Staphylococcus*, a category of bacteria that can infect the skin and other organs, sometimes seriously

Stensen duct (STEN-sen dukt) the duct of the parotid gland that enters the mouth cavity

sternoclavicular joint (ster-no-klah-VIK-yoo-lar joynt) the direct point of attachment between the bones of the upper extremity and the axial skeleton

sternocleidomastoid (stern-oh-klye-doh-MAS-toyd) "strap" muscle located on the anterior aspect of the neck

steroid hormones (STEH-royd HOR-mohnz) lipid-soluble hormones that pass intact through the cell membrane of the target cell and influence cell activity by acting on specific genes

stimulus (STIM-yoo-lus) agent that causes a change in the activity of a structure

stoma (STOH-mah) an opening, such as the opening created in a colostomy procedure

stomach an expansion of the digestive tract between the esophagus and small intestine

stratum corneum (STRAH-tum KOR-nee-um) the tough outer layer of the epidermis; cells are filled with keratin

stratum germinativum (STRAH-tum JER-mi-nah-tiv-um) the innermost of the tightly packed epithelial cells of the epidermis; cells in this layer are able to reproduce themselves

strength training contracting muscles against resistance to enhance muscle hypertrophy

striated muscle (STRYE-ay-ted MUSS-el) see **skeletal muscle**

stroke volume the amount of blood that is ejected from the ventricles of the heart with each beat

subcutaneous tissue (sub-kyoo-TAY-nee-us) tissue below the layers of skin; made up of loose connective tissue and fat

sublingual gland (sub-LING-gwal) either of a pair of salivary glands that drain saliva into the floor of the mouth

submandibular gland (sub-man-DIB-yoo-lar) either of a pair of salivary glands that drain saliva into the mouth on either side of the lingual frenulum

submucosa (sub-myoo-KOH-sah) connective tissue layer containing blood vessels and nerves in the wall of the digestive tract

sudoriferous gland (soo-doh-RIF-er-us) glands that secrete sweat; also referred to as *sweat glands*

sulcus (SUL-kus) furrow or groove

superficial near the body surface

superior higher; opposite of inferior

superior vena cava (VEE-nah KAY-vah) one of two large veins returning deoxygenated blood to the right atrium

supinate (SOO-pih-nate) to turn the palm of the hand upward; opposite of pronate

supination (soo-pin-AY-shen) see **supinate**

supine (SOO-pine) used to describe the body lying in a horizontal position facing upward

supraclavicular (soo-prah-klah-VIK-yoo-lar) area above the clavicle

surfactant (sur-FAK-tant) a substance covering the surface of the respiratory membrane inside the alveolus, which reduces surface tension and prevents the alveoli from collapsing

suture (SOO-chur) immovable joint

sweat transparent, watery liquid released by glands in the skin that eliminates ammonia and uric acid and helps maintain body temperature; also known as **perspiration**

sympathetic nervous system (sim-pah-THEH-tik NER-vus SIS-tem) part of the autonomic nervous system; ganglia are connected to the thoracic and lumbar regions of the spinal cord; functions as an emergency system

sympathetic postganglionic neuron (sim-pah-THET-ik post-gang-lee-ON-ik NOO-ron) dendrites and cell body are in a sympathetic ganglion, and axon travels to a variety of visceral effectors

sympathetic preganglionic neuron (sim-pah-THET-ik pree-gang-lee-ON-ik NOO-ron) dendrites and cell body are located in the gray matter of the thoracic and lumbar segments of the spinal cord; axon leaves the cord through an anterior root of a spinal nerve and terminates in a collateral ganglion

synapse (SIN-aps) junction between adjacent neurons

synaptic cleft (si-NAP-tik kleft) the space between a synaptic knob and the plasma membrane of a postsynaptic neuron

synaptic knob (si-NAP-tik nob) a tiny bulge at the end of a terminal branch of a presynaptic neuron's axon that contains vesicles with neurotransmitters

synarthrosis (sin-ar-THROH-sis) a joint in which fibrous connective tissue joins bones and holds them together tightly; commonly called **suture**

synergist (SIN-er-jist) muscle that assists a prime mover

synergist muscle (SIN-er-jist MUSS-el) see **synergist**

synovial fluid (si-NO-vee-al) the thick, colorless lubricating fluid secreted by the synovial membrane

synovial membrane (si-NO-vee-al) connective tissue membrane lining the spaces between bones and joints that secretes synovial fluid

system group of organs arranged so that the group can perform a more complex function than any one organ can perform alone

systemic circulation blood flow from the left ventricle to all parts of the body and back to the right atrium

systole (SIS-toh-lee) contraction of the heart muscle

systolic pressure (sis-TOL-ik) force with which blood pushes against artery walls when ventricles contract

T

target cell (TAR-get sell) cell acted on by a particular hormone and responding to it

tarsals (TAR-salz) seven bones of the heel and back part of the foot; the calcaneus is the largest

taste bud any of the chemical receptors that generate nerve impulses, resulting in the sense of taste

T cell another name for **T lymphocyte**

telemetry (tel-EM-et-ree) technology by which data, such as heart activity monitored by an electrocardiograph, can be sent to a remote location through telephone wires, radio waves, or other communication pathway

telophase (TEL-oh-fayz) last stage of mitosis in which the cell divides

temporal (TEM-poh-ral) muscle that assists the masseter in closing the jaw

tendon (TEN-don) a band or cord of fibrous connective tissue that attaches a muscle to a bone or other structure

tendon sheath (TEN-don sheeth) tube-shaped structure lined with synovial membrane that encloses certain tendons

tenosynovitis (ten-oh-sin-oh-VYE-tis) inflammation of a tendon sheath

teratogen (TAYR-ah-toh-jen) any environmental factor that causes a birth defect (abnormality present at birth); common teratogens include radiation (e.g., x rays), chemicals (e.g., drugs, cigarettes, or alcohol), and infections in the mother (e.g., herpes or rubella)

testes (TES-teez) (*pl.,* testis) pair of male gonads that produce the male sex cells or sperm

testosterone (tes-TOS-teh-rohn) male sex hormone produced by the interstitial cells in the testes; the "masculinizing hormone"

tetanic contraction (teh-TAN-ik) sustained contraction

tetanus (TET-ah-nus) sustained muscular contraction

thalamus (THAL-ah-muss) located just above the hypothalamus; its functions are to help produce sensations and associate sensations with emotions; plays a part in the arousal mechanism

theory an explanation of a scientific principle that has been tested experimentally and found to be true; compare to **hypothesis** and **law**

thermoregulation (ther-moh-reg-yoo-LAY-shun) maintaining homeostasis of body temperature

third-degree burn involves complete destruction of both epidermis and dermis with injury extending into subcutaneous tissue; see **full-thickness burn**

thoracic (thoh-RAS-ik) pertaining to the chest area of the body (upper trunk)

thoracic duct (thoh-RAS-ik) largest lymphatic vessel in the body

thorax (THOR-aks) chest

threshold stimulus (THRESH-hold STIM-yoo-lus) minimal level of stimulation required to cause a muscle fiber to contract

thrombin (THROM-bin) protein important in blood clotting

thrombocyte (THROM-boh-sytes) also called a *platelet*; plays a role in blood clotting

thrombosis (throm-BOH-sis) formation of a clot in a blood vessel

thrombus (THROM-bus) stationary blood clot

thymosin (THY-moh-sin) hormone produced by the thymus that is vital to the development and functioning of the body's immune system

thymus gland (THY-muss) endocrine gland located in the mediastinum; vital part of the body's immune system

thyroid gland (THY-royd) endocrine gland located in the neck that stores its hormones until needed; thyroid hormones regulate cellular metabolism

thyroid-stimulating hormone (TSH) (THY-royd STIM-yoo-lay-ting HOR-mohn) a tropic hormone secreted by the anterior pituitary gland that stimulates the thyroid gland to increase its secretion of thyroid hormone

thyroxine (T_4) (thy-ROK-sin) thyroid hormone that stimulates cellular metabolism

tibia (TIB-ee-ah) shinbone

tibialis anterior (tib-ee-AL-is an-TEER-ee-or) dorsiflexor of the foot

tidal volume (TV) (TYE-dal) amount of air breathed in and out with each breath

tinea pedis (TIN-ee-ah PED-is) athlete's foot, a fungal infection of the skin characterized by redness and itching

tissue group of similar cells that perform a common function

tissue fluid a dilute saltwater solution that bathes every cell in the body

tissue hormone (HOR-mohn) prostaglandins; produced in a tissue and diffuses only a short distance to act on cells within the tissue

tissue typing a procedure used to identify tissue compatibility before an organ transplant

T lymphocytes (T LIM-foh-sytes) cells that are critical to the function of the immune system; produce cell-mediated immunity

tonic contraction (TON-ik) special type of skeletal muscle contraction used to maintain posture

tonsillectomy (tahn-sih-LEK-toh-mee) surgical procedure used to remove the tonsils

tonsillitis (tahn-sih-LYE-tis) an inflammation of the tonsils

tonsils (TAHN-silz) masses of lymphoid tissue; protect against bacteria; three types: palatine tonsils, located on each side of the throat; pharyngeal tonsils (adenoids), near the posterior opening of the nasal cavity; and lingual tonsils, near the base of the tongue

total metabolic rate (TMR) (met-ah-BOL-ik) total amount of energy used by the body per day

total WBC count the total number of WBCs per cubic millimeter of blood

trabecula (trah-BEK-yoo-la) (*pl.,* trabeculae) tiny branchlike threads in a tissue, such as the beams of spongy (cancellous) bone, that surround a network of spaces

trachea (TRAY-kee-ah) the windpipe; the tube extending from the larynx to the bronchi

tract a single nerve pathway made up of several bundles of axons and extending through the central nervous system; compare to **nerve**

transcription (trans-KRIP-shun) occurs when the double-stranded DNA molecules unwind and form mRNA

transitional epithelium (tranz-IH-shen-al ep-ih-THEE-lee-um) type of epithelial tissue that forms membranes capable of stretching without breaking, as in the urinary bladder; cells in this type of tissue can stretch from a roughly columnar shape out to a flattened shape (squamous) and back without damage

translation the synthesis of a protein by ribosomes

transverse arch (TRANS-vers) see **metatarsal arch**

transversus abdominis (trans-VER-sus ab-DOM-i-nis) the innermost layer of the anterolateral abdominal wall

trapezium (trah-PEE-zee-um) the carpal bone of the wrist that forms the saddle joint that allows the opposition of the thumb

trapezius (trah-PEE-zee-us) triangular muscle in the back that elevates the shoulder and extends the head backwards

triceps brachii (TRY-seps BRAY-kee-eye) extensor of the elbow

tricuspid valve (try-KUSS-ped) the valve located between the right atrium and ventricle

triglyceride (try-GLISS-er-yde) lipid that is synthesized from fatty acids and glycerol or from excess glucose or amino acids; stored mainly in adipose tissue cells

trigone (TRY-gon) triangular area on the wall of the urinary bladder

triiodothyronine (T₃) (try-eye-oh-doh-THY-roh-neen) thyroid hormone that stimulates cellular metabolism

tropic hormone (TROH-pik HOR-mohn) hormone that stimulates another endocrine gland to grow and secrete its hormones

true rib any of the first seven pairs of ribs that are attached to the sternum

tumor (TOO-mer) growth of tissues in which cell proliferation is uncontrolled and progressive

tunica adventitia (TOO-nih-kah ad-ven-TISH-ah) the outermost layer found in blood vessels

tunica albuginea (TOO-nih-kah al-byoo-JIN-ee-ah) a tough, whitish membrane that surrounds each testis and enters the gland to divide it into lobules

tunica externa (TOO-nih-kah eks-TER-nah) the outermost layer found in blood vessels; also called **tunica adventitia**

tunica intima (TOO-nih-kah IN-tih-mah) endothelium that lines the blood vessels

tunica media (TOO-nih-kah MEE-dee-ah) the muscular middle layer found in blood vessels; the tunica media of arteries is more muscular than that of veins

T wave deflection on an electrocardiogram that occurs with repolarization of the ventricles

twitch a quick, jerky response to a single stimulus

tympanic membrane (tim-PAN-ik) drumlike membrane; also called **eardrum**

type 1 diabetes mellitus (dye-ah-BEE-teez mell-EYE-tus) a condition resulting when the pancreatic islets secrete too little insulin, resulting in increased levels of blood glucose; formerly known as *juvenile-onset diabetes* or *insulin-dependent diabetes mellitus*

type 2 diabetes mellitus (dye-ah-BEE-teez mell-EYE-tus) a condition resulting when cells of the body become less sensitive to the hormone insulin and perhaps the pancreatic islets secrete too little insulin, resulting in increased levels of blood glucose; formerly known as *maturity-onset diabetes* or *insulin-independent diabetes mellitus*

U

ulcer (UL-ser) a necrotic open sore or lesion

ulna (UL-nah) one of the two forearm bones; located on the little finger side

ultrasonogram (ul-trah-SOHN-oh-gram) a technique using sound to produce images

umbilical artery (um-BIL-i-kul AR-ter-ee) two small arteries that carry oxygen-poor blood from the developing fetus to the placenta

umbilical cord (um-BIL-i-kul) flexible structure connecting the fetus with the placenta, which allows the umbilical arteries and vein to pass

umbilical region (um-BIL-ik-al) center region of nine regions of the abdominopelvic cavity, as identified by a "tic-tac-toe" grid laid out over the abdominopelvic area; located beneath the umbilicus (navel)

umbilical vein (um-BIL-i-kul) a large vein carrying oxygen-rich blood from the placenta to the developing fetus

upper respiratory tract (res-PYE-rah-tor-ee) division of respiratory tract outside the thorax that is composed of the nose, pharynx, and larynx

urea (yoo-REE-ah) nitrogen-containing waste product

uremia (yoo-REE-mee-ah) high levels of nitrogen-containing waste products in the blood; also referred to as **uremic poisoning**

uremic poisoning (yoo-REE-mik POY-zon-ing) see **uremia**

ureter (YOOR-eh-ter) long tube that carries urine from kidney to bladder

urethra (yoo-REE-thrah) passageway for elimination of urine; in males, also acts as a genital duct that carries sperm to the exterior

urinary meatus (YOOR-i-nair-ee mee-AY-tus) external opening of the urethra

urinary retention (YOOR-i-nair-ee ree-TEN-shun) condition in which no urine is voided

urinary suppression (YOOR-i-nair-ee supp-PRESH-un) condition in which kidneys do not produce urine

urinary system (YOOR-i-nair-ee) system responsible for excreting liquid waste from the body

urination (yoor-i-NAY-shun) passage of urine from the body; emptying of the bladder

urine (YOOR-in) fluid waste excreted by the kidneys

uterine tube (YOO-ter-in) either of the pair of tubes that conduct the ovum from the ovary to the uterus; also called **fallopian tube**

uterus (YOO-ter-us) hollow, muscular organ where a fertilized egg implants and grows

uvula (YOO-vyoo-lah) cone-shaped process hanging down from the soft palate that helps prevent food and liquid from entering the nasal cavities

V

vagina (vah-JYE-nah) internal tube from the uterus to the vulva

vas deferens (vas DEF-er-enz) see **ductus deferens**

vasomotor mechanism (vay-soh-MOH-tor MEK-ah-niz-em) factors that control changes in the diameter of arterioles by changing the tension of smooth muscles in the vessel walls

vastus (VAS-tus) wide; of great size

vein vessel carrying blood toward the heart

ventral (VEN-tral) of or near the belly; in humans, front or anterior; opposite of dorsal or posterior

ventral body cavity (VEN-trul BOD-ee KAV-it-ee) organ-containing space in the anterior trunk of the body that includes the thoracic and abdominopelvic cavities; compare with **dorsal body cavity**

ventricle (VEN-tri-kulz) small cavity, such as the pumping chambers of the heart

venule (VEN-yool) any of the small blood vessels that collect blood from the capillaries and join to form veins

vermiform appendix (VERM-i-form ah-PEN-diks) a tubular structure attached to the cecum; composed of lymphatic tissue

vertebra (VER-teh-brah) (*pl.,* vertebrae [VER-teh-bray]) bone that makes up the spinal column

vertebral column (ver-TEE-bral) the spinal column, made up of a series of separate vertebrae that form a flexible, curved rod

vestibular nerve (ves-TIB-yoo-lar) a division of the vestibulocochlear nerve (the eighth cranial nerve)

vestibule (VES-ti-byool) located in the inner ear; the portion adjacent to the oval window between the semicircular canals and the cochlea

villus (VIL- us) (*pl.,*villi [VIL-eye]) fingerlike fold covering the plicae of the small intestines

visceral effector (VIS-er-al ee-FEK-ter) see **autonomic effector**

visceral pericardium (VIS-er-al pair-i-KAR-dee-um) the pericardium that covers the heart; also called **epicardium**

visceral portion (VIS-er-al) serous membrane that covers the surface of organs found in the body cavity

vital capacity (VC) (VYE-tal kah-PAS-i-tee) largest amount of air that can be moved in and out of the lungs in one inspiration and expiration

vitamin a type of organic molecule needed in small quantities to help enzymes operate effectively

vitreous humor (VIT-ree-us HYOO-mor) the jellylike fluid found in the eye, posterior to the lens

vocal cord one of the bands of tissue in larynx responsible for production of sound (speech)

voiding (VOYD-ing) emptying of the bladder; also called **micturition** and **urination**

volar (VOH-lar) palm or sole

voluntary muscle see **skeletal muscle**

vulva (VUL-vah) external genitals of the female

W

wart raised bump that is a benign neoplasm (tumor) of the skin; caused by viruses

white matter nerves covered with white myelin

withdrawal reflex a reflex that moves a body part away from an irritating stimulus

Y

yellow bone marrow (MARE-oh) fatty tissue found inside the medullary cavity of a long bone

yolk sac in humans, involved with the production of blood cells in the developing embryo

Z

zona fasciculata (ZOH-nah fas-sic-yoo-LAY-tah) middle zone of the adrenal cortex; secretes glucocorticoids

zona glomerulosa (ZOH-nah gloh-mare-yoo-LOH-sah) outer zone of the adrenal cortex; secretes mineralocorticoids

zona reticularis (ZOH-nah reh-tik-yoo-LAIR-is) inner zone of the adrenal cortex; secretes small amounts of sex hormones

zygomaticus (zye-goh-MAT-i-kus) muscle that elevates the corners of the mouth and lips; also known as the *smiling muscle*

zygote (ZYE-goht) a fertilized ovum

b indicates boxes, *f* indicates illustrations, and *t* indicates tables.